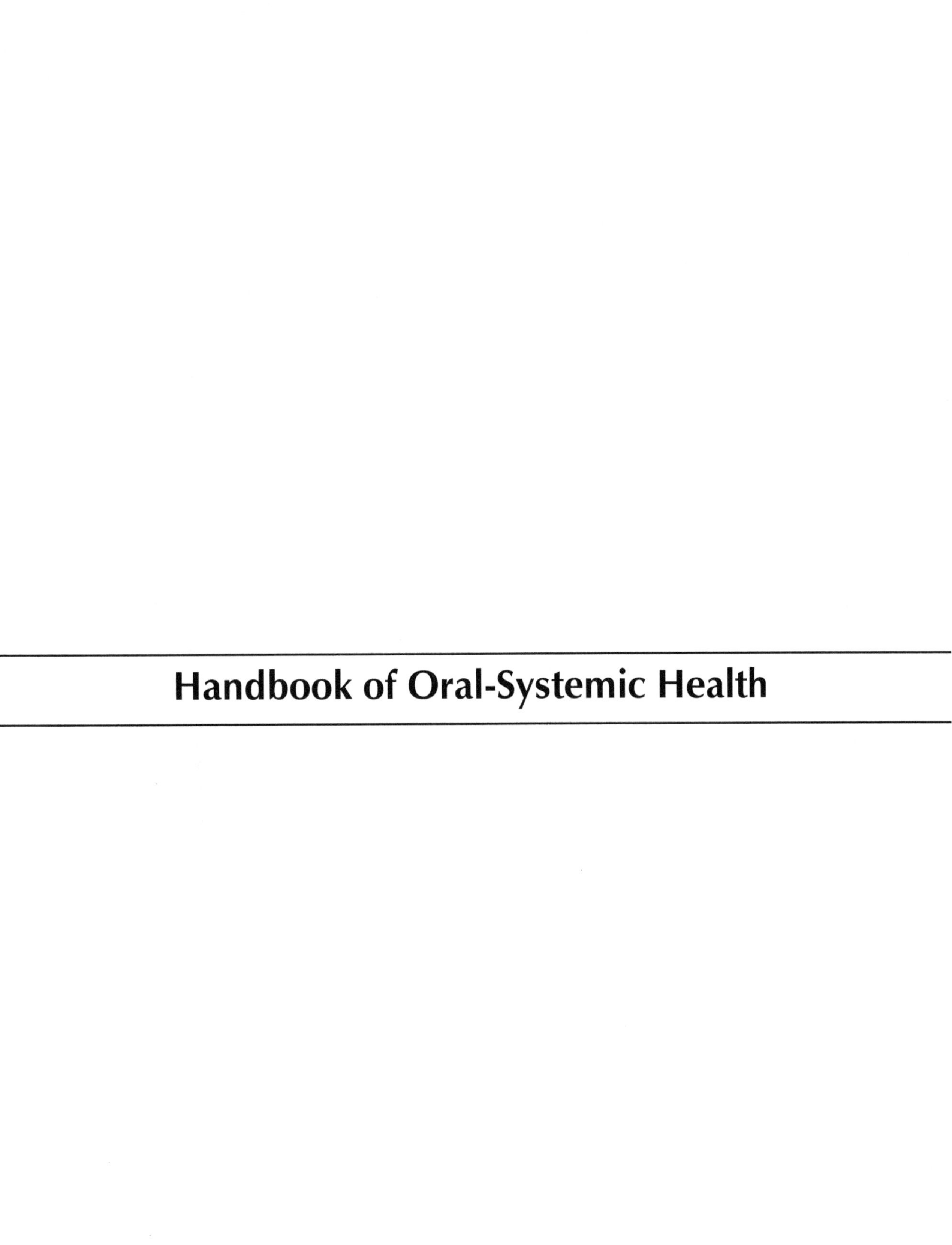

Handbook of Oral-Systemic Health

Handbook of Oral-Systemic Health

Editor: Herman Caleb

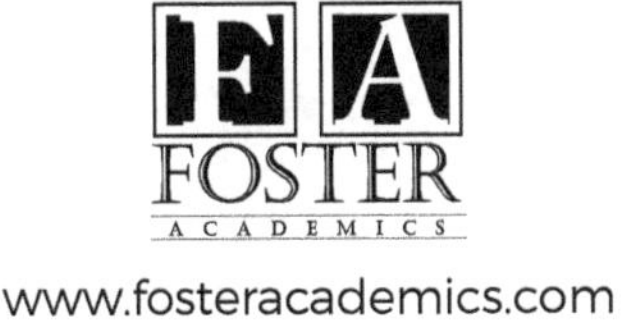

www.fosteracademics.com

www.fosteracademics.com

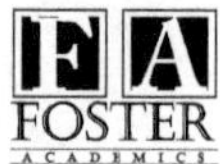

Cataloging-in-Publication Data

Handbook of oral-systemic health / edited by Herman Caleb.
p. cm.
Includes bibliographical references and index.
ISBN 978-1-64646-588-0
1. Oral manifestations of general diseases. 2. Mouth--Diseases--Complications.
3. Mouth--Infections--Complications. 4. Mouth--Care and hygiene.
5. Dental hygiene. 6. Oral medicine. I. Caleb, Herman.
RK61 .H36 2023
617.522--dc23

Foster Academics,
118-35 Queens Blvd., Suite 400,
Forest Hills, NY 11375, USA

ISBN 978-1-64646-588-0 (Hardback)

Contents

Preface

This book has been an outcome of determined endeavour from a group of educationists in the field. The primary objective was to involve a broad spectrum of professionals from diverse cultural background involved in the field for developing new researches. The book not only targets students but also scholars pursuing higher research for further enhancement of the theoretical and practical applications of the subject.

The oral cavity acts as an intersection between dentistry and medicine, and provides an overview of the overall health of a person. Oral bacteria can contribute to diseases in other parts of the body. A number of systemic diseases have been associated with oral health including Alzheimer's disease and dementia, cardiovascular diseases, obesity, rheumatoid arthritis, diabetes, and various types of cancers. The associations between oral and systematic health can be understood using two mechanisms. The first one is associated with the chronic inflammation in the oral cavity. This leads to an increase in inflammatory markers in the blood that affects the immune response or supplements to the overall disease burden on the body. Secondly, the oral cavity may serve as a source for pathogenic bacteria to enter the bloodstream which can affect systemic pathologies. This book aims to shed light on some of the unexplored aspects of oral and systemic health, and the recent researches in this area of study. It presents researches and studies performed by experts across the globe. The book will serve as a valuable source of reference for graduate and postgraduate students.

It was an honour to edit such a profound book and also a challenging task to compile and examine all the relevant data for accuracy and originality. I wish to acknowledge the efforts of the contributors for submitting such brilliant and diverse chapters in the field and for endlessly working for the completion of the book. Last, but not the least; I thank my family for being a constant source of support in all my research endeavours.

Editor

1

A Perspective: Integrating Dental and Medical Research Improves Overall Health

Wendy Mouradian[1,2], *Janice Lee*[3], *Joan Wilentz*[4] *and Martha Somerman*[3,5*]

[1] *School of Dentistry, University of Washington, Seattle, WA, United States,* [2] *The Santa Fe Group, New York, NY, United States,* [3] *National Institute of Dental and Craniofacial Research, National Institutes of Health, Bethesda, MD, United States,* [4] *Independent Researcher, New York, NY, United States,* [5] *National Institute of Arthritis and Musculoskeletal and Skin Diseases, National Institutes of Health, Bethesda, MD, United States*

Correspondence:
Martha Somerman
martha.somerman@nih.gov

The past decade has seen marked increases in research findings identifying oral-systemic links. Yet, much of dental research remains poorly integrated with mainstream biomedical research. The historic separation of dentistry from medicine has led to siloed approaches in education, research and practice, ultimately depriving patients, providers, and policy makers of findings that could benefit overall health and well-being. These omissions amount to lost opportunities for risk assessment, diagnosis, early intervention and prevention of disease, increasing cost and contributing to a fragmented and inefficient healthcare delivery system. This perspective provides examples where fostering interprofessional research collaborations has advanced scientific understanding and yielded clinical benefits. In contrast are examples where failure to include dental research findings has limited progress and led to adverse health outcomes. The impetus to overcome the dental-medical research divide gains further urgency today in light of the coronavirus pandemic where contributions that dental research can make to understanding the pathophysiology of the SARS-CoV-2 virus and in diagnosing and preventing infection are described. Eliminating the research divide will require collaborative and trans-disciplinary research to ensure incorporation of dental research findings in broad areas of biomedical research. Enhanced communication, including interoperable dental/medical electronic health records and educational efforts will be needed so that the public, health care providers, researchers, professional schools, organizations, and policymakers can fully utilize oral health scientific information to meet the overall health needs of the public.

Keywords: medical-dental integration, oral-systemic research, clinical trials, interoperable electronic health records, microbiome

INTRODUCTION

Biomedical research grew dramatically after World War II with the generation of new antibiotics, the unraveling of the genetic code, the birth of molecular biology, and the first successful organ transplants, among major milestones. The National Institutes of Health (NIH) expanded accordingly, but in ways reflecting traditional clinical specialties that divide the body into disparate organs and systems, a division that perpetuates the sharp divide between dentistry and medicine.

But the very discoveries and technologies that are rapidly transforming our understanding of life and life processes demand we put the body back together again (**Table 1**). For example, we know that a gene associated with a particular organ can manifest in other organs, or turn other genes on or off, and we know that a drug targeted to a particular pathogen can wreak havoc elsewhere in the body. But what is also now clear is that the body is even more extensively and deeply connected than had been thought. The coronavirus pandemic is a case in point. A member of a family of viruses typically associated with respiratory symptoms, severe acute respiratory syndrome coronavirus 2 (SARS-CoV-2), which is responsible for the coronavirus disease 2019 (COVID-19), can result in fatigue, loss of smell and taste, gastrointestinal problems, cognitive deficits, depression, life-threatening pneumonia, neurological disorders and symptoms that can persist in some individuals long after initial infection (15–18). Yet the mouth and oral health considerations continue to be treated as a class by themselves, separate from the rest of the body, ignored and omitted from research studies large and small. This gap results in missed opportunities to reveal important oral-systemic interactions or explain how other parts of the body regulate functions in the mouth. This perspective provides examples of the consequences resulting from the lack of integration and the benefits gained when oral-systemic integration is in place. This is a perspective, not a review, but we provide additional references to a few scientific papers and reviews within the last 6 years, which expand on the examples provided here (19–27).

THE FAILURE TO CONNECT

Not Really All Parts of Us, but Getting Close

The goal of this innovative Precision Medicine initiative, launched by the NIH in 2015, named *All of Us*, is to build one of the most diverse health databases in history by inviting one million Americans, 18 and older, of all backgrounds, to voluntarily submit biologic samples and personal information to enable investigators to learn how biology, lifestyle and environment affect health (28). Participants are asked to answer surveys; they can submit data from wearable measuring devices and allow researchers access to their electronic health records (29). Early on, to get the program going, they were not able to include dental questions in the survey. More recently, two dental questions were added i.e., have you seen a dentist in the last 12 months and do you have access to dental care, with plans to include a more comprehensive oral-dental history, plus collecting salivary samples within the coming year, behind schedule due to the pandemic. We are optimistic that oral-dental health data will be included within the context of total health. On another positive note, UK Biobank now includes collecting salivary samples along with an oral health survey (30).

Incompatible EHRs

The goal of integrated oral and overall health data from *All of Us* is exacerbated by the general lack of interoperability between medical and dental electronic health records making it difficult to obtain an individual's inclusive dental and medical history. Exclusion of oral health data can delay diagnoses and treatment by missing characteristic oral signs of particular conditions, syndromes and diseases, with repercussions on overall health over the lifetime. Establishing a fully integrated dental-medical electronic health record must be a priority to ensure research advances provide optimal clinical care and guidance (28, 29). We recognize the current siloed approaches are on both the medical and dental side. Many dental communities have not fully embraced interprofessional models of teaching and clinical practice, favoring the technical aspects of dentistry. We need buy-in from all healthcare teams to be successful in delivering the concepts discussed in this perspective.

Childhood Caries Risk

Failure to include oral health in other large genomic-phenomic studies also limits understanding of oral conditions directly. For example, childhood dental caries remains the number one chronic disease in children, more prevalent than asthma (30). This state of affairs is amplified by health disparities that disproportionately affect poorer groups, minorities and other underserved and vulnerable populations who lack access to care (31). While some progress has been made toward identifying genetic contributions to periodontal disease and caries (2), failure to include oral health research in large-scale genomic-phenomic initiatives of gene-environment interactions impedes mechanistic understanding of caries risk in children.

Oral Health in Aging

Biological aging is considered a normal physiological process known to be influenced by an individual's risk to include, but not limited to, hormonal changes, chronic inflammatory diseases, diet (nutrition/sugar intake/alcohol), and smoking. There is increasing evidence that periodontal disease, as a chronic infection with persistent inflammation locally and systemically, may contribute to unhealthy aging (32–35). The increasing evidence that severity of periodontal disease has a negative effect on telomere length, where decrease in telomere length is a measure of biological aging, highlights the importance of including oral health status as part of determination of one's total health across a life span (36). Another area needing attention relates to salivary flow with aging. Studies have demonstrated that even though there is some decrease in salivation and a change in salivary composition with aging, it is adequate in healthy aging individuals (37, 38). However, the onset of systemic diseases and the addition of many commonly used drugs as well as radiation therapies can irritate oral tissues and directly cause xerostomia, raising the risk of caries. Yet, how many providers recognize these risks or ask their patients if their various therapies or drug regimens have had any effects on their oral/dental tissues? The inclusion of oral health in aging research is critical to better serve older individuals and develop therapies to preserve oral health.

THE NEED FOR DENTAL SCIENTISTS IN CLINICAL TRIALS

The knowledge dental scientists bring to characteristics of oral tissues can provide valuable clues in diagnosing systemic diseases as well as predicting and elucidating the impact of new therapies

TABLE 1 | Tools and technologies informing clinical practice and oral health outcomes.

Artificial Intelligence and Machine Learning: New technologies are being applied to craniofacial disease detection, including advanced imaging and the use of artificial intelligence/machine learning. The exciting area of facial recognition has exploded with the common use of personal smart phones, security cameras, and social media. These technologies are being applied for identifying rare and undiagnosed diseases that have a craniofacial phenotype. The ability to link a 3D graphic phenotype to a mutation variant is only possible with ongoing research in quantitative imaging modalities and large-scale application to genetic data, such as the efforts of Face2Gene[1]. Importantly, and with growing attention, is the need to establish careful guidelines for appropriate use of A.I. and machine learning, where improvements made in patient care do not compromise an individual's privacy (1, 2). Further, dental educators need to incorporate information in their curricula to ensure graduates are prepared to execute these and other emerging tools and technologies.

Imaging Advancements: The increasing use of cone-beam computed tomography, particularly by oral and maxillofacial surgeons and orthodontists, for evaluation of craniofacial growth, skeletal malocclusions and placement of dental implants has added an important tool to the expanding technology for research. The development of 3D craniofacial landmarks (3), deep learning segmentation and malocclusion classification methods (4–6) and application of geometric morphometric analysis to 3D skeletal imaging in disease cohorts such as cleft lip/palate (7) has opened the possibility of understanding developmental biological processes in patients and overcoming limitations of animal models that often do not reflect the human disease. The addition of 3D oral scans can improve the quantification of oral anomalies typically associated with many systemic diseases (8, 9). Very often, oral manifestations may be the earliest signs of disease or genetic anomaly and the easiest to quantify, biopsy or collect as biospecimens for detailed analysis.

Regenerative Medicine: New scaffold designs, improved imaging and technologies to track genes, cells and proteins during development and regeneration, and use of organoids as 3D miniatured models derived from stem cells are among major innovations that are advancing regenerative medicine in the quest to replace tissues/organs lost to trauma or disease. Some ongoing activities in this space include the National Academy of Medicine Regenerative Medicine Forum started in 2016[2] and Armed Forces Institute of Regenerative Medicine (AFIRM), a multi-institutional, interdisciplinary network[3], with opportunities for funding projects focused on wounded servicemen and women, e.g., repair of muscles, nerves and body parts (10–13).

Electronic Health Records: As the value of Precision Medicine/Individualized Healthcare has become more apparent the need for interoperable electronic health records has emerged as a key element needed for establishing accurate databases linking genomics data with other data about an individual, e.g., health history, race/ethnicity, demographics. This has resulted in significant improvements in EHR, however there have been limited attempts in the dental arena to have electronic dental records interoperable and even less related to developing platforms so that medical-dental records are interoperable. Importantly, initiatives to date indicate that interoperable electronic records result in increased preventive care visits and decreased costs associated with medical-dental diseases.

Genetics/Genomics/Proteomics: The development of sophisticated tools and technologies has resulted in an exponential growth in studies focused on identifying genes, proteins, cells, factors (host-immune responses) and microbes and in new knowledge toward understanding health and disease over a person's life span. The ability to use systematic genetic mapping in families and communities has assisted researchers in identifying genetic variants and thus, improve diagnosis and treatment, including new drugs and some gene therapy (14). Fortunately, as presented in this perspective, oral-dental researchers, in collaborations across disciplines, have taken advantage of these tools and technologies to include: improved/earlier diagnosis of certain genetic disorders, better understanding of microbial-host interactions, locally and systemically and development of salivary diagnostics for COVID-19.

[1] *https://www.face2gene.com/clinic-deep-phenotypingof-genetic-disorder-dysmorphic-features/*
[2] *http://www.nationalacademies.org/hmd/Activities/Research/RegenerativeMedicine.aspx*
[3] *https://www.afirm.mil/*

on the oral cavity. Recent examples of clinical trials conducted without input from dental scientists illustrate the delays in diagnosis and potential harms in patient outcomes.

Dental Phenotypes

Individuals with genetic mutations often exhibit specific dental phenotypes (observable traits), which may be seen on oral examination. For example, individuals with hypophosphatasia (HPP), caused by mutations in the alkaline phosphatase gene, often have defects in the formation of tooth root cementum, dentin and enamel. Yet clinical trials using alkaline phosphatase enzyme replacement therapy for HPP failed to include an examination of participants' teeth (39). The effects of such therapies on the teeth are just now being analyzed. Several other disorders where oral tissues are now included in the research study have resulted in recognition of substantial oral tissue phenotypes that can lead to more rapid and earlier diagnosis and treatment (8, 40–42).

New Immuno-Cancer Treatments

Other examples of dental contributions to clinical studies and trials are related to broader effects of new therapies on oral tissues. For example, many drugs may affect salivary gland function, alter tooth color, affect mucosal function or cause oral lesions—at times so severe that patients must discontinue therapy. As a result, new drug treatments for a variety of serious disorders require the involvement of oral health scientists as key members of the research team at the outset. The development of immune checkpoint inhibitors (ICI) to treat cancers has identified the concerning side effect of profound xerostomia after a few weeks or months of treatment (43). While this has encouraged research on how ICI disrupts salivary gland function, it underscores why inclusion of dentist scientists is critical.

Osteonecrosis of the Jaw

Without dental-medical integration the oral side effects of new therapies can take years to fathom. This was the case for medication-related osteonecrosis of the jaw (44). It has now been established that anti-resorptive drugs used not only to treat osteoporosis but also some cancers, can result in severe jaw problems as well as other anomalies of bone metabolism. The research confirming cause and effect was the result of intense cross collaboration between dental and non-dental researchers including animal studies, case reports and patient records. It is currently part of clinical endocrinology guidelines to consult a dentist when initiating these therapies, especially cancer therapies (45). Similar best clinical practices include obtaining early dental consultation prior to the initiation of head and neck radiation therapy (for oral cancers). This integration of dental with medical care has lowered the risk of the devastating side effect of osteoradionecrosis of the jaw and improved the quality of life for patients undergoing radiation therapy.

Hospital Acquired Pneumonia

Hospital acquired pneumonia (HAP) accounts for 25 percent of all hospital-acquired infections (46) and presents a serious risk for patients hospitalized with COVID-19 (47). Studies conducted in a veterans' hospital setting have supplied evidence that non-ventilator-associated HAP was reduced significantly by providing standard oral health care (48), improving patient outcomes while lowering costs of care. This study has been expanded to include eight VA hospitals with plans for national VA deployment. While substantial evidence exists that oral health care is a modifiable risk factor for HAP and other infectious diseases, it has not been adopted universally (49, 50).

Human Papillomavirus Virus (HPV) Vaccine

This is an example where dental patient evaluation was omitted in clinical trials to evaluate the effectiveness of HPV vaccines. HPV vaccines are now recognized for their potential to prevent HPV-related oropharyngeal cancers, which have risen dramatically in recent years, especially in younger-aged groups (51). It took collaborative research efforts to reveal that this sexually transmitted disease can cause devastating manifestation in the oral cavity, and to increase research support to better understand the biologic implications of HPV +/− oral cancers. Since research has shown that some individuals are more likely to seek dental care (including for cosmetic reasons) compared with medical care, dental professionals need appropriate training so they can counsel their patients appropriately and even administer HPV and other vaccines, including COVID-19 (52). In fact, several states have approved providing vaccines in the dental setting, a view supported by the American Dental Association (53, 54).

GAINS WHEN DENTAL SCIENTISTS ARE PART OF THE TEAM

Several areas of research are benefiting from new broad-based initiatives, cross-collaborations and multidisciplinary teamwork, specifically: microbiology, salivary studies, and craniofacial anomalies.

The Human Microbiome

From the initial discoveries that dental caries and periodontal disease were associated with specific bacterial species, oral health scientists have analyzed the complex microbial communities lining oral and dental surfaces in what were called biofilms. These complex microbial communities continue to be explored for relationships with many other diseases, including malignancies (55–57). With availability of newer tools and technologies researchers have expanded their horizons beyond mapping the human genome with its 20,000 genes to explore the much larger domain of the human microbiome, including previously uncultivable microbes. The Human Microbiome Project (HMP) was launched by NIH in 2007 (58) to map the human microbiome, choosing five sites: mouth, nasal, skin, gastrointestinal and urogenital tract. It is a stunning example of the information that can be gleaned when the dental domain is included in transdisciplinary research projects (59). One of the HMP outcomes has been a deeper awareness that microbes have a major influence on the host in health and disease, a story which is just beginning to unfold (60–68). As far as the mouth is concerned, it is a domain where oral scientists have been pioneers (69).

The *immune-microbiome complex* has become an area of intense investigation comparing the effects of a healthy vs. a diseased microbiome on the host-immune response. Intriguingly, Klebsiella can induce an inflammatory response in the gut, but not in the oral mucosa (60), while Fusobacterium nucleatum, an oral bacterium associated with severe periodontal disease, is linked to colon cancer (70). Porphyromonas gingivalis, a keystone pathogen in chronic periodontal disease, has been identified in amyloid plaques of individuals with Alzheimer's disease (71, 72).

The Periodontitis-Diabetes Story

The observation that patients with uncontrolled diabetes often have severe periodontitis inspired yet another major success story of the payoff when dental and non-dental researchers work together. Initial observations among the Pima tribe (73, 74) led to a focus on host-immune-microbial interactions and the key observation that in cases of uncontrolled diabetes, oral tissues, along with other tissues in the body, exhibit a hyperinflammatory response to local insults, such as infection or trauma. Addressing the hyperinflammatory issues early proved to be effective in managing, and in some cases preventing, the periodontal disease consequences of diabetes. Provision of non-surgical treatment has been associated with reductions in metabolic markers of dysglycemia, primarily glycated hemoglobin (75–77). Further, analyses of insurance databases have suggested that the provision of non-surgical periodontal treatment to persons with diabetes is associated with improved health outcomes, including reduced utilization and costs (78–80). So persuasive have been the findings from these studies that a number of U.S. insurance companies now offer additional dental care for their diabetic clients as a way to forestall more serious complications and hospitalizations. The establishment of the diabetes-periodontitis connection has important implications for addressing health disparities. Diabetes and obesity (a risk factor for diabetes) disproportionately occur in poor and minority groups. If they lack access to dental care, the impact of the two diseases will be more severe.

Salivary Diagnostics

The attractiveness of using saliva, known to contain, among other things, viral pathogens, shed cellular material (including genetic), and circulating antibodies, coupled with ease of sampling, has resulted in research targeted at detecting specific diseases or disorders and some success in the commercial development of diagnostic kits for this purpose. However, as saliva is a diluted exudate compared with blood, the amount of a given biomarker in saliva may be inadequate to detect with current tools and

TABLE 2 | Approaches toward achieving integration of oral health within the context of total health.

Collaborative and trans-disciplinary efforts are needed to integrate dental science research into broad areas of biomedical research in both the public and private sectors, where its omission has limited progress and in some cases led to adverse health outcomes (97).
Implementation science programs and learning health care systems should be deployed to ensure that the biomedical knowledge generated by an integrated research enterprise is translated into clinical practice, public policies, and consumer-directed applications, including programs to improve health literacy (19, 98). Educational efforts, along with policies that ensure equitable access to oral health care for all communities, locally, nationally and globally, can help eliminate the health disparities that persist in our nation.
The development of interoperable electronic health records (EHRs) that collectively track medical and dental health histories for patients and providers is essential to further understanding of an individual's health profile over the life span, noting risk factors, acute and chronic illnesses, and other critical information (28).
Advance Communications/Networking across disciplines: Several communities over the last few years have developed initiatives highlighting the importance of attending to all aspects of the body, including the oral region, in research, clinical care, education and policy development, in order to improve total health for all. Yet interactions and the exchange of ideas among the various constituencies are often lacking and consequently possibilities for advancing transdisciplinary approaches to health improvement are missed. Perhaps an "Oral-Systemic Health Hub" is needed where events and publications of importance to the larger community are posted regularly. For example, the Santa Fe Group has organized a *Continuum on the Benefits of Integrating Oral Health into Overall Health* [a series of webinars, a Salon and other resources on this topic (www.santafegroup.org/events)], and other groups are working on initiatives with a similar focus. And at the time of submission of this *Perspective* a Resource Library for the Integration of Primary Care and Oral Health was announced: https://resourcelibrary.hsdm.harvard.edu/. This site has already been populated with many publications and events. These and similar efforts reflect the mounting interest in integration and transdisciplinary approaches to health improvement which it is hoped *Frontiers in Dental Medicine* and *Frontiers in Oral Health* will continue to seed.

technologies Advanced technologies may improve that situation and indeed the advent of the coronavirus pandemic has already led to the development of safe and effective salivary test kits to detect SARS-CoV-2 in an individual (81). Symptomatic and asymptomatic spread of this virus is likely from saliva droplets and respiratory fluids (82, 83). Additionally, saliva may serve as a better source for detection of oral conditions such as oral pharyngeal HPV cancer than currently used blood tests and may be an ideal source for a "liquid biopsy" for point of care application (84–87).

Craniofacial Conditions

One of the best examples of comprehensive, collaborative care that includes dental specialists in a multidisciplinary setting is the craniofacial anomalies team. The American Cleft Palate-Craniofacial Association (ACPA) recognizes craniofacial teams who meet standards based on parameters of care that have been shown through research to provide optimal care for children with cleft lip and palate or other craniofacial anomalies. Dental specialists are integral to these teams with a direct impact on improved quality and outcomes of treatment. Several areas of research have advanced the care of children with congenital craniofacial anomalies and the understanding of disease processes leading to potential novel therapeutics for ectodermal dysplasia (88–90), promising intrauterine therapies to rescue cleft palate in mouse models (91–95), and better understanding of post-natal craniofacial development in patients with cleft lip and palate (7).

THE PANDEMIC AND DENTAL RESEARCH

While the dental community has long implemented safe practices of infection control and personalized protective equipment (PPE) resulting in very low infection rates among dentists during the pandemic (96), the potential for engaging the dental community in enhanced testing and sampling technologies is huge. Through the simple act of touching a dental mirror to the inside cheek of a patient, a dentist can be the "point of contact" for sampling saliva as a diagnostic fluid. Additionally, biosensors incorporated in a dental mirror or toothbrush can record vital signs, including temperature fluctuations and oxygen saturation, which could detect the early presence of disease in a community. Realtime data collection from such smart tools can protect the US population by predicting early hotspots of disease, as noted by Kinsa smart thermometers during the early phase of the SARS-CoV-2 pandemic[1].

CONCLUSIONS: A CALL TO ACTION FOR RESEARCHERS, EDUCATORS AND CLINICIANS

The goal of this perspective is to increase awareness of these issues and to activate researchers, healthcare providers, economists, policy drivers, advocacy groups and the communities we serve, locally and globally, to advance collaborations across all disciplines/communities. We cannot afford to ignore data from the dental, oral and craniofacial part of the body. A few suggested action items are presented in **Table 2**.

AUTHOR CONTRIBUTIONS

All authors listed have made a substantial, direct and intellectual contribution to the work, and approved it for publication.

ACKNOWLEDGMENTS

Special thanks are extended to the FDEM staff and to the Santa Fe Group.

[1]https://www.nytimes.com/2020/03/18/health/coronavirus-fever-thermometers.html

REFERENCES

1. Bender EM, McMillan-Major A, Shmitchell S. On the dangers of stochastic parrots: can language models be too big? In: *FAccT '21: Proceedings of the 2021 ACM Conference on Fairness, Accountability, and Transparency*. (2021). p. 610–23. doi: 10.1145/3442188.3445922
2. Matheny M, Thadaney Israni S, Ahmed M, Whicher D, editors. *Artificial Intelligence in Health Care: The Hope, the Hype, the Promise, the Peril.* NAM Special Publication. Washington, DC: National Academy of Medicine (2019). Available online at: https://nam.edu/artificial-intelligence-special-publication/
3. Liberton DK, Verma P, Contratto A, Lee JS. Development and validation of novel three-dimensional craniofacial landmarks on cone-beam computed tomography scans. *J Craniofac Surg.* (2019) 30:e611–15. doi: 10.1097/SCS.0000000000005627
4. Torosdagli N, Liberton DK, Verma P, Sincan M, Lee JS, Bagci U. Deep geodesic learning for segmentation and anatomical landmarking. *IEEE Trans Med Imaging.* (2019) 38:919–31. doi: 10.1109/TMI.2018.2875814
5. Kim, Misra D, Rodriguez L, Gill M, Liberton DK, Almpani K, et al. Malocclusion classification on 3d cone-beam CT craniofacial images using multi-channel deep learning models. *Annu Int Conf IEEE Eng Med Biol Soc.* (2020) 2020:1294–8. doi: 10.1109/EMBC44109.2020.9176672
6. Misra DG, Lee MJS, Antani S. Segmentation of anterior tissues in craniofacial cone-beam CT images. In: *IEEE 33rd International Symposium on Computer-Based Medical Systems.* (2020). p. 71–6. doi: 10.1109/CBMS49503.2020.00021
7. Liberton DK, Verma P, Almpani K, Fung PW, Mishra R, Oberoi S, et al. Craniofacial analysis may indicate co-occurrence of skeletal malocclusions and associated risks in development of cleft lip and palate. *J Dev Biol.* (2020) 8:2. doi: 10.3390/jdb8010002
8. Jani P, Nguyen QC, Almpani K, Keyvanfar C, Mishra R, Liberton D, et al. Severity of oro-dental anomalies in Loeys-Dietz syndrome segregates by gene mutation. *J Med Genet.* (2020) 57:699–707. doi: 10.1136/jmedgenet-2019-106678
9. Daich Varela M, Jani P, Zein WM, D'Souza P, Wolfe L, Chisholm J, et al. The peroxisomal disorder spectrum and Heimler syndrome: deep phenotyping and review of the literature. *Am J Med Genet C Semin Med Genet.* (2020) 184:618–30. doi: 10.1002/ajmg.c.31823
10. Liu J, Kim YS, Richardson CE, Tom A, Ramakrishnan C, Birey F, et al. Genetically targeted chemical assembly of functional materials in living cells, tissues, and animals. *Science.* (2020) 367:1372–6. doi: 10.1126/science.aay4866
11. Lumelsky N, O'Hayre M, Chander P, Shum L, Somerman MJ. Autotherapies: enhancing endogenous healing and regeneration. *Trends Mol Med.* (2018) 24:919–30. doi: 10.1016/j.molmed.2018.08.004
12. Nagai K, Ideguchi H, Kajikawa T, Li X, Chavakis T, Cheng J, et al. An injectable hydrogel-formulated inhibitor of prolyl-4-hydroxylase promotes T regulatory cell recruitment and enhances alveolar bone regeneration during resolution of experimental periodontitis. *FASEB J.* (2020) 34:13726–40. doi: 10.1096/fj.202001248R
13. Kim J, Koo BK, Knoblich JA. Human organoids: model systems for human biology and medicine. *Nat Rev Mol Cell Biol.* (2020) 21:571–84. doi: 10.1038/s41580-020-0259-3
14. Collins FS, Doudna JA, Lander ES, Rotimi CN. Human molecular genetics and genomics - important advances and exciting possibilities. *N Engl J Med.* (2021) 384:1–4. doi: 10.1056/NEJMp2030694
15. Gupta A, Madhavan MV, Sehgal K, Nair N, Mahajan S, Sehrawat TS, et al. Extrapulmonary manifestations of COVID-19. *Nat Med.* (2020) 26:1017–32. doi: 10.1038/s41591-020-0968-3
16. da Rosa Mesquita R, Francelino Silva Junior LC, Santos Santana FM, Farias de Oliveira T, Campos Alcântara R, Monteiro Arnozo G, et al. Clinical manifestations of COVID-19 in the general population: systematic review. *Wien Klin Wochenschr.* (2020) 133:377–82. doi: 10.1007/s00508-020-01760-4
17. Pierron D, Pereda-Loth V, Mantel M, Moranges M, Bignon E, Alva O, et al. Smell and taste changes are early indicators of the COVID-19 pandemic and political decision effectiveness. *Nat Commun.* (2020) 11:5152. doi: 10.1038/s41467-020-18963-y
18. Coke CJ, Davison B, Fields N, Fletcher J, Rollings J, Roberson L, et al. SARS-CoV-2 infection and oral health: therapeutic opportunities and challenges. *J Clin Med.* (2021) 10:156. doi: 10.3390/jcm10010156
19. Chambers DA, Feero WG, Khoury MJ. Convergence of implementation science, precision medicine, and the learning health care system: a new model for biomedical research. *JAMA.* (2016) 315:1941–2. doi: 10.1001/jama.2016.3867
20. Wang CJ, McCauley LK. Osteoporosis and periodontitis. *Curr Osteoporos Rep.* (2016) 14:284–91. doi: 10.1007/s11914-016-0330-3
21. Siddiqi, Zafar S, Sharma A, Quaranta A. Diabetes mellitus and periodontal disease: the call for interprofessional education and interprofessional collaborative care - A systematic review of the literature. *J Interprof Care.* (2020) 1–9. doi: 10.1080/13561820.2020.1825354
22. Kitamoto S, Nagao-Kitamoto H, Jiao Y, Gillilland MG, 3rd, Hayashi A, Imai J, et al. The intermucosal connection between the mouth and gut in commensal pathobiont-driven colitis. *Cell.* (2020) 182:447–62 e14. doi: 10.1016/j.cell.2020.05.048
23. Kleinstein SE, Nelson KE, Freire M. Inflammatory networks linking oral microbiome with systemic health and disease. *J Dent Res.* (2020) 99:1131–9. doi: 10.1177/0022034520926126
24. Dioguardi M, Crincoli V, Laino L, Alovisi M, Sovereto D, Mastrangelo F, et al. The role of periodontitis and periodontal bacteria in the onset and progression of Alzheimer's disease: a systematic review. *J Clin Med.* (2020) 9:495. doi: 10.3390/jcm9020495
25. Ling MR, Chapple IL, Matthews JB. Peripheral blood neutrophil cytokine hyper-reactivity in chronic periodontitis. *Innate Immun.* (2015) 21:714–25. doi: 10.1177/1753425915589387
26. Delbove T, Gueyffier F, Juillard L, Kalbacher E, Maucort-Boulch D, Nony P, et al. Effect of periodontal treatment on the glomerular filtration rate, reduction of inflammatory markers and mortality in patients with chronic kidney disease: a systematic review. *PLoS One.* (2021) 16:e0245619. doi: 10.1371/journal.pone.0245619
27. Nguyen QC, Duverger O, Mishra R, Mitnik GL, Jani P, Frischmeyer-Guerrerio PA, et al. Oral health-related quality of life in Loeys-Dietz syndrome, a rare connective tissue disorder: an observational cohort study. *Orphanet J Rare Dis.* (2019) 14:291. doi: 10.1186/s13023-019-1250-y
28. Mosen DM, Banegas MP, Dickerson JF, Fellows JL, Brooks NB, Pihlstrom DJ, et al. Examining the association of medical-dental integration with closure of medical care gaps among the elderly population. *J Am Dent Assoc.* (2021) 152:302–8. doi: 10.1016/j.adaj.2020.12.010
29. Tenuta LMA, Canady C, Eber RM, Johnson L. Agreement in medications reported in medical and dental electronic health records. *JDR Clin Trans Res.* (2021). doi: 10.1177/23800844211004525. [Epub ahead of print].
30. Benjamin RM. Oral health: the silent epidemic. *Public Health Rep.* (2010) 125:158–9. doi: 10.1177/003335491012500202
31. Eke PI, Dye BA, Wei L, Slade GD, Thornton-Evans GO, Borgnakke WS, et al. Update on prevalence of periodontitis in adults in the United States: NHANES 2009 to 2012. *J Periodontol.* (2015) 86:611–22. doi: 10.1902/jop.2015.140520
32. Sen S, Redd K, Trivedi T, Moss K, Alonso A, Soliman EZ, et al. Periodontal disease, atrial fibrillation and stroke. *Am Heart J.* (2021) 235:36–43. doi: 10.1016/j.ahj.2021.01.009
33. Romandini M, Baima G, Antonoglou G, Bueno J, Figuero E, Sanz M. Periodontitis, edentulism, and risk of mortality: a systematic review with meta-analyses. *J Dent Res.* (2021) 100:37–49. doi: 10.1177/0022034520952401
34. Monsarrat P, Blaizot A, Kemoun P, Ravaud P, Nabet C, Sixou M, et al. Clinical research activity in periodontal medicine: a systematic mapping of trial registers. *J Clin Periodontol.* (2016) 43:390–400. doi: 10.1111/jcpe.12534
35. Van Dyke TE, Kholy KE, Ishai A, R.Takx AP, Mezue K, Abohashem SM, et al. Inflammation of the periodontium associates with risk of future cardiovascular events. *J Periodontol.* (2021) 92:348–58. doi: 10.1002/JPER.19-0441
36. Nguyen LM, Chon JJ, Kim EE, Cheng JC, Ebersole JL. Biological aging and periodontal disease: analysis of NHANES. (2001-2002). *JDR Clin Trans Res.* (2021). doi: 10.1177/2380084421995812. [Epub ahead of print].
37. Baum BJ. Salivary gland fluid secretion during aging. *J Am Geriatr Soc.* (1989) 37:453–8. doi: 10.1111/j.1532-5415.1989.tb02644.x
38. Ship JA, Pillemer SR, Baum BJ. Xerostomia and the geriatric patient. *J Am Geriatr Soc.* (2002) 50:535–43. doi: 10.1046/j.1532-5415.2002.50123.x
39. Whyte MP. Hypophosphatasia - aetiology, nosology, pathogenesis, diagnosis and treatment. *Nat Rev Endocrinol.* (2016) 12:233–46. doi: 10.1038/nrendo.2016.14

40. Thumbigere-Math V, Alqadi A, Chalmers NI, Chavez MB, Chu EY, Collins MT, et al. Hypercementosis associated with ENPP1 mutations and GACI. *J Dent Res.* (2018) 97:432–41. doi: 10.1177/0022034517744773
41. Chavez MB, Kramer K, Chu EY, Thumbigere-Math V, Foster BL. Insights into dental mineralization from three heritable mineralization disorders. *J Struct Biol.* (2020) 212:107597. doi: 10.1016/j.jsb.2020.107597
42. Lee AE, Chu EY, Gardner PJ, Duverger O, Saikali A, Wang SK, et al. A cross-sectional cohort study of the effects of FGF23 deficiency and hyperphosphatemia on dental structures in hyperphosphatemic familial tumor calcinosis. *JBMR Plus.* (2021) 5:e10470. doi: 10.1002/jbm4.10470
43. Warner BM, Baer AN, Lipson EJ, Allen C, Hinrichs C, Rajan A, et al. Sicca syndrome associated with immune checkpoint inhibitor therapy. *Oncologist.* (2019) 24:1259–69. doi: 10.1634/theoncologist.2018-0823
44. Wan JT, Sheeley DM, Somerman MJ, Lee JS. Mitigating osteonecrosis of the jaw (ONJ) through preventive dental care and understanding of risk factors. *Bone Res.* (2020) 8:14. doi: 10.1038/s41413-020-0088-1
45. Foster BL, Nociti FH Jr, Somerman MJ. The rachitic tooth. *Endocr Rev.* (2014) 35:1–34. doi: 10.1210/er.2013-1009
46. Magill SS, Edwards JR, Bamberg W, Beldavs ZG, Dumyati G, Kainer MA, et al. Multistate point-prevalence survey of health care-associated infections. *N Engl J Med.* (2014) 370:1198–208. doi: 10.1056/NEJMoa1306801
47. Botros N, Iyer P, Ojcius DM. Is there an association between oral health and severity of COVID-19 complications? *Biomed J.* (2020) 43:325–7. doi: 10.1016/j.bj.2020.05.016
48. Munro S, Baker D. Reducing missed oral care opportunities to prevent non-ventilator associated hospital acquired pneumonia at the department of veterans affairs. *Appl Nurs Res.* (2018) 44:48–53. doi: 10.1016/j.apnr.2018.09.004
49. Kaneoka, Pisegna JM, Miloro KV, Lo M, Saito H, Riquelme LF, et al. Prevention of healthcare-associated pneumonia with oral care in individuals without mechanical ventilation: a systematic review and meta-analysis of randomized controlled trials. *Infect Control Hosp Epidemiol.* (2015) 36:899–906. doi: 10.1017/ice.2015.77
50. Baker D, Quinn B. Hospital acquired pneumonia prevention initiative-2: incidence of nonventilator hospital-acquired pneumonia in the United States. *Am J Infect Control.* (2018) 46:2–7. doi: 10.1016/j.ajic.2017.08.036
51. Gillison ML, Chaturvedi AK, Anderson WF, Fakhry C. Epidemiology of human papillomavirus-positive head and neck squamous cell carcinoma. *J Clin Oncol.* (2015) 33:3235–42. doi: 10.1200/JCO.2015.61.6995
52. Strauss SM, Alfano MC, Shelley D, Fulmer T. Identifying unaddressed systemic health conditions at dental visits: patients who visited dental practices but not general health care providers in 2008. *Am J Public Health.* (2012) 102:253–5. doi: 10.2105/AJPH.2011.300420
53. Villa, Chmieliauskaite M, Patton LL. Including vaccinations in the scope of dental practice: the time has come. *J Am Dent Assoc.* (2021) 152:184–6. doi: 10.1016/j.adaj.2020.09.025
54. Wright JT. COVID-19 vaccination: science, politics and public health. *J Am Dent Assoc.* (2021) 152:181–3. doi: 10.1016/j.adaj.2021.01.009
55. F.Teles RF, Alawi F, Castilho RM, Wang Y. Association or causation? Exploring the oral microbiome and cancer links. *J Dent Res.* (2020) 99:1411–24. doi: 10.1177/0022034520945242
56. Bornigen D, Ren B, Pickard R, Li J, Ozer E, Hartmann EM, et al. Alterations in oral bacterial communities are associated with risk factors for oral and oropharyngeal cancer. *Sci Rep.* (2017) 7:17686. doi: 10.1038/s41598-017-17795-z
57. Kitamoto S, Nagao-Kitamoto H, Hein R, Schmidt TM, Kamada N. The bacterial connection between the oral cavity and the gut diseases. *J Dent Res.* (2020) 99:1021–9. doi: 10.1177/0022034520924633
58. Turnbaugh PJ, Ley RE, Hamady M, Fraser-Liggett CM, Knight R, Gordon JI. The human microbiome project. *Nature.* (2007) 449:804–10. doi: 10.1038/nature06244
59. Gevers D, Knight R, Petrosino JF, Huang K, McGuire AL, Birren BW, et al. The human microbiome project: a community resource for the healthy human microbiome. *PLoS Biol.* (2012) 10:e1001377. doi: 10.1371/journal.pbio.1001377
60. Atarashi K, Suda W, Luo C, Kawaguchi T, Motoo I, Narushima S, et al. Ectopic colonization of oral bacteria in the intestine drives TH1 cell induction and inflammation. *Science.* (2017) 358:359–65. doi: 10.1126/science.aan4526
61. Tsukasaki M, Komatsu N, Nagashima K, Nitta T, Pluemsakunthai W, Shukunami C, et al. Host defense against oral microbiota by bone-damaging T cells. *Nat Commun.* (2018) 9:701. doi: 10.1038/s41467-018-03147-6
62. Willis JR, Gabaldon T. The human oral microbiome in health and disease: from sequences to ecosystems. *Microorganisms.* (2020) 8:308. doi: 10.3390/microorganisms8020308
63. Genco RJ, Sanz M. Clinical and public health implications of periodontal and systemic diseases: an overview. *Periodontol 2000.* (2020) 83:7–13. doi: 10.1111/prd.12344
64. Aquino-Martinez R, Hernandez-Vigueras S. Severe COVID-19 lung infection in older people and periodontitis. *J Clin Med.* (2021) 10:279. doi: 10.3390/jcm10020279
65. Paul O, Arora P, Mayer M, Chatterjee S. Inflammation in periodontal disease: possible link to vascular disease. *Front Physiol.* (2020) 11:609614. doi: 10.3389/fphys.2020.609614
66. Chung M, Zhao N, Meier R, Koestler DC, Wu G, de Castillo E, et al. Comparisons of oral, intestinal, and pancreatic bacterial microbiomes in patients with pancreatic cancer and other gastrointestinal diseases. *J Oral Microbiol.* (2021) 13:1887680. doi: 10.1080/20002297.2021.1887680
67. Helenius-Hietala J, Suominen AL, Ruokonen H, Knuuttila M, Puukka P, Jula A, et al. Periodontitis is associated with incident chronic liver disease-A population-based cohort study. *Liver Int.* (2019) 39:583–91. doi: 10.1111/liv.13985
68. Acharya, Bajaj JS. Gut microbiota and complications of liver disease. *Gastroenterol Clin North Am.* (2017) 46:155–69. doi: 10.1016/j.gtc.2016.09.013
69. Hajishengallis G, Chavakis T. Local and systemic mechanisms linking periodontal disease and inflammatory comorbidities. *Nat Rev Immunol.* (2021). doi: 10.1038/s41577-020-00488-6
70. Mima K, Nishihara R, Qian ZR, Cao Y, Sukawa Y, Nowak JA, et al. Fusobacterium nucleatum in colorectal carcinoma tissue and patient prognosis. *Gut.* (2016) 65:1973–80. doi: 10.1136/gutjnl-2015-310101
71. Dominy SS, Lynch C, Ermini F, Benedyk M, Marczyk A, Konradi A, et al. Porphyromonas gingivalis in Alzheimer's disease brains: evidence for disease causation and treatment with small-molecule inhibitors. *Sci Adv.* (2019) 5:eaau3333. doi: 10.1126/sciadv.aau3333
72. Costa MJF, de Araújo IDT, da Rocha Alves L, da Silva RL, Dos Santos Calderon P, Borges BCD, et al. Relationship of Porphyromonas gingivalis and Alzheimer's disease: a systematic review of pre-clinical studies. *Clin Oral Investig.* (2021) 25:797–806. doi: 10.1007/s00784-020-03764-w
73. Shlossman M, Knowler WC, Pettitt DJ, Genco RJ. Type 2 diabetes mellitus and periodontal disease. *J Am Dent Assoc.* (1990) 121:532–6. doi: 10.14219/jada.archive.1990.0211
74. Nelson RG, Shlossman M, Budding LM, Pettitt DJ, Saad MF, Genco RJ, et al. Periodontal disease and NIDDM in Pima Indians. *Diabetes Care.* (1990) 13:836–40. doi: 10.2337/diacare.13.8.836
75. D'Aiuto F, Gkranias N, Bhowruth D, Khan T, Orlandi M, Suvan J, et al. Systemic effects of periodontitis treatment in patients with type 2 diabetes: a 12 month, single-centre, investigator-masked, randomised trial. *Lancet Diabetes Endocrinol.* (2018) 6:954–65. doi: 10.1016/S2213-8587(18)30038-X
76. Cao R, Li Q, Wu Q, Yao M, Chen Y, Zhou H. Effect of non-surgical periodontal therapy on glycemic control of type 2 diabetes mellitus: a systematic review and Bayesian network meta-analysis. *BMC Oral Health.* (2019) 19:176. doi: 10.1186/s12903-019-0829-y
77. Baeza M, Morales A, Cisterna C, Cavalla F, Jara G, Isamitt Y, et al. Effect of periodontal treatment in patients with periodontitis and diabetes: systematic review and meta-analysis. *J Appl Oral Sci.* (2020) 28:e20190248. doi: 10.1590/1678-7757-2019-0248
78. Nasseh K, Vujicic M, Glick M. The relationship between periodontal interventions and healthcare costs and utilization. Evidence from an Integrated Dental, Medical, and Pharmacy Commercial Claims Database. *Health Econ.* (2017) 26:519–27. doi: 10.1002/hec.3316
79. Smits KPJ, Listl S, Plachokova AS, Van der Galien O, Kalmus O. Effect of periodontal treatment on diabetes-related healthcare costs: a retrospective study. *BMJ Open Diabetes Res Care.* (2020) 8:e001666. doi: 10.1136/bmjdrc-2020-001666
80. Alfano MC. The economic impact of periodontal inflammation. In: Glick M, editor. *The Oral-Systemic Health Connection, 2nd ed.* Batavia, IL: Quintessence Publishing Co, Inc. p. 358–69.

81. Wyllie AL, Fournier J, Casanovas-Massana A, Campbell M, Tokuyama M, Vijayakumar P, et al. Saliva or nasopharyngeal swab specimens for detection of SARS-CoV-2. *N Engl J Med.* (2020) 383:1283–6. doi: 10.1056/NEJMc2016359
82. Fernandes LL, Pacheco VB, Borges L, Athwal HK, de Paula Eduardo F, Bezinelli L, et al. Saliva in the diagnosis of COVID-19: a review and new research directions. *J Dent Res.* (2020) 99:1435–43. doi: 10.1177/0022034520960070
83. Huang N, Perez P, Kato T, Mikami Y, Okuda K, Gilmore RC, et al. SARS-CoV-2 infection of the oral cavity and saliva. *Nat Med.* (2021) 27:892–903. doi: 10.1038/s41591-021-01296-8
84. Tang KD, Baeten K, Kenny L, Frazer IH, Scheper G, Punyadeera C. Unlocking the potential of saliva-based test to detect HPV-16-driven oropharyngeal cancer. *Cancers.* (2019) 11:473. doi: 10.3390/cancers11040473
85. Ahn SM, Chan JY, Zhang Z, Wang H, Khan Z, Bishop JA, et al. Saliva and plasma quantitative polymerase chain reaction-based detection and surveillance of human papillomavirus-related head and neck cancer. *JAMA Otolaryngol Head Neck Surg.* (2014) 140:846–54. doi: 10.1001/jamaoto.2014.1338
86. Fakhry, Blackford AL, Neuner G, Xiao W, Jiang B, Agrawal A, et al. Association of oral human papillomavirus DNA persistence with cancer progression after primary treatment for oral cavity and oropharyngeal squamous cell carcinoma. *JAMA Oncol.* (2019) 5:985–92. doi: 10.1001/jamaoncol.2019.0439
87. Aro K, Wei F, Wong DT, Tu M. Saliva liquid biopsy for point-of-care applications. *Front Public Health.* (2017) 5:77. doi: 10.3389/fpubh.2017.00077
88. Margolis CA, Schneider P, Huttner K, Kirby N, Houser TP, Wildman L, et al. Prenatal treatment of X-linked hypohidrotic ectodermal dysplasia using recombinant ectodysplasin in a canine model. *J Pharmacol Exp Ther.* (2019) 370:806–13. doi: 10.1124/jpet.118.256040
89. Schneider H, Faschingbauer F, Schuepbach-Mallepell S, Korber I, Wohlfart S, Dick A, et al. Prenatal correction of X-linked hypohidrotic ectodermal dysplasia. *N Engl J Med.* (2018) 378:1604–10. doi: 10.1056/NEJMoa1714322
90. Marchegiani S, Davis T, Tessadori F, van Haaften G, Brancati F, Hoischen A, et al. Recurrent Mutations in the Basic Domain of TWIST2 Cause Ablepharon Macrostomia and Barber-Say Syndromes. *Am J Hum Genet.* (2015) 97:99–110. doi: 10.1016/j.ajhg.2015.05.017
91. Jia S, Zhou J, Wee Y, Mikkola ML, Schneider P, D'Souza RN. Anti-EDAR agonist antibody therapy resolves palate defects in Pax9(-/-) mice. *J Dent Res.* (2017) 96:1282–9. doi: 10.1177/00220345177 26073
92. Jia S, Zhou J, D'Souza RN. Pax9's dual roles in modulating Wnt signaling during murine palatogenesis. *Dev Dyn.* (2020) 249:1274–84. doi: 10.1002/dvdy.189
93. Jia S, Zhou J, Fanelli C, Wee Y, Bonds J, Schneider P, et al. Small-molecule Wnt agonists correct cleft palates in Pax9 mutant mice *in utero*. *Development.* (2017) 144:3819–3828. doi: 10.1242/dev.1 57750
94. Oliver JD, Turner EC, Halpern LR, Jia S, Schneider P, D'Souza RN. Molecular diagnostics and *in utero* therapeutics for orofacial clefts. *J Dent Res.* (2020) 99:1221–7. doi: 10.1177/00220345209 36245
95. Oliver JD, Jia S, Halpern LR, Graham EM, Turner EC, Colombo JS, et al. Innovative molecular and cellular therapeutics in cleft palate tissue engineering. *Tissue Eng Part B Rev.* (2020). doi: 10.1089/ten.teb.20 20.0181
96. Estrich CG, Mikkelsen M, Morrissey R, Geisinger ML, Ioannidou E, Vujicic M, et al. Estimating COVID-19 prevalence and infection control practices among US dentists. *J Am Dent Assoc.* (2020) 151:815–24. doi: 10.1016/j.adaj.2020.09.005
97. Somerman MJ, Mouradian WE. Integrating oral and systemic health: innovations in transdisciplinary science, health care and policy. *Front Dent Med.* (2020) 1:599214. doi: 10.3389/fdmed.2020.599214
98. Atchinson KA, Weintraub JA. *Discussion Paper - Integration of Oral Health and Primary Care: Communication, Coordination, and Referral.* National Academy of Medicine, Perspectives: Expert Voices in Health and Health Care (2018). doi: 10.31478/201810e

2

Characterization of the Oral Microbiome Among Children with Type 1 Diabetes Compared with Healthy Children

Moti Moskovitz[1], Mira Nassar[1,2], Nadav Moriel[3], Avital Cher[3], Sarit Faibis[1], Diana Ram[1], David Zangen[4], Moran Yassour[3] and Doron Steinberg[2]*

[1] *Department of Pediatric Dentistry, Faculty of Dental Medicine, Hadassah Medical Center, The Hebrew University of Jerusalem, Jerusalem, Israel,* [2] *Biofilm Research Laboratory, Faculty of Dental Medicine, Institute of Dental Sciences, The Hebrew University of Jerusalem, Jerusalem, Israel,* [3] *Microbiology and Molecular Genetics Department, Faculty of Medicine, The Hebrew University of Jerusalem, Jerusalem, Israel,* [4] *Division of Pediatric Endocrinology, Hadassah Medical Center, The Hebrew University of Jerusalem, Jerusalem, Israel*

Correspondence:
Moti Moskovitz
motim@md.huji.ac.il

Aim: Current microbiome profiling of type 1 diabetes mellitus (T1D) patients is mostly limited to gut microbiome. We characterized the oral microbiome associated with T1D in children after the onset of the disease and explored its relationship with oral physiological factors and dental status.

Methods: This cohort study comprised 37 children aged 5–15 years with T1D and 29 healthy children matched in age and gender. Unstimulated whole saliva was collected from diabetic and non-diabetic children, in the morning after brushing their teeth and a fasting period of at least 1 h before sampling. 16S rRNA gene-based analysis was performed by Powersoil Pro kit by Qiagen and Phusion High-Fidelity PCR Master Mix. Oral physiological and dental parameters studied included decayed, missing, and filled teeth index, salivary flow rate, and salivary pH, glucose, calcium, phosphate, and urea levels.

Results: Of the identified 105 different genera and 211 different species, the most abundant genera were *Streptococcus*, *Prevotella*, *Veillonella*, *Haemophilus*, and *Neisseria*. *Streptococcus* was more abundant in T1D children. The diabetes group had 22 taxa at the genus level and 33 taxa at the species level that were not present in the control group and the control group exhibited 6 taxa at the genus level and 9 taxa at the species level that did not exist in the diabetes group. In addition, *Catonella*, *Fusobacterium*, and *Mogibacterium* differed between healthy and T1D subjects. Eight species and eight subspecies were significantly more abundant among healthy children than in T1D children. *Porphyromonas* and *Mogibacterium* genera were significantly correlated with salivary parameters. We found similarities between taxa revealed in the present study and those found in gut microbiome in type 1 diabetes mellitus according to gutMDisorder database.

Conclusions: Salivary microbiome analysis revealed unique microbial taxa that differed between T1D children and healthy subjects. Several genera found in the saliva of T1D children were associated with gut microbiome in T1D individuals.

Keywords: type 1 diabetes, children, 16S rRNA gene sequencing, salivary microbiome, periodontitis

INTRODUCTION

Oral microbiome represents an important part of the human microbiome and can have detrimental consequences on both our general and oral health. The genetic setup of the host may affect the microbial composition and function, the activation of intrinsic and adaptive immunity, and susceptibility to various diseases (Zhou et al., 2020). Accumulating evidence links oral bacteria to several systemic diseases including diabetes (Genco et al., 2005). Type 1 diabetes (T1D), also known as insulin-dependent diabetes, is a chronic autoimmune-mediated disease in which the insulin-producing pancreatic beta cells are destroyed. Although it can be diagnosed at any age, it is one of the most common chronic diseases of childhood and adolescence (Maahs et al., 2010; Hong et al., 2017). T1D accounts for 5–10% of diabetic patients worldwide (Maahs et al., 2010; World Health Organization, 2018) and is the second most frequent autoimmune disease in childhood; its incidence has tripled in the last 30 years (de Groot et al., 2017). Worldwide, 1.1 million children and adolescents under the age of 20 live with T1D (International Diabetes Federation, 2019).

The increasing disease rate cannot be explained merely by genetic factors but implies that these changes are an outcome of interactions between the environment and predisposing genes (Siljander et al., 2019).

Diabetes is associated with several soft-tissue abnormalities in the oral cavity secondary to the disease that have a significant effect on the quality of life of diabetic patients (Ferizi et al., 2018). Patients with T1D are more susceptible to periodontal diseases and tooth loss and such problems might be aggravated with aging (Sadeghi et al., 2017). Quantitative and qualitative salivary changes in diabetics have also been confirmed (Angus and Richard, 2008).

The oral microbiome is known to vary in response to oral and systemic diseases (Simpson and Thomas, 2016). Diabetes has a significant impact on the gut microbial composition, stability, and connectivity, which in turn can alter the development of T1D by influencing the immune response of hosts (Han et al., 2018). Oral microbiome of adults has been implicated in the development of type 2 diabetes (T2D), but has been rarely explored in T1D. Long et al. (2017) analyzed the oral microbiome of T2D patients and discovered that the relative abundance of *Actinobacteria*, which associates with a lower risk of developing T2D, decreased (Long et al., 2017). On the contrary, a study in T1D subjects showed significantly higher abundance of taxa belonging to the phyla *Actinobacteria* and *Firmicutes*, including *Streptococcus* spp., *Actinomyces* spp., and *Rothia* spp. (de Groot et al., 2017).

The complex etiology of T1D is underlined by the fact that several years may pass between initial β-cell damage to manifestation of clinical diabetes (Størling and Pociot, 2017). Thus, early diagnosis of diabetes by targeting the microbiota at the latent period could potentially enable early treatment and postpone T1D development in children with β-cell autoimmunity.

The aim of the present study was to profile the salivary microbiome of children with T1D based on 16S ribosomal RNA (16S rRNA) gene community profiling, and to compare it with healthy children, while considering additional aspects of the oral environment. We also analyzed the impact of oral and salivary parameters including DMFT index, salivary flow rate, glucose, pH, calcium, phosphate, and urea on the salivary microbiome.

MATERIALS AND METHODS

Study Population

Ethical Considerations

All procedures performed were in accordance with the study protocol [ClinicalTrials.gov (NCT03908021)] that was approved by the Institutional Human Subjects Ethics Committee of Hadassah Medical Organization (0714-18-HMO). No compensation was provided for the participating patients. The study was conducted in the period from 2019 to 2020.

Because this was an initial study examining the differences in oral microbiome between children with T1D and non-diabetic children, no power calculation was performed. It was decided to collect saliva from all attendants to the division of Pediatric Endocrinology, Hadassah Medical Center, Hebrew University of Jerusalem, Israel, who met the inclusion criteria and were willing to participate in the study during a period of 1 year. Those children were matched in age and gender with healthy children attending the postgraduate program in Orthodontics of the Hebrew University–Hadassah Faculty of Dental Medicine. Control group saliva collection was terminated after a year.

The study was conducted on 66 children, including 37 with diabetes aged 5–15 years, during a routine follow-up visit at the Pediatric Endocrinology Clinic, Hadassah Hebrew University Medical Center (Jerusalem, Israel). All diabetic children were treated with but not with any other therapy at least a week prior to checkup. The control group, matched in age and gender, included

29 healthy children who were attending the Orthodontic Clinic at the same medical center. All healthy children were without functional orthodontic appliances and no history of drug therapy at least a week prior to checkup. Exclusion criteria for both groups were diseases other than T1D and known oral disease. All patients were medication free apart from insulin if needed at the day of sample collection and at least a week before.

Clinical Examination and Collection of Saliva Samples

Clinical dental health status was measured using the Decayed, Missing and Filled Teeth (DMFT) Index according to the WHO caries diagnostic criteria for epidemiological studies (World Health Organization, 1997). All dental examinations were performed by a single qualified dentist from the department of Pediatric Dentistry, Faculty of Dental Medicine, Hebrew University of Jerusalem, Israel, in accordance with the clinic checkup procedures.

Access to dental care, parents' dental education, and the quality of diet were provided through patients' and parents' interview.

Unstimulated whole saliva was collected from diabetic and non-diabetic children, in the morning after brushing their teeth and a fasting period of at least 1 h before sampling. The children were asked to spit saliva into a 15-ml sterile tube over a measured period of time and sufficient for salivary parameter measurement. Only the liquid of the saliva was allocated and collected for the analysis (He et al., 2015).

Before centrifugation, 350 μl of saliva was stored at −80°C for microbiome analysis, and pH and salivary glucose were determined. The saliva samples were then centrifuged at 1,500 RCF (relative centrifugal force) for 15 min at 4°C to reduce salivary debris and viscosity. Salivary calcium, phosphate, and urea were evaluated later in the supernatant fluid, stored at −20°C.

Measurement of Salivary Flow Rate, pH, and Glucose

The salivary flow rate was defined without the foam as the volume (in ml) of saliva secreted per minute of collection. Salivary pH was measured using color-coded pH-indicator strips (pH 0–14 Universal indicator, MQuant; Sigma-Aldrich, Israel). Glucose test strips (Medi-Test Combi 3A; Praxisdienst, Germany) measured salivary glucose.

Measurement of Salivary Calcium, Phosphate, and Urea

Salivary calcium, phosphate, and urea concentrations were calorimetrically measured from the stored clear salivary supernatant fluid and according to the manufacturer's instructions. The following kits were used, respectively: Calcium Colorimetric Assay Kit (MAK022—Sigma-Aldrich, St. Louis, MO 63103, United States), Phosphate Colorimetric Assay Kit (MAK030—Sigma-Aldrich), and Amplite Colorimetric Urea Assay Kit *Blue Color* (10058—AAT Bioquest, Sunnyvale, CA 94085, United States).

Microbiome Analysis and 16S Ribosomal RNA Gene-Based Analysis

DNA extraction was performed by the Powersoil Pro kit by Qiagen (47016), following the company's protocol, with mild modifications. All saliva samples were centrifuged at 14,000 × *g* for 10 min at 4°C. The supernatant fluid was discarded and the pellet was re-suspended in 800 μl of CD1 and then added to the PowerBead Pro tube. Samples were also treated in a bead beaten beater (TissueLyzer; QIAGEN) at 20 Hz for 10 min. 16S rRNA libraries were prepared according to the published protocol (Poyet et al., 2019) with mild modifications. First, qPCR was used to normalize template concentrations and determine the optimal cycle number needed for amplification of the V4 region of the 16S rRNA gene. In the qPCR, each sample was amplified in two 25-μl reactions using iTaq Universal SYBR Green Supermix (#17525124) and the primers 515 F (AATGATACGGCGA CCACCGAGATCTACACTATGGTAATTGT GTGCCAGCMG CCGCGGTAA) and 806rcbc0 (CAAGCAGAAGACGGCATAC GAGAT TCCCTTGTCTCC AGTCAGTCAG CC GGACTACH VGGGTWTCTAAT). Samples were quantified using the formula $1.75^{\Delta Ct}$. To minimize over-amplification, each sample was diluted to the lowest concentration sample, and the Ct value of this lowest concentration sample was used as the cycle number in the PCR reaction for library construction.

For library construction, four 25-μl reactions were prepared per sample using Phusion High-Fidelity PCR Master Mix with HF buffer (M0531L) and the primer 515F and 806R. Each sample was given a unique reverse barcode primer from the Golay primer set (see "Ultra-high-throughput microbial community analysis on the Illumina HiSeq and MiSeq platforms"; Caporaso et al., 2012). The replicates were then pooled and cleaned using Agencourt AMPure XP beads. Purified libraries were diluted 1:100 and quantified via qPCR, again using two reactions of 25 μl with iTaq Universal SYBR Green Supermix, but with the primers Read 1 and Read 2. The undiluted samples were normalized by way of pooling using the formula mentioned previously, and the pools were quantified by Qubit, as well as analyzed on the TapeStation. The pools were then normalized into a final pool based on the concentration calculated by Qubit, the average library size determined by TapeStation results, and the number of samples in the pool.

Final pools were sequenced on an Illumina MiSeq using the custom index 5′-ATTAGAWACCCBDGTAGTCCGGCTGA CTGACT-3′ and custom Read 1 and Read 2, mentioned previously, and using 30% PhiX.

16S Ribosomal RNA Analysis

All sequences passed fastQC using default parameters and had an average of 11,500 reads (with a minimum of 5,876 reads per sequence). BURST v0.99 (Al-Ghalith and Knights, 2017) was applied to the raw reads using default parameters, and with the burst_linux_DB12 database,[1] which is based on the RefSeq Targeted Loci Project.[2]

[1] https://github.com/knights-lab/BURST/releases/download/v0.99.7f/burst_linux_DB12

[2] https://www.ncbi.nlm.nih.gov/refseq/targetedloci/

Results were then divided according to taxonomic level. For family, genus, species, and subspecies level, a threshold of reads was set to 25. Thus, only taxa which had more than 25 reads throughout all the samples were further analyzed. Following the removal of the bacteria that did not meet the threshold, the relative abundance of each bacterium in each sample was re-normalized. A taxon was considered abundant if it had a relative abundance greater than 5% in at least one sample.

Statistically Significant Differential Taxonomic Analysis

To find differential bacterial taxa in which the relative abundance was statistically different between T1D patients and control subjects, we used MaAsLin 2 (Microbiome Multivariable Associations with Linear Models) (Mallick et al., 2021) multivariate linear regression along with an annotation of whether the sample belonged to a case or control. MaAslin2 results were considered statistically significant in case q-value < 0.25. Relevant taxa were then plotted using the ggplot2 package v3.3.3 (Wickham, 2016) in R v4.0.3. The plots include annotation of the coefficient, p-value, and q-value as calculated by MaAslin2.

Taxa Appearing Only in the Study or Control Group

To find bacteria at a certain taxonomic level that appeared only in one of the groups, we took the data table of the relevant taxonomic level and selected only the bacteria that were completely missing in one study group. The value represented by the axis refers to the sum of the relative abundances of the bacteria, within the samples of the axis's population.

Microbial Taxa Association With Various Variables

To find significant associations between various subject parameters and specific bacteria, the data of the relevant taxonomic level was given as input to MaAslin2 alongside a table containing the various metadata variables. Results were considered significant if they had a q-value smaller than 0.25.

Heatmap of Abundant Taxa

A genus was considered abundant if it had a relative abundance greater than 5% in at least one sample across all analyzed samples. This added up to 23 abundant genera in our analysis. The relative abundance of each genus within each sample was plotted into a heatmap, along with an annotation at the top of the plot designating if the sample belonged to a case or control. The heatmap plot was created using the pheatmap package v1.0.12 (Raivo, 2019) in R v4.0.3.

Alpha Diversity Analysis

Alpha diversity measurement was done using the Shannon diversity index that was calculated using the diversity function within the vegan v2.5.7 R package.[3] A Wilcoxon test was applied between the two population groups using the ggpubr v0.4 package.[4]

[3]https://CRAN.R-project.org/package=vegan

[4]https://CRAN.R-project.org/package=ggpubr

Principal Coordinate Analysis

Beta diversity was calculated using the Bray–Curtis dissimilarity index as calculated using the vegan 2.5.7 and ape 5.4.1 R packages (Paradis and Schliep, 2019).

Data Analysis

The average and standard error (SE) of DMFT index, salivary flow rate, pH, glucose, calcium, phosphate, and urea between the two groups were analyzed using Student's t-test and $p < 0.05$ was considered statistically significant.

Microbiome data were analyzed by the "Burst Analyzer" software (Burst-Analyzer—knights-lab)[5] and MaAslin2 comprehensive R package (Maaslin2—Bioconductor)[6] for efficiently determining specific genus and families in which considerable differences were found between study and control samples. Data visualization was performed by ggplot2 in R package (Wickham, 2016).

RESULTS

Population

The study group included 37 children with T1D (17 males) with a mean age (±SD) of 13 ± 2.69 years, and the control group included 29 (11 males) healthy children with a mean age (±SD) of 10 ± 2.38 years with no other relevant differences noted between the groups. All study group participants were using insulin since diagnosed as having T1D; 81.1% of them used insulin pumps with continuous delivery of short-acting insulin. The mean (±SD) time since diagnosis of diabetes was 2 ± 2.58 years. According to the patients' files, 70.3% of diabetic children were metabolically stable at the time of sample collection.

As looking into caries risk factors is beyond the scope of this preliminary study, we used only a general interview that is accepted for initial checkup in the department of Pediatric Dentistry, Faculty of Dental Medicine, Hebrew University of Jerusalem, Israel. A more comprehensive study that will address this issue is planned as a future project. Interviews revealed that children with T1D visited the dentist only when necessary, while children in the control group were orthodontic patients who kept high standards of oral care. The level of parents' education regarding dental care in T1D group was medium and low, whereas the control group dominated with the medium and higher levels of parents' education.

Salivary Microbiome

Sequencing Data

A total of 762,156 reads were obtained from sequencing with an average of ~11.5 thousand reads per sample (ranging from 5,876 to 42,528 reads). Sequencing data passed quality check using FastQC[7] with default parameters. Following BURST taxonomic alignments 690,143 raw reads were mapped with an average of 10,456 reads per sample (ranging from 5,482 to 26,107 reads per

[5]https://github.com/knights-lab/BURST

[6]https://www.bioconductor.org/packages/release/bioc/html/Maaslin2.html

[7]https://www.bioinformatics.babraham.ac.uk/projects/fastqc/

sample). After removing bacteria with less than 25 reads across all samples at the genus level, 689,850 reads remained for further analysis with an average of 10,452 reads per sample (ranging from 5,478 to 26,106 reads). After similar filtering at the species level, 689,399 reads remained for further analysis with an average of 10,445 reads per sample (ranging between 5,474 and 26,101 reads per sample).

Microbiome Characterization

We found 105 different genera and 211 different species in the oral microbiome of the tested children. Most abundant genera in the saliva of both groups were *Streptococcus*, *Prevotella*, *Veillonella*, *Haemophilus*, and *Neisseria*. We first wanted to check whether the bacterial communities of the two study populations were similar or not. Overall, there are no strong shifts between the two sample types, and the most abundant genera in the saliva of both groups are *Streptococcus*, *Prevotella*, *Veillonella*, *Haemophilus*, and *Neisseria* (**Figure 1A**). Performing a principal coordinate analysis (PCoA) on these samples did not reveal any clear separation between the groups (**Figure 1B**). However, when we examined the microbial richness of each sample, we found that control samples had a significantly higher diversity (calculated using Shannon diversity index, **Figure 1C**).

We next searched for differential taxa between the T1D and control samples. Using a multivariate linear regression model, we identified eight differential species and three differential genera (see section "Materials and Methods). Eight species had significantly higher values among healthy children than in T1D children (**Table 1** and **Figure 2A**), and at the subspecies level, eight taxa were higher in the control group than T1D group

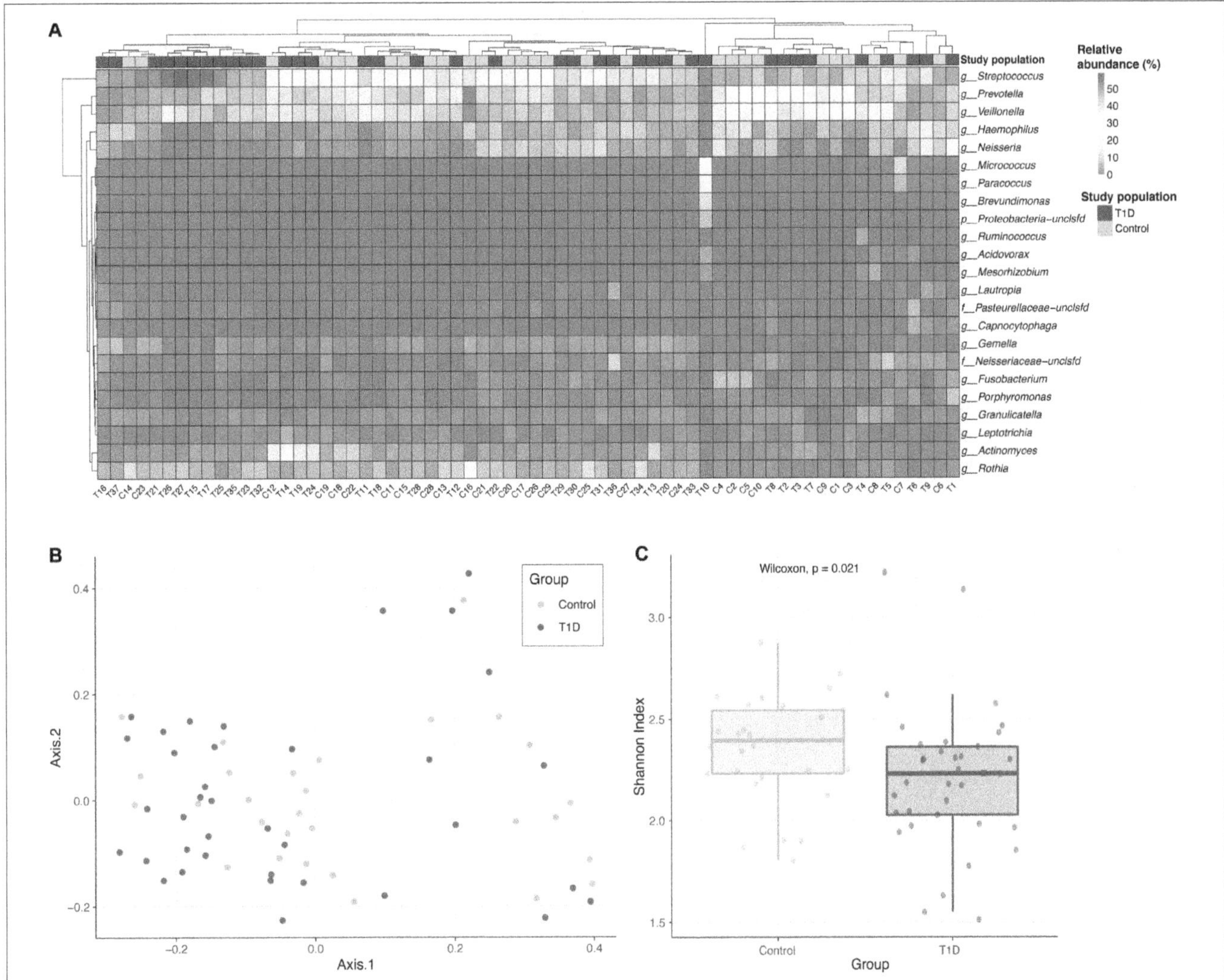

FIGURE 1 | Overall microbial composition in the two population groups. **(A)** Relative abundance of the most abundant genera in the saliva of T1D group (red) and the control group (yellow). The color of each cell in the heatmap is related to the abundance level of each genera per sample. **(B)** PCoA of the Bray–Curtis dissimilarity between study samples. Samples from T1D and controls are colored in red and yellow, respectively. Samples that are closer in their microbiome composition will be closer in this 2D plot. No clear distinction between the groups is identified. **(C)** Alpha diversity comparison of microbial communities of saliva samples from T1D group (red) and control group (yellow). Shannon diversity index was calculated as the metric for alpha diversity. The boxes represent the interquartile range (IQR) between the first and third quartiles (25th and 75th percentiles, respectively) and the vertical line inside the box defines the median. *P*-value calculated using Wilcoxon test.

TABLE 1 | Eight species and eight subspecies had significantly higher values among healthy children than in T1D children.

Species	*p*	*q*
Granulicatella-unclassified	0.00537	0.162
Mogibacterium-unclassified	0.00391	0.137
Alloprevotella rava	0.00154	0.118
Catonella morbi	0.00171	0.118
Fusobacterium periodonticum	0.00101	0.118
Oribacterium parvum	0.00701	0.185
Prevotella melaninogenica	0.00223	0.118
Prevotella pallens	0.00374	0.137
Subspecies	***p***	***q***
Granulicatella-unclassified	0.00537	0.165
Mogibacterium-unclassified	0.00390	0.140
Alloprevotella rava-unclassified	0.00154	0.120
Fusobacterium periodonticum-unclassified	0.00101	0.120
Catonella morbi atcc 51271	0.00171	0.120
Oribacterium parvum acb1	0.00701	0.188
Prevotella melaninogenica atcc 25845	0.00223	0.120
Prevotella pallens atcc 700821	0.00374	0.140

(**Table 1**). Three bacterial genera were higher in the control group than in T1D (**Figure 2B**) including *Catonella* ($p = 0.0017$, $q = 0.0894$), *Fusobacterium* ($p = 0.0007$, $q = 0.0798$), and *Mogibacterium* ($p = 0.0056$, $q = 0.1986$).

To clarify the relationship between the changes in the salivary microbiome and other salivary parameters, we analyzed the correlations between metadata and different microbes. We found that some physiological parameters (salivary pH and DMFT index) were associated with two genera of microbes (*Porphyromonas* and *Mogibacterium*; **Figure 2C**).

Finally, the diabetes group presented 22 taxa at the genus level and 33 taxa at the species level that were not presented in the control group, and the control group exhibited six taxa at the genus level and nine taxa at the species level that were not present in the diabetes group (**Figure 2D** and **Supplementary Table 1**).

The five most abundant genera in the T1D group were *Brevundimonas*, *Ruminococcus*, *Micrococcaceae-unclassified*, *Blautia*, and *Faecalibacterium* with sum of values 13.79, 5.60, 3.70, 2.57, and 2.0, respectively. The most abundant species in the T1D group were *Brevundimonas-unclassified*, *Micrococcaceae-unclassified*, *Lactobacillus salivarius*, *Ruminococcus bromii*, *Prevotella copri*, *Ruminococcus champanellensis*, *Faecalibacterium prausnitzii* with sum of values 13.79, 3.70, 3.65, 3.27, 2.43, 2.33, and 2.10, respectively. The most abundant genera in the control group were *Hymenobacter*, *Xanthomonadaceae-unclassified*, *Dietzia*, *Microbacterium*, and *Erythromicrobium* with sum of values 2.76, 0.50, 0.46, 0.43, and 0.34. The most abundant species in the control group were *Hymenobacter qilianensis*, *Flavobacterium columnare*, *Brevibacterium daeguense*, *Xanthomonadaceae-unclassified*, *Methanobrevibacter olleyae*, *Bacteroides vulgatus*, and *Dietzia-unclassified* with sum of values 2.76, 0.91, 0.76, 0.50, 0.47, 0.46, and 0.42.

Physiological Measures

Salivary Flow Rate

The average (±SE) of diabetic and healthy children were 0.50 ± 0.04 ml/min and 0.53 ± 0.03 ml/min, respectively, with no difference between the groups ($p = 0.47$) (**Table 2**).

Salivary pH. Salivary pH showed no difference between the two groups ($p > 0.05$), with an average (±SE) 6.88 ± 0.11 and 7.14 ± 0.10 of the experimental and control group, respectively.

Salivary Glucose

The percentage of salivary glucose concentrations showed 95 and 100% negative results in diabetic and healthy children, respectively (**Table 3**).

Salivary Calcium, Phosphate, and Urea

There were no differences in the average (±SE) values of salivary calcium (1.37 ± 0.11 and 1.12 ± 0.08 nmol/μl, $p = 0.10$), phosphate (4.72 ± 0.25 and 4.71 ± 0.22 nmol/μl, $p = 0.98$), and urea (4.30 ± 0.17 and 4.23 ± 0.18 nmol/μl, $p = 0.77$) in diabetic and healthy children, respectively.

Decayed, Missing, and Filled Teeth Index

Clinical examination showed higher caries incidence in diabetic children. The average (±SE) values with respect to DMFT index were 6.08 ± 0.61 and 3.76 ± 0.67 in the experimental and control group, respectively ($p < 0.05$). Furthermore, diabetic females had more tooth decay with no statistically significant difference between the groups (DMFT = 6.45 compared with 5.65 among diabetic males, $p = 0.52$). As reported from the data gathered while interviewing patients and parents, diabetic patients had poor quality diet, poor oral hygiene, less access to dental care, and less parents' dental education compared with the control group.

DISCUSSION

Only a limited number of studies have investigated the oral microbial composition of patients with T1D. We examined the oral microbiome in children with T1D and healthy children and found significant differences between the oral microbiota of diabetic children and the oral microbiota of healthy children. This is in accordance with de Groot et al. (2017) who found a markedly difference in oral microbiota in T1D (e.g., abundance of Streptococci) compared with healthy controls.

A recently published study by Pachoński et al. (2021) using classical methods routinely used in microbiological diagnostics confirmed quantitative and qualitative significant difference between the oral microbiome of children with T1D and healthy children. The present study used salivary samples, which according to Pachoński et al. (2021) are much more diverse than the samples they acquired with swab technique in the soft tissue of the oral cavity.

As in Pachoński et al. (2021)'s study, *Streptococcus* genus was also one of the largest groups of isolated microorganisms in the present study. However, we additionally found a large amount of *Prevotella*, *Veillonella*, *Haemophilus*, and *Neisseria*. Significantly higher number of bacteria from the *Streptococcus*

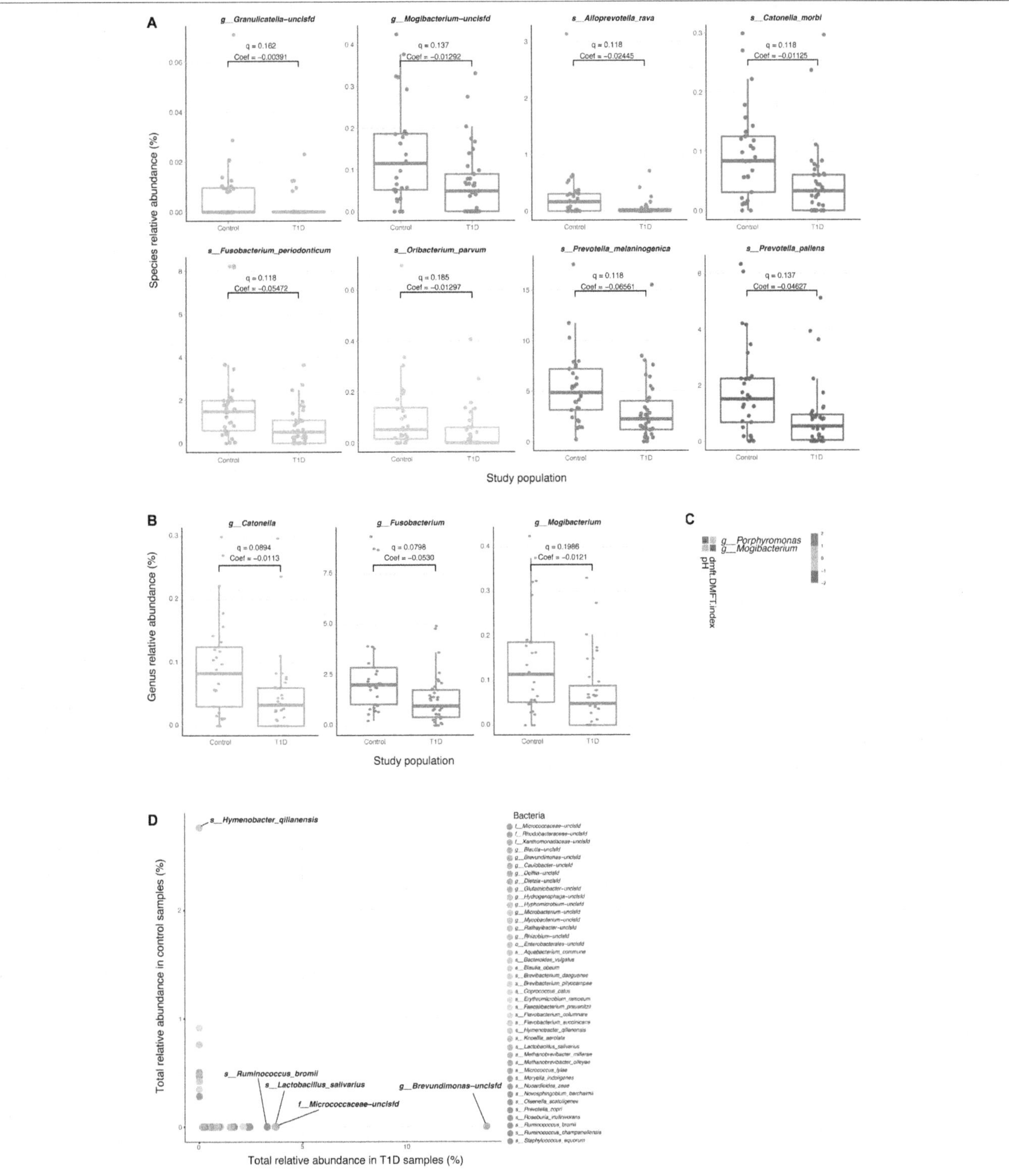

FIGURE 2 | Differential microbial taxa between T1D samples and controls. **(A,B)** Relative abundance of the significant taxa at the species **(A)** and genus **(B)** level, in T1D samples and control samples. Q-values and coefficients calculated using a multivariate linear regression model (MaAsLin, see section "Materials and Methods). The boxes represent the interquartile range (IQR) between the first and third quartiles (25th and 75th percentiles, respectively) and the vertical line inside the box defines the median. **(C)** Significant associations between microbial taxa and clinical parameters of the oral cavity. Only salivary pH and DMFT index are shown in the vertical axis as significantly correlated parameters ($q < 0.25$), and two genera; *Porphyromonas* and *Mogibacterium*, are shown in the horizontal axis. The variations in color are the magnitude of correlation between both variables. Correlation coefficient values range between −1.0 and 1.0; a correlation coefficient that is greater than zero indicates a positive relationship between two variables, a value that is less than zero signifies a negative relationship between two variables. **(D)** Relative abundance species apparent in only one type of population. The horizontal axis represents the sum of the relative abundance of the bacteria in T1D samples. The vertical axis represents the sum of the relative abundance of the bacteria in control samples.

TABLE 2 | Salivary parameters in children with type 1 diabetes mellitus and healthy children.

Parameters	Diabetics		Non-diabetics		*P*-value
	N	**Average ± SE**	**N**	**Average ± SE**	
Salivary flow rate (ml/min)	37	0.50 ± 0.04	29	0.53 ± 0.03	0.47
DMFT index	37	6.08 ± 0.61	29	3.76 ± 0.67	0.01*
pH	37	6.88 ± 0.11	29	7.14 ± 0.10	0.24
Calcium (nmol/ml)	37	1.37 ± 0.11	29	1.12 ± 0.08	0.10
Phosphate (nmol/ml)	37	4.72 ± 0.25	29	4.71 ± 0.22	0.98
Urea (nmol/ml)	37	4.30 ± 0.17	29	4.23 ± 0.18	0.77

**Significant differences.*

genus were found in the group of children with well-controlled diabetes mellitus compared with healthy children in Pachoński et al. (2021) and in the present study. Our study shows that 16S rRNA gene-based analysis enables the identification of a very broad scope of organisms: 105 different genera and 211 different species. The present study was also able to establish a unique group of bacteria (taxon) at the genus level and at the species level that either appeared or were absent in the saliva of T1D children. In addition to species and subspecies, clinical microbiologists study bacterial genera and families, so we concentrated on the differences between healthy and diabetic children in those taxonomic groups. The present data exhibited significant increase of the genera *Catonella, Fusobacterium,* and *Mogibacterium* in the control group. At the species level, *Granulicatella* spp., *Alloprevotella rava, Catonella morbi, Fusobacterium periodonticum, Oribacterium parvum, Prevotella melaninogenica,* and *Prevotella pallens* were significantly more abundant in the control group, in addition to *Catonella morbi ATCC 51271, Oribacterium parvum ACB1,* and *Prevotella melaninogenica ATCC 25845* at the subspecies level. *Brevundimonas, Ruminococcus, Micrococcaceae* spp., *Blautia,* and *Faecalibacterium* were predominant genera only in the T1D group.

According to the literature, three of these subspecies—*Blautia, Ruminococcus* (of family Lachnospiraceae), and *Faecalibacterium*—were enriched in women with gestational diabetes (Crusell et al., 2018).

TABLE 3 | Salivary glucose percentage in children with type 1 diabetes mellitus and healthy children.

Parameters	Diabetics		Non-diabetics	
		Percentage		**Percentage**
Glucose	Negative*	95	Negative	100
	Normal*	5	Normal	0

**Using Medi-Test Combi 3A where the color fields correspond to the following ranges of glucose concentrations: neg. (yellow), neg. or normal (greenish), 2.8, 8.3, 27.8 ≥ 55.5 mmol/L.*

As reported in the Results section, several unique taxa were identified in T1D: *Lactobacillus salivarius, Ruminococcus bromii, Prevotella copri, Ruminococcus champanellensis,* and *Faecalibacterium prausnitzii.* The identification of those unique taxa can be partly clarified by the quality of diet consumed by diabetic patients, in addition to the increase of periodontal inflammation among T1D children (Novotna et al., 2015). Diet has an important role in composition and metabolism of the oral microbiome. We report poor-quality diet among T1D children, which is in line with previous reports (Patton, 2011) of high saturated fat consumption and low intake of fruits, vegetables, and whole grain foods. Such diets are rich in advanced glycation end products (AGEs), which are complex heterogeneous compounds derived from non-enzymatic glycation reactions. While dietary advanced glycation end products (dAGEs) are formed during industrial processing and home cooking, high plasma glucose, as in diabetes (Rhee and Kim, 2018), accelerates the formation of endogenous AGEs. AGE-modified proteins accumulate within the body and are thought to play a role in a number of age-related diseases including diabetes. Long-term glycemic control regime decreased AGE levels in patients with T1D (Kostolanská et al., 2009).

As the absorption of dietary AGEs is limited, the majority of protein-bound AGEs pass through the gastrointestinal tract to the colon, where they can serve as substrates for the gut microbiota. Conflicting evidence on how dietary AGEs influence the composition of the microbiome include reduced levels of *Prevotella copri,* found here to be predominant genera only in the T1D group in peritoneal dialysis patients who underwent a 4-week low-dAGE regime (Yacoub et al., 2017) and that an AGE-rich diet in rats reduced the abundance of *Ruminococcaceae* and *Alloprevotella,* genera that we found to be both predominant and exclusive to the T1D group. The same diet increased the levels of *Bacteroides* (found in our study only in the control group) (Qu et al., 2017).

Elaboration on the unique taxa found in T1d patients in our study:

(1) *Brevundimonas* spp. are non-fermenting Gram-negative bacteria considered of minor clinical importance infection. Many of these non-fermenting Gram-negative bacteria are opportunistic pathogens that affect patients suffering from underlying medical conditions (Ryan and Pembroke, 2018) including diabetes (Lee et al., 2011). In the oral cavity, *Brevundimonas diminuta* was detected in refractory periodontitis (Krishnan et al., 2017).

(2) *Blautia* and *Faecalibacterium prausnitzii* are members of the human gut microbiome producing butyrate as fermentation end product. A high concentration of butyrate could result in apoptosis in human gingival epithelial cells and play an essential role in the initiation of periodontitis (Guan et al., 2021). Abundances of *Faecalibacterium* were negatively correlated with HbA1c levels in T1D (Huang et al., 2018). Moreover, a relative overabundance of the genus *Blautia* was found in the gut microbiome in the prediabetes and progressive stage of T1D (Kostic et al., 2015).

(3) *Prevotella copri* is by far the most abundant member of the genus *Prevotella* inhabiting the human large intestines. *P. copri* is strictly dependent on a sugar source partly elucidating its detection in T1D individuals in our cohort, who reported poor quality and high sugar diet. In the oral cavity, the proportion of *P. copri* was relatively higher in T2D patients with periodontitis (Sun et al., 2020). Thus, the detection of *Brevundimonas*, *Blautia*, *Faecalibacterium prausnitzii*, and *P. copri* in the oral cavity of T1D children may be associated with altered periodontal state among the study group.

(4) *Ruminococcus* is a genus of gut microbiome. Experimental evidence has confirmed its significant difference in the gut of diabetic mice may contribute to the pathogenesis of T1D by decreasing FOXP3-positive regulatory T cells (Tregs) that protect against diabetes (Krych et al., 2015). *R. bromii* possesses an exceptional ability to colonize and degrade starch particles in the human colon (Crost et al., 2018). *R. champanellensis* is a cellulose-degrading bacterium from human gut microbiota, in which fermentable carbohydrates are required for growth of this species (Chassard et al., 2012). Thus, the presence of *Ruminococcus* species in the saliva of T1D children in our cohort might be due to high intake of starch and sugars fermented by these bacteria.

(5) *Lactobacillus* is an indigenous member of human gut and oral microbiota. *L. salivarius* was found to be more highly associated with caries in children than the other *lactobacilli* because it is acidogenic and can produce lactate, acetate, and hydrogen peroxide (Piwat et al., 2010). Thus, we suggest that the elevated caries incidence among T1D children could induce increase of *L. salivarius* in the study group.

When checking the taxa found in the present study against data on T1D in gutMDisorder,[8] a manually curated database of comprehensive dysbiosis of the gut microbiota (Cheng et al., 2020), the genus *Blautia* increased in the gut microbiome of T1D patient and was present only in the T1D group in our study. Genus *Haemophilus* and family *Veillonellaceae* were abundant in both groups in the present study compared with a decrease in the gut microbiome of T1D patients. *Fusobacteria* phyla were more abundant in the control group of the present study and were decreased in gut microbiome. *Porphyromonadacea* species were increased in the gut of T1D patients and appeared to be correlated with oral parameters in the present study. Genus *Prevotella* was abundant in both groups in the present study compared with a decrease in the gut microbiome of T1D patients. Genus *Bacteroides* was increased in T1D gut microbiome, but *Bacteroides vulgatus* was found only in the saliva of the control group in the present study. Being part of the typical westernized pattern, *Bacteroides*, *Faecalibacterium*, and *Prevotella* were the predominant genera in gut microbiota composition of both women with gestational diabetes and normal glucose regulation (Crusell et al., 2018). Although we find similarities between gut and oral microbiome, there appear to be multifaceted relations that are determined by the environment; genera *Porphyromonas* and *Mogibacterium* were correlated with both pH and DMFT index parameters and were both classified as microbial signatures of periodontitis in the oral microbiome (How et al., 2016; Hunter et al., 2016). There are studies that show a lower incidence of dental caries in diabetic children compared with their healthy peers (Orbak et al., 2008), differing from our study and from others (Ferizi et al., 2018) who presented a significantly higher DMFT index in children with T1D than that in the control. This can be related to the fact that in both studies children with T1D rarely visited the dentist. In addition, in the present study children in the control group were orthodontic patients who kept high standards of oral care.

No differences in unstimulated salivary flow rate and salivary glucose calcium and phosphate levels were detected between the two groups. Furthermore, no significant difference was observed between diabetic and healthy children with respect to salivary urea, in disagreement with López et al. (2003) who found greater salivary urea levels in T1D children than in controls.

Study Limitation

Like Pachoński et al. (2021), the present study was a preliminary one and was not aimed to link between quality of dental care and oral hygiene and differentiating the dental health status between the children with T1D and healthy controls. Differentiating the oral microbiome in this case will be targeted by a more specific future study. Because this was an initial study examining the differences in oral microbiome between children with type 1 diabetes and non-diabetes children no power calculation was performed. It was decided to collect saliva from all attendants to the division of Pediatric Endocrinology, Hadassah Medical Center, Hebrew University of Jerusalem, Israel, who met the inclusion criteria and were willing to participate in the study during a period of 1 year.

CONCLUSION

We have established a unique microbial taxon that either appeared or were absent in the saliva of T1D children.

Many of the bacteria identified belong to the gut microbiome, indicating the complex interplay between the oral and gut microbiome in the pathogenesis of T1D.

In addition, some microbial taxa were linked to other parameters in the oral cavity of T1D individuals, such as higher incidence of dental caries.

ACKNOWLEDGMENTS

This project is part of the thesis of MN. We would like to thank the Department of Orthodontics of the Faculty of Dental Medicine, Hebrew University of Jerusalem, and Hadassah Medical Center, Jerusalem, Israel, for their help.

[8]http://bio-annotation.cn/gutMDisorder/browse.dhtml

AUTHOR CONTRIBUTIONS

MM, SF, DZ, DR, and DS conceived and designed the study. MN collected the samples. MN and AC performed laboratory assays. MY and NM performed bioinformatics analysis. MN and MM performed statistical analysis and wrote the draft of the manuscript. MM, DS, and MN interpreted the results. MM and DS supervised the work and revised and contributed to the final manuscript. DR contributed with resources and funding. All authors read and approved the final article.

REFERENCES

1. Al-Ghalith, G., and Knights, D. (2017). *Knights-Lab/BURST: BURST v0.99.4a.Technical Report, Zenodo*. Available online at: https://zenodo. org/record/836859#.YQoxOku_paQ (accessed May, 2019).
2. Angus, C. C., and Richard, P. W. (2008). *Handbook of Pediatric Dentistry*. London: Mosby, Elsevier Health Sciences.
3. Caporaso, J., Lauber, C., Walters, W., Berg-Lyons, D., Huntley, J., Fierer, N., et al. (2012). Ultra-high-throughput microbial community analysis on the Illumina HiSeq and MiSeq platforms. *ISME J.* 6, 1621–1624. doi: 10.1038/ismej. 2012.8
4. Chassard, C., Delmas, E., Robert, C., Lawson, P. A., and Bernalier-Donadille,A. (2012). *Ruminococcus champanellensis* sp. nov., a cellulose-degrading bacterium from human gut microbiota. *Int. J. Syst. Evol. Microbiol.* 62(Pt 1), 138–143. doi: 10.1099/ijs.0.027375-0
5. Cheng, L., Qi, C., Zhuang, H., Fu, T., and Zhang, X. (2020). gutMDisorder: a comprehensive database for dysbiosis of the gut microbiota in disorders and interventions. *Nucleic Acids Res.* 48, D554–D560. doi: 10.1093/nar/gkz843
6. Crost, E. H., Le Gall, G., Laverde-Gomez, J. A., Mukhopadhya, I., Flint, H. J., and Juge, N. (2018). Mechanistic insights into the cross-feeding of *Ruminococcus gnavus* and *Ruminococcus bromii* on host and dietary carbohydrates. *Front. Microbiol.* 9:2558. doi: 10.3389/fmicb.2018.02558
7. Crusell, M. K. W., Hansen, T. H., Nielsen, T., Allin, K. H., Rühlemann, M. C., Damm, P., et al. (2018). Gestational diabetes is associated with change in the gut microbiota composition in third trimester of pregnancy and postpartum. *Microbiome* 6:89. doi: 10.1186/s40168-018-0472-x
8. de Groot, P. F., Belzer, C., Aydin, Ö, Levin, E., Levels, J. H., Aalvink, S., et al. (2017). Distinct fecal and oral microbiota composition in human type 1 diabetes, an observational study. *PLoS One* 12:e0188475. doi: 10.1371/journal.pone. 0188475
9. Ferizi, L., Dragidella, F., Spahiu, L., Begzati, A., and Kotori, V. (2018). The Influence of Type 1 diabetes mellitus on dental caries and salivary composition. *Int. J. Dent.* 2018:5780916. doi: 10.1155/2018/5780916
10. Genco, R. J., Grossi, S. G., Ho, A., Nishimura, F., and Murayama, Y. (2005). A proposed model linking inflammation to obesity, diabetes, and periodontal infections. *J. Periodontol.* 76(11 Suppl), 2075–2084. doi: 10.1902/jop.2005.76.11-S.2075
11. Guan, X., Li, W., and Meng, H. (2021). A double-edged sword: role of butyrate in the oral cavity and the gut. *Mol. Oral Microbiol.* 36, 121–131. doi: 10.1111/omi. 12322
12. Han, H., Li, Y., Fang, J., Liu, G., Yin, J., Li, T., et al. (2018). Gut microbiota and type 1 diabetes. *Int. J. Mol. Sci.* 19:995. doi: 10.3390/ijms19040995
13. He, J., Li, Y., Cao, Y., Xue, J., and Zhou, X. (2015). The oral microbiome diversity and its relation to human diseases. *Folia Microbiol. (Praha)* 60, 69–80. doi: 10.1007/s12223-014-0342-2
14. Hong, Y. H. J., Hassan, N., Cheah, Y. K., Jalaludin, M. Y., and Kasim, Z. M. (2017). Management of T1DM in children and adolescents in primary care. *Malays. Fam. Physician* 31, 18–22.
15. How, K. Y., Song, K. P., and Chan, K. G. (2016). *Porphyromonas gingivalis*: an Overview of periodontopathic pathogen below the gum line. *Front. Microbiol.* 7:53. doi: 10.3389/fmicb.2016.00053
16. Huang, Y., Li, S. C., Hu, J., Ruan, H. B., Guo, H. M., Zhang, H. H., et al. (2018). Gut microbiota profiling in Han Chinese with type 1 diabetes. *Diabetes Res. Clin. Pract.* 141, 256–263. doi: 10.1016/j.diabres.2018.04.032
17. Hunter, M. C., Pozhitkov, A. E., and Noble, P. A. (2016). Microbial signatures of oral dysbiosis, periodontitis and edentulism revealed by gene meter methodology. *J. Microbiol. Methods* 131, 85–101. doi: 10.1016/j.mimet.2016. 09.019
18. International Diabetes Federation (2019). *IDF Diabetes Atlas*, 9th Edn. Brussels: International Diabetes Federation.
19. Kostic, A. D., Gevers, D., Siljander, H., Vatanen, T., Hyötyläinen, T., Hämäläinen, A. M., et al. (2015). DIABIMMUNE Study Group, Xavier RJ. The dynamics of the human infant gut microbiome in development and in progression toward type 1 diabetes. *Cell Host Microbe* 17, 260–273. doi: 10.1016/j.chom.2015. 01.001
20. Kostolanská, J., Jakus, V., and Barák, L. (2009). HbA1c and serum levels of advanced glycation and oxidation protein products in poorly and well controlled children and adolescents with type 1 diabetes mellitus. *J. Pediatr. Endocrinol. Metab.* 22, 433–442. doi: 10.1515/JPEM.2009.22.5.433
21. Krishnan, K., Chen, T., and Paster, B. J. (2017). A practical guide to the oral microbiome and its relation to health and disease. *Oral Dis.* 23, 276–286. doi: 10.1111/odi.12509
22. Krych, Ł, Nielsen, D. S., Hansen, A. K., and Hansen, C. H. F. (2015). Gut microbial markers are associated with diabetes onset, regulatory imbalance, and IFN-γ level in NOD Mice. *Gut Microbes* 6, 101–109. doi: 10.1080/19490976.2015. 1011876
23. Lee, M. R., Huang, Y. T., Liao, C. H., Chuang, T. Y., Lin, C. K., Lee, S. W., et al. (2011). Bacteremia caused by *Brevundimonas* species at a tertiary care hospital in Taiwan, 2000–2010. *Eur. J. Clin. Microbiol. Infect. Dis.* 30, 1185–1191. doi: 10.1007/s10096-011-1210-5
24. Long, J., Cai, Q., Steinwandel, M., Hargreaves, M. K., Bordenstein, S. R., Blot, W. J., et al. (2017). Association of oral microbiome with type 2 diabetes risk. *J. Periodontal Res.* 52, 636–643. doi: 10.1111/jre.12432
25. López, M., Colloca, M., Páez, R., Schallmach, J., Koss, M., and Chervonagura, A. (2003). Salivary characteristics of diabetic children. *Braz. Dent. J.* 14, 26–31. doi: 10.1590/S0103-64402003000100005
26. Maahs, D. M., West, N. A., Lawrence, J. M., and Mayer-Davis, E. J. (2010). Epidemiology of Type 1 Diabetes. *Endocrinol. Metab. Clin. North Am.* 39, 481–497. doi: 10.1016/j.ecl.2010.05.011
27. Mallick, H., Rahnavard, A., McIver, L. J., Ma, S., Zhang, Y., Nguyen, L. H., et al. (2021). Multivariable association discovery in population-scale meta-omics studies. *bioRxiv* [Preprint] doi: 10.1101/2021.01.20.427420 bioRxiv 2021.01.20.427420,
28. Novotna, M., Podzimek, S., Broukal, Z., Lencova, E., and Duskova, J. (2015). Periodontal diseases and dental caries in children with type 1 diabetes mellitus. *Mediators Inflamm.* 51:379626. doi: 10.1155/2015/379626
29. Orbak, R., Simsek, S., Orbak, Z., Kavrut, F., and Colak, M. (2008). The influence of type-1 diabetes mellitus on dentition and oral health in children and adolescents. *Yonsei Med. J.* 49, 357–365. doi: 10.3349/ymj.2008.49.3.357
30. Pachon´ski, M., Koczor-Rozmus, A., Mocny-Pachon´ska, K., Łanowy, P., Mertas, A., and Jarosz-Chobot, P. (2021). Oral microbiota in children with type 1 diabetes mellitus. *Pediatr. Endocrinol. Diabetes Metab.* 27, 100–108. doi: 10.5114/pedm. 2021.104343
31. Paradis, E., and Schliep, K. (2019). ape 5.0: an environment for modern phylogenetics and evolutionary analyses in R. *Bioinformatics.* 35, 526–528. doi: 10.1093/bioinformatics/bty633
32. Patton, S. R. (2011). Adherence to diet in youth with type 1 diabetes. *J. Am. Diet. Assoc.* 111, 550–555. doi: 10.1016/j.jada.2011.01.016
33. Piwat, S., Teanpaisan, R., Thitasomakul, S., Thearmontree, A., and Dahlén, G. (2010). *Lactobacillus* species and genotypes associated with dental caries in Thai preschool children. *Mol. Oral Microbiol.* 25, 157–164.
34. Poyet, M., Groussin, M. S., Gibbons, M., Avila-Pacheco, J., Jiang, X., Kearney, S. M., et al. (2019). A library of human gut bacterial isolates paired with longitudinal multiomics data enables mechanistic microbiome research. *Nature Medicine* 25, 1442–1452. doi: 10.1038/s41591-019-0559-3
35. Qu, W., Yuan, X., Zhao, J., Zhang, Y., Hu, J., Wang, J., et al. (2017). Dietary advanced glycation end products modify gut microbial composition and partially increase colon permeability in rats. *Mol. Nutr. Food Res.* 61:1700118.
36. Raivo, K. (2019). *pheatmap: Pretty Heatmaps. R package version 1.0.12.* Available online at: https://CRAN.R-project.org/package=pheatmap (accessed 01 04, 2019).

37. Rhee, S. Y., and Kim, Y. S. (2018). The role of advanced glycation end products in diabetic vascular complications. *Diabetes Metab. J.* 42, 188–195. doi: 10.4093/ dmj.2017.0105

38. Ryan, M. P., and Pembroke, J. T. (2018). *Brevundimonas* spp: emerging global opportunistic pathogens. *Virulence* 9, 480–493.

39. Sadeghi, R., Taleghani, F., Mohammadi, S., and Zohri, Z. (2017). The effect of diabetes mellitus type i on periodontal and dental status. *J. Clin. Diagn. Res.* 11, ZC14–ZC17. doi: 10.7860/JCDR/2017/25742.10153

40. Siljander, H., Honkanen, J., and Knip, M. (2019). Microbiome and type 1 diabetes. *EBioMedicine* 46, 512–521.

41. Simpson, K., and Thomas, J. (2016). Oral microbiome: contributions to local and systemic infections. *Curr. Oral Health Rep.* 3, 45–55. doi: 10.1007/ s40496-016- 0079-x

42. Størling, J., and Pociot, F. (2017). Type 1 diabetes candidate genes linked to pancreatic islet cell inflammation and beta-cell apoptosis. *Genes (Basel)* 8:72. doi: 10.3390/genes8020072

43. Sun, X., Li, M., Xia, L., Fang, Z., Yu, S., Gao, J., et al. (2020). Alteration of salivary microbiome in periodontitis with or without type-2 diabetes mellitus and metformin treatment. *Sci. Rep.* 10:15363. doi: 10.1038/s41598-020-72035-1

44. Wickham, H. (2016). *ggplot2: Elegant Graphics for Data Analysis.* New York, NY: Springer-Verlag. doi: 10.1007/978-3-319-24277-4

45. World Health Organization (2018). *Diabetes.* Geneva: World Health Organization. World Health Organization (1997). *Oral Health Surveys: Basic Methods*, 4th Edn. Geneva: World Health Organization.

46. Yacoub, R., Nugent, M., Cai, W., Nadkarni, G. N., Chaves, L. D., Abyad, S., et al. (2017). Advanced glycation end products dietary restriction effects on bacterial gut microbiota in peritoneal dialysis patients; a randomized open label controlled trial. *PLoS One* 12:e0184789. doi: 10.1371/journal.pone. 0184789

47. Zhou, H., Sun, L., Zhang, S., Zhao, X., Gang, X., and Wang, G. (2020). Evaluating the causal role of gut microbiota in type 1 diabetes and its possible pathogenic mechanisms. *Front. Endocrinol. (Lausanne)* 11:125. doi: 10.3389/ fendo.2020. 00125

3

Longitudinal Observation of Outcomes and Patient Access to Integrated Care Following Point-of-Care Glycemic Screening in Community Health Center Dental Safety Net Clinics

Ingrid Glurich[1], *Richard Berg*[2], *Aloksagar Panny*[1], *Neel Shimpi*[1], *Annie Steinmetz*[1], *Greg Nycz*[3] *and Amit Acharya*[1,3,4*]

[1] *Center for Oral and Systemic Health, Marshfield Clinic Research Institute, Marshfield, WI, United States,* [2] *Office of Research Computing and Analytics, Marshfield Clinic Research Institute, Marshfield, WI, United States,* [3] *Family Health Center of Marshfield, Inc., Marshfield Clinic Health System, Marshfield, WI, United States,* [4] *Advocate Aurora Research Institute, LLC, Advocate Aurora Health, Inc., Downers Grove, IL, United States*

Correspondence:
Amit Acharya
amit.acharya@aah.org

Introduction: Rates of diabetes/prediabetes continue to increase, with disparity populations disproportionately affected. Previous field trials promoted point-of-care (POC) glycemic screening in dental settings as an additional primary care setting to identify potentially at-risk individuals requiring integrated care intervention. The present study observed outcomes of POC hemoglobin A1c (HbA1c) screening at community health center (CHC) dental clinics (DC) and compliance with longitudinal integrated care management among at-risk patients attending dental appointments.

Materials and Methods: POC HbA1c screening utilizing Food and Drug Administration (FDA)-approved instrumentation in DC settings and periodontal evaluation of at-risk dental patients with no prior diagnosis of diabetes/prediabetes and no glycemic testing in the preceding 6 months were undertaken. Screening of patients attending dental appointments from October 24, 2017, through September 24, 2018, was implemented at four Wisconsin CHC-DCs serving populations with a high representation of disparity. Subjects meeting at-risk profiles underwent POC HbA1c screening. Individuals with measures in the diabetic/prediabetic ranges were advised to seek further medical evaluation and were re-contacted after 3 months to document compliance. Longitudinal capture of glycemic measures in electronic health records for up to 2 years was undertaken for a subset ($n = 44$) of subjects with available clinical, medical, and dental data. Longitudinal glycemic status and frequency of medical and dental access for follow-up care were monitored.

Results: Risk assessment identified 224/915 (24.5%) patients who met inclusion criteria following two levels of risk screening, with 127/224 (57%) qualifying for POC HbA1c screening. Among those tested, 62/127 (49%) exhibited hyperglycemic measures: 55 in the prediabetic range and seven in the diabetic range. Moderate-to-severe periodontitis was more prevalent in patients with prediabetes/diabetes than in individuals with measures in the normal range. Participant follow-up compliance at 3 months was 90%. Longitudinal follow-up documented high rates of consistent access (100 and 89%, respectively), to the integrated medical/DC environment over 24 months for individuals with hyperglycemic screening measures.

Conclusion: POC glycemic screening revealed elevated HbA1c measures in nearly half of at-risk CHC-DC patients. Strong compliance with integrated medical/dental management over a 24-month interval was observed, documenting good patient receptivity to POC screening in the dental setting and compliance with integrated care follow-up by at-risk patients.

Keywords: diabetes mellitus, prediabetic state, point-of-care testing, general practice, dental, glycated hemoglobin A, risk assessment, delivery of healthcare

BACKGROUND

Overview of Problem

The Centers for Disease Control and Prevention (CDC) projected that over 10.5% of individuals in the USA have diabetes mellitus (DM), with 21% undiagnosed [1]. Moreover, ~34.5% of the US adult population has prediabetes, with >80% unaware of their glycemic status (CDC, 2020) [2]. Between 2015 and 2030, diabetes prevalence in the USA is projected to increase by 54%, annual diabetes-associated mortality by 38%, and annual overall cost associated with diabetes to exceed $620 billion [3]. These data project that diabetes remains on track for continued escalation of its epidemic status.

Similarly, recently updated projections of periodontal disease (PD) reported increasing prevalence, currently estimated in excess of 40%, with higher rates projected among the elderly and in association with race and ethnicity, projected by population-based screening [4]. Because recent systematic review and meta-analysis of the evidence base surrounding bidirectional associations between PD and diabetes continues to support potential interactions between these conditions [5], there is an increased need to expand and promote integration of interdisciplinary efforts across primary dental and medical settings to identify and manage high-risk individuals.

Whereas, current US Preventive Services Task Force (USPSTF) guidelines recommends screening for type 2 DM (T2DM) for individuals with hypertension, aged 40–70 years who meet obesity status definitions [6], glycemic screening in the dental setting has remained controversial (reviewed by Glurich et al. [7]). Biological screening in the dental setting was not recommended at the time USPSTF guidelines were issued because diabetes is not managed in the dental domain and an adequate evidence base to support screening was lacking. However, alignment of recent key developments supports timeliness of re-evaluation of dental clinic (DC) settings as primary care settings where at-risk patients can be identified. These key developments include (a) epidemiological evidence of the burgeoning epidemic status of T2DM and PD cited above; (b) evidence demonstrating substantive prevalence of undiagnosed T2DM/prediabetes in the DC setting [8, 9]; (c) publication of an expert consensus report and clinical guidelines recommending integrated T2DM and PD management issued by 2018 Joint Workshop International Diabetes Federation and European Federation of Periodontology following systematic examination of the evidence [10]; (d) findings of systematic review of meta meta-analyses surrounding bidirectional relationships between T2DM and PD, which continue to support value in integrated interventional approaches to prevention and treatment [11]; and (e) updated guidelines and issuance of Current Dental Terminology (CDT) codes (2019) to support point-of-care (POC) glycemic assessment in dental settings to inform patient management [12].

Study Rationale

Implementation of POC hemoglobin A1c (HbA1c) screening across four community health center DCs (CHC-DC) in Wisconsin described herein was supported by a systematic review undertaken to examine outcomes of clinical and field trials published since 2007 exploring POC screening of patients attending dental visits [8]. Eligibility criteria for subjects enrolled in these field trials included the following: (1) no pre-existing diagnosis of T2DM/prediabetes, (2) no biological glycemic measure in a defined period, and (3) documentation that patients had known risk factors for diabetes [8]. These studies sought to estimate prevalence of undiagnosed T2DM/prediabetes in their dental patient population. Substantial rates of putative T2DM (1–14%) and prediabetes (19–90%) were detected across a range of dental practices with highest rates observed in dental practices serving a higher proportion of patients meeting disparity population definitions [13, 14]. However, studies that reported on re-evaluation of glycemic measures in the medical setting on patients testing into hyperglycemic ranges mainly did so only within 24–48 h following the POC screening test and failed to establish the true rate of diabetes diagnosis based on the prevailing clinical practice guidelines effective in the temporal window of these studies. These guidelines stated requirements for confirmatory glycemic measures in the diabetic range within 6 months. Longitudinal follow-up of further glycemic evaluation or concordance between the screening measures and further biological glycemic assessment across time was also not an objective of the field trials. Furthermore, instrumentation to conduct biological glycemic screening varied across studies and included glucometers not approved by the Food and Drug Administration (FDA) for global screening in 7/10 studies systematically reviewed [8]. Finally, the glycemic measure used to screen glycemic levels at POC also varied across studies with 7/10 employing HbA1c [8]. Findings of the systematic review underlined a need for appropriately designed protocols to support further assessment of the relative clinical value in conducting POC screening in the DC setting. Emphasis was placed on targeting of undiagnosed patients with risk factors for DM and no glycemic measures within a defined temporal window in order to evaluate the value of designating the DC setting as an additional interdisciplinary primary care setting.

Analysis of longitudinal patient engagement in integrated care delivery following POC screening was also of interest to CHC-DC operationalizing safety net operations. In lieu of population-based screening, targeted screening was posited to identify potentially undiagnosed individuals who require further medical assessment and appropriate follow-up in both the medical and dental settings. Notably, regression modeling of candidate variables contributing to diabetic risk by authors of previous field trials screening for undiagnosed hyperglycemia in DC settings identified PD prevalence and missing teeth as novel independent risk factors [13, 14]. Detection of T2DM/prediabetes risk, ideally at early stages, was targeted positing that intervention during early development could slow or prevent progression in activated patients and potentially reduce risk for onset of diabetic complications and chronicity of PD.

The focus of the current study was to implement POC HbA1c testing to detect rates of T2DM and prediabetes across patients of four CHC-DC in Wisconsin with targeted screening only of the subset of patients with risk factors for hyperglycemia and observe patient behavior relative to seeking medical–dental access if glycemic screening measures were elevated. The study design included questionnaire-based screening, in combination with Clinical Laboratory Improvement Act (CLIA)-waived HbA1c testing utilizing Federal FDA-approved instrumentation in the DC settings targeting only dental patients with high-risk profiles. Observational longitudinal follow-up was further planned to monitor patient compliance with triage and follow-up testing by medical providers 3 months post-screening. Finally, a subset of patients across three of four centers where data were accessible in the electronic health records (EHRs) was monitored for glycemic follow-up and evidence of periodontal evaluation within a minimum time frame of 1 year and up to 2 years post-POC screening in order to more accurately observe concordance of screening outcome, true biological status, and access to available integrated medical/dental care delivery models in CHC settings.

DESIGN AND METHODS

Study Design and Objectives

This observational community case study evaluated clinical utility of identifying the subset of eligible dental patients potentially at risk for T2DM/prediabetes in the context of scheduled dental visits at participating CHC-DC sites where a POC HbA1c screening protocol was implemented. Specifically, the study focused on the subset of individuals attending dental care appointments with no existing diagnosis or history of DM/prediabetes and no glycemic screening within the past 6 months to document glycemic status but who exhibit risk factors for diabetes and met inclusion criteria as outlined in the study flow diagram in **Figure 1**.

The study objectives included observational characterization of (1) undiagnosed dysglycemia prevalence detected; (2) tracking of compliance with triage to medical evaluation and follow-up; and (3) longitudinal tracking of individuals to observe access to medical and dental care for individuals found to be at high risk for T2DM/prediabetes following POC screening in the dental setting.

Population and Setting

This community case study was undertaken across three CHC-DC serving largely rural populations in Wisconsin including 2 of 10 CHC-DC operated by Family Health Center of Marshfield, Inc. (FHC-M) and Marshfield Clinic Health System (MCHS) in the following: (1) Marshfield, Wisconsin (WI); (2) Medford, WI; and (3) Bridge Community Dental Center serving the regional population of Wausau, WI. The fourth DC that enrolled patients was St. Elizabeth Ann Seton Dental Clinic, a walk-in clinic serving an urban population in Milwaukee, WI. Study enrollment was undertaken over 11 months from October 24, 2017, through September 24, 2018. Longitudinal follow-up was carried out for a minimum additional 12 to up to 24 months through October 1, 2019, on subjects with available data in order to observe patient longitudinal access for follow-up glycemic measures in the medical setting and periodontal assessments in the dental setting. All of the participating sites represent DCs designated as dental safety nets established largely in rural settings to serve disparity populations who otherwise have limited access to dental care [15]. Over 85% of patients seeking care at FHC-M dental centers alone are on Medicaid [16] and other CHCs similarly provide dental care to a high volume of the Medicaid population and to those with no dental insurance coverage largely due to poverty status. The majority of patients seen at St. Elizabeth Ann Seton Dental Clinic in Milwaukee, as a "walk-in" clinic, have no dental home. Their operations largely target provision of dental care to individuals experiencing acute dental conditions. While periodontal assessment and longitudinal tracking data on these patients were not available, patient enrollment at this fourth site was included mainly to explore rates of hyperglycemia in their patient population and gauge receptivity of clientele of this clinic to HbA1c screening in the dental setting.

Overview of Participant Screening Procedures

The study and all study forms were reviewed and approved by the Institutional Review Board of the MCHS. Participating DCs applied for and were issued CLIA waivers to support conduct of HbA1c screening in the dental setting using Siemens DCA Vantage HbA1c Analyzer (Siemens Healthineers, USA). This analyzer uses an immuno-assay to determine

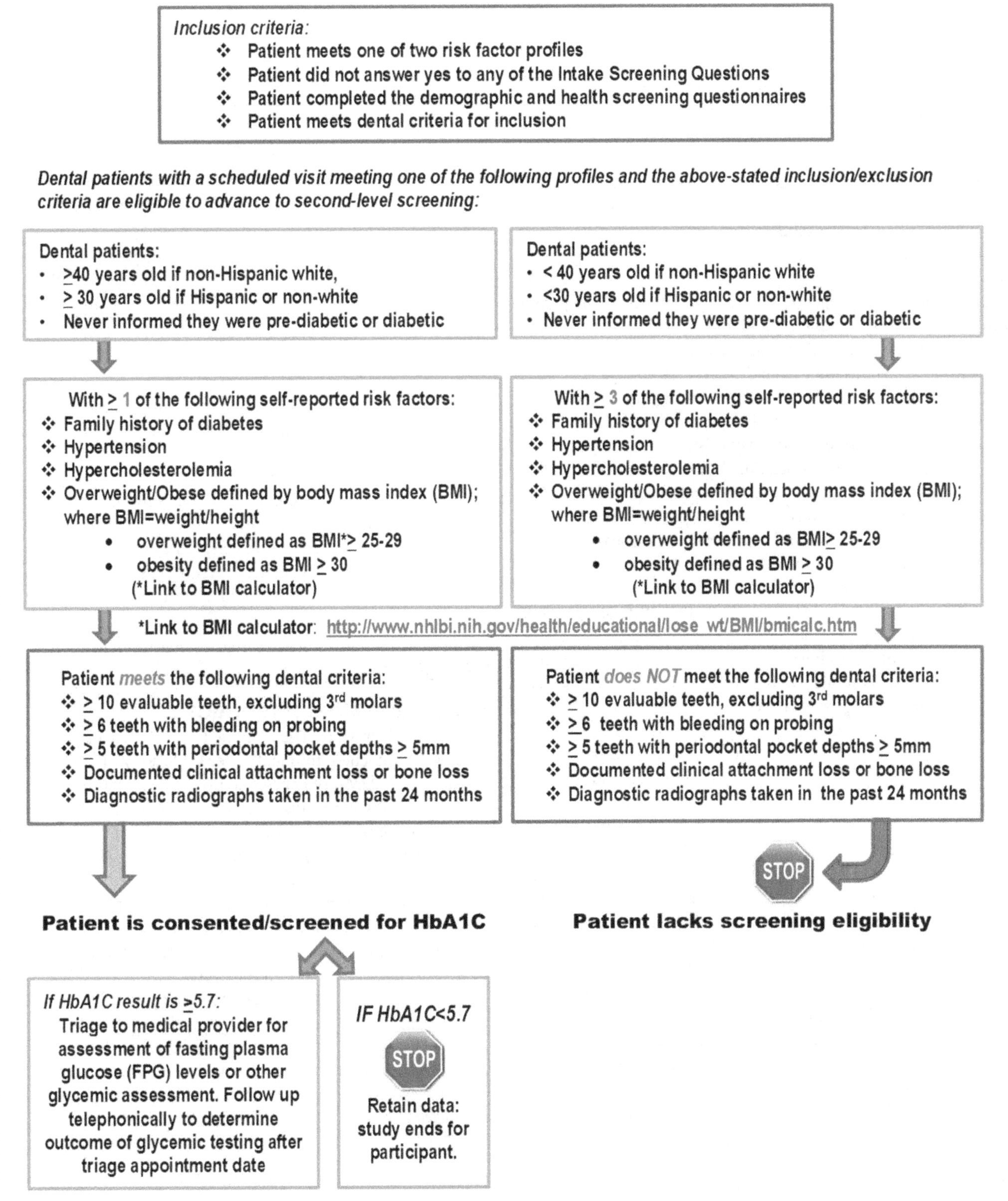

Inclusion criteria:

- Patient meets one of two risk factor profiles
- Patient did not answer yes to any of the Intake Screening Questions
- Patient completed the demographic and health screening questionnaires
- Patient meets dental criteria for inclusion

Dental patients with a scheduled visit meeting one of the following profiles and the above-stated inclusion/exclusion criteria are eligible to advance to second-level screening:

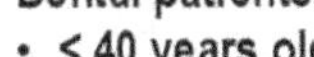

Dental patients:

- >40 years old if non-Hispanic white,
- > 30 years old if Hispanic or non-white
- Never informed they were pre-diabetic or diabetic

Dental patients:

- < 40 years old if non-Hispanic white
- <30 years old if Hispanic or non-white
- Never informed they were pre-diabetic or diabetic

With > 1 of the following self-reported risk factors:

- Family history of diabetes
- Hypertension
- Hypercholesterolemia
- Overweight/Obese defined by body mass index (BMI); where BMI=weight/height
  - overweight defined as BMI*> 25-29
  - obesity defined as BMI > 30
  (*Link to BMI calculator)

With > 3 of the following self-reported risk factors:

- Family history of diabetes
- Hypertension
- Hypercholesterolemia
- Overweight/Obese defined by body mass index (BMI); where BMI=weight/height
  - overweight defined as BMI> 25-29
  - obesity defined as BMI > 30
  (*Link to BMI calculator)

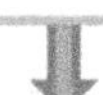

*Link to BMI calculator: http://www.nhlbi.nih.gov/health/educational/lose_wt/BMI/bmicalc.htm

Patient *meets* the following dental criteria:

- > 10 evaluable teeth, excluding 3rd molars
- > 6 teeth with bleeding on probing
- > 5 teeth with periodontal pocket depths > 5mm
- Documented clinical attachment loss or bone loss
- Diagnostic radiographs taken in the past 24 months

Patient *does NOT* meet the following dental criteria:

- > 10 evaluable teeth, excluding 3rd molars
- > 6 teeth with bleeding on probing
- > 5 teeth with periodontal pocket depths > 5mm
- Documented clinical attachment loss or bone loss
- Diagnostic radiographs taken in the past 24 months

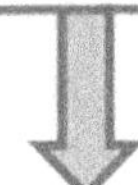

Patient is consented/screened for HbA1C

STOP

Patient lacks screening eligibility

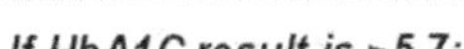

If HbA1C result is >5.7:
Triage to medical provider for assessment of fasting plasma glucose (FPG) levels or other glycemic assessment. Follow up telephonically to determine outcome of glycemic testing after triage appointment date

IF HbA1C<5.7

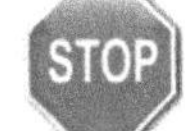

Retain data: study ends for participant.

FIGURE 1 | Study flow diagram for study-eligible dental patients.

HbA1c measurement, has FDA approval for CLIA-waived POC HbA1c screening in the clinical setting, and reproduces results of the validated laboratory reference method HA 8160 cationic exchange high-performance liquid chromatography with high fidelity and accuracy [17]. The instrument was supplied to the study team through the 17VNPL DCA

Vantage Analyzer Placement Program [18]. All testing supplies, reagents, and normal/abnormal controls were purchased from the manufacturer.

Sample size estimates were based on targeting of 1,000 patients for initial screening to identify patients with undiagnosed diabetes/prediabetes based on rates reported in earlier field trials examining POC glycemic testing in the dental setting [8] and estimated patient census across the four sites. Enrollment of ~200 undiagnosed cases was conservatively projected. Enrollment was terminated at 11 months following screening of 915 patients and enrollment of the study-eligible cohort (n = 224). Screening was accomplished in two steps. The *Intake Screening Questionnaire* consisting of nine questions was completed by all patients presenting at the participating dental centers to determine eligibility for POC HbA1c screening in the dental setting (Appendix 1). Those who answered "no" to all questions met eligibility criteria and gave written informed consent for enrollment in the study. Enrolled subjects next completed the demographic and comorbidity profile questionnaire (Appendix 2), which consisted of 12 questions, and the American Diabetes Association Diabetes risk test (https://www.diabetes.org/risk-test), which generated a risk score. The final screening step involved capillary collection of blood following a finger stick and analysis of the HbA1c measure by the Siemens DCA Vantage HbA1c Analyzer. Enrolled subjects with measures < 5.7% exited the study, while those with measures ≥ 5.7% were continued for longitudinal observational follow-up for at least 12 months. These subjects first received telephonic follow-up 3 months following HbA1c screening to determine whether they had complied with recommended triage to medical providers for further monitoring of their glycemic status. Follow-up included longitudinal tracking of glycemic measure outcomes or identification of a new prescription for medications associated with glycemic regulation in the medical setting and observation of periodontal assessments and/or other dental procedures in the dental setting. Patients also either underwent periodontal assessment at time of enrollment or had clinical assessments abstracted from the EHRs if they had been evaluated within 3 months of study enrollment. Assessment criteria included documentation of bone loss, attachment loss, and moderate-to-severe PD based on updated definitions of PD classification defined by the American Academy of Periodontology (AAP) Task Force [19]. **Figure 1** summarizes parameters applied to ensure stringency regarding documentation of PD. Patients were required to have a minimum of 10 evaluable teeth excluding third molars. Further requirements included documentation of the following: ≥6 with bleeding on probing, ≥5 teeth with periodontal pocket depth (PPD) ≥ 5 mm, and evidence of clinical attachment loss ≥ 3 mm or >16% (≥3-mm bone loss) based on diagnostic radiographs captured within the past 24 months as defined by AAP classification definitions [18]. Data on number of missing teeth were also collected.

Analytical Approach

Data were summarized to characterize participant characteristics and study outcomes relative to glycemic measures. HbA1c values defined by American Diabetes Association were used to classify normal range (<5.7%), prediabetic range (≥5.7–6.4%), and diabetic range (>6.4%) [20]. Outcomes of study subjects with measures ≥ 5.7% and rate of access to medical and dental care and glycemic measures captured in the EHR were also tracked over time to determine integrated care access. Due to small numbers of subjects with measures in the diabetic range, these patients were pooled with those in the prediabetic range for statistical comparisons Fisher's exact test was used for comparisons of categorical characteristics (e.g., gender), and the Wilcoxon rank sum test was used for comparisons of numerical characteristics (e.g., age).

TABLE 1 | Descriptive characteristics of screened cohort.

	Study eligible?	
	No (*n* = 93)	**Yes (*n* = 127)**
Mean age (years)	32.3 ± 9.5	51.1 ± 13.3
Male	30.1%	35.4%
White race	76.3%	68.5%
Hispanic	6.5%	19.7%
Hypertension	6.5%	35.4%
Hypercholesterolemia	2.2%	36.2%
Mean BMI	28.5 ± 8	30.9 ± 7.9
History of smoking	59.1%	49.6%

BMI, body mass index.

RESULTS

Population Characteristics

Across the four CHC-DC sites, a total of 915 patients were initially approached to identify 224 (24%) with no existing diagnosis of T2DM/prediabetes or glycemic evaluation in the past 6 months. Following exclusion of four individuals, 127/220 (58%) met criteria for potential risk for undiagnosed T2DM/prediabetes and underwent further screening and POC HbA1c testing. Characteristics of the screened cohort are summarized in **Table 1**. Screening for risk factors selected a cohort characterized by older age and higher frequency of Hispanic ethnicity.

Among study-eligible subjects (n = 127), 100% underwent POC HbA1c screening. Results of HbA1c shown in **Table 2** found that 62/127 (49%) of the subset of potentially at-risk patients had POC screening HbA1c values ≥ 5.7%, with 55/62 (89%) and 7/62 (11%), exhibiting measures in the prediabetic and diabetic ranges, respectively. Subjects with HbA1c measures above normal ranges were somewhat older and showed some differences in established risk factors, but our numbers in the diabetic range were too small (n = 7, with HbA1c > 6.4%) for definitive comparisons.

Observations Across Dental Variables

Among enrolled subjects, periodontal assessments within 3 months or at time of enrollment were captured for 100/127 (79%) of at-risk subjects who underwent POC HbA1c screening in dental settings. **Table 3** shows outcomes of the periodontal assessment stratified by glycemic status indicated by outcome of POC HbA1c screening measures, including percent of subjects with bone loss, attachment loss, and moderate-to-severe PD

TABLE 2 | Outcomes of POC HbA1c screening summarized by participant characteristics.

	Normal[#] ($n = 65$)	Pre-DM[##] ($n = 55$)	DM[###] ($n = 7$)	*P*-value[a]
Mean age (years)	48.9 ± 13.3	53.5 ± 13.5	51.9 ± 9.5	0.035
Male	30.8%	34.5%	85.7%	0.273
White race	70.8%	65.5%	71.4%	0.703
Hispanic	18.5%	20.0%	28.6%	0.824
Hypertension	36.9%	30.9%	57.1%	0.853
Hypercholesterolemia	35.4%	34.5%	57.1%	0.856
Mean BMI	29.9 ± 8.5	31.8 ± 7.3	32.8 ± 6.0	0.091
History of smoking	58.5%	40.0%	42.9%	0.051

[a]Test result comparing normal to pre-DM pooled with DM. Percentage of participants meeting PD definitions is shown for each subset of patients classified by HbA1c screening outcomes reflecting glycemic status as defined by the American Diabetes Association: normal range[#] (<5.7%), prediabetic range[##] (≥5.7–6.4%), and diabetic range[###] (>6.4%) [19]. Data in this table were based on self-reported responses completed by eligible participants at time of enrollment in response to the questionnaires (see Appendices).
POC, point-of-care; HbA1c, hemoglobin A1c; DM, diabetes mellitus.

TABLE 3 | Dental measures as available for cohort with POC HbA1c screening data.

	Normal[#] ($n = 50$)	Pre-DM[##] ($n = 45$)	DM[###] ($n = 5$)	*P*-value[a]
Attachment loss	76.6%	82.5%	100%	0.434
Bone loss	70.2%	85.7%	80.0%	0.136
Moderate/severe PD	31.1%	43.6%	80.0%	0.132
Mean number of missing teeth	5.4 ± 6.4	5.7 ± 6.0	3 ± 2.2	0.777
Mean bleeding on probing	5 ± 6.8	4.4 ± 5.3	11 ± 9.0	0.660

[a]Results of statistical evaluations comparing normal with pre-DM pooled with DM. Definitions of criteria used to define moderate-to-severe PD for study participants: patients were required to have a minimum of 10 evaluable teeth excluding third molars. Furthermore, documentation of the following parameters was required: ≥6 teeth with bleeding on probing, ≥5 teeth with periodontal pocket depths (PPDs) of ≥5 mm, evidence of clinical attachment loss ≥ 3 mm, or ≥16% (≥3 mm) bone loss based on diagnostic radiographs captured within the past 24 months, as defined by AAP classification definitions [18]. Data on number of missing teeth were also captured. Percentage of participants meeting PD definitions is shown for each subset of patients classified by HbA1c screening outcomes reflecting glycemic status as defined by the American Diabetes Association: normal range[#] (<5.7%); prediabetic range[##] (≥5.7–6.4%); and diabetic range[###] (>6.4%) [19].
POC, point of care; HbA1c, hemoglobin A1c; DM, diabetes mellitus; AAP, American Academy of Periodontology; PD, periodontal disease.

based on updated definitions of PD classification defined by the AAP Task Force [19]. Although the differences were not statistically significant, subjects with elevated HbA1c measures showed higher levels of PD than those with normal measures across all three periodontal parameters assessed.

Longitudinal Follow-Up

At 3 months, 90% of subjects who had undergone biological screening with HbA1c measures ≥ 5.7% participated in telephonic follow-up. At follow-up, 79% reported having attended or scheduled appointments with medical providers. Longitudinal follow-up for ≥12 months (range: >12–24 months) by monitoring glycemic measures and prescription data for pharmaceuticals targeting glycemic control was possible for 44/127 (35%) of subjects enrolled at FHC-M dental centers or the Bridge Community site, who also accessed medical care through MCHS. As shown in **Figure 2A**, mean glycemic measures determined in the medical setting in patients with HbA1c measures in the normal range captured at POC in the dental setting were lower than mean of measures for those subjects whose screening measure captured at POC in the dental setting was ≥5.7% (5.6 vs. 6.2%, respectively). A trend toward higher prevalence of missing teeth was also noted among those with POC HbA1c measures ≥ 5.7% (**Figure 2B**).

The integrated medical–dental EHR (iEHR) was screened from time of enrollment to up to 24 months to capture any new laboratory data indicating glycemic screening. During the 24 months of follow-up, 153 glucose measures across the 42 patients were documented in the iEHR (mean = 3.6 measures per patient; range: 1-16 measures). Comparing results of POC HbA1c measures at time of enrollment and at time of first follow-up glycemic measure (HbA1c or fasting plasma glucose), elevated glycemic status at screening was corroborated in 32/44 (73%) of subjects. Notably, fasting and random glucose measures were more routinely performed to monitor at-risk patients and were available for 42/44 patients. For two patients, only pharmaceutical exposures to medications indicating glycemic management were available for follow-up. Observation of glycemic data for >12 months (up to 24 months) was possible for 29/42 (69%) of subjects being followed up for whom laboratory values were available. Among 4/127 participants (3.1%), a new diagnosis of T2DM was validated based on confirmation of glycemic measures during longitudinal follow-up, assignment of new diagnostic code, and/or newly prescribed medications for glycemic control. Among the 23/44 patients with screening measures in the prediabetic range for whom longitudinal follow-up was possible, prediabetic/diabetic status was validated in 18/23 (78%) of subjects during longitudinal follow-up. An additional six patients who had exhibited high-normal values for POC HbA1c screening measures were found to have measures in the prediabetic range during follow-up.

A trend toward improved glycemic status over time was noted in 20% of subjects in response to pharmacological management and/or lifestyle changes. Patient access for dental management was also trackable for 80% of 44 patients with available data in the EHR. Among these patients, 88% underwent at least one periodontal examination during the 2-year observational follow-up window.

DISCUSSION

Findings Regarding Rate of Hyperglycemic Risk in the Community Health Center Dental Clinic Population

A growing evidence base continues to support that onset and progression of chronic systemic and oral diseases are driven by integrated pathophysiological processes and impact on health outcomes in a holistic manner. In this scenario, simultaneous

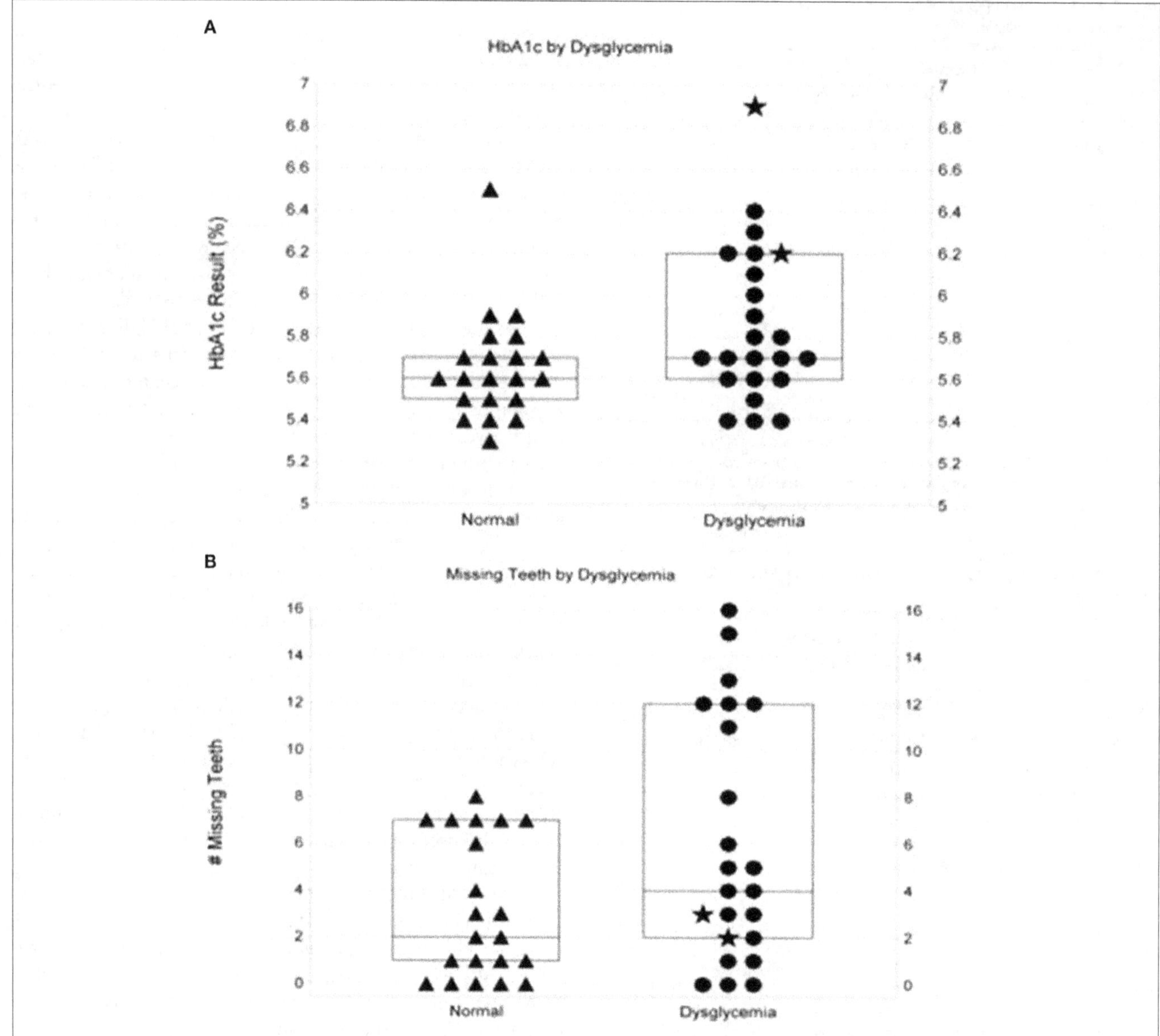

FIGURE 2 | Characteristics of at-risk dental patients with normo-glycemic point-of-care screening outcomes vs. those with outcomes in the pre-diabetic/diabetic range. **(A)** shows distribution of follow-up glycemic measures performed by a commercial laboratory in the medical setting on at-risk patients with normoglycemic vs. elevated glycemic measures when screened at point-of-care. Box plot in **(A)** show the median and interquartile range. Two patients screening in the diabetic range are denoted by ★. The figure shows a trend ($p = 0.054$) for more follow-up measures in hyperglycemic ranges (defined as HbA1c measures $\geq$ 5.7% or fasting plasma glucose measures $\geq$ 100 mg/dL. **(B)** illustrates observations surrounding numbers of missing teeth documented in at-risk patients with initial elevated HbA1c screening measures ($\geq$5.7%) vs. number of missing teeth in those with point-of-care HbA1c measures in the normoglycemic range (p-value = 0.094). Box plots in **(B)** show the median and interquartile range. Two patients screening in the diabetic range are denoted by ★.

exacerbation may occur with bidirectional contributions impacting both oral and systemic disease severity especially in the absence of effective integrated intervention. Increasingly, re-evaluation of our health-care delivery models has been advocated with emphasis on evolution of improved integrated medical–dental care delivery models supported by systematic examination to show evidence that such models are cost-effective and actually leverage improved patient outcomes [21]. In the absence of medical–dental integration across the entire spectrum of stakeholders, which may be further confounded by disparities in access experienced by some segments of the population, the potential for contribution to the epidemic escalation of diabetes and PD remains. The current study sought to examine whether one targeted intervention, namely, biological testing for glycemic status in the unconventional primary DC setting that provides health care to populations with overrepresentation of disparity populations, could activate patients to access care by providers practicing in an integrated care delivery environment. Among study-eligible, high-risk subjects with a low track record for glycemic monitoring attending dental visits at CHC-DC who underwent HbA1c screening at POC, the rate of hyperglycemia was 49%. Notably, as seen in **Table 1**, a higher percentage of study-eligible subjects reported comorbidities [hypertension, hypercholesterolemia, and body mass index (BMI) > 30] compared with the screened population whose risk profile did not meet eligibility requirements for POC screening, corroborating previously reported findings regarding high prevalence of multiple comorbidities among patients with diabetes [22]. Moreover, in the subpopulation with elevated glycemic screening measures where longitudinal follow-up was possible, screening results were corroborated for 78% of participants.

Outcomes of Longitudinal Follow-Up

This case study examined longitudinal follow-up in the longest temporal window reported to date (up to 2 years) following implementation of POC glycemic screening in four CHC dental primary care settings to determine impact on patient care-seeking behavior in health-care environments offering integrated care delivery access in the context of dental safety net operations. Implementation of biological screening for hyperglycemia at POC using FDA-approved glucometers in the subpopulation of appointed dental patients meeting high-risk profiles detected a 24% rate of at-risk individuals based on patient survey responses alone. Among this subset, 58% qualified for POC HbA1c screening in the dental primary care setting. Notably, differences surrounding periodontal prevalence in this relatively small study between patients screening in the normoglycemic and hyperglycemic were not statistically significant. Nonetheless, a trend toward higher rates of more advanced PD was noted among subjects with POC HbA1c measures in the prediabetic and diabetic ranges as compared with patients with normoglycemic measures as evidenced by percent of bone loss, attachment loss, and PD severity level across the glycemic strata. Telephonic follow-up at 3 months to monitor subjects' planned compliance with recommended triage for follow-up with a medical provider was possible for 90% of all study participants. Among these participants, all but one patient indicated compliance or planned follow-up. Notably, among the subset of participants where investigators could access data in the iEHR, semi-annual or annual glycemic assessments for up to 2 years post the date of POC screening were documented for 100% of subjects. Moreover, attendance for annual periodontal assessments up to 24 months post-POC testing was also documented for 80% of the subset. Taken together, longitudinal observation documented a change in patient behavior relative to accessing integrated care for glycemic and periodontal assessment, and a high level of patient activation following POC glycemic screening in the CHC-DC setting was observed.

Comparisons With Historical Field Trials Examining Point-of-Care Glycemic Testing in Community Health Center Dental Clinic Settings

In a field trial conducted by Genco et al. [23] that examined feasibility of POC glycemic screening across a range of dental settings, the authors similarly observed that compliance with triage for glycemic monitoring in the medical setting was highest in the CHCs compared with private dental practices (79 vs. 22% ($p = 0.001$). Furthermore, 85% compliance was noted in a CHC with an integrated care delivery model participating in their field trial [23]. Data from the current study corroborate initial findings reported by Genco et al. Notably, Greenberg et al. [24] also found higher rates of acceptance for triage to the medical setting by dental providers among patients attending DCs (86%) vs. private dental practices (76%). A systematic review examining the role of diabetic screening in the dental setting by various stakeholders similarly reported that five studies examining patient opinion surrounding acceptability of diabetic screening in the dental setting unanimously reported high rates of acceptability [25].

PD represents an early complication and harbinger of diabetes/prediabetes [9], emphasizing the need for cross-disciplinary integrated care delivery models. A 2015 study conducted in an outpatient clinic serving low- to mid-income population in Amsterdam treating patients with diabetes in a non-integrated setting conducted a trial targeting improved communication between medical and dental professionals. An alternative model explored in an additional study by these authors included provision of an oral health questionnaire completed by the dentist, and periodontal screening index (PSI) score was supplied to the physician during patient visits to inform patient management as an alternative approach to POC testing. Notably, among patients with moderate-to-high PSI scores, 65% had untreated PD. The study reported that moderate-to-high PSI was moderately more prevalent in 54% of the population with T2DM and in 57% of patients exhibiting obesity, but response rate for questionnaire completion was reported as 41% [26].

These data suggest that some populations may be more responsive to accessing integrated care delivery, although reasons for this are currently unclear and would require further investigation. Given that CHC-DC serve disparity populations with among the highest rates of PD and diabetes, data from the current study and other initial field trials suggest that the clientele of CHC-DC operating as safety nets are motivated to access integrated care delivery that offers affordable access to both medical and dental care for this population. Moreover, such populations are likely to derive the greatest level of benefit given the high prevalence of PD and diabetes documented among disparity populations. However, due to limited sample sizes of studies to date that have been able to observe integrated care access, studies in larger populations across more diverse populations are needed to further test this premise.

Study Limitations

Some study limitations are noteworthy. Longitudinal glycemic and dental follow-up was possible for approximately one third of 44/127 (35%) of study participants who underwent HbA1c screening and was not possible for an additional 35% of patients seen mainly for treatment of dental emergencies at the walk-in St. Elizabeth Ann Seton Dental Clinic in Milwaukee Wisconsin, which does not provide routine dental care to these patients or track their dental history. However, the walk-in St. Elizabeth Ann Seton Dental Clinic patients were responsive to study participation, and 20/44 (45%) of them indicated intent to comply with recommendation for medical follow-up. For the remaining 30% of patients, access to longitudinal follow-up data was not available, although these patients may have sought care in other health-care systems where EHR access was not possible. Whereas, glycemic evaluation for fasting or random glucose measure in the medical setting was available for 95% of patients, follow-up HbA1c measures were only available for 62% of participants. Finally, due to constraints in the sample size in which longitudinal follow-up was possible, further data modeling was precluded.

AUTHOR CONTRIBUTIONS

IG contributed to study design, drafted the study protocol, data analysis, regulatory paperwork, implemented point-of-care glycemic testing and protocols, and drafted the manuscript. RB performed biostatistical analyses, informed statistical aspects of study design, and edited the manuscript. AP assisted with data management, data set preparation, data analysis, and reviewed manuscript. NS contributed to strategic design of all study objectives, final review, final editing of manuscript, and figure development. AS provided day-to-day oversight of study activities, tracked enrollment, quality checked data entry, developed reports, provided oversight of multi-site project management, fiscal oversight, and review the final manuscript. GN participated in study design relative to operational aspects occurring in the dental clinical setting, facilitated establishment and integration of point-of-care glycemic testing and research activities involving patient examinations into clinical operations, championed the study with dentists and hygienists, and participated in final editing of manuscript. AA initiated the study, obtained and oversaw funding for study support, provided study oversight, lead the study design and activities of the research team, prepared study reports, and participated in final editing of the manuscript. All authors contributed to the article and approved the submitted version.

ACKNOWLEDGMENTS

The authors wish to acknowledge the 17VNPL DCA Vantage Analyzer Placement Program for supplying the HbA1c analyzer for the study. The authors further acknowledge assistance from the following research coordinators with patient enrollment and data collection and entry into REDcap: Rebecca Pilsner, Linda Heeren, Emily Redmond, and DeeAnn Polacek. The authors further acknowledge assistance from Jackie Salzwedel for completing the 3-month follow-up phone calls. We also wish to acknowledge efforts of Georgia Fischer and Maika Lee as site study managers; Michael Stroik for data retrieval at Bridge Community Dental Center, Wausau, WI; and Robyn Kibler as site project manager at St. Elizabeth Ann Seton Dental Clinic, Milwaukee, WI.

REFERENCES

1. *Centers for Disease Control and Prevention National Diabetes Statistics Report.* (2020). Available online at: https://www.cdc.gov/diabetes/library/features/diabetes-stat-report.html-report.html (accessed October 2, 2021).
2. Centers for Disease Control and Prevention. *Prevalence of Prediabetes Among Adults.* Available online at: https://www.cdc.gov/diabetes/data/statistics-report/prevalence-of-prediabetes.html#:~:text=An%20estimated%2088%20million%20adults,A1C%20level%20(Table%203) (accessed October 2, 2021).
3. Rowley WR, Bezold C, Arikan Y, Byrne E, Krohe S. Diabetes 2030: insights from yesterday, today and future trends. *Popul Health Manag.* (2017) 20:6-12. doi: 10.1089/pop.2015.0181
4. Eke PI, Thornton-Evans GO, Wei L, Borgnakke WS, Dye BA, Genco RJ. Periodontitis in US adults: national health and nutrition examination survey 2009-2014. *J Am Dent Assoc.* (2018) 149:576–88.e6. doi: 10.1016/j.adaj.2018.04.023
5. Nascimento GG, Leite FRM, Vestergaard P, Scheutz F, Lopez R. Does diabetes increase the risk of periodontitis? A systematic review and meta-regression analysis of longitudinal prospective studies. *Acta Diabetol.* (2018) 55:653-67. doi: 10.1007/s00592-018-1120-4
6. Siu AL, USPSTF. Screening for abnormal blood glucose and type 2 diabetes mellitus: U.S. preventive services task force recommendation statement. *Annal Intern Med.* (2015) 163:861-8. doi: 10.7326/M15-2345
7. Glurich I, Nycz G, Acharya A. Status update on translation of integrated primary dentalmedical care delivery for management of diabetic patients. *Clin Med Res.* (2017) 15:21-32. doi: 10.3121/cmr.2017.1348
8. Glurich I, Bartkowiak B, Berg RL, Acharya A. Screening for dysglycaemia in dental primary care practice settings: systematic review of the evidence. *Int Dent J.* (2018) 68:369-77. doi: 10.1111/idj.12405
9. Teeuw WJ, Kosho MX, Poland DC, Gerdes VE, Loos BG. Periodontitis as a possible early sign of diabetes mellitus. *BMJ Open Diabetes Res Care.* (2017) 5:e000326. doi: 10.1136/bmjdrc-2016-000326
10. Sanz M, Ceriello A, Buysschaert M, Chapple I, Demmer RT, Graziani F, et al. Scientific evidence on the links between periodontal disease and diabetes: consensus report and guidelines of the joint workshop on periodontal diseases and diabetes by the International Diabetes Federation and the European Federation of Periodontology. *Diab Res Clin Prac.* (2018) 137:231–41. doi: 10.1016/j.diabres.2017.12.001
11. Glurich I, Acharya A. Updates from the evidence base examining association between periodontal disease and type 2 diabetes mellitus: current status and clinical relevance. *Curr Diab Rep.* (2019) 19:121. doi: 10.1007/s11892-019-1228-0
12. American Dental Association. *D0411 and D0412-ADA Quick Guide to in-Office Monitoring and Documenting Patient Blood Glucose and HbA1C level.* Available online at: https://www.ada.org/~/media/ADA/Publications/Files/CDT_D0411_D0412_Guide_v1_2019Jan02.pdf?la=en~9Jan02.pdf?la$=$en (accessed October 2, 2021).
13. Lalla E, Kunzel C, Burkett S, Chenchg B, Lamster IB. Identification of unrecognized diabetes and prediabetes in a dental setting. *J Dent Res.* (2011) 90:855-60. doi: 10.1177/0022034511407069
14. Lalla E, Cheng B, Kunzel C, Burkett S, Lamster IB. Dental findings and identification of undiagnosed hyperglycemia. *J Dent Res.* (2013) 92:888-92. doi: 10.1177/0022034513502791
15. Nycz G, Acharya A, Glurich I. Solutions to dental access disparity: blueprint of an innovative community health center-based model for rurally-based communities. *J Public Health Dent.* (2020) 80:4-8. doi: 10.1111/jphd.12347
16. Nycz G, Shimpi N, Glurich I, Ryan M, Sova G, Weiner S, et al. Positioning operations in the dental safety net to enhance value-based care delivery in an integrated health-care setting. *J Public Health Dent.* (2020) 80(Suppl 2):S71-6. doi: 10.1111/jphd.12392
17. Sanchez-Mora C, Rodriguez-Oliva MS, Fernandez-Riejos P, Mateo J, Polo-Padillo J, Goberna R, et al. Evaluation of two HbA1c point-of-care analyzers. *Clin Chen Lab Med.* (2011) 49:653-7. doi: 10.1515/CCLM.2011.101
18. Whitley HP, Yong EV, Rasinen C. Selecting an A1C point-of-care instrument. *Diabetes Spectr.* (2015) 28:201-8. doi: 10.2337/diaspect.28.3.201
19. American academy of periodontology task force report on the update to the 1999 classification of periodontal diseases and conditions *J Periodontol* (2015) 86:835–8. doi: 10.1902/jop.2015.157001

20. American Diabetes Association. Standards of medical care in diabetes. *Diabetes Care.* (2018) 41(Suppl 1):S1-59. doi: 10.2337/dc18-S015
21. Somerman M, Mouradian WE. Integrating oral and systemic health: innovations in science, health care and policy. *Front Dent Med.* (2020) 1:599214. doi: 10.3389/fdmed.2020.599214
22. Lin PJ, Kent DM, Winn A, Cohen JT, Neumann PJ. Multiple chronic conditions in type 2 diabetes mellitus: prevalence and consequences. *Am J Manag Care.* (2015) 21:e23-34.
23. Genco RJ, Schifferle RE, Dunford RG, Falkner KL, Hsu WC, Balukjian J. Screening for diabetes mellitus in dental practices: a field trial. *J Am Dent Assoc.* (2014) 145:57-64. doi: 10.14219/jada.2013.7
24. Greenberg BL, Kantor ML, Jiang SS, Glick M. Patients' attitudes toward screening for medical conditions in a dental setting. *J Public Health Dent.* (2012) 72:28-35. doi: 10.1111/j.1752-7325.2011.00280.x
25. Yonel Z, Cerullo E, Kröger AT, Gray LJ. Use of dental practices for the identification of adults with undiagnosed type 2 diabetes mellitus or non-diabetic hyperglycaemia: a systematic review. *Diabet Med.* (2020) 37:1443-53. doi: 10.1111/dme.14324
26. Ahdi M, Teeuw WJ, Meeuwissen HG, Hoekstra JB, Gerdes VE, Loos BG, et al. Oral health information from the dentist to the diabetologist. *Eur J Intern Med.* (2015) 26:498-503. doi: 10.1016/j.ejim.2015.06.006

4

Oral *Prevotella* Species and their Connection to Events of Clinical Relevance in Gastrointestinal and Respiratory Tracts

Eija Könönen and Ulvi K. Gursoy*

Institute of Dentistry, University of Turku, Turku, Finland

***Correspondence:**
Eija Könönen
eija.kononen@utu.fi

Prevotella is recognized as one of the core anaerobic genera in the oral microbiome. In addition, members of this genus belong to microbial communities of the gastrointestinal and respiratory tracts. Several novel *Prevotella* species, most of them of oral origin, have been described, but limited knowledge is still available of their clinical relevance. *Prevotella melaninogenica* is among the anaerobic commensals on oral mucosae from early months of life onward, and other early colonizing *Prevotella* species in the oral cavity include *Prevotella nigrescens* and *Prevotella pallens*. Oral *Prevotella* species get constant access to the gastrointestinal tract via saliva swallowing and to lower airways via microaspiration. At these extra-oral sites, they play a role as commensals but also as potentially harmful agents on mucosal surfaces. The aim of this narrative review is to give an updated overview on the involvement of oral *Prevotella* species in gastrointestinal and respiratory health and disease.

Keywords: anaerobic bacteria, commensalism, dysbiosis, inflammation, microbiology, *Prevotella*, systemic disease, taxonomy

INTRODUCTION

Anaerobic bacteria constitute a significant part of oral microbial communities. In the oral cavity, Bacteroidetes is one of the major phyla and *Prevotella* its largest genus (Dewhirst et al., 2010). This genus, which has expanded significantly during the past decades, consists of gram-negative, strictly anaerobic, mainly short rod-shaped bacteria. In healthy adults, detection rates of *Prevotella* organisms are high in saliva and dental plaque (Keijser et al., 2008; Xu et al., 2015). In saliva, richness of the diversity within this genus is especially high (Keijser et al., 2008). At the species level, however, the majority of data currently available deals with *Prevotella intermedia* and/or *Prevotella nigrescens* due to their clinical relevance in oral pathologies but also ignorance of commensals. A study looking for intraoral distribution of bacterial species in 225 systemically healthy individuals showed *Prevotella melaninogenica* in high proportions in saliva and at the dorsum and lateral sites of the tongue (Mager et al., 2003).

In the context of this review, human habitats exposed to oral bacteria to be colonized outside the oral cavity are presented in **Figure 1**. There are obvious differences in the microbial communities between body habitats and between individual metabolic niches (Costello et al., 2009; Segata et al., 2012). At the genus level, *Prevotella* is frequent and widespread all over on the surfaces of the human body; however, a species-level identification methodology is necessary for revealing whether

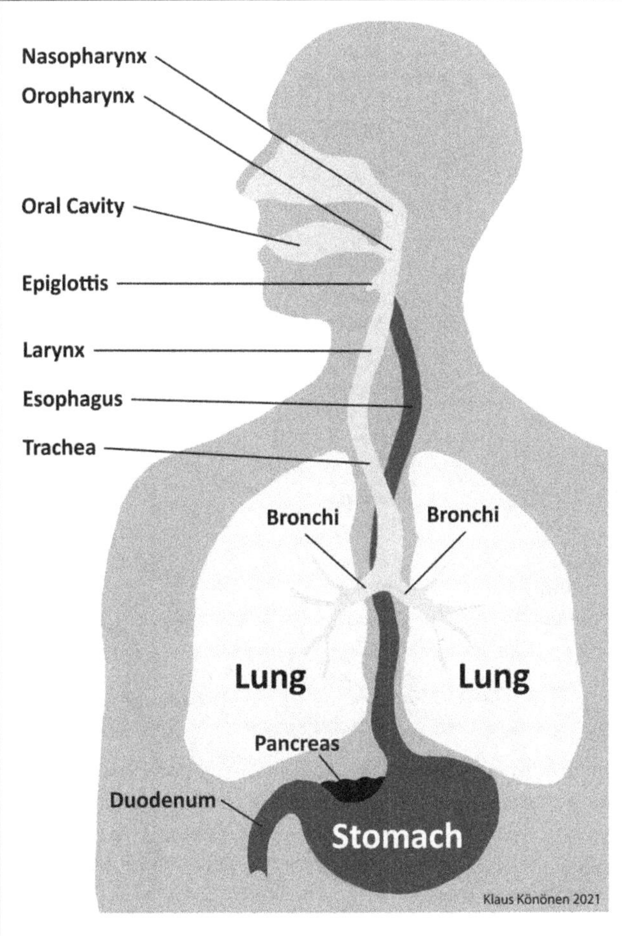

FIGURE 1 | The anatomy and potential habitats in the aerodigestive tract in humans.

same species colonize throughout the gastrointestinal tract and whether their relative abundance varies among the habitats as well as inter-individually (Segata et al., 2012; Schmidt et al., 2019). *Prevotella* strains present in saliva are of particular interest. Due to constant saliva swallowing of approximately 1.5 L daily (Humphrey and Williamson, 2001), this oral fluid is the most plausible vehicle for oral microorganisms and their biologically active components to be translocated to other parts of the digestive tract (Schmidt et al., 2019). Oral bacteria surviving to pass acidic circumstances of the stomach get access to the small intestine and colon, where they can interfere with intestinal bacteria (Schmidt et al., 2019; Kitamoto et al., 2020). At the genus level, *Prevotella* is a common colonizer of these distant habitats. However, at the species level, distinct bacterial populations occupy the oral and intestinal microenvironments. Also immune cells involved in chronic inflammatory processes in the mouth end up via saliva to the gut, sometimes resulting in pathological consequences (Byrd and Gulati, 2021).

In the respiratory tract, potential routes for bacterial translocation from the oral cavity include (micro)aspiration, in particular, and hematogenous spread. Indeed, recent studies have shaken our views on the oral source of bacteria for the composition of microbial communities of the lower respiratory tract (Bassis et al., 2015; Dickson et al., 2016). Currently, *Prevotella* is considered one of the major genera colonizing mucosal surfaces of the aerodigestive tract, including the lungs, which were long seen as a sterile site in the human body.

In this narrative review, the purpose is to give an updated overview on the presence of oral *Prevotella* species as members of the gastrointestinal and respiratory microbiota and on their involvement in diseases at these sites above the waistline.

TAXONOMICAL OVERVIEW OF ORAL *PREVOTELLA*

In 1990, the genus *Prevotella* was described by reclassifying a group of moderately saccharolytic and bile-susceptible *Bacteroides* species as members of this novel genus (Shah and Collins, 1990). The name *Prevotella* came after A. R. Prévot, who was a French microbiologist with pioneering expertise in anaerobic bacteriology. Most of these reclassified *Prevotella* organisms were recovered from the oral cavity of humans, *P. melaninogenica* being the type species of the genus. At that time, pigment production of colonies on blood agar was seen as an important feature to divide the organisms into pigmented and non-pigmented *Prevotella* species (Jousimies-Somer et al., 2002). In addition to *P. melaninogenica*, the pigmented group included *Prevotella loescheii*, *Prevotella denticola* (part of strains), *P. intermedia*, and *Prevotella corporis*, their color intensity varying from light brown to black. Some years later, the pigmented group within *Prevotella* was expanded by two phylogenetically closely related species, *P. nigrescens* (Shah and Gharbia, 1992) and *Prevotella pallens* (Könönen et al., 1998). During the 1990s, there was a notable research interest in black-pigmented gram-negative anaerobes, including *Porphyromonas* and *Prevotella* species, due to their link to various pathologies in humans (Finegold et al., 1993).

After the creation of the genus *Prevotella* and reclassification of moderately saccharolytic *Bacteroides* as *Prevotella* species by Shah and Collins (1990), there has been a great expansion of the genus with novel species, most of them of oral origin. **Table 1** presents the validly published *Prevotella* species that have been primarily isolated from the oral cavity: 12 species formerly classified as *Bacteroides* and 18 novel *Prevotella* species described after 1990. On the other hand, a couple of reclassifications were made; while the former *Mitsuokella dentalis* is now *Prevotella dentalis* (Willems and Collins, 1995), *Prevotella tannerae* was removed to a novel, closely related genus *Alloprevotella*, also including a novel oral species, *Alloprevotella rava* (Downes et al., 2013). Two species with a distant phylogeny, *Prevotella heparinolytica* and *Prevotella zoogleoformans*, remain "on the waiting list" to be removed from the genus *Prevotella* (Dewhirst et al., 2010).

In addition to the above-mentioned species principally isolated from the oral cavity, several novel *Prevotella* species have been described based on a few strains, or even a single strain, from various clinical specimens. Origins of these strains were as follows: two *Prevotella amnii* strains from amniotic fluid

TABLE 1 | Validly published *Prevotella* and *Alloprevotella* species with the primary isolation from the human oral cavity.

Year/Reference	Former *Bacteroides* sp. reclassified as *Prevotella* sp.	Year/References	Novel *Prevotella* and *Alloprevotella* spp.	Comments
Shah and Collins, 1990	*P. melaninogenica* (type species)	Shah and Gharbia, 1992	*P. nigrescens*	
	P. buccae	Moore et al., 1994	*P. enoeca* *P. tannerae*	
	P. buccalis	Willems and Collins, 1995	*P. dentalis*	*Mitsuokella dentalis*
	P. denticola	Könönen et al., 1998	*P. pallens*	
	P. heparinolytica	Sakamoto et al., 2004	*P. salivae* *P. shahii*	
	P. intermedia	Sakamoto et al., 2005a	*P. multiformis*	
	P. loescheii	Sakamoto et al., 2005b	*P. multisaccharivorax*	
	P. oralis	Downes et al., 2005	*P. baroniae* *P. marshii*	
	P. oris	Downes et al., 2007	*P. maculosa*	
	P. oulorum	Downes et al., 2008	*P. histicola*	
	P. veroralis	Downes et al., 2009	*P. micans*	
	P. zoogleoformans	Sakamoto et al., 2010	*P. aurantiaca*	
		Downes et al., 2010	*P. saccharolytica*	
		Downes and Wade, 2011	*P. fusca* *P. scopos*	
		Downes et al., 2013	*A. rava* *A. tannerae*	*Alloprevotella* gen. nov., reclassification of *P. tannerae*

(Lawson et al., 2008), eight *Prevotella bergensis* strains from skin and soft tissue infections (Downes et al., 2006), one *Prevotella brunnea* strain from a wound at foot (Buhl et al., 2019), one *Prevotella colorans* strain from a wound (Buhl et al., 2016), three *Prevotella jejuni* strains from the jejunum of a celiac child (Hedberg et al., 2013), three *Prevotella nanceiensis* strains from bronchial fluid, lung abscess, or blood (Alauzet et al., 2007), one *Prevotella pleuritidis* strain from pleural fluid (Sakamoto et al., 2007), one *Prevotella timonensis* strain from breast abscess (Glazunova et al., 2007), and one *Prevotella vespertina* strain from an abscess locating at the upper respiratory tract (Buhl and Marschal, 2020). With this limited information given, the knowledge of their preferred habitat remains open.

Three former *Bacteroides* species, reclassified as *Prevotella bivia*, *Prevotella corporis*, and *Prevotella disiens* (Shah and Collins, 1990) come mainly from the human urogenital tract but there are also occasional recoveries from the mouth. In the current literature, several novel *Prevotella* species from stool specimens have been described as colonizers of the colon. Of those, *Prevotella copri* has drawn remarkable attention due to its potential beneficial effects on human well-being (Tett et al., 2021), although its connections to chronic inflammatory conditions of the gut have been recognized, too (Ley, 2016).

Besides biochemical and physiological testing, methods for *Prevotella* classification have traditionally included DNA–DNA hybridization, measuring of G + C content, and multilocus enzyme electrophoresis, however, classification gradually changes toward genomic methods. Full-sequencing of the 16S rRNA gene is a routine, but also comparison to whole-genome sequence databases is available and has been used in recent *Prevotella* descriptions (Buhl et al., 2016, 2019; Buhl and Marschal, 2020). Tett et al. (2021) recently described genomic characteristics of 25 named human *Prevotella* species, among those 17 species with genomes of multiple oral isolates in the analysis. Varying genome lengths between 2.37–4.26 Mb and G + C contents between 36.4–56.1% as well as the high number of core genes speak for the wide diversity within this genus.

PREVOTELLA IN BACTERIAL COMMUNITIES OF THE DIGESTIVE TRACT

Prevotella as Members of the Core Microbiota in the Gastrointestinal Tract

Concerning the alimentary tract from the oropharynx downward above the waistline, it was for long considered of being without a resident microbiota until advanced molecular methods allowed to challenging these earlier beliefs, which were based on negative cultures by routine microbiology methods from the esophagus and stomach (Pei et al., 2004; Bik et al., 2006). Pei et al. (2004) tested their hypotheses on the presence of indigenous bacteria on esophageal mucosa and on their fastidious nature, i.e., mainly being uncultivable. Biopsy specimens from the distal esophagus of four healthy individuals were examined with 16S rDNA sequencing-based techniques, and the results showed Bacteroidetes as the second most common phylum and *Prevotella* as the second most common genus after *Streptococcus*. *P. pallens* was among the 14 bacterial taxa found in all individuals, while many other named *Prevotella* species were also recovered: *Prevotella veroralis* from three individuals, *P. intermedia* and *P. melaninogenica* from two individuals, and *P. denticola*,

P. nigrescens, and *Prevotella oris* each from one individual. In addition, several not-yet-named *Prevotella* clones were among the findings (Pei et al., 2004). To increase the understanding of the esophageal microbiome and its function in the host, Deshpande et al. (2018) studied the esophageal microbiome of over 100 individuals, with special emphasis on age, gender, proton pump inhibitor use, host genetics, and development of esophageal disease. They demonstrated that the esophageal microbiome clusters into functionally distinct bacterial community types. Cluster 3 was dominated by *P. melaninogenica* and *P. pallens*, and cluster 2 by mitis group streptococci, while cluster 1 was an intermediate type with respect to abundances of *Streptococcus* and *Prevotella*, indicating their ratio of being a significant factor in defining esophageal community types (Deshpande et al., 2018). It was shown that various, distinct pathways are increased in each community type. Age was observed to affect relative abundances within these two major genera; age positively correlated with *Streptococcus parasanguinis* (but not with mitis group streptococci), whereas age had an inverse correlation with *P. melaninogenica* (but not with *P. pallens*). Interestingly, there was a co-exclusion relationship between mitis group streptococci and *Prevotella* species across all esophageal disease stages (Deshpande et al., 2018).

Bik et al. (2006) collected gastric biopsy specimens from 23 adults, suffering from symptomatic upper gastrointestinal disease and being positive or negative for *Helicobacter pylori*. Advanced sensitive methods were used to reveal the bacterial composition of the gastric microbiota and the impact of *H. pylori* on its composition. There was a much larger bacterial diversity in gastric biopsies than was expected, but the sequence collection was also different from those of the mouth and esophagus presented in other studies. Interestingly, especially Bacteroidetes phylotypes were often absent from *H. pylori*-positive individuals (Bik et al., 2006). However, several recognized oral *Prevotella* species (and several *Prevotella* clones) were detected in individuals who were *H. pylori*-negative by conventional methods. Among the findings were, in descending order in their abundance, *P. melaninogenica* and *P. pallens*, in particular, and few *P. oris*, *P. intermedia*, *P. nigrescens*, *Prevotella oralis*, *Prevotella oulorum*, and *P. denticola*. It was emphasized that bacterial DNA may not indicate the presence of resident bacteria but, instead, could reflect the presence of bacterial cell remnants or transient flow of these bacteria in the specimens (Bik et al., 2006). Recently, it was confirmed that *H. pylori*, if present, dominates the bacterial community composition of the stomach, lowering the diversity and evenness of phylotypes (Schulz et al., 2018). Similarly to the study by Bik et al. (2006), two genera, *Streptococcus* and *Prevotella*, proved to dominate in bacterial communities of the upper gastrointestinal tract in *H. pylori*-negative individuals. By analyzing saliva, and stomach and duodenal aspirates and biopsies from a cohort of 24 individuals with chronic gastritis by high-throughput sequencing, Schulz et al. (2018) identified the oral cavity (saliva) of being the main source of active bacteria for the gastric microbiota, indicating a continuous migration of oral bacteria through the upper gastrointestinal tract. In individuals without *H. pylori*, no difference was seen in relative abundance of *Prevotella* and *Alloprevotella* between saliva and stomach aspirates, while reduced abundance for both genera was detected between the stomach and duodenum. In general, no significant difference at the genus level was observed in oral communities between individuals with or without *H. pylori*, but three phylotypes, among those *P. oris*, had significantly higher abundance in individuals without *H. pylori* (Schulz et al., 2018). Each individual harbored own specific bacterial communities throughout the upper gastrointestinal tract.

Saliva has been suggested as a key driver for the composition of bacterial communities in various habitats of the upper digestive tract, and as another key driver, a shared epithelial lining of their mucosae (Segata et al., 2012). Vasapolli et al. (2019) looked thoroughly for bacterial community changes in 21 healthy individuals throughout their gastrointestinal tract, including a wide selection of specimens: saliva, stomach (antrum and corpus), duodenum, terminal ileum, ascending and descending colon, and feces. They demonstrated that bacterial communities detected in samples from saliva, stomach, and duodenum formed 1 cluster and those from the lower gastrointestinal tract another cluster, while fecal communities differed from mucosa-associated findings of the gut (Vasapolli et al., 2019). The highest phylotype richness, including the genus *Prevotella*, was found in saliva, staying rather steady across the upper body sites, whereas in samples from lower parts of the body, a significantly reduced phylotype richness was observed. Among the phylum Bacteroidetes, abundance of *Prevotella* organisms present in saliva gradually decreased downward up to the duodenum, the decrease being drastic thereafter, whereas an opposite occurred to abundance of *Bacteroides* organisms (Vasapolli et al., 2019). In line were the results of a thorough culture-based study, performed in a homologous group of beagle dogs (Mentula et al., 2005), showing clear differences between jejunal and fecal samples and where a unique bacterial composition for each dog was found in small-intestinal fluid with a few species only at a time and fluctuating counts. Smoking seems to be a lifestyle factor affecting the mucosa-associated microbiota of the duodenum; in current smokers, a significantly reduced abundance of the phylum Bacteroidetes and the genus *Prevotella* was observed, and this reduction was only partially restored after quitting of smoking (Shanahan et al., 2018). *P. nanceiensis* was suggested to be a discriminatory species for previous smokers.

A few *Prevotella* species isolated from feces are considered having their habitat in the intestine. According to the current knowledge, especially *P. copri* is both a prevalent and abundant organism in the gut [see an excellent review by Tett et al. (2021)]. Interestingly, lifestyle factors, diet in particular, have a significant impact on its abundance. In non-Westernized populations with diets rich of carbohydrates and fibers, the *P. copri* complex is a common inhabitant of the gut, while different bacterial taxa dominate in populations with Western-type diets. On one hand, the *P. copri* complex seems to possess beneficial metabolic effects on human health but, on the other hand, potential detrimental effects may also exist (Ley, 2016; Tett et al., 2021). The impact of diet on oral *Prevotella* species is not known.

Prevotella Involvement in Gastrointestinal Diseases

In the human esophagus, gastroesophageal reflux disease is a rather common pathological condition, where the relaxation of the sphincter muscle at the lower esophagus allows acidic stomach contents frequently flow back into the esophagus and further into the pharynx[1]. This constant leakage irritates the epithelial surface, causing reflux symptoms or esophagitis, which may lead to Barrett's esophagus with a disturbed epithelium structure. The potential role of changes in the esophageal and/or salivary microbiota has been studied and, in this context, the genus *Prevotella* is of interest (Liu et al., 2013; Kawar et al., 2021). Bacterial communities of the distal esophagus were examined at the phylum and genus levels in biopsy samples collected from Japanese patients with either normal esophagus, reflux esophagitis, or Barrett's esophagus (Liu et al., 2013). The study revealed Bacteroidetes among the major phyla, and the proportions of *Prevotella* clones in the samples were 3, 5, and 12%, respectively. Of the six patients in each group, the number of *Prevotella*-positive patients was three, four, and six, respectively. A distinct bacterial composition seen between the groups was assumed to indicate an association with an esophageal health status and disease type (Liu et al., 2013). Recently, Kawar et al. (2021) compared the bacterial composition of salivary samples collected from reflux patients treated with proton pump inhibitors to that from non-medicated reflux patients and healthy controls. Abundant taxa present in the samples from the latter two groups differed considerably, including reduced abundances of *P. melaninogenica* and *P. pallens* in saliva of reflux patients. It was assumed that a lowered pH in the oral cavity of non-medicated patients explains this difference, since no significant difference was found between saliva of medicated reflux patients and healthy controls (Kawar et al., 2021).

Bacterial compositions of the stomach and duodenum were examined in 98 Korean patients with symptomatic gastritis (Han et al., 2019). It was demonstrated that the gastric and duodenal microbiota differ from each other. Symptom scores only weakly correlated with abundance of gastric *H. pylori* but, instead, correlated more strongly with the duodenal microbiota. An interesting gender-related finding was the higher relative abundance of *P. pallens* in the stomach of women than in that of men. There was a negative correlation with relative abundance of *P. pallens* and the severity of symptoms in the stomach. Positive correlations were found with *P. nanceiensis* and *A. rava* in the duodenum. According to the authors, other factors than *H. pylori* need to be taken into account in symptomatic gastritis (Han et al., 2019).

A novel *Prevotella* species was detected for the first time in a biopsy taken from the jejunum of a child with celiac disease and was named as *P. jejuni* due to its localization in this part of the small intestine (Hedberg et al., 2013). However, this species seems to be a common inhabitant of the oral cavity and especially in saliva, similarly to its close relative, *P. melaninogenica* (own unpublished data). Alterations in the salivary microbiota and metabolome in celiac children, who had been under glutein-free diet at least for 2 years, were examined and compared to those of healthy control children (Francavilla et al., 2014). The number of total cultivable anaerobes differed between the groups, with reduced amounts found in children with celiac disease. Members of the phylum Bacteroidetes, among those *P. nanceiensis*, dominated in saliva, with increased abundance in celiac children. It was concluded that the diet change of 2 years may not be enough to restore the salivary microbiota (Francavilla et al., 2014).

Although the relation of the oral microbiota to inflammatory bowel diseases (IBD) is still controversial, there is evidence on their connection to dysbiotic bacterial communities in saliva (Said et al., 2014; Xun et al., 2018; Qi et al., 2021). Dysbiosis with an increased relative abundance of Bacteroidetes, in turn, causes an elevated inflammatory response, which is also seen in saliva as increased levels of cytokines like interleukin-1β (Said et al., 2014). No alterations were observed in the richness and diversity of bacterial communities between saliva from IBD patients and healthy controls, whereas the bacterial composition in saliva varied (Said et al., 2014; Qi et al., 2021). While abundance of *Streptococcus* decreased, that of *Prevotella* (besides *Veillonella*) and *P. melaninogenica* significantly increased in both Crohn's disease and ulcerative colitis patients. The genus *Prevotella* was suggested as a potential indicator related to Crohn's disease (Qi et al., 2021). Moreover, the dysbiotic salivary composition contributed to aggravated immune disorders in IBD patients.

Prevotella in Cancers of the Digestive Tract Above the Waistline

In the esophagus, cancer types differ depending on the geographical location; in the East, squamous cell carcinoma (SCC) dominates, whereas adenocarcinoma is more common in Western countries (Sung et al., 2021). In the first study to examine bacterial infection as a background factor for esophageal SCC and to identify bacteria that could predict the cancer prognosis, the genus *Prevotella* came up as a potential prognostic indicator for this cancer type (Liu et al., 2018). Patients with lymph node metastasis had higher abundance of *Prevotella* and *Treponema* than patients without metastatic findings, while increased abundance of *Prevotella* combined with *Streptococcus* affected survival rates, predicting poor prognosis. Alterations of the esophageal microbiota have also been studied in connection to Barrett's esophagus and esophageal adenocarcinoma (Lopetuso et al., 2020). The former condition with changes in the epithelial structure with acid stress and inflammation is considered to expose to metaplastic mucosa. Again, abundance of *Prevotella* was significantly increased, however, species-level shifts showed decreased proportions of *P. melaninogenica* in samples from Barrett's esophageal mucosa with or without cancer but increased proportions of unclassified *Prevotella*. *P. histicola* was common on mucosae of Barrett's esophagus, while *P. nigrescens* proportions on metaplastic mucosa were slightly increased (Lopetuso et al., 2020). The authors reported a co-exclusion association between *Streptococcus* and *Prevotella*; a significant reduction in relative abundance of *Streptococcus* and

[1]https://www.hopkinsmedicine.org/gastroenterology_hepatology/_pdfs/esophagus_stomach/gastroesophageal_reflux_disease.pdf

corresponding increase in abundance of *Prevotella* were observed on mucosae of both Barrett's esophagus and adenocarcinoma.

A decade ago, bacterial communities of the stomach in gastric cancer patients were described for the first time by molecular techniques and compared to those in dyspeptic patients with normal mucosa as controls (Dicksved et al., 2009). The second most dominant phylum proved to be Bacteroidetes, composing mainly of *Prevotella* taxa; among known species, *Prevotella multiformis*, *P. nigrescens*, *P. oris*, and *A. tannerae* were recognized in gastric cancer patients. It can be speculated whether changed conditions due to an increased use of acid-reducing drugs or neoplastic mucosa would allow the colonization of atypical bacteria in the stomach and progression of cancer (Dicksved et al., 2009; Coker et al., 2018). Coker et al. (2018) investigated mucosal biopsy specimens collected from superficial gastritis, atrophic gastritis, intestinal metaplasia, and gastric cancer patients, and detected highest abundance of several oral bacteria, among those *P. intermedia* and *P. oris*, in gastric cancer samples. It was emphasized, however, that it remains to be elucidated in targeted studies whether bacteria enriched are passengers or drivers of carcinogenesis (Coker et al., 2018).

Poor oral hygiene is suggested as a moderate risk factor for pancreatic cancer (Huang et al., 2016). This may be connected to increased amounts of microbial biofilms on oral surfaces and activation of host inflammatory response. In a recent study, a large variety of samples from the gastrointestinal tract, including oral (saliva and swabs from tongue, buccal mucosa, and gingiva), upper intestinal (duodenum tissue and swabs from jejunum and bile duct), and pancreatic (tumor or normal tissue and pancreatic duct) samples were examined to clarify the microbiota in patients with pancreatic cancer or other diseases of the pancreas or the foregut (Chung et al., 2021). *Streptococcus*, *Veillonella*, and *Prevotella* were the most shared genera between oral and gut or pancreatic samples, and *P. veroralis* among the most frequently shared species. Amplicon Sequence Variants had some overlaps between the close sites within the mouth and within the pancreas. In co-abundance analyses, distinct strain-level cluster patterns were observed among microbial findings in buccal swabs, saliva, duodenal tissue, jejunal swabs, and pancreatic tumor tissue. In the latter sample site, *P. nigrescens* was found among dominating species in one cluster (Chung et al., 2021).

PREVOTELLA IN BACTERIAL COMMUNITIES OF THE RESPIRATORY TRACT

Prevotella as Members of the Core Microbiota in the Respiratory Tract

A gradual maturation of the early microbiota of the lower respiratory tract occurs within less than 2 months after birth in full-term infants (Pattaroni et al., 2018). Three distinct colonization patterns were recognized in tracheal aspirates and were explained by distinct microenvironments in preterm and term infants. Of those, a mixed microbial profile consisted of a balanced composition of six genera, including *Streptococcus* and *Neisseria* as keystone genera, and anaerobic *Prevotella*, *Veillonella*, *Porphyromonas*, and *Fusobacterium*. This combination stayed stable across the first year of life (Pattaroni et al., 2018). Interestingly, this is a typical bacterial composition for the early microbiota established in the mouth during the first year of life (Könönen et al., 1999; Könönen, 2005). It also resembles the composition of the lung microbiota of adults during health (Bassis et al., 2015).

Similar interacting consortia as seen in the oral cavity (but not in the nasal cavity) can be observed in the lower respiratory tract, even though relative abundance and diversity richness are lower in the lungs (Bassis et al., 2015). Indeed, the oropharynx is considered the principal origin for the lung bacteriome during health (Bassis et al., 2015; Dickson et al., 2016). At the genus level, *Prevotella* is consistently among the core bacterial communities of the respiratory tract (Bassis et al., 2015; Einarsson et al., 2019). However, methodologies assessing the bacterial taxa at the species level, and even at the strain level, are necessary for discovering their source and role as beneficial, harmless or potentially harmful members of the bacterial communities at a specific body site. Noteworthy is that the *Prevotella* genus accommodates a high number of species with distinct clinical significance.

Valuable, detailed species-level oropharyngeal data assessed by in-depth sequencing are available from a study where tonsillar crypts in 2- to 4-year-old children and young adults were examined during recurrent tonsillitis and were compared to tonsillar crypts in children with tonsillar hyperplasia but without inflammation and those in healthy adult controls (Jensen et al., 2013). *Streptococcus* and *Prevotella* were found in all 20 samples from children and high *Prevotella* abundance was observed. Recurrent tonsillitis associated with a shift in the bacterial composition, especially with increased *P. melaninogenica/P. histicola* in adults. Typical oral *Prevotella* species, including *Prevotella buccae*, *P. dentalis*, *P. denticola*, *Prevotella fusca*, *Prevotella micans*, *P. oralis*, *P. oris*, *P. pallens*, *Prevotella salivae*, and *P. veroralis*, were more abundant in adults but *Prevotella saccharolytica* in children. *P. intermedia* was absent, except for a healthy adult with a high quantity. The recoveries of *P. nanceiensis* and *P. pleuritidis* from the oropharynx give support for their oral habitat. These study results indicate that a core microbiome, with a few significant genera, is present in tonsillar crypts regardless of individuals' age and health status (Jensen et al., 2013).

Recently, a potential link between the microbial community composition and lung homeostasis was examined by analyzing bronchoalveolar lavage samples from a longitudinally followed post-transplant study population (Das et al., 2021). Although the lung microbiota proved to be highly variable, there were a few bacterial taxa with high prevalence and/or abundance, and the majority of them were either obligate or facultative anaerobes. Among the most prevalent species were *P. melaninogenica*, *Veillonella atypica*, *Veillonella dispar*, *Streptococcus mitis*, and *Granulicatella adiacens* (all typical recoveries from the oral cavity). The microbiota was categorized into four distinct compositional states (pneumotypes) where the balanced pneumotype represented a diverse bacterial community, resembling that in the oropharynx and including

P. melaninogenica, which occurred in 97.4% of the samples (Das et al., 2021). In addition, this pneumotype had a high immune-modulatory activity and preserved lung stability.

Although oral bacteria get access to proximal airways via microaspiration, their growth at high densities is prevented by the continuous mucociliary clearance (Bassis et al., 2015). A recent study using a mouse model (Wu et al., 2021) demonstrated that the episodic aspiration of oral commensals, such as *P. melaninogenica*, *Veillonella parvula*, and *S. mitis*, leads to dysbiosis and low-dose inflammation in the lower airways; the consequence is a reduced susceptibility to pathogenic *Streptococcus pneumoniae* via activation of pulmonary Th17 cells. The shift in the human lung microbiome from the phylum Bacteroidetes in health to Gammaproteobacteria in disease indicates that *Prevotella*-activated Th17 response is an essential part of the pathogen recognition and suppression system of a healthy lung environment (Huffnagle et al., 2017). Anaerobic bacteria, especially *Prevotella*, are frequent recoveries from clinical respiratory specimens; however, understanding of their contribution to lung diseases is not clear yet.

Prevotella Involvement in Acute Diseases of the Respiratory Tract

Along with high research interest targeted to the COVID-19 pandemic, an increasing number of reports on the potential involvement of oral bacteria in the disease persistence and treatment outcome are available in the current literature. Interestingly, also *Prevotella* organisms, being analyzed from salivary, oropharyngeal, and bronchoalveolar lavage samples examined for SARS-CoV-2, have come up recently in this context. The microbiome and SARS-CoV-2 viral loads in saliva were compared between hospitalized COVID-19 and control patients (Miller et al., 2021). Although no significant difference in their bacterial compositions was found, the abundance of some taxa associated with the viral load in saliva; here, of special interest is enriched *P. pallens* but reduced *P. denticola* and *P. oris* in saliva of COVID-19 patients (Miller et al., 2021). Xiong et al. (2021) examined the difference in the microbial composition between SARS-CoV-2-positive and -negative pharyngeal swab samples collected from symptomatic patients with cough and fever. A significantly reduced species richness was seen in COVID-19 samples. The top-3 genera enriched were *Streptococcus, Prevotella,* and *Campylobacter*. Changes in abundance were seen also for several *Prevotella* species, such as *P. denticola, P. oris, P. jejuni, P. intermedia, P. melaninogenica, P. fusca*, and *P. scopos*, which were among the 37 species distinctive for the healthy and diseased individuals, and most of them separated the symptomatic COVID-19 and non-COVID groups from each other (Xiong et al., 2021). A dysbiotic oropharyngeal microbiota with gram-negative commensals, considered pathobionts due to their lipopolysaccharide production, has been connected to a so-called long-COVID disease (Haran et al., 2021). Among 164 patients with various types of symptoms, increased abundances of several *Prevotella* species were among the top predicting taxa from swabs of the posterior oropharynx: *P. denticola, P. nigrescens, P. histicola*, and *P. oulorum* in the patient group with ongoing symptoms, and *P. denticola, P. melaninogenica, P. jejuni*, and *P. nigrescens* in the determined long-COVID group (Haran et al., 2021). Sulaiman et al. (2021) examined a hospitalized cohort of 589 critically ill COVID-19 patients, characterizing their lung microbiome from bronchoalveolar lavage samples. Especially interesting were the findings of two oral commensals, *P. oris* and *Mycoplasma salivarium*, among the most dominant, functionally active microbial taxa. While *M. salivarium* was enriched in the deceased and >28-day mechanically ventilated groups, *P. oris* was enriched in the ≤28-day group. It was suggested that dissimilar microbial pressures related to host factors could explain the difference between the groups (Sulaiman et al., 2021). These studies indicate that the microbiome of the host plays a role in COVID-19 outcome.

Oral bacteria present in saliva can promote aspiration pneumonia via colonizing on mucosal surfaces, affecting immune response of epithelial cells, and producing proinflammatory cytokines and degradative enzymes, but dispersal via hematogenous route is also an option (Scannapieco, 2021). Older age and supine position as well as poor oral hygiene increase the risk for aspiration of bacteria from the oral cavity to lower parts of the respiratory tract (Hasegawa et al., 2014; Scannapieco, 2021). In pneumonias as well as pleural empyema, both anaerobes and oral bacteria, which can be missed by conventional culture, are more frequent findings by molecular methods (Yamasaki et al., 2013; Dyrhovden et al., 2019; Aoki et al., 2021). In community-acquired pneumonia, approximately 8% of bronchoalveolar lavage specimens from 64 hospitalized pneumonia patients were positive for *Prevotella/Alloprevotella*, three with *P. veroralis*, and *P. melaninogenica* and *A. tannerae* one each (Yamasaki et al., 2013). These findings came from mild cases, however, their pathogenic role remained unknown. Attempts to recover bacterial taxa regardless of their expected pathogenicity or quantity from respiratory specimens revealed *Prevotella* species in the majority of 17 aspiration pneumonias and eight lung abscesses (Aoki et al., 2021). Only occasional *Prevotella* recoveries, including *P. buccae, P. oris, P. pleuritidis*, and *A. tannerae*, came from 27 pleural empyema with poorly described etiology but potentially of oral origin (Dyrhovden et al., 2019).

Prevotella Involvement in Chronic Diseases of the Respiratory Tract

Chronic diseases of the airways are characterized by a reduced capability of eliminating microbes (Dickson et al., 2016). This may allow a persistent colonization of opportunistic pathogens, such as *Pseudomonas aeruginosa* or *Haemophilus influenzae*, with harmful consequences for respiratory health. During exacerbation, there are acute periods resulting in both local and systemic inflammation and worsened lung function. Due to culture-independent methods and increased research interest in the role of anaerobic bacteria and their function, it has been shown that dysbiotic bacterial compositions are, indeed, involved in inflammation of the respiratory airways (Dickson et al., 2016; Huffnagle et al., 2017). The presence of *Prevotella* in the lower respiratory tract is related to the Th17 activation and differentiation, as defined by Th17-chemoattractant chemokine concentrations and STAT3 expression, respectively (Segal et al., 2016). However, the role of *Prevotella*-mediated Th17 activation in the maintenance of lung health is not fully elucidated yet. A recent mouse-model study demonstrated that the episodic aspiration of oral commensals (*P. melaninogenica*, *V. parvula*, and *S. mitis*) leads to dysbiosis and low-dose inflammation in lower airways, decreasing the susceptibility to the respiratory pathogen *S. pneumoniae* via activation of pulmonary Th17 cells (Wu et al., 2021).

Reduced abundances of the phylum Bacteroidetes and the genus *Prevotella* have been observed in the oropharynx of patients with asthma and chronic obstructive pulmonary disease (COPD) as well as in bronchial washings in COPD patients (Hilty et al., 2010; Park et al., 2014; Einarsson et al., 2016). A recent study examined pediatric asthma-associated alterations in the respiratory microbiota connected to host metabolism and responses, showing that several *Prevotella* species were enriched in the control group as well as *P. pallens* and *Prevotella* oral taxon 306 having an inverse correlation with total and allergen-specific IgE levels (Chiu et al., 2020). In the oropharynx of 13 adult asthma patients, *Prevotella* proved to be the most abundant genus and *P. melaninogenica*, *P. pallens*, and *P. nigrescens*, in descending order, most abundant *Prevotella* species (Lopes Dos Santos Santiago et al., 2017). Although *P. melaninogenica* and *S. mitis/S. pneumoniae* were the most abundant species, the bacterial compositions did not differ from those found in non-asthmatic individuals. As regards COPD, a recent study characterizing a potential association between the microbiota and risk for exacerbation or airflow limitation revealed significantly reduced proportions of *P. histicola*, *Gemella morbillorum*, and *Streptococcus gordonii* in sputum of patients with high risk of COPD exacerbation (Yang et al., 2021). The authors assumed that this kind of alteration in the resident microbiota to a dysbiotic direction could enhance inflammation in respiratory mucosae. In a mouse model, *P. melaninogenica*, *P. nanceiensis*, and *P. salivae* strains were shown to induce COPD-like symptoms via activation of neutrophils and elevating cytokine expression in a TLR-2 dependent manner (Larsen et al., 2014). An interesting finding was that only whole cells but not lipopolysaccharide of *Prevotella* initiated these symptoms, indicating that TLR-4 does not take part in the cellular response against *Prevotella* seen in healthy airways of humans. In a previous study, the authors demonstrated that the same *Prevotella* strains were able to reduce the expression of *Haemophilus*-induced human dendritic cell IL-12p70, but not IL-23 and IL-10 expressions (Larsen et al., 2012). Later, it was demonstrated that *Prevotella* outer membrane proteins (OMPs) are responsible for the Th17 development, activation, and IL-17B and IL-17A expression, which eventually promote pulmonary fibrosis (Yang et al., 2019). Noteworthy is that OMPs of *Prevotella* contain lipopolysaccharides and lipoproteins, which stimulate IL-17 expression via the TLR-Myd88 signaling pathway (Yang et al., 2019). These results indicate that commensal *Prevotella* organisms not only contribute to the aggravation of airway immune response, but also enable the regulation of pathogen-induced immune response.

Also in other chronic diseases of the lower respiratory tract, like bronchiectasis and cystic fibrosis, *Prevotella* is among the predominant findings (Tunney et al., 2013; Renwick et al., 2014; Muhlebach et al., 2018; Einarsson et al., 2019). For example, a multi-center study, including over 200 participants with age ranging from childhood to mid-adulthood and with different genetic and geographic backgrounds, examined whether there is a link between strict anaerobes and the severity of cystic fibrosis (Muhlebach et al., 2018). Across all ages, *Streptococcus* and *Prevotella* had the highest detection rates in sputum samples, 82 and 51%, respectively. Contrasting to the high prevalence of *Prevotella*, its abundance appeared to be low. Interestingly, the presence of anaerobes associated with phenotypically milder disease, whereas *Pseudomonas* (*P. aeruginosa*), the typical pathogen in cystic fibrosis, associated with severe disease (Muhlebach et al., 2018). Recently, Einarsson et al. (2019) assessed microbial community structures within the airways and clarified how various taxa are distributed in communities representing health or chronic disease (here: bronchiectasis and cystic fibrosis). The "core" community was composed of members of the genera *Streptococcus*, *Veillonella*, *Prevotella*, *Granulicatella*, and *Fusobacterium*, while skewed community structures were found in cystic fibrosis and bronchiectasis samples. Notably, anaerobic bacteria, e.g., *Prevotella* and *Veillonella*, proved to affect the variance within the airways, interacting with opportunistic lower airway pathogens (Einarsson et al., 2019).

Some species-level data are available on *Prevotella* in cystic fibrosis. A recent multi-center study (O'Connor et al., 2021), looking for bacterial communities in bronchoalveolar lavage fluid of 63 diseased and 128 control individuals from infancy to young adulthood, demonstrated the *S. mitis* group (52%) and *P. melaninogenica* (44%) as being the most prevalent bacterial taxa. However, distinct abundance patterns were recognized between the study groups; while the abundance of the *S. mitis* group was high regardless of age in controls, *Staphylococcus aureus* dominated in cystic fibrosis. Low abundance of *P. histicola* was found in part of diseased and control individuals across the age spectrum, and interestingly, *P. oris* was detected at high abundance in some diseased individuals (O'Connor et al., 2021). Based on the comparison of bronchoalveolar fluid and oropharyngeal swab samples, overall diversity of the upper and lower airway microbiome is similar in clinically stable children with cystic fibrosis (Renwick et al., 2014). However, bacterial communities in lower airways significantly differed between cystic fibrosis and control children; while *P. veroralis* was absent in cystic fibrosis, it was common in controls. Pulsed-field gel electrophoresis patterns were produced in a study targeting to reveal the degree of clonal similarity of 42 *Prevotella* isolates collected from sputum samples during stable, exacerbated, and post-exacerbation periods (Gilpin et al., 2017). Initial sampling was performed during clinical stability, and the *Prevotella* findings included *P. denticola*, *P. histicola*, *P. melaninogenica*, *P. nigrescens*, and *P. salivae*. Seven isolates could not be definitely identified but remained as *P. veroralis/P. histicola* or *P. melaninogenica/P. histicola*. Genotyping analysis allowed recognizing similar banding patterns (genotypes) during the follow-up. It was suggested that, instead of repeated acquisition, a persistent colonization of *Prevotella* species had occurred in patients with cystic fibrosis (Gilpin et al., 2017). In an experimental study, cystic fibrosis bronchial epithelial cells were exposed to *P. histicola* or *P. nigrescens* (Bertelsen et al., 2021). Both strains were able to induce disrupted NF-κB(p65) and MAPK activations via suppressing TLR-4 and stimulating TLR-2 in epithelial cells. Infection with a *P. nigrescens* strain induced only low levels of p65-mediated inflammation compared to inflammatory response of a *P. aeruginosa* strain from the same patient (Bertelsen et al., 2020). The authors speculated that by TLR-2 signaling, and by reducing TLR-4 release and IL-6 and IL-8 production, *Prevotella* may inhibit the growth of the major pathogen, *P. aeruginosa*, and have a beneficial effect on immune response in the lungs affected by cystic fibrosis.

SUMMARY

Due to increased research interest in commensal bacteria in humans, there is now considerable evidence on the complex nature of commensal bacterial communities in the lower airways as well as gastrointestinal tract above the waistline, including the esophagus, stomach, and upper part of the small intestine. It is obvious that oral members of the genus *Prevotella* play an important role in health and disease at these body sites. In the gastrointestinal tract, the presence of *Prevotella* may influence, positively or negatively, the severity of disease, such as reflux disease, gastritis, IBD, and different cancer types. In the respiratory tract, current research has brought information on the potential involvement of oral bacteria, including some *Prevotella* organisms, in COVID-19 persistence and treatment outcome. As regards *Prevotella* species in chronic respiratory diseases, the current data report on reduced abundance of anaerobes, especially *Prevotella*, which indicates a disruption of homeostatic respiratory microbiota, potentially exposing to lung disease progression. To date, there is only a limited number of mechanistic studies to explain the relation between specific *Prevotella* species involved in diseases in the respiratory and gastrointestinal tracts. The wide intra-genus variation and distinct properties of individual species within the genus *Prevotella* call for further studies on oral *Prevotella* species and their involvement inside and outside the oral cavity to clarify their impact on human health and disease.

AUTHOR CONTRIBUTIONS

EK conceptualized the manuscript and was responsible for the content dealing with microbes. UKG was responsible for immune-inflammatory aspects. Both authors read and approved the final manuscript.

ACKNOWLEDGMENTS

We thank Klaus Könönen for generating the anatomical illustration for this article.

REFERENCES

1. Alauzet, C., Mory, F., Carlier, J. P., Marchandin, H., Jumas-Bilak, E., and Lozniewski, A. (2007). *Prevotella nanceiensis* sp. nov., isolated from human clinical samples. *Int. J. Syst. Evol. Microbiol.* 57, 2216–2220. doi: 10.1099/ijs.0.65173-0
2. Aoki, K., Ishii, Y., and Tateda, K. (2021). Detection of associated bacteria in aspiration pneumonia and lung abscesses using partial 16S rRNA gene amplicon sequencing. *Anaerobe* 69:102325. doi: 10.1016/j.anaerobe.2021.102325
3. Bassis, C. M., Erb-Downward, J. R., Dickson, R. P., Freeman, C. M., Schmidt, T. M., Young, V. B., et al. (2015). Analysis of the upper respiratory tract microbiotas as the source of the lung and gastric microbiotas in healthy individuals. *mBio* 6:e00037. doi: 10.1128/mBio.00037-15
4. Bertelsen, A., Elborn, J. S., and Schock, B. C. (2020). Infection with *Prevotella nigrescens* induces TLR2 signalling and low levels of p65 mediated inflammation in Cystic Fibrosis bronchial epithelial cells. *J. Cyst. Fibros.* 19, 211–218. doi: 10.1016/j.jcf.2019.09.005
5. Bertelsen, A., Elborn, J. S., and Schock, B. C. (2021). Microbial interaction: *Prevotella* spp. reduce *P. aeruginosa* induced inflammation in cystic fibrosis bronchial epithelial cells. *J. Cyst. Fibros.* 20, 682–691. doi: 10.1016/j.jcf.2021. 04.012
6. Bik, E. M., Eckburg, P. B., Gill, S. R., Nelson, K. E., Purdom, E. A., Francois, F., et al. (2006). Molecular analysis of the bacterial microbiota in the human stomach. *Proc. Natl. Acad. Sci. U.S.A.* 103, 732–737. doi: 10.1073/pnas.050665 5103
7. Buhl, M., and Marschal, M. (2020). *Prevotella vespertina* sp. nov., isolated from an abscess of a hospital patient. *Int. J. Syst. Evol. Microbiol.* 70, 4576–4582. doi: 10.1099/ijsem.0.004316
8. Buhl, M., Dunlap, C., and Marschal, M. (2019). *Prevotella brunnea* sp. nov., isolated from a wound of a patient. *Int. J. Syst. Evol. Microbiol.* 69, 3933–3938. doi: 10.1099/ijsem.0.003715
9. Buhl, M., Willmann, M., Liese, J., Autenrieth, I. B., and Marschal, M. (2016). *Prevotella colorans* sp. nov., isolated from a human wound. *Int. J. Syst. Evol. Microbiol.* 66, 3005–3009. doi: 10.1099/ijsem.0.001134
10. Byrd, K. M., and Gulati, A. S. (2021). The "Gum-Gut" axis in inflammatory bowel diseases: a hypothesis-driven review of associations and advances. *Front. Immunol.* 12:620124. doi: 10.3389/fimmu.2021.620124
11. Chiu, C. Y., Chou, H. C., Chang, L. C., Fan, W. L., Dinh, M. C. V., Kuo, Y. L., et al. (2020). Integration of metagenomics-metabolomics reveals specific signatures and functions of airway microbiota in mite-sensitized childhood asthma. *Allergy* 75, 2846–2857.
12. Chung, M., Zhao, N., Meier, R., Koestler, D. C., Wu, G., de Castillo, E., et al. (2021). Comparisons of oral, intestinal, and pancreatic bacterial microbiomes in patients with pancreatic cancer and other gastrointestinal diseases. *J. Oral Microbiol.* 13:1887680. doi: 10.1080/20002297.2021.1887680
13. Coker, O. O., Dai, Z., Nie, Y., Zhao, G., Cao, L., Nakatsu, G., et al. (2018). Mucosal microbiome dysbiosis in gastric carcinogenesis. *Gut* 67, 1024–1032. doi: 10.1136/gutjnl-2017-314281
14. Costello, E. K., Lauber, C. L., Hamady, M., Fierer, N., Gordon, J. I., and Knight, R. (2009). Bacterial community variation in human body habitats across space and time. *Science* 326, 1694–1697. doi: 10.1126/science.1177486
15. Das, S., Bernasconi, E., Koutsokera, A., Wurlod, D. A., Tripathi, V., Bonilla-Rosso, G., et al. (2021). A prevalent and culturable microbiota links ecological balance to clinical stability of the human lung after transplantation. *Nat. Commun.* 12:2126. doi: 10.1038/s41467-021-22344-4
16. Deshpande, N. P., Riordan, S. M., Castaño-Rodríguez, N., Wilkins, M. R., and Kaakoush, N. O. (2018). Signatures within the esophageal microbiome are associated with host genetics, age, and disease. *Microbiome* 6:227. doi: 10.1186/ s40168-018-0611-4
17. Dewhirst, F. E., Chen, T., Izard, J., Paster, B. J., Tanner, A. C., Yu, W. H., et al. (2010). The human oral microbiome. *J. Bacteriol.* 192, 5002–5017. doi: 10.1128/ JB.00542-10

18. Dickson, R. P., Erb-Downward, J. R., Martinez, F. J., and Huffnagle, G. B. (2016). The microbiome and the respiratory tract. *Annu. Rev. Physiol.* 78, 481–504. doi: 10.1146/annurev-physiol-021115-105238
19. Dicksved, J., Lindberg, M., Rosenquist, M., Enroth, H., Jansson, J. K., and Engstrand, L. (2009). Molecular characterization of the stomach microbiota in patients with gastric cancer and in controls. *J. Med. Microbiol.* 58, 509–516. doi: 10.1099/jmm.0.007302-0
20. Downes, J., and Wade, W. G. (2011). *Prevotella fusca* sp. nov. and *Prevotella scopos* sp. nov., isolated from the human oral cavity. *Int. J. Syst. Evol. Microbiol.* 61, 854–858. doi: 10.1099/ijs.0.023861-0
21. Downes, J., Dewhirst, F. E., Tanner, A. C. R., and Wade, W. G. (2013). Description of *Alloprevotella rava* gen. nov., sp. nov., isolated from the human oral cavity, and reclassification of *Prevotella tannerae* Moore et al., 1994 as *Alloprevotella tannerae* gen. nov., comb. nov. *Int. J. Syst. Evol. Microbiol.* 63, 1214–1218. doi: 10.1099/ijs.0.041376-0
22. Downes, J., Hooper, S. J., Wilson, M. J., and Wade, W. G. (2008). *Prevotella histicola* sp. nov., isolated from the human oral cavity. *Int. J. Syst. Evol. Microbiol.* 58, 1788–1791. doi: 10.1099/ijs.0.65656-0
23. Downes, J., Liu, M., Kononen, E., and Wade, W. G. (2009). *Prevotella micans* sp. nov., isolated from the human oral cavity. *Int. J. Syst. Evol. Microbiol.* 59, 771–774. doi: 10.1099/ijs.0.002337-0
24. Downes, J., Sutcliffe, I. C., Booth, V., and Wade, W. G. (2007). *Prevotella maculosa* sp. nov., isolated from the human oral cavity. *Int. J. Syst. Evol. Microbiol.* 57, 2936–2939. doi: 10.1099/ijs.0.65281-0
25. Downes, J., Sutcliffe, I. C., Hofstad, T., and Wade, W. G. (2006). *Prevotella bergensis* sp. nov., isolated from human infections. *Int. J. Syst. Evol. Microbiol.* 56, 609–612. doi: 10.1099/ijs.0.63888-0
26. Downes, J., Sutcliffe, I., Tanner, A. C. R., and Wade, W. G. (2005). *Prevotella marshii* sp. nov. and *Prevotella baroniae* sp. nov., isolated from the human oral cavity. *Int. J. Syst. Evol. Microbiol.* 55, 1551–1555. doi: 10.1099/ijs.0.63634-0
27. Downes, J., Tanner, A. C. R., Dewhirst, F. E., and Wade, W. G. (2010). *Prevotella saccharolytica* sp. nov., isolated from the human oral cavity. *Int. J. Syst. Evol. Microbiol.* 60, 2458–2461. doi: 10.1099/ijs.0.014720-0
28. Dyrhovden, R., Nygaard, R. M., Patel, R., Ulvestad, E., and Kommedal, Ø (2019). The bacterial aetiology of pleural empyema. A descriptive and comparative metagenomic study. *Clin. Microbiol. Infect.* 25, 981–986. doi: 10.1016/j.cmi. 2018.11.030
29. Einarsson, G. G., Comer, D. M., McIlreavey, L., Parkhill, J., Ennis, M., Tunney, M. M., et al. (2016). Community dynamics and the lower airway microbiota in stable chronic obstructive pulmonary disease, smokers and healthy non-smokers. *Thorax* 71, 795–803. doi: 10.1136/thoraxjnl-2015-207235
30. Einarsson, G. G., Zhao, J., LiPuma, J. J., Downey, D. G., Tunney, M. M., and Elborn, J. S. (2019). Community analysis and co-occurrence patterns in airway microbial communities during health and disease. *ERJ Open Res.* 5, 00128–2017. doi: 10.1183/23120541.00128-2017
31. Finegold, S. M., Strong, C. A., McTeague, M., and Marina, M. (1993). The importance of black-pigmented gram-negative anaerobes in human infections. *FEMS Immunol. Med. Microbiol.* 6, 77–82. doi: 10.1111/j.1574-695X.1993. tb00306.x
32. Francavilla, R., Ercolini, D., Piccolo, M., Vannini, L., Siragusa, S., De Filippis, F., et al. (2014). Salivary microbiota and metabolome associated with celiac disease. *Appl. Environ. Microbiol.* 80, 3416–3425. doi: 10.1128/AEM.00362-14
33. Gilpin, D. F., Nixon, K. A., Bull, M., McGrath, S. J., Sherrard, L., Rolain, J. M., et al. (2017). Evidence of persistence of *Prevotella* spp. in the cystic fibrosis lung. *J. Med. Microbiol.* 66, 825–832. doi: 10.1099/jmm.0.000500
34. Glazunova, O. O., Launay, T., Raoult, D., and Roux, V. (2007). *Prevotella timonensis* sp. nov., isolated from a human breast abscess. *Int. J. Syst. Evol. Microbiol.* 57, 883–886. doi: 10.1099/ijs.0.64609-0
35. Han, H. S., Lee, S. Y., Oh, S. Y., Moon, H. W., Cho, H., and Kim, J. H. (2019). Correlations of the gastric and duodenal microbiota with histological, endoscopic, and symptomatic gastritis. *J. Clin. Med.* 8:312. doi: 10.3390/jcm8030312
36. Haran, J. P., Bradley, E., Zeamer, A. L., Cincotta, L., Salive, M. C., Dutta, P., et al. (2021). Inflammation-type dysbiosis of the oral microbiome associates with the duration of COVID-19 symptoms and long-COVID. *JCI Insight* 17:152346. doi: 10.1172/jci.insight.152346
37. Hasegawa, A., Sato, T., Hoshikawa, Y., Ishida, N., Tanda, N., Kawamura, Y., et al. (2014). Detection and identification of oral anaerobes in intraoperative bronchial fluids of patients with pulmonary carcinoma. *Microbiol. Immunol.* 58, 375–381. doi: 10.1111/1348-0421.12157
38. Hedberg, M. E., Israelsson, A., Moore, E. R. B., Svensson-Stadler, L., Wai, S. N., Pietz, G., et al. (2013). *Prevotella jejuni* sp. nov., isolated from the small intestine of a child with coeliac disease. *Int. J. Syst. Evol. Microbiol.* 63, 4218–4223. doi: 10.1099/ijs.0.052647-0
39. Hilty, M., Burke, C., Pedro, H., Cardenas, P., Bush, A., Bossley, C., et al. (2010). Disordered microbial communities in asthmatic airways. *PLoS One* 5:e8578. doi: 10.1371/journal.pone.0008578
40. Huang, J., Roosaar, A., Axéll, T., and Ye, W. (2016). A prospective cohort study on poor oral hygiene and pancreatic cancer risk. *Int. J. Cancer* 138, 340–347. doi: 10.1002/ijc.29710
41. Huffnagle, G. B., Dickson, R. P., and Lukacs, N. W. (2017). The respiratory tract microbiome and lung inflammation: a two-way street. *Mucosal. Immunol.* 10, 299–306. doi: 10.1038/mi.2016.108
42. Humphrey, S. P., and Williamson, R. T. (2001). A review of saliva: normal composition, flow, and function. *J. Prosthet. Dent.* 85, 162–169. doi: 10.1067/mpr.2001.113778
43. Jensen, A., Fagö-Olsen, H., Sørensen, C. H., and Kilian, M. (2013). Molecular mapping to species level of the tonsillar crypt microbiota associated with health and recurrent tonsillitis. *PLoS One* 8:e56418. doi: 10.1371/journal. pone. 0056418
44. Jousimies-Somer, H., Summanen, P., Citron, D. M., Baron, E. J., Wexler, H. M., and Finegold, S. M. (2002). *Wadsworth-KTL Anaerobic Bacteriology Manual*. Belmont, CA: Star Publishing.
45. Kawar, N., Park, S. G., Schwartz, J. L., Callahan, N., Obrez, A., Yang, B., et al. (2021). Salivary microbiome with gastroesophageal reflux disease and treatment. *Sci. Rep.* 11:188. doi: 10.1038/s41598-020-80170-y
46. Keijser, B. J., Zaura, E., Huse, S. M., van der Vossen, J. M., Schuren, F. H., Montijn, R. C., et al. (2008). Pyrosequencing analysis of the oral microflora of healthy adults. *J. Dent. Res.* 87, 1016–1020. doi: 10.1177/154405910808701104
47. Kitamoto, S., Nagao-Kitamoto, H., Hein, R., Schmidt, T. M., and Kamada, N. (2020). The bacterial connection between the oral cavity and the gut diseases. *J. Dent. Res.* 99, 1021–1029. doi: 10.1177/0022034520924633
48. Könönen, E. (2005). Anaerobes in the upper respiratory tract in infancy. *Anaerobe* 11, 131–136. doi: 10.1016/j.anaerobe.2004.11.001
49. Könönen, E., Eerola, E., Frandsen, E. V., Jalava, J., Mättö, J., Salmenlinna, S., et al. (1998). Phylogenetic characterization and proposal of a new pigmented species to the genus *Prevotella*: *Prevotella pallens* sp. nov. *Int. J. Syst. Bacteriol.* 48, 47–51. doi: 10.1099/00207713-48-1-47
50. Könönen, E., Kanervo, A., Takala, A., Asikainen, S., and Jousimies-Somer, H. (1999). Establishment of oral anaerobes during the first year of life. *J. Dent. Res.* 78, 1634–1639. doi: 10.1177/00220345990780100801
51. Larsen, J. M., Musavian, H. S., Butt, T. M., Ingvorsen, C., Thysen, A. H., and Brix, S. (2014). Chronic obstructive pulmonary disease and asthma-associated *Proteobacteria*, but not commensal *Prevotella* spp., promote Toll-like receptor 2-independent lung inflammation and pathology. *Immunology* 144, 333–342. doi: 10.1111/imm.12376
52. Larsen, J. M., Steen-Jensen, D. B., Laursen, J. M., Søndergaard, J. N., Musavian, H. S., Butt, T. M., et al. (2012). Divergent pro-inflammatory profile of human dendritic cells in response to commensal and pathogenic bacteria associated with the airway microbiota. *PLoS One* 7:e31976.
53. Lawson, P. A., Moore, E., and Falsen, E. (2008). *Prevotella amnii* sp. nov., isolated from human amniotic fluid. *Int. J. Syst. Evol. Microbiol.* 58, 89–92. doi: 10.1099/ ijs.0.65118-0
54. Ley, R. E. (2016). Gut microbiota in 2015: *Prevotella* in the gut: choose carefully. *Nat. Rev. Gastroenterol. Hepatol.* 13, 69–70. doi: 10.1038/nrgastro.2016.4
55. Liu, N., Ando, T., Ishiguro, K., Maeda, O., Watanabe, O., Funasaka, K., et al. (2013). Characterization of bacterial biota in the distal esophagus of Japanese patients with reflux esophagitis and Barrett's esophagus. *BMC Infect. Dis.* 13:130. doi: 10.1186/1471-2334-13-130
56. Liu, Y., Lin, Z., Lin, Y., Chen, Y., Peng, X. E., He, F., et al. (2018). *Streptococcus* and *Prevotella* are associated with the prognosis of oesophageal squamous cell carcinoma. *J. Med. Microbiol.* 67, 1058–1068. doi: 10.1099/jmm.0.000754
57. Lopes Dos Santos Santiago, G., Brusselle, G., Dauwe, K., Deschaght, P., Verhofstede, C., Vaneechoutte, D., et al. (2017). Influence of chronic azithromycin treatment on the composition of the oropharyngeal microbial community in patients with severe asthma. *BMC Microbiol.* 17:109. doi: 10. 1186/s12866-017-1022-6
58. Lopetuso, L. R., Severgnini, M., Pecere, S., Ponziani, F. R., Boskoski, I., Larghi, A., et al. (2020). Esophageal microbiome signature in patients with

Barrett's esophagus and esophageal adenocarcinoma. *PLoS One* 15:e0231789. doi: 10. 1371/journal.pone.0231789

59. Mager, D. L., Ximenez-Fyvie, L. A., Haffajee, A. D., and Socransky, S. S. (2003). Distribution of selected bacterial species on intraoral surfaces. *J. Clin. Periodontol.* 30, 644–654. doi: 10.1034/j.1600-051x.2003.00376.x
60. Mentula, S., Harmoinen, J., Heikkilä, M., Westermarck, E., Rautio, M., Huovinen, P., et al. (2005). Comparison between cultured small-intestinal and fecal microbiotas in beagle dogs. *Appl. Environ. Microbiol.* 71, 4169–4175. doi: 10. 1128/AEM.71.8.4169-4175.2005
61. Miller, E. H., Annavajhala, M. K., Chong, A. M., Park, H., Nobel, Y. R., Soroush, A., et al. (2021). Oral microbiome alterations and SARS-CoV-2 saliva viral load in patients with COVID-19. *Microbiol. Spectr.* 13:e0005521. doi: 10.1128/ Spectrum.00055-21
62. Moore, L. V., Johnson, J. L., and Moore, W. E. (1994). Descriptions of *Prevotella tannerae* sp. nov. and *Prevotella enoeca* sp. nov. from the human gingival crevice and emendation of the description of *Prevotella zoogleoformans*. *Int. J. Syst. Bacteriol.* 44, 599–602. doi: 10.1099/00207713-44-4-599
63. Muhlebach, M. S., Hatch, J. E., Einarsson, G. G., McGrath, S. J., Gilipin, D. F., Lavelle, G., et al. (2018). Anaerobic bacteria cultured from cystic fibrosis airways correlate to milder disease: a multisite study. *Eur. Respir. J.* 52:1800242. doi: 10.1183/13993003.00242-2018
64. O'Connor, J. B., Mottlowitz, M. M., Wagner, B. D., Boyne, K. L., Stevens, M. J., Robertson, C. E., et al. (2021). Divergence of bacterial communities in the lower airways of CF patients in early childhood. *PLoS One* 16:e0257838. doi: 10.1371/journal.pone.0257838
65. Park, H., Shin, J. W., Park, S. G., and Kim, W. (2014). Microbial communities in the upper respiratory tract of patients with asthma and chronic obstructive pulmonary disease. *PLoS One* 9:e109710. doi: 10.1371/journal.pone.0109710
66. Pattaroni, C., Watzenboeck, M. L., Schneidegger, S., Kieser, S., Wong, N. C., Bernasconi, E., et al. (2018). Early-life formation of the microbial and immunological environment of the human airways. *Cell Host Microbe* 24, 857–865.e4. doi: 10.1016/j.chom.2018.10.019
67. Pei, Z., Bini, E. J., Yang, L., Zhou, M., Francois, F., and Blaser, M. J. (2004). Bacterial biota in the human distal esophagus. *Proc. Natl. Acad. Sci. U.S.A.* 101, 4250–4255. doi: 10.1073/pnas.0306398101
68. Qi, Y., Zang, S. Q., Wei, J., Yu, H. C., Yang, Z., Wu, H. M., et al. (2021). High-throughput sequencing provides insights into oral microbiota dysbiosis in association with inflammatory bowel disease. *Genomics* 113, 664–676. doi: 10.1016/j.ygeno.2020.09.063
69. Renwick, J., McNally, P., John, B., DeSantis, T., Linnane, B., Murphy, P., et al. (2014). The microbial community of the cystic fibrosis airway is disrupted in early life. *PLoS One* 9:e109798. doi: 10.1371/journal.pone.0109798
70. Said, H. S., Suda, W., Nakagome, S., Chinen, H., Oshima, K., Kim, S., et al. (2014). Dysbiosis of salivary microbiota in inflammatory bowel disease and its association with oral immunological biomarkers. *DNA Res.* 21, 15–25. doi: 10.1093/dnares/dst037
71. Sakamoto, M., Huang, Y., Umeda, M., Ishikawa, I., and Benno, Y. (2005a). *Prevotella multiformis* sp. nov., isolated from human subgingival plaque. *Int. J. Syst. Evol. Microbiol.* 55, 815–819. doi: 10.1099/ijs.0.63451-0
72. Sakamoto, M., Ohkusu, K., Masaki, T., Kako, H., Ezaki, T., and Benno, Y. (2007). *Prevotella pleuritidis* sp. nov., isolated from pleural fluid. *Int. J. Syst. Evol. Microbiol.* 57, 1725–1728. doi: 10.1099/ijs.0.64885-0
73. Sakamoto, M., Suzuki, M., Huang, Y., Umeda, M., Ishikawa, I., and Benno, Y. (2004). *Prevotella shahii* sp. nov. and *Prevotella salivae* sp. nov., isolated from the human oral cavity. *Int. J. Syst. Evol. Microbiol.* 54, 877–883. doi: 10.1099/ ijs. 0.02876-0
74. Sakamoto, M., Suzuki, N., and Okamoto, M. (2010). *Prevotella aurantiaca* sp. nov., isolated from the human oral cavity. *Int. J. Syst. Evol. Microbiol.* 60, 500–503. doi: 10.1099/ijs.0.012831-0
75. Sakamoto, M., Umeda, M., Ishikawa, I., and Benno, Y. (2005b). *Prevotella multisaccharivorax* sp. nov., isolated from human subgingival plaque. *Int. J. Syst. Evol. Microbiol.* 55, 1839–1843. doi: 10.1099/ijs.0.63739-0
76. Scannapieco, F. A. (2021). Poor oral health in the etiology and prevention of aspiration pneumonia. *Dent. Clin. North Am.* 65, 307–321. doi: 10.1016/j. cden. 2020.11.006
77. Schmidt, T. S., Hayward, M. R., Coelho, L. P., Li, S. S., Costea, P. I., Voigt, A. Y., et al. (2019). Extensive transmission of microbes along the gastrointestinal tract. *eLife* 8:e42693. doi: 10.7554/eLife.42693
78. Schulz, C., Schütte, K., Koch, N., Vilchez-Vargas, R., Wos-Oxley, M. L., Oxley, A. P. A., et al. (2018). The active bacterial assemblages of the upper GI tract in individuals with and without *Helicobacter* infection. *Gut* 67, 216–225. doi: 10.1136/gutjnl-2016-312904
79. Segal, L. N., Clemente, J. C., Tsay, J. C., Koralov, S. B., Keller, B. C., Wu, B. G., et al. (2016). Enrichment of the lung microbiome with oral taxa is associated with lung inflammation of a Th17 phenotype. *Nat. Microbiol.* 1:16031. doi: 10.1038/nmicrobiol.2016.31
80. Segata, N., Haake, S. K., Mannon, P., Lemon, K. P., Waldron, L., Gevers, D., et al. (2012). Composition of the adult digestive tract bacterial microbiome based on seven mouth surfaces, tonsils, throat and stool samples. *Genome Biol.* 13:R42. doi: 10.1186/gb-2012-13-6-r42
81. Shah, H. N., and Collins, D. M. (1990). *Prevotella*, a new genus to include *Bacteroides melaninogenicus* and related species formerly classified in the genus *Bacteroides*. *Int. J. Syst. Bacteriol.* 40, 205–208. doi: 10.1099/00207713-40-2-205 Shah, H. N., and Gharbia, S. E. (1992). Biochemical and chemical studies on strains designated *Prevotella intermedia* and proposal of a new pigmented species, *Prevotella nigrescens* sp. nov. *Int. J. Syst. Bacteriol.* 42, 542–546. doi: 10.1099/00207713-42-4-542
82. Shanahan, E. R., Shah, A., Koloski, N., Walker, M. M., Talley, N. J., Morrison, M., et al. (2018). Influence of cigarette smoking on the human duodenal mucosa-associated microbiota. *Microbiome* 6:150. doi: 10.1186/ s40168-018- 0531-3
83. Sulaiman, I., Chung, M., Angel, L., Tsay, J. J., Wu, B. G., Yeung, S. T., et al. (2021). Microbial signatures in the lower airways of mechanically ventilated COVID- 19 patients associated with poor clinical outcome. *Nat. Microbiol.* 6, 1245–1258. doi: 10.1038/s41564-021-00961-5
84. Sung, H., Ferlay, J., Siegel, R. L., Laversanne, M., Soerjomataram, I., Jemal, A., et al. (2021). Global Cancer Statistics 2020: GLOBOCAN estimates of incidence and mortality worldwide for 36 cancers in 185 countries. *CA Cancer J. Clin.* 71, 209–249. doi: 10.3322/caac.21660
85. Tett, A., Pasolli, E., Masetti, G., Ercolini, D., and Segata, N. (2021). *Prevotella* diversity, niches and interactions with the human host. *Nat. Rev. Microbiol.* 19, 585–599. doi: 10.1038/s41579-021-00559-y
86. Tunney, M. M., Einarsson, G. G., Wei, L., Drain, M., Klem, E. R., Cardwell, C., et al. (2013). Lung microbiota and bacterial abundance in patients with bronchiectasis when clinically stable and during exacerbation. *Am. J. Respir. Crit. Care Med.* 187, 1118–1126. doi: 10.1164/rccm.201210-1937OC
87. Vasapolli, R., Schütte, K., Schulz, C., Vital, M., Schomburg, D., Pieper, D. H., et al. (2019). Analysis of transcriptionally active bacteria throughout the gastrointestinal tract of healthy individuals. *Gastroenterology* 157, 1081–1092.e3. doi: 10.1053/j.gastro.2019.05.068
88. Willems, A., and Collins, M. D. (1995). 16S rRNA gene similarities indicate that *Hallella seregens* (Moore and Moore) and *Mitsuokella dentalis* (Haapsalo et al.) are genealogically highly related and are members of the genus *Prevotella*: emended description of the genus *Prevotella* (Shah and Collins) and description of *Prevotella dentalis* comb. nov. *Int. J. Syst. Bacteriol.* 45, 832–836. doi: 10.1099/ 00207713-45-4-832
89. Wu, B. G., Sulaiman, I., Tsay, J. J., Perez, L., Franca, B., Li, Y., et al. (2021). Episodic aspiration with oral commensals induces a MyD88-dependent, pulmonary T-helper cell type 17 response that mitigates susceptibility to *Streptococcus pneumoniae*. *Am. J. Respir. Crit. Care Med.* 203, 1099–1111. doi: 10.1164/rccm. 202005-1596OC
90. Xiong, D., Muema, C., Zhang, X., Pan, X., Xiong, J., Yang, H., et al. (2021). Enriched opportunistic pathogens revealed by metagenomic sequencing hint potential linkages between pharyngeal microbiota and COVID-19. *Virol. Sin.* 12, 1–10. doi: 10.1007/s12250-021-00391-x
91. Xu, X., He, J., Xue, J., Wang, Y., Li, K., Zhang, K., et al. (2015). Oral cavity contains distinct niches with dynamic microbial communities. *Environ. Microbiol.* 17, 699–710. doi: 10.1111/1462-2920.12502
92. Xun, Z., Zhang, Q., Xu, T., Chen, N., and Chen, F. (2018). Dysbiosis and ecotypes of the salivary microbiome associated with inflammatory bowel diseases and the assistance in diagnosis of diseases using oral bacterial profiles. *Front. Microbiol.* 9:1136. doi: 10.3389/fmicb.2018.01136
93. Yamasaki, K., Kawanami, T., Yatera, K., Fukuda, K., Noguchi, S., Nagata, S., et al. (2013). Significance of anaerobes and oral bacteria in community-acquired pneumonia. *PLoS One* 8:e63103. doi: 10.1371/journal.pone.0063103

94. Yang, C. Y., Li, S. W., Chin, C. Y., Hsu, C. W., Lee, C. C., Yeh, Y. M., et al. (2021). Association of exacerbation phenotype with the sputum microbiome in chronic obstructive pulmonary disease patients during the clinically stable state. *J. Transl. Med.* 19:121. doi: 10.1186/s12967-021-02 788-4

95. Yang, D., Chen, X., Wang, J., Lou, Q., Lou, Y., Li, L., et al. (2019). Dysregulated lung commensal bacteria drive interleukin-17b production to promote pulmonary fibrosis through their outer membrane vesicles. *Immunity* 19, 692–706. doi: 10.1016/j.immuni.2019.02.001

5

The Advent of COVID-19; Periodontal Research has Identified Therapeutic Targets for Severe Respiratory Disease: An Example of Parallel Biomedical Research Agendas

Elaine O. C. Cardoso[1,2], *Noah Fine*[1], *Michael Glogauer*[1,2,3], *Francis Johnson*[4], *Michael Goldberg*[1,2], *Lorne M. Golub*[5] *and Howard C. Tenenbaum*[1,2*]

[1] Faculty of Dentistry, University of Toronto, Toronto, ON, Canada, [2] Department of Dentistry, Centre for Advanced Dental Research and Care, Mount Sinai Hospital, University of Toronto, Toronto, ON, Canada, [3] University Health Network (UHN), Toronto, ON, Canada, [4] Department of Pharmacological Sciences, School of Medicine, Stony Brook University, Stony Brook, NY, United States, [5] Department of Oral Biology and Pathology, School of Dental Medicine, Stony Brook University, Stony Brook, NY, United States

***Correspondence:**
Howard C. Tenenbaum
howard.tenenbaum@sinaihealth.ca

The pathophysiology of SARS-CoV-2 infection is characterized by rapid virus replication and aggressive inflammatory responses that can lead to acute respiratory distress syndrome (ARDS) only a few days after the onset of symptoms. It is suspected that a dysfunctional immune response is the main cause of SARS-CoV-2 infection-induced lung destruction and mortality due to massive infiltration of hyperfunctional neutrophils in these organs. Similarly, neutrophils are recruited constantly to the oral cavity to combat microorganisms in the dental biofilm and hyperfunctional neutrophil phenotypes cause destruction of periodontal tissues when periodontitis develops. Both disease models arise because of elevated host defenses against invading organisms, while concurrently causing host damage/disease when the immune cells become hyperfunctional. This represents a clear nexus between periodontal and medical research. As researchers begin to understand the link between oral and systemic diseases and their potential synergistic impact on general health, we argue that translational research from studies in periodontology must be recognized as an important source of information that might lead to different therapeutic options which can be effective for the management of both oral and non-oral diseases. In this article we connect concepts from periodontal research on oral inflammation while exploring host modulation therapy used for periodontitis as a potential strategy for the prevention of ARDS a deadly outcome of COVID-19. We suggest that host modulation therapy, although developed initially for management of periodontitis, and which inhibits proteases, cytokines, and the oxidative stress that underlie ARDS, will provide an effective and safe treatment for COVID-19.

Keywords: COVID-19, SARS-CoV-2, periodontal research, ARDS, PMN hyperactivation

INTRODUCTION

The outbreak of viral pneumonia cases from SARS-CoV-2 was first reported by the Chinese government in December 2019 (1). As with other viral diseases SARS-CoV-2 can cause various respiratory infections, including multifocal interstitial pneumonia which was leading to admission to intensive care and death in infected patients (2). This infection, named Coronavirus disease 2019 (COVID-19) (3), can cause complications including the development of acute respiratory distress syndrome (ARDS); an often fatal disorder (2, 4).

ARDS is caused by many pathogens including influenza and coronavirus. Although its precise pathophysiologic mechanisms are not completely clear, it could be the result of direct damage caused by the viral pathogen and then, more importantly, the triggering of a complex dysregulation of the inflammatory environment (5, 6). Indeed, it has been argued that the host-mediated lung and other tissue damage has more to do with the massive infiltration of polymorphonuclear neutrophils (PMNs) in the lungs rather than purely direct viral effects in relation to morbidity and mortality (4, 6, 7).

Immuno-Inflammatory Pathogenesis of COVID-19

Data from cohorts of critically ill patients with COVID-19-related pneumonia provide evidence of cytokine profiles like those of hyperinflammatory states seen in bacterial and viral pneumonias (4, 8). SARS-CoV-2 invades the host cell by binding of its viral spike glycoprotein to the host's cellular receptor for ACE2. Once in the cell, the virus may "deceive" the immune system through strategies that prevent pattern recognition receptors (PRRs) such as toll-like receptors (TLRs) from recognizing pathogen-associated molecular patterns (PAMPs) and will start replicating freely within the infected cells using their own organelles and other cellular components (9). In addition, SARS- CoV-2 has also evolved strategies that interfere in the production of type I/III IFN which are essential for the development of effective immunity (9). As a result of this state of unchecked replication, SARS-CoV-2 can reach high titres shortly after initial infection that leads to an exponential production of PAMPS, cell damage and release of damage-associated molecular patterns (DAMPS), all of which triggering a hyperactive inflammatory responses (10).

The attachment of SARS-CoV-2 to ACE2 for host cell entry leads to down-regulation of ACE2 and a subsequent increase of angiotensin II (ANGII) (11–16) which dysregulate the renin-angiotensin system (RAS) (17). In elevated levels, ANGII acts as a pro-inflammatory mediator that ultimately activates NFκB, disintegrin, and metalloprotease 17 (ADAM17) (18). This activated pro-inflammatory environment triggers the production of reactive oxygen species (ROS), fibrosis, matrix metalloproteinases (MMPs), production of cytokines such as IL-6 and IL-8 by macrophages and recruitment of PMNs. The virus also activates NFκB (11, 15) that amplifies downstream signaling for cytokine production (14, 15). The release of cytokines activates pathogenic T helper type 1 (Thl) cells rapidly which then secrete additional pro-inflammatory cytokines (11, 12, 19). This is followed by additional infiltration of macrophages and PMNs into alveolar cavities where they begin to contribute to the hyper-inflammatory response (11, 14, 15). ANGII is also known to trigger the coagulation cascade by activating platelets through surface AngII receptors binding and inducing platelet shape change (20) both of which associated with thrombosis (21). In summary, SARS-CoV-2 binding to ACE2 for cell invasion is likely the first step for activation of the cytokine storm which releases uncontrolled levels of cytokines, including IL-1β, 1L-6, IL-8, and IL-10 (22), that prime the host for development of hyperactive inflammatory responses. Manifestation of the cytokine storm is extremely complex but in general in addition to virus-induced infiltration of inflammatory cells to the lungs causing oxidative stress and initial inflammation it relies on even more PMN infiltration into the lung whereby cytokines, MMPs, PMN elastase, ROS, and nitric oxide (NO) are released into the inflamed tissue (22, 23) causing diffuse alveolar damage, pulmonary edema, pulmonary fibrosis, acute lung tissue destruction, multiple organ failure and death. These developments essentially describe ARDS as seen in patients suffering from COVID-19 (11–16).

PMNs are the first and most numerous innate immune cells to reach the infection site and therefore play a central role in the resolution of inflammation through specific mechanisms of virus inactivation including the release of MMPs, cytokines, ROS, peroxidases and PMN extracellular traps (NETs) (24). This is of course protective. But PMNs can also become "hyperactive," and when this happens, PMNs contribution to antiviral defense can cause harmful effects to the host including the development of pneumonia and ARDS (25–27). Paradoxically then, despite the critical roles played by PMN cells insofar as clearance of viral pathogens and other infectious disease is concerned it's recognized that excessively sensitized/activated PMN responses promote a vicious cycle of inflammatory damage to the very tissues to which they were dispatched as a consequence of a PMN-induced cytokine storm (24). Notably, MMP-2 and−9 destroy the extracellular matrix in the lungs by degrading collagen found in the basement membrane comprising their parenchymal architecture (22). The virucidal effects of ROS and the recruitment and activation of even more PMNs through the production of cytokines can perpetuate the hyperinflammatory response thereby leading to lung and other tissue injuries including the development of vasculitides and thrombotic conditions characteristic of ARDS (24, 27). In addition, ROS production further increases vascular and epithelial permeability, allowing for continuous infiltration of PMNs and serosanguinous exudates into the alveolar space (27). Finally, the formation of NETs aided by activated platelets in response to endothelial damage, ROS and IL-1β production and virus replication may increase the risk of thromboembolic events in COVID-19 patients by triggering complement activation and further fuelling the coagulation cascade (9) (**Figure 1**).

A summary of the role of PMNs on the severity of COVID-19 in recent studies is shown in **Table 1**.

To prevent this, we hypothesize that any treatment which could prevent excess PMN infiltration and hyperactivation while also blocking excessive levels of MMP activity, elastase activities

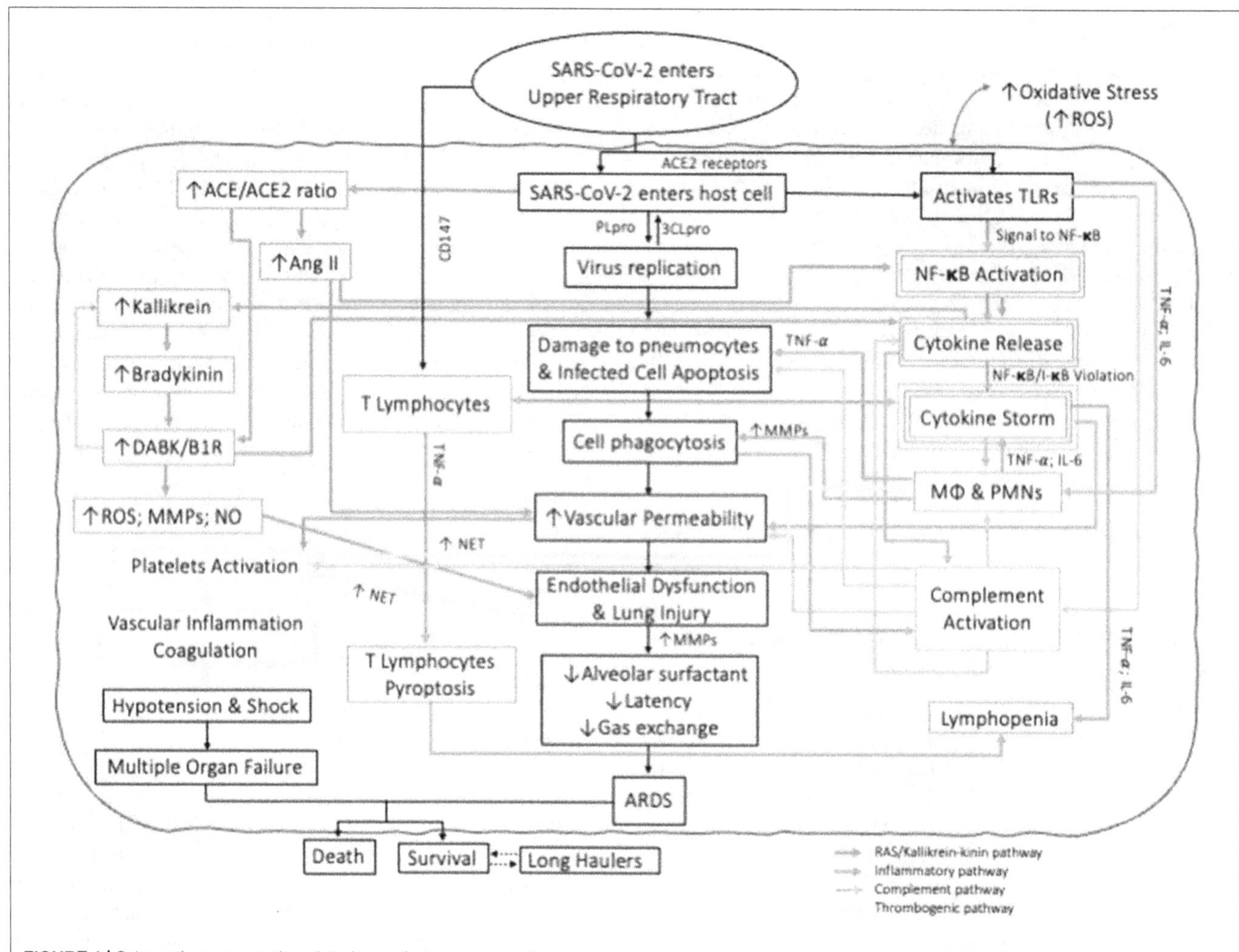

FIGURE 1 | Schematic representation of the interactions amongst and between four independent pathophysiologic pathways involved in the cytokine storm cascade during COVID-19. Note mechanisms for COVID parallel those also described for periodontal diseases.

and simultaneously reducing excessive ROS levels or activity might represent a useful approach to the prevention and/or amelioration of the morbidity and mortality associated with the cytokine storm/ARDS in patients with COVID-19.

Links Between Oral Inflammation and Systemic Disease

As researchers begin to understand the link between oral and systemic diseases more clearly and their potential synergistic impact on general health, we argue that translational research from studies in periodontology must be recognized as an important source of information that might lead to new and different therapeutic options which can be effective for the management of both oral and non-oral diseases.

While evidence of associations between periodontal diseases and systemic conditions have long been noted (36), there has been increased interest in determining the underlying mechanisms that might explain the oral-systemic pathophysiology. We suggest that a causal and indeed bidirectional link may exist between periodontitis and systemic non-communicable diseases. However, we also have to recognize that they could also be manifestations of common underlying pathophysiological mechanisms. This said, these two concepts are not mutually exclusive, and therefore we must emphasize that both putative mechanisms could be involved in those associations, as demonstrated by studies that show bidirectionality of association. For instance, early epidemiological studies have demonstrated the bidirectional adverse interrelationship between an altered host inflammatory response in PD and the metabolic imbalance in diabetes (37) while more recently, a causal association was demonstrated between periodontitis and chronic kidney diseases mediated *via* oxidative stress (38), which seems highly relevant to this argument. We also point out that oxidative stress is a key element of PMN hyperfunctionality related to overproduction of ROS and downregulation of endogenous antioxidants such as NrF2 mediated expression of superoxide dismutase (39). Inflammation is therefore the common factor amongst periodontitis and the chronic diseases of aging, or simply "the disease" (40). Insofar the individual's susceptibility to systemic diseases, our research support the hypothesis that PD sensitizes or primes the peripheral innate immune system, and predominantly the

TABLE 1 | Summary of the role of PMNs on the severity of COVID-19 in recent studies.

As predictors of poor outcomes	Higher PMN counts in non- survivors than in survivors (4)
	Increased NET formation associated with COVID-19–related ARDS (28)
	Increased NET formation as a potential biomarker for disease severity (28)
	PMN-to-lymphocyte ratio as the most promising predictive factor for critical illness incidence of COVID-19 pneumonia (29)
	Markers of PMN activation amongst the most potent discriminators of critical illness (30)
	PMN activation preceding the onset of critical illness and predicting mortality (30)
	Higher levels of specific markers of NETs in patients receiving mechanical ventilation than in those breathing room air (31)
	Neutrophilia observed In the last 24 h preceding death (32)
	NETs infiltrate in lungs of patients with a fatal outcome (32)
	Dramatic increase of PMNs with COVID-19 severity and ARDS (33)
	Increased number of circulating PMNs as an indicator of worse outcomes (2)
Linked to dysregulated immune response	Blood PMNs produce high levels of NETs; NETs are highly detected in the tracheal aspirate and lung tissue (34)
	SARS-CoV-2–activated PMNs induce lung epithelial cell death through the release of NETs (34)
	PMN activation-associated signatures prominently enriched in severe patient groups (35)
	Dysregulated NET formation in lungs (6)

PMNs in such a manner as to allow those cells to trigger and/or exacerbate inflammatory diseases in distant organ systems (41).

Periodontal Disease-Induced Immunopathology and COVID-19

The oral cavity is unique in that the teeth are the only structures in the body that *de facto* protrude through the lining epithelium, in this case the gingival tissues. As such a unique seal exists between the gingiva and tooth surfaces and therefore between the oral cavity and its contents thereby preventing ingress of microbial or other pathogens into the body (42). This biologic seal, specifically a connective tissue and epithelial attachment to cementum, is not perfect and is permeable even in health but moreso in states of inflammation. To enhance protection from pathogens, cells of the innate immune system such as PMNs, are recruited constantly to the oral cavity as part of a healthy and self-limiting inflammatory response against the challenges imposed by the oral microorganisms found in the dental biofilm (43). Interestingly, while bacteria or their by-products may lead to periodontal tissue damage, the host immunoinflammatory response to microorganisms in dental biofilms, when uncontrolled, is considered the main cause of periodontal pathogenesis (40, 44), something akin to destruction of lung tissues observed in ARDS. In parallel to what is seen in ARDS, the initial host immune response starts when PRRs expressed in the membrane of epithelial cells and gingival fibroblasts interact with PAMPs, including lipopolysaccharide (LPS) found in the cell wall of specific periodontal bacteria (45). LPS is considered a potent ligand for TLR4 (46) and activation of both the TLR2 and TLR4 pathways has been described in studies with *Porphyromonas gingivalis* (47). PAMP-TLRs binding and MyD88 signaling results in the activation of the downstream signaling pathways associated with inflammation and upregulation of pro-inflammatory transcription factors, such as NFκB (48), leading to the release of inflammatory cytokines and chemokines (49, 50). The most common cytokines involved in this process are TNF-α, IL- 1β, IL-6, and IL-8 (51, 52), while chemokines include CXCL8/IL-8, CCL2, CCL3, and CCL5 (49, 50) and their release causes vasodilation and chemical gradients that facilitate the migration of leukocytes, mostly PMNs from the vasculature to the site of injury (53). Infiltration of such inflammatory cells leads to release of ROS, MMPs and NETs, as well as to chemotaxis and phagocytosis as defense mechanisms against infection and inflammation (54–58). However, as periodontal diseases are not considered as a classic bacterial infection but rather a dysbiotic disease such mechanisms are necessary but possibly not sufficient to cause disease (59). Periodontal dysbiosis leads to a disturbance of the local homeostasis and immune subversion that increases microbial colonization, virulence, and persistence to disease, and result in persistent recruitment of PMNs (60) with hyperfunctional or hyperactive phenotypes (43, 54–56, 61–63). Similar to what happens in patients with COVID-19, these now hyperactivated PMNs pour out high levels of ROS and degradative enzymes along with ever increasing levels of proinflammatory cytokines (55, 56, 62). These actions lead to severe destruction of the connective tissues about the affected teeth leading to pain, bleeding and ultimately tooth loss (58, 64).

This phenotype of hyperinflammatory PMNs has also been observed to play an important role in the pathogenesis of systemic diseases such as diabetes and cardiovascular disease, suggesting an epidemiological association between periodontal diseases and systemic conditions (65, 66). More importantly, these hyperactivated phenotypes have been observed in severe cases of COVID-19 (67, 68), as well as in aging-related conditions (69). Therefore, the presence of periodontitis in patients who are infected with SARS-CoV-2 could represent an as yet unrecognized comorbidity that could contribute to more severe symptoms of COVID-19. While there are now emerging scientific publications that align with this suggestion (70, 71), it still stands in the grounds of scientific inference. Two plausible mechanisms may explain this association: one being related to the periodontitis-induced inflammatory response; a pre-existing pro-inflammatory state. This could act synergistically and therefore amplify the systemic inflammatory response induced by infection with SARS-CoV-2. Another possibility includes the notion there could be a genetic predisposition of the host to develop hyperinflammatory conditions that are favorable to both the development of PD or COVID-19. Regarding the former, our team's previous research has shown that an increase in the level of hyperactivated PMNs in bone marrow and blood can be caused by periodontal inflammation and that this predisposes to an exacerbated PMN response to distant inflammatory conditions. In other words, PD primes the immune system and thus intensifies the overall innate immune response, thus exacerbating general inflammatory disease (41) including COVID-19.

Similarly, in an experimental study of the respiratory mucosa before, during, and after respiratory syncytial virus (RSV) infection in humans, participants who succumbed to infection had more activated PMNs in their airways before exposure to the virus than those who staved off infection. After viral exposure, a reduction in antiviral response in the neutrophilic mucosal environment was observed, more specifically suppression of interleukin-17 (IL-17), followed by disease onset. The authors hypothesized that primed PMNs, typically associated with immune response to previous bacterial infections might increase the individual's susceptibility to symptomatic viral infections and potentially even COVID-19 (72). A strong hyperactivation phenotype in peripheral PMNs has already been directly associated with severe cases of COVID-19, including increased phagocytosis, degranulation and chemotaxis, and increased expression of genes involved in pro-inflammatory cytokine release. Within these severe cases, the emergence of an immature PMN population, characteristic of emergency myelopoiesis, was the main difference observed between the immune responses in fatal and non-fatal cases of COVID-19 (73). NET formation in tissue injury and thrombotic complications are additional pathogenic mechanisms whereby circulating PMNs can lead to more severe COVID-19 (6, 28, 31, 32, 34). This highlights another potential mechanisms linking PD as a potential comorbidity in COVID-19 cases: the pro-thrombotic state as a result of PD-associated haemodynamic, endothelial, and inflammatory triggers that may lead to an abnormality in the coagulation or fibrinolysis system (74).

From Bench to Chairside With a Bridge to the Bedside—Host Modulation Therapy (HMT)

We suggest that the SARS-CoV-2 pandemic has highlighted the need for a greater understanding of the role of PMNs in combating viral infections, as COVID-19-related PMN-mediated inflammation in the lungs can be life-threatening (6). While supporting the potential role of PD-related innate immune response in systemic inflammatory conditions, our team proposes the use of host modulation therapy (HMT), as designed initially for treatment of PD for treatment of systemic inflammatory diseases that interact with PD (41), as well as in the prevention and treatment of ARDS, given the similarity of the underlying inflammatory mechanisms. Hereunder we describe the tenets of HMT.

HMT has been established in periodontology as a successful therapeutic approach for management of chronic periodontal and refractory periodontal diseases, all of which are PMN-mediated disorders. This therapy, pioneered by our group (notably Dr. Golub's group), was a paradigm shift in periodontal therapy for using tetracycline-based molecules and *not* reliant on their antimicrobial properties, to downregulate the activities of PMN-derived MMPs, suppression of inflammatory cytokines, and for quenching of ROS (75–78). In relation to periodontitis, work has focused on the use of subantimicrobial dose doxycycline (Periostat®), but higher dose use over a short term is certainly feasible when treating extreme cases of inflammation as in the acute stage of COVID-19. This has also led to the development of effective treatment for rosacea using sub-antimicrobial-dose doxycycline slow release form (Oracea®/Aprillon®) (79) More recently, this concept was boosted by Serhan's studies on pro-resolving lipid mediators in which he argues that a failure in resolution of inflammation rather than its hyperactivation leads to chronic inflammation (80, 81). Pre-clinical studies have shown that treatment with lipid mediators after experimentally induced periodontitis in animals was associated with bone loss prevention, regeneration of periodontal tissues and bacterial shifts in the subgingival microbiota (82–84). In humans, differences in pro-resolving lipid mediator profiles were observed between periodontally healthy and periodontitis participants and thus associated with the state of periodontal inflammation (85). These targets are important factors contributing to the breakdown of periodontal tissues, but also to other tissues being attacked by dysregulated inflammation-mediated destruction observed in periodontitis and ARDS (including stimulation of the vasculitides). Along similar lines, our group has shown that the flavonoids, resveratrol, and curcumin, downregulate ROS-mediated oxidative stress, inhibit ROS production/activity, and inhibit pro-inflammatory cytokine formation in animal model studies of periodontitis, which should protect tissues under inflammatory attack (86, 87). In animals subjected to cigarette smoke inhalation, we showed that resveratrol effectively blocks the harmful effects of aryl hydrocarbons found in cigarette smoke and the environment, which could be very important inasmuch as smoking represents a significant comorbidity for COVID-19 and is also a major risk factor for periodontitis and favor healing (88, 89). There is also evidence animal model data showing that by using HMT, the development of ARDS can be blocked (90, 91).

We suggest that the effectiveness of HMT could be independent of the type of infectious virus because it targets the host's cellular mechanisms that propagate ARDS (and of course PD) and not only the virus itself. Therefore, we suggest that mutations of the virus should be equally less material insofar as the putative effectiveness of HMT in prevention and treatment of ARDS. Recent evidence showed that tetracyclines have *in vitro* activity in post-entry stages of the infection with SARS-CoV-2 (92) and resveratrol blocks replication of coronavirus and other respiratory viruses (93, 94). We propose that the use of drug/nutraceutical HMT described initially for periodontitis could reduce morbidity, mortality, and possibly longer-term sequelae of COVID-19.

The concept of HMT emerged for the treatment of periodontitis almost 40 years ago, after the identification of host-response mechanisms as the mediators of the destruction

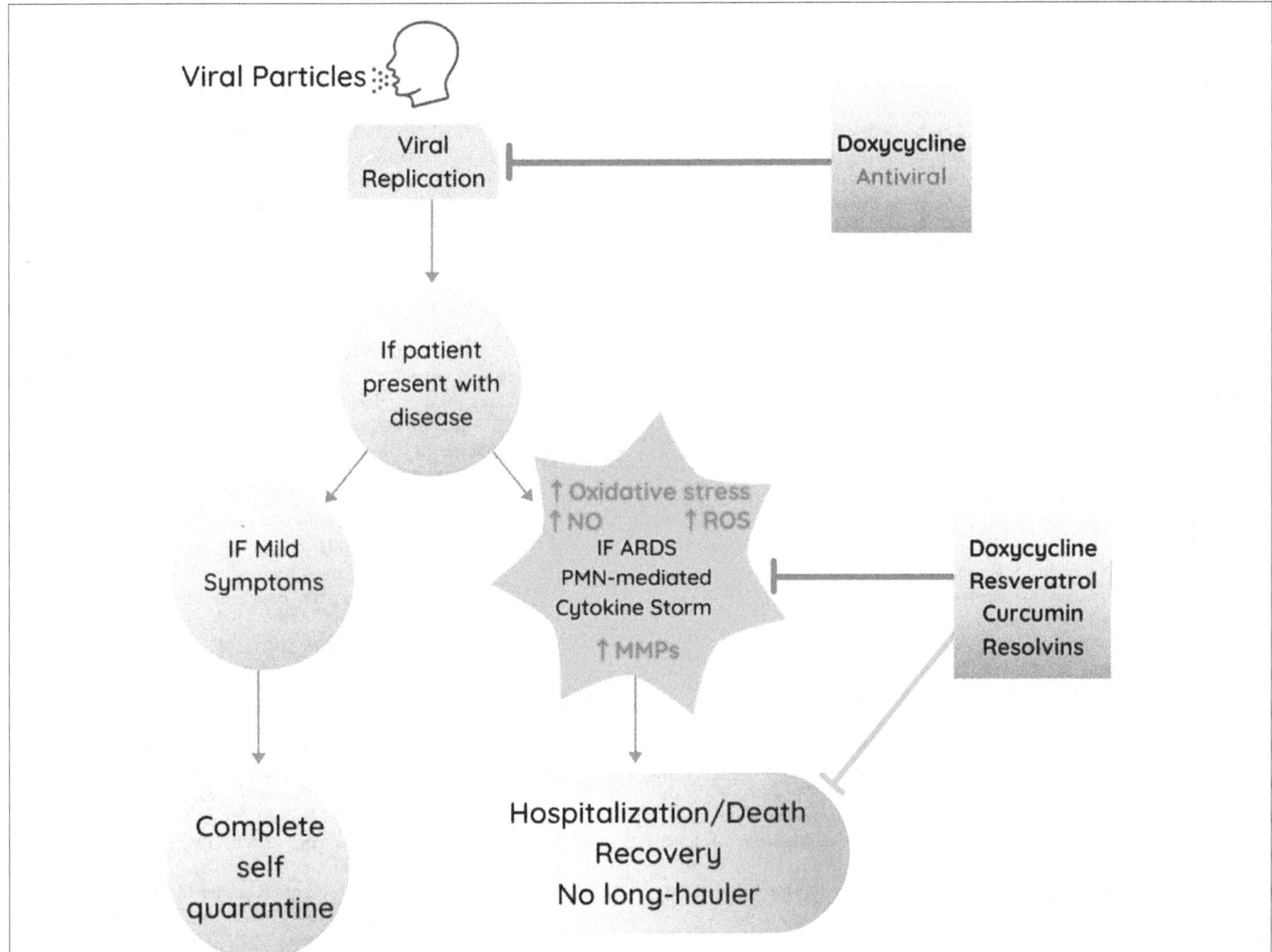

FIGURE 2 | Proposed multidrug treatment approach, developed in part from therapeutic targets identified for management of periodontal diseases for each phase of Covid-19 presenting both inhibitory (in red) and stimulating or improvement-associated effects (in green). Note also that the use of antivirals (other than doxycycline) is depicted in a slightly faded font to delineate that these other therapeutics were not developed from or based on periodontal research investigations.

of the collagen-rich periodontal tissues and subsequent experiments with systemic drugs that inhibited collagen- and bone-destructive enzymes. Around the same time HMT was shown to be effective for downregulation of pathologically elevated levels of inflammation in systemic conditions such as arthritis, cancer, lung and cardiovascular diseases and rosacea (95). Based on this concept, we have presented evidence, described initially in the periodontal research literature, about the protective properties of a new approach to therapy, HMT, that fits precisely the treatment needs of patients with COVID-19/SARS-CoV-2 infection. And, unlike other medications being investigated for the treatment of COVID-19-mediated lung disease there are virtually no concerns about potential toxicity.

The rationale for this proposed treatment approach is based on the use of some or all the compounds identified above to inhibit the cytokine storm/ARDS, including PMN-mediated hyperinflammatory responses and tissue destruction and including the development of thromboembolic disorders. This approach should reduce hospitalization, ICU admissions, and death associated with COVID-19 markedly as suggested in **Figure 2**.

CONCLUSION

We suggest that we've demonstrated how research focused initially on oral inflammatory diseases has illuminated therapeutic targets that can be attacked by relatively simple and safe compounds, thereby reducing hospitalization, morbidity and mortality associated with COVID-19.

AUTHOR CONTRIBUTIONS

HT, LG, MGo, and MGl contributed to conception and design of the study. NF, LG, HT, and MGl, contributed to the experimental analyses and performance. EC and HT wrote the first draft of the manuscript while all others wrote or edited sections of the manuscript. All authors contributed to manuscript revision, read, and approved the submitted version.

REFERENCES

1. Zhu N, Zhang D, Wang W, Li X, Yang B, Song J, et al. A novel coronavirus from patients with pneumonia in China, 2019. *N Engl J Med.* (2020) 382:727–33. doi: 10.1056/NEJMoa2001017
2. Huang C, Wang Y, Li X, Ren L, Zhao J, Hu Y, et al. Clinical features of patients infected with 2019 novel coronavirus in Wuhan, China. *Lancet.* (2020) 395:497–506. doi: 10.1016/S0140-6736(20)30183-5
3. *WHO Director-General's Remarks at the Media Briefing on 2019-nCoV on 11 February 2020.* World Health Organization. Available online at: https://www.who.int/director-general/speeches/detail/who-director-general-s-remarks-at-the-media-briefing-on-2019-ncov-on-11-february-2020
4. Wang D, Hu B, Hu C, Zhu F, Liu X, Zhang J, et al. Clinical characteristics of 138 hospitalized patients with 2019 novel coronavirus-infected pneumonia in Wuhan, China. *JAMA.* (2020) 323:1061–9. doi: 10.1001/jama.2020.1585
5. Wang QW, Su Y, Sheng JT, Gu LM, Zhao Y, Chen XX, et al. Anti-influenza A virus activity of rhein through regulating oxidative stress, TLR4, Akt, MAPK, and NF-κB signal pathways. *PLoS ONE.* (2018) 13:e0191793. doi: 10.1371/journal.pone.0191793
6. Barnes BJ, Adrover JM, Baxter-Stoltzfus A, Borczuk A, Cools-Lartigue J, Crawford JM, et al. Targeting potential drivers of COVID-19: neutrophil extracellular traps. *J Exp Med.* (2020) 217:e20200652. doi: 10.1084/jem.20200652
7. Teijaro JR, Walsh KB, Rice S, Rosen H, Oldstone MB. Mapping the innate signaling cascade essential for cytokine storm during influenza virus infection. *Proc Natl Acad Sci USA.* (2014) 111:3799–804. doi: 10.1073/pnas.1400593111
8. Qin C, Zhou L, Hu Z, Zhang S, Yang S, Tao Y, et al. Dysregulation of Immune Response in Patients With Coronavirus 2019 (COVID-19) in Wuhan, China. *Clin Infect Dis.* (2020) 71:762–8. doi: 10.1093/cid/ciaa248
9. Amor S, Fernández Blanco L, Baker D. Innate immunity during SARS-CoV-2: evasion strategies and activation trigger hypoxia and vascular damage. *Clin Exp Immunol.* (2020) 202:193–209. doi: 10.1111/cei.13523
10. Domingo P, Mur I, Pomar V, Corominas H, Casademont J, de Benito N. The four horsemen of a viral apocalypse: the pathogenesis of SARS-CoV-2 infection (COVID-19). *EBioMedicine.* (2020) 58:102887. doi: 10.1016/j.ebiom.2020.102887
11. Hu B, Huang S, Yin L. The cytokine storm and COVID-19. *J Med Virol.* (2020) 93:250–6. doi: 10.1002/jmv.26232
12. Ragab D, Salah Eldin H, Taeimah M, Khattab R, Salem R. The COVID-19 cytokine storm; what we know so far. *Front Immunol.* (2020) 11:1446. doi: 10.3389/fimmu.2020.01446
13. Sun X, Wang T, Cai D, Hu Z, Chen J, Liao H, et al. Cytokine storm intervention in the early stages of COVID-19 pneumonia. *Cytokine Growth Factor Rev.* (2020) 53:38–42. doi: 10.1016/j.cytogfr.2020.04.002
14. Hussman JP. Cellular and molecular pathways of Covid-19 and potential points of therapeutic intervention. *Front Pharmacol.* (2020) 11:1169. doi: 10.3389/fphar.2020.01169
15. Mahmudpour M, Roozbeh J, Keshavarz M, Farrokhi S, Nabipour I. COVID-19 cytokine storm: the anger of inflammation. *Cytokine.* (2020) 133:155151. doi: 10.1016/j.cyto.2020.155151
16. Soy M, Keser G, Atagündüz P, Tabak F, Atagündüz I, Kayhan S. Cytokine storm in COVID-19: pathogenesis and overview of anti-inflammatory agents used in treatment. *Clin Rheumatol.* (2020) 39:2085–94. doi: 10.1007/s10067-020-05190-5
17. Ingraham NE, Barakat AG, Reilkoff R, Bezdicek T, Schacker T, Chipman JG, et al. Understanding the renin-angiotensin-aldosterone-SARS-CoV axis: a comprehensive review. *Eur Respir J.* (2020) 56:2000912. doi: 10.1183/13993003.00912-2020
18. Devaux CA, Rolain JM, Raoult D. ACE2 receptor polymorphism: susceptibility to SARS-CoV-2, hypertension, multi-organ failure, and COVID-19 disease outcome. *J Microbiol Immunol Infect.* (2020) 53:425–35. doi: 10.1016/j.jmii.2020.04.015
19. Ye Q, Wang B, Mao J. The pathogenesis and treatment of the 'Cytokine Storm' in COVID-19. *J Infect.* (2020) 80:607–13. doi: 10.1016/j.jinf.2020.03.037
20. Jagroop IA, Mikhailidis DP. Angiotensin II can induce and potentiate shape change in human platelets: effect of losartan. *J Hum Hypertens.* (2000) 14:581–5. doi: 10.1038/sj.jhh.1001102
21. Nachman RL, Rafii S. Platelets, petechiae, and preservation of the vascular wall. *N Engl J Med.* (2008) 359:1261–70. doi: 10.1056/NEJMra0800887
22. Roy SK, Kendrick D, Sadowitz BD, Gatto L, Snyder K, Satalin JM, et al. Jack of all trades: pleiotropy and the application of chemically modified tetracycline-3 in sepsis and the acute respiratory distress syndrome (ARDS). *Pharmacol Res.* (2011) 64:580–9. doi: 10.1016/j.phrs.2011.06.012
23. Zhou X, Wang D, Ballard-Croft CK, Simon SR, Lee HM, Zwischenberger JB. A tetracycline analog improves acute respiratory distress syndrome survival in an ovine model. *Ann Thorac Surg.* (2010) 90:419–26. doi: 10.1016/j.athoracsur.2010.04.052
24. Galani IE, Andreakos E. Neutrophils in viral infections: current concepts and caveats. *J Leukoc Biol.* (2015) 98:557–64. doi: 10.1189/jlb.4VMR1114-555R
25. Abraham E. Neutrophils and acute lung injury. *Crit Care Med.* (2003) 31(4 Suppl.):S195–9. doi: 10.1097/01.CCM.0000057843.47705.E8
26. Sideras P, Apostolou E, Stavropoulos A, Sountoulidis A, Gavriil A, Apostolidou A, et al. Activin, neutrophils, and inflammation: just coincidence? *Semin Immunopathol.* (2013) 35:481–99. doi: 10.1007/s00281-013-0365-9
27. Potey PM, Rossi AG, Lucas CD, Dorward DA. Neutrophils in the initiation and resolution of acute pulmonary inflammation: understanding biological function and therapeutic potential. *J Pathol.* (2019) 247:672–85. doi: 10.1002/path.5221
28. Middleton EA, He XY, Denorme F, Campbell RA, Ng D, Salvatore SP, et al. Neutrophil extracellular traps contribute to immunothrombosis in COVID-19 acute respiratory distress syndrome. *Blood.* (2020) 136:1169–79. doi: 10.1182/blood.2020007008
29. Liu J, Liu Y, Xiang P, Pu L, Xiong H, Li C, et al. Neutrophil-to-lymphocyte ratio predicts critical illness patients with 2019 coronavirus disease in the early stage. *J Transl Med.* (2020) 18:206. doi: 10.1186/s12967-020-02374-0
30. Meizlish ML, Pine AB, Bishai JD, Goshua G, Nadelmann ER, Simonov M, et al. A neutrophil activation signature predicts critical illness and mortality in COVID-19. *Blood Adv.* (2021) 5:1164–77. doi: 10.1182/bloodadvances.2020003568
31. Zuo Y, Yalavarthi S, Shi H, Gockman K, Zuo M, Madison JA, et al. Neutrophil extracellular traps in COVID-19. *JCI Insight.* (2020) 5:e138999. doi: 10.1172/jci.insight.138999
32. Radermecker C, Detrembleur N, Guiot J, Cavalier E, Henket M, d'Emal C, et al. Neutrophil extracellular traps infiltrate the lung airway, interstitial, and vascular compartments in severe COVID-19. *J Exp Med.* (2020) 217:e20201012. doi: 10.1084/jem.20201012
33. Gong J, Dong H, Xia QS, Huang ZY, Wang DK, Zhao Y, et al. Correlation analysis between disease severity and inflammation-related parameters in patients with COVID-19: a retrospective study. *BMC Infect Dis.* (2020) 20:963. doi: 10.1186/s12879-020-05681-5
34. Veras FP, Pontelli MC, Silva CM, Toller-Kawahisa JE, de Lima M, Nascimento DC, et al. SARS-CoV-2-triggered neutrophil extracellular traps mediate COVID-19 pathology. *J Exp Med.* (2020) 217:e20201129. doi: 10.1084/jem.20201129
35. Aschenbrenner AC, Mouktaroudi M, Krämer B, Oestreich M, Antonakos N, Nuesch-Germano M, et al. Disease severity-specific neutrophil signatures in blood transcriptomes stratify COVID-19 patients. *Genome Med.* (2021) 13:7. doi: 10.1186/s13073-020-00823-5
36. U.S. Department of Health and Human Services. *Oral Health in America: A Report of the Surgeon General.* Services USDoHaH, editor. Rockville, MD: National Institute of Dental and Craniofacial Research; National Institutes of Health (2000).
37. Taylor GW. Bidirectional interrelationships between diabetes and periodontal diseases: an epidemiologic perspective. *Ann Periodontol.* (2001) 6:99–112. doi: 10.1902/annals.2001.6.1.99
38. Sharma P, Fenton A, Dias IHK, Heaton B, Brown CLR, Sidhu A, et al. Oxidative stress links periodontal inflammation and renal function. *J Clin Periodontol.* (2021) 48:357–67. doi: 10.1111/jcpe.13414
39. Chiu AV, Saigh MA, McCulloch CA, Glogauer M. The role of NrF2 in the regulation of periodontal health and disease. *J Dent Res.* (2017) 96:975–83. doi: 10.1177/0022034517715007
40. Van Dyke TE. Inflammation and periodontal diseases: a reappraisal. *J Periodontol.* (2008) 79(8 Suppl):1501–2. doi: 10.1902/jop.2008.080279

41. Fine N, Chadwick JW, Sun C, Parbhakar KK, Khoury N, Barbour A, et al. Periodontal inflammation primes the systemic innate immune response. *J Dent Res.* (2020) 100:318–25. doi: 10.1177/0022034520963710
42. Nanci A. *Ten Cate's Oral Histology - E-Book: Development, Structure, and Function.* Philadelphia, PA: Elsevier (2017).
43. Fine N, Hassanpour S, Borenstein A, Sima C, Oveisi M, Scholey J, et al. Distinct oral neutrophil subsets define health and periodontal disease states. *J Dent Res.* (2016) 95:931–8. doi: 10.1177/0022034516645564
44. Van Dyke TE. The management of inflammation in periodontal disease. *J Periodontol.* (2008) 79(8 Suppl):1601–8. doi: 10.1902/jop.2008.080173
45. Hanada T, Yoshimura A. Regulation of cytokine signaling and inflammation. *Cytokine Growth Factor Rev.* (2002) 13:413–21. doi: 10.1016/S1359-6101(02)00026-6
46. Zeng XZ, Zhang YY, Yang Q, Wang S, Zou BH, Tan YH, et al. Artesunate attenuates LPS-induced osteoclastogenesis by suppressing TLR4/TRAF6 and PLCγ1-Ca. *Acta Pharmacol Sin.* (2020) 41:229–36. doi: 10.1038/s41401-019-0289-6
47. Hajishengallis G, Sojar H, Genco RJ, DeNardin E. Intracellular signaling and cytokine induction upon interactions of *Porphyromonas gingivalis* fimbriae with pattern-recognition receptors. *Immunol Invest.* (2004) 33:157–72. doi: 10.1081/IMM-120030917
48. Song B, Zhang YL, Chen LJ, Zhou T, Huang WK, Zhou X, et al. The role of Toll-like receptors in periodontitis. *Oral Dis.* (2017) 23:168–80. doi: 10.1111/odi.12468
49. Cavalla F, Araujo-Pires AC, Biguetti CC, Garlet GP. Cytokine networks regulating inflammation and immune defense in the oral cavity. *Curr Oral Health Rep.* (2014) 1:104–13. doi: 10.1007/s40496-014-0016-9
50. Souto GR, Queiroz CM, Costa FO, Mesquita RA. Relationship between chemokines and dendritic cells in human chronic periodontitis. *J Periodontol.* (2014) 85:1416–23. doi: 10.1902/jop.2014.130662
51. Garlet GP. Destructive and protective roles of cytokines in periodontitis: a re-appraisal from host defense and tissue destruction viewpoints. *J Dent Res.* (2010) 89:1349–63. doi: 10.1177/0022034510376402
52. Han X, Lin X, Seliger AR, Eastcott J, Kawai T, Taubman MA. Expression of receptor activator of nuclear factor-kappaB ligand by B cells in response to oral bacteria. *Oral Microbiol Immunol.* (2009) 24:190–6. doi: 10.1111/j.1399-302X.2008.00494.x
53. Kolaczkowska E, Kubes P. Neutrophil recruitment and function in health and inflammation. *Nat Rev Immunol.* (2013) 13:159–75. doi: 10.1038/nri3399
54. Fredriksson M, Gustafsson A, Asman B, Bergström K. Periodontitis increases chemiluminescence of the peripheral neutrophils independently of priming by the preparation method. *Oral Dis.* (1999) 5:229–33. doi: 10.1111/j.1601-0825.1999.tb00306.x
55. Matthews JB, Wright HJ, Roberts A, Cooper PR, Chapple IL. Hyperactivity and reactivity of peripheral blood neutrophils in chronic periodontitis. *Clin Exp Immunol.* (2007) 147:255–64. doi: 10.1111/j.1365-2249.2006.03276.x
56. Matthews JB, Wright HJ, Roberts A, Ling-Mountford N, Cooper PR, Chapple IL. Neutrophil hyper-responsiveness in periodontitis. *J Dent Res.* (2007) 86:718–22. doi: 10.1177/154405910708600806
57. Gustafsson A, Asman B. Increased release of free oxygen radicals from peripheral neutrophils in adult periodontitis after Fc delta-receptor stimulation. *J Clin Periodontol.* (1996) 23:38–44. doi: 10.1111/j.1600-051X.1996.tb00502.x
58. Chapple IL, Matthews JB. The role of reactive oxygen and antioxidant species in periodontal tissue destruction. *Periodontol 2000.* (2007) 43:160–232. doi: 10.1111/j.1600-0757.2006.00178.x
59. Hajishengallis G, Lamont RJ. Beyond the red complex and into more complexity: the polymicrobial synergy and dysbiosis (PSD) model of periodontal disease etiology. *Mol Oral Microbiol.* (2012) 27:409–19. doi: 10.1111/j.2041-1014.2012.00663.x
60. Lamont RJ, Hajishengallis G. Polymicrobial synergy and dysbiosis in inflammatory disease. *Trends Mol Med.* (2015) 21:172–83. doi: 10.1016/j.molmed.2014.11.004
61. Fredriksson M, Gustafsson A, Asman B, Bergström K. Hyper-reactive peripheral neutrophils in adult periodontitis: generation of chemiluminescence and intracellular hydrogen peroxide after *in vitro* priming and FcgammaR-stimulation. *J Clin Periodontol.* (1998) 25:394–8. doi: 10.1111/j.1600-051X.1998.tb02461.x
62. Ling MR, Chapple IL, Matthews JB. Peripheral blood neutrophil cytokine hyper-reactivity in chronic periodontitis. *Innate Immun.* (2015) 21:714–25. doi: 10.1177/1753425915589387
63. Wright HJ, Matthews JB, Chapple IL, Ling-Mountford N, Cooper PR. Periodontitis associates with a type 1 IFN signature in peripheral blood neutrophils. *J Immunol.* (2008) 181:5775–84. doi: 10.4049/jimmunol.181.8.5775
64. Figueredo CM, Fischer RG, Gustafsson A. Aberrant neutrophil reactions in periodontitis. *J Periodontol.* (2005) 76:951–5. doi: 10.1902/jop.2005.76.6.951
65. Hatanaka E, Monteagudo PT, Marrocos MS, Campa A. Neutrophils and monocytes as potentially important sources of proinflammatory cytokines in diabetes. *Clin Exp Immunol.* (2006) 146:443–7. doi: 10.1111/j.1365-2249.2006.03229.x
66. Yasunari K, Watanabe T, Nakamura M. Reactive oxygen species formation by polymorphonuclear cells and mononuclear cells as a risk factor of cardiovascular diseases. *Curr Pharm Biotechnol.* (2006) 7:73–80. doi: 10.2174/138920106776597612
67. Reyes L, Sanchez-Garcia MA, Morrison T, Howden AJM, Watts ER, Arienti S, et al. A type I IFN, prothrombotic hyperinflammatory neutrophil signature is distinct for COVID-19 ARDS. *Wellcome Open Res.* (2021) 6:38. doi: 10.12688/wellcomeopenres.16584.1
68. Morrissey S, Geller A, Hu X, Tieri D, Cooke E, Ding C, et al. Emergence of low-density inflammatory neutrophils correlates with hypercoagulable state and disease severity in COVID-19 patients. *medRxiv*, (2020). doi: 10.1101/2020.05.22.20106724
69. Tseng CW, Liu GY. Expanding roles of neutrophils in aging hosts. *Curr Opin Immunol.* (2014) 29:43–8. doi: 10.1016/j.coi.2014.03.009
70. Aquino-Martinez R, Hernández-Vigueras S. Severe COVID-19 lung infection in older people and periodontitis. *J Clin Med.* (2021) 10:279. doi: 10.3390/jcm10020279
71. Marouf N, Cai W, Said KN, Daas H, Diab H, Chinta VR, et al. Association between periodontitis and severity of COVID-19 infection: a case-control study. *J Clin Periodontol.* (2021) 48:483–91. doi: 10.1111/jcpe.13435
72. Habibi MS, Thwaites RS, Chang M, Jozwik A, Paras A, Kirsebom F, et al. Neutrophilic inflammation in the respiratory mucosa predisposes to RSV infection. *Science.* (2020) 370:eaba9301. doi: 10.1126/science.aba9301
73. Wilk AJ, Lee MJ, Wei B, Parks B, Pi R, Martínez-Colón GJ, et al. Multi-omic profiling reveals widespread dysregulation of innate immunity and hematopoiesis in COVID-19. *bioRxiv.* (2020). doi: 10.1101/2020.12.18.423363
74. Bizzarro S, van der Velden U, ten Heggeler JM, Leivadaros E, Hoek FJ, Gerdes VE, et al. Periodontitis is characterized by elevated PAI-1 activity. *J Clin Periodontol.* (2007) 34:574–80. doi: 10.1111/j.1600-051X.2007.01095.x
75. Golub LM, McNamara TF, D'Angelo G, Greenwald RA, Ramamurthy NS. A non-antibacterial chemically-modified tetracycline inhibits mammalian collagenase activity. *J Dent Res.* (1987) 66:1310–4. doi: 10.1177/00220345870660080401
76. Golub LM, Ramamurthy NS, McNamara TF, Greenwald RA, Rifkin BR. Tetracyclines inhibit connective tissue breakdown: new therapeutic implications for an old family of drugs. *Crit Rev Oral Biol Med.* (1991) 2:297–321. doi: 10.1177/10454411910020030201
77. Golub LM, Suomalainen K, Sorsa T. Host modulation with tetracyclines and their chemically modified analogues. *Curr Opin Dent.* (1992) 2:80–90.
78. Golub LM, Wolff M, Roberts S, Lee HM, Leung M, Payonk GS. Treating periodontal diseases by blocking tissue-destructive enzymes. *J Am Dent Assoc.* (1994) 125:163–9; discussion: 9–71. doi: 10.14219/jada.archive.1994.0261
79. Monk E, Shalita A, Siegel DM. Clinical applications of non-antimicrobial tetracyclines in dermatology. *Pharmacol Res.* (2011) 63:130–45. doi: 10.1016/j.phrs.2010.10.007
80. Serhan CN, Chiang N, Van Dyke TE. Resolving inflammation: dual anti-inflammatory and pro-resolution lipid mediators. *Nat Rev Immunol.* (2008) 8:349–61. doi: 10.1038/nri2294
81. Serhan CN. Controlling the resolution of acute inflammation: a new genus of dual anti-inflammatory and proresolving mediators. *J Periodontol.* (2008) 79(8 Suppl):1520–6. doi: 10.1902/jop.2008.080231
82. Lee CT, Teles R, Kantarci A, Chen T, McCafferty J, Starr JR, et al. Resolvin E1 reverses experimental periodontitis and dysbiosis. *J Immunol.* (2016) 197:2796–806. doi: 10.4049/jimmunol.1600859

83. Van Dyke TE, Hasturk H, Kantarci A, Freire MO, Nguyen D, Dalli J, et al. Proresolving nanomedicines activate bone regeneration in periodontitis. *J Dent Res.* (2015) 94:148–56. doi: 10.1177/0022034514557331
84. Hasturk H, Kantarci A, Goguet-Surmenian E, Blackwood A, Andry C, Serhan CN, et al. Resolvin E1 regulates inflammation at the cellular and tissue level and restores tissue homeostasis *in vivo. J Immunol.* (2007) 179:7021–9. doi: 10.4049/jimmunol.179.10.7021
85. Ferguson B, Bokka NR, Maddipati KR, Ayilavarapu S, Weltman R, Zhu L, et al. Distinct profiles of specialized pro-resolving lipid mediators and corresponding receptor gene expression in periodontal inflammation. *Front Immunol.* (2020) 11:1307. doi: 10.3389/fimmu.2020.01307
86. Corrêa MG, Pires PR, Ribeiro FV, Pimentel SZ, Casarin RC, Cirano FR, et al. Systemic treatment with resveratrol and/or curcumin reduces the progression of experimental periodontitis in rats. *J Periodontal Res.* (2017) 52:201–9. doi: 10.1111/jre.12382
87. Ikeda E, Ikeda Y, Wang Y, Fine N, Sheikh Z, Viniegra A, et al. Resveratrol derivative-rich melinjo seed extract induces healing in a murine model of established periodontitis. *J Periodontol.* (2018) 89:586–95. doi: 10.1002/JPER.17-0352
88. Ribeiro FV, Pino DS, Franck FC, Benatti BB, Tenenbaum H, Davies JE, et al. Resveratrol inhibits periodontitis-related bone loss in rats subjected to cigarette smoke inhalation. *J Periodontol.* (2017) 88:788–98. doi: 10.1902/jop.2017.170025
89. Corrêa MG, Absy S, Tenenbaum H, Ribeiro FV, Cirano FR, Casati MZ, et al. Resveratrol attenuates oxidative stress during experimental periodontitis in rats exposed to cigarette smoke inhalation. *J Periodontal Res.* (2019) 54:225–32. doi: 10.1111/jre.12622
90. Steinberg J, Halter J, Schiller H, Gatto L, Carney D, Lee HM, et al. Chemically modified tetracycline prevents the development of septic shock and acute respiratory distress syndrome in a clinically applicable porcine model. *Shock.* (2005) 24:348–56. doi: 10.1097/01.shk.0000180619.06317.2c
91. Steinberg J, Halter J, Schiller HJ, Dasilva M, Landas S, Gatto LA, et al. Metalloproteinase inhibition reduces lung injury and improves survival after cecal ligation and puncture in rats. *J Surg Res.* (2003) 111:185–95. doi: 10.1016/S0022-4804(03)00089-1
92. Gendrot M, Andreani J, Jardot P, Hutter S, Delandre O, Boxberger M, et al. *In vitro* antiviral activity of doxycycline against SARS-CoV-2. *Molecules.* (2020) 25:5064. doi: 10.3390/molecules25215064
93. Campagna M, Rivas C. Antiviral activity of resveratrol. *Biochem Soc Trans.* (2010) 38(Pt 1):50–3. doi: 10.1042/BST0380050
94. Lin SC, Ho CT, Chuo WH, Li S, Wang TT, Lin CC. Effective inhibition of MERS-CoV infection by resveratrol. *BMC Infect Dis.* (2017) 17:144. doi: 10.1186/s12879-017-2253-8
95. Golub LM, Lee HM. Periodontal therapeutics: current host-modulation agents and future directions. *Periodontol 2000.* (2020) 82:186–204. doi: 10.1111/prd.12315

6

Characterization of Supragingival Plaque and Oral Swab Microbiomes in Children with Severe Early Childhood Caries

Vivianne Cruz de Jesus[1,2], *Mohd Wasif Khan*[2,3], *Betty-Anne Mittermuller*[1,2,4], *Kangmin Duan*[1,2], *Pingzhao Hu*[2,3,5]*, *Robert J. Schroth*[1,2,4,6]* *and Prashen Chelikani*[1,2]*

[1] *Manitoba Chemosensory Biology Research Group, Department of Oral Biology, University of Manitoba, Winnipeg, MB, Canada,* [2] *Children's Hospital Research Institute of Manitoba (CHRIM), Winnipeg, MB, Canada,* [3] *Department of Biochemistry and Medical Genetics, University of Manitoba, Winnipeg, MB, Canada,* [4] *Department of Preventive Dental Science, University of Manitoba, Winnipeg, MB, Canada,* [5] *Department of Computer Science, University of Manitoba, Winnipeg, MB, Canada,* [6] *Department of Pediatrics and Child Health, University of Manitoba, Winnipeg, MB, Canada*

***Correspondence:**
Pingzhao Hu
pingzhao.hu@umanitoba.ca
Robert J. Schroth
robert.schroth@umanitoba.ca
Prashen Chelikani
prashen.chelikani@umanitoba.ca

The human oral cavity harbors one of the most diverse microbial communities with different oral microenvironments allowing the colonization of unique microbial species. This study aimed to determine which of two commonly used sampling sites (dental plaque vs. oral swab) would provide a better prediction model for caries-free vs. severe early childhood caries (S-ECC) using next generation sequencing and machine learning (ML). In this cross-sectional study, a total of 80 children (40 S-ECC and 40 caries-free) < 72 months of age were recruited. Supragingival plaque and oral swab samples were used for the amplicon sequencing of the V4-16S rRNA and ITS1 rRNA genes. The results showed significant differences in alpha and beta diversity between dental plaque and oral swab bacterial and fungal microbiomes. Differential abundance analyses showed that, among others, the cariogenic species *Streptococcus mutans* was enriched in the dental plaque, compared to oral swabs, of children with S-ECC. The fungal species *Candida dubliniensis* and *C. tropicalis* were more abundant in the oral swab samples of children with S-ECC compared to caries-free controls. They were also among the top 20 most important features for the classification of S-ECC vs. caries-free in oral swabs and for the classification of dental plaque vs. oral swab in the S-ECC group. ML approaches revealed the possibility of classifying samples according to both caries status and sampling sites. The tested site of sample collection did not change the predictability of the disease. However, the species considered to be important for the classification of disease in each sampling site were slightly different. Being able to determine the origin of the samples could be very useful during the design of oral microbiome studies. This study provides important insights into the differences between the dental plaque and oral swab bacteriome and mycobiome of children with S-ECC and those caries-free.

Keywords: dental plaque, oral swab, bacteria, fungi, microbiota, machine learning, case-control, artificial intelligence

INTRODUCTION

The oral cavity harbors one of the most diverse microbial communities within the human body (Stearns et al., 2011). A variety of oral niches (non-shedding tooth surfaces, tongue, cheek, hard and soft palates, and gingival sulcus) provide different levels of oxygen, nutrients, salivary flow, and masticatory forces (Hall et al., 2017). Each of these different microenvironments allow the colonization of unique and adapted microbial communities. Therefore, it is expected that the microbial composition of each oral site differs significantly from each other.

Usually, the oral microbiota exists in a homeostatic balance with the host and contributes to the development of the immune system. However, once this balance is disturbed, some microbial species can overgrow and diseases associated with site-specific microbes such as periodontitis (subgingival microbiota), dental caries (supragingival microbiota), and oral candidiasis (oral mucosal and salivary microbiota) may occur (Lamont et al., 2018; Vila et al., 2020). Therefore, it is important to select the most appropriate site of sampling for the study and/or diagnosis of each oral infectious diseases. Recent studies have shown that the SARS-CoV-2 virus, which causes the coronavirus disease 19 (COVID-19), can be detected in saliva (Fernandes et al., 2020). It has been reported that salivary glands can be important reservoir of the virus (Xu et al., 2020b). Consequently, the presence of high SARS-CoV-2 viral load in saliva could make it a suitable diagnostic tool for COVID-19. Therefore, this also validates the importance of exploring different sampling options for diagnosis of infectious diseases (Fernandes et al., 2020; Sapkota et al., 2020; Xu et al., 2020a).

Since the nineteenth century, it is known that the oral microbes play a crucial role in the development of dental caries (Russell, 2009). However, the establishment of new technologies, such as next generation sequencing (NGS) and machine learning algorithms, has provided a unique opportunity to an enhanced understanding of the role of oral microbes (bacteria, fungi, and viruses) on caries development and progression.

As dental caries continues to be one of the most prevalent chronic diseases among children worldwide, there is a clear need for a deeper understanding of how oral microbial communities and their interactions could impact children's oral health. The terms early childhood caries (ECC) and severe ECC (S-ECC) were first introduced in the 1990s (Ismail and Sohn, 1999). ECC is described as any caries experience in the primary dentition of children younger than 6 years of age. S-ECC is the severe form of ECC and has an important effect on children's development and well-being (Pierce et al., 2019; Folayan et al., 2020).

We hypothesized that the microbial (bacterial and fungal) profile of dental plaque significantly differs from that of oral swabs, and because the dental biofilm is in closer contact with the tooth surface, it would provide a better prediction model for caries onset. To test this hypothesis, first we characterized the differences between the dental plaque and oral swab bacterial and fungal microbiota in children with S-ECC and those caries-free. Second, we analyzed which of those commonly used sampling sites (dental plaque and oral swab) would provide a better model for the classification of S-ECC vs. caries-free, using machine learning approaches. Third, we further evaluated whether the observed differences between the microbial profiles of the samples could be used for the differentiation between the sampling sites (dental plaque vs. oral swab) to assist researchers during the design of oral microbiome studies. This is one of the first studies to explore the oral microbiome profiles to classify oral sites.

Abbreviations: ASVs, Amplicon Sequence Variants; FDR, False Discovery Rate; HOMD, Human Oral Microbiome database; ITS1, Internal Transcribed Spacer 1; PCoA, Principal Coordinates Analysis; PERMANOVA, Permutational Multivariate Analysis of Variance using distance matrices; S-ECC, Severe Early Childhood Caries.

MATERIALS AND METHODS

Study Population

In this cross-sectional study, eighty children < 72 months of age were recruited between December 2017 and August 2018. Among those, 40 had S-ECC, according to the American Academy of Pediatric Dentistry definition (AAPD, 2020), and 40 were caries-free. Children with S-ECC were recruited at the Misericordia Health Centre (MHC), Winnipeg-MB, Canada, on the day of their full-mouth rehabilitative dental surgery under general anesthesia. Caries-free children were recruited from the community. Caries-free children had a dmft (cumulative score of the number of decayed, missing, or filled primary teeth) index equal to zero and had no incipient lesions. To confirm the caries-free status, a dental examination was performed by R.J.S. at the Children's Hospital Research Institute of Manitoba by means of visual/tactile examination using artificial light and no radiographs. Inclusion criteria: children less than 72 months of age who were caries-free (dmft = 0) or have been diagnosed with S-ECC (based on the American Academy of Pediatric Dentistry definition). Exclusion criteria: children older than 72 months of age, use of antibiotics, and children who did not satisfy the case definition of S-ECC.

Based on the power analysis published by La Rosa et al. (2012) at 5% significance level, with 40 samples per group and the average number of reads of 50,000 per sample our study would achieve a power > 97%. This study protocol was approved by the University of Manitoba's Health Research Ethics Board (HREB # HS20961–H2017:250) and by the MHC, Winnipeg, MB, Canada. Written informed consent was provided by the parents or legal caregivers (de Jesus et al., 2020). This work follows the STROBE guidelines checklist for cross-sectional studies (**Supplementary Table**).

Sample Collection

Due to the young age of the participants and their inability to spit saliva, oral swab samples were collected with a sterile polyester-tipped applicator (Fisher Scientific) by swabbing the buccal mucosa and anterior floor of the mouth under the tongue. The oral swabs were stored in RNAprotect Reagent (Qiagen, Cat. # 74324, Hilden, Germany) at −80°C until further analysis. Supragingival plaque samples were collected from all available tooth surfaces with a sterile interdental brush (Agnello et al., 2017; de Jesus et al., 2020). They were dislodged into the RNAprotect Reagent (Qiagen, Cat. # 76506, Hilden, Germany) and stored at −80°C until further analysis. For simplicity, supragingival plaque samples are referred to as dental plaque.

DNA Extraction and 16S and ITS1 rRNA Amplicon Sequencing

Total DNA was extracted from 160 samples (80 oral swabs and 80 dental plaque samples) using QIAamp DNA mini kit (Qiagen, Hilden, Germany) following manufacturer's protocol. An additional enzymatic digestion step with lysozyme treatment (20 μg/ml lysozyme in a buffer containing 20 mM Tris HCl, pH 8; 1.2% Triton X 100; 2 mM EDTA) was performed before DNA extraction from dental plaque samples.

The total DNA was sent on dry ice to McGill University-Génome Québec Innovation Center (Montreal, Canada) for paired-end Illumina MiSeq PE250 sequencing. The primers 515F, (5′-GTGCCAGCMGCCGCG GTAA-3′) and 806R (5′-GGACTACHVGGGTWTCTAAT-3′), targeting the V4 hypervariable region of the bacterial 16S rRNA gene and the primers ITS1-30 (5′-GTCCCTGCCCTTTGTACACA-3′) and ITS1-217 (5′-TTTCGCTGCGTTCTTCATCG-3′), targeting the Internal Transcribed Spacer 1 (ITS1) of the fungal rRNA gene were used for amplification (Usyk et al., 2017; de Jesus et al., 2020).

Bioinformatics and Statistical Analysis

The sequences were received as demultiplexed, barcode removed, paired ends fastq files. The quality control analysis was performed with FastqC v0.11.8 (Andrews, 2010). The sequences were then imported and analyzed with QIIME2 2018.11 (Bolyen et al., 2019). The 16S pair-end sequences were quality trimmed, filtered to remove ambiguous and chimeric sequences, and merged using DADA2 implemented in QIIME2, resulting in the amplicon sequence variant (ASV) table (Callahan et al., 2016). The ITS1 pair-end sequences were trimmed using the Q2-ITSxpress QIIME2 plugin prior to the DADA2 step, with default parameters (Rivers et al., 2018). The taxonomic assignment of ASVs was performed using the Human Oral Microbiome Database (HOMD, version 15.1) for bacteria and the UNITE database (version 8.2; QIIME developer release) for fungi at 99% sequence similarity (Dewhirst et al., 2010; Agnello et al., 2017; Abarenkov et al., 2020b; de Jesus et al., 2020). Due to the presence of many fungal ASVs that were assigned only at kingdom level, further fungal ASV curation was performed with the R package LULU (Frøslev et al., 2017). The remaining ASVs assigned as *Fungi* at kingdom level only, or with unidentified phylum were manually assessed using the program BLASTN in NCBI (Zhang et al., 2000). The ASVs with non-fungal BLASTN results were discarded and the remaining were repeatedly assigned to new taxonomic assignments using different UNITE databases threshold levels (Abarenkov et al., 2020a,b,c) and taxonomy classification methods (q2-feature-classifier classify-sklearn and classify-consensus-blast) in QIIME2, as described previously (Martinsen et al., 2021). The data was imported into R using the R package "qiime2R" (version 0.99.13) and additional filtering was performed using "phyloseq" (version 1.30.0) to remove singletons and samples with less than 1,000 reads (McMurdie and Holmes, 2013; Bisanz, 2018; Depner et al., 2020). The ASV counts were then normalized using the cumulative-sum scaling (CSS) approach from the R package "metagenomeSeq" version 1.28.2 (Paulson et al., 2013).

The alpha diversity analyses (within-samples) were performed using the Chao1 and Shannon indices to estimate richness and diversity, respectively, using raw ASV count data from QIIME2 in "phyloseq". Pairwise comparisons of alpha diversity were done by the paired Wilcoxon signed rank test. Beta diversity measures were calculated on CSS normalized ASV data. This analysis was performed to compare the structure of the bacterial and fungal microbial communities between samples, using the permutational analysis of variance (PERMANOVA) test with 999 permutations in the R package "vegan" (adonis function; version 2.5.6) (Anderson, 2001). It was visualized using principle coordinate analysis (PCoA) with Bray-Curtis dissimilarity index in the R package "ggplot2" (version 3.3.3) (Beals, 1984; Wickham, 2016).

Differentially abundant species were identified using the DESeq2 negative binomial Wald test, controlling the false discovery rate (FDR) for multiple comparison, within "phyloseq" (Love et al., 2014). For this, the raw ASV counts were collapsed to the species level. For comparisons between dental plaque vs. oral swab, a paired DESeq2 analysis was performed. FDR adjusted $P < 0.05$ was considered significant.

Machine Learning Analysis

Machine learning methods were used to train multivariable classification models to identify the caries status, S-ECC and caries-free. To generate the machine learning models, taxonomic features were used in the form of ASV tables collapsed to species-level. For the classification, we used the workflow provided in "Siamcat," which provides a machine learning toolbox for metagenome analysis through state-of-the-art machine learning methods (Wirbel et al., 2019, 2021). The data were separately processed for fungi and bacteria and sample-wise relative abundance for the microbiome quantitative profiles was used as input data to maintain the uniformity.

To process the data in "Siamcat," features with a prevalence of less than five percent across samples were removed and the

TABLE 1 | Characteristics of study participants*.

	Caries status	
	S-ECC (*N* = 40)	**Caries-free (*N* = 40)**
Age (months), mean ± SD	45.6 ± 11.4	46.2 ± 14.2
Sex, n(%)		
Female	25 (62.5)	21 (52.5)
Male	15 (37.5)	19 (47.5)

**Other demographics of the study participants have been previously published (de Jesus et al., 2020).*

remaining features were normalized by centered log-ratio (CLR) transformation. The data was then prepared for cross-validation with eightfold and 5 repeats. After this, the models were trained using Lasso, Ridge, Elastic Net (Enet), and RandomForest classification methods in Siamcat, which uses the "mlr" package for machine learning based classification (Bischl et al., 2016). The models' performance for cross validation was evaluated using the area under the receiver operating characteristic (AUROC) value. To show the importance of the model features, the model feature weights were converted to relative weights and up to the top 20 features were selected, based on their median values, to generate a heatmap using the R package "ggplot2" (Wickham, 2016).

For the machine-learning based classification of plaque and swab samples, a pairwise sample analysis was performed using a boosting conditional logistic regression from R package "clogitboost," which takes the paired nature of the dental plaque and oral swab samples into account (Shi and Yin, 2015). The model was fitted using component-wise smoothing spline. The caries-free and S-ECC samples were divided into training and test sets using three-quarters of the data for training and the remaining for test in a way that paired samples for plaque and swab should be together in either training or test sets. For the features (species) selection in training dataset, we obtained the p-values from the differential abundance analysis described above. The top features selected by the p-values were used to train the classification models. Since we have only 30 independent samples in the training set, we considered only top 5, 10, 15, 20, and 25 features to build the model, respectively. The models' performance was evaluated using AUROC. Each of the trained models were then tested on the test set. The

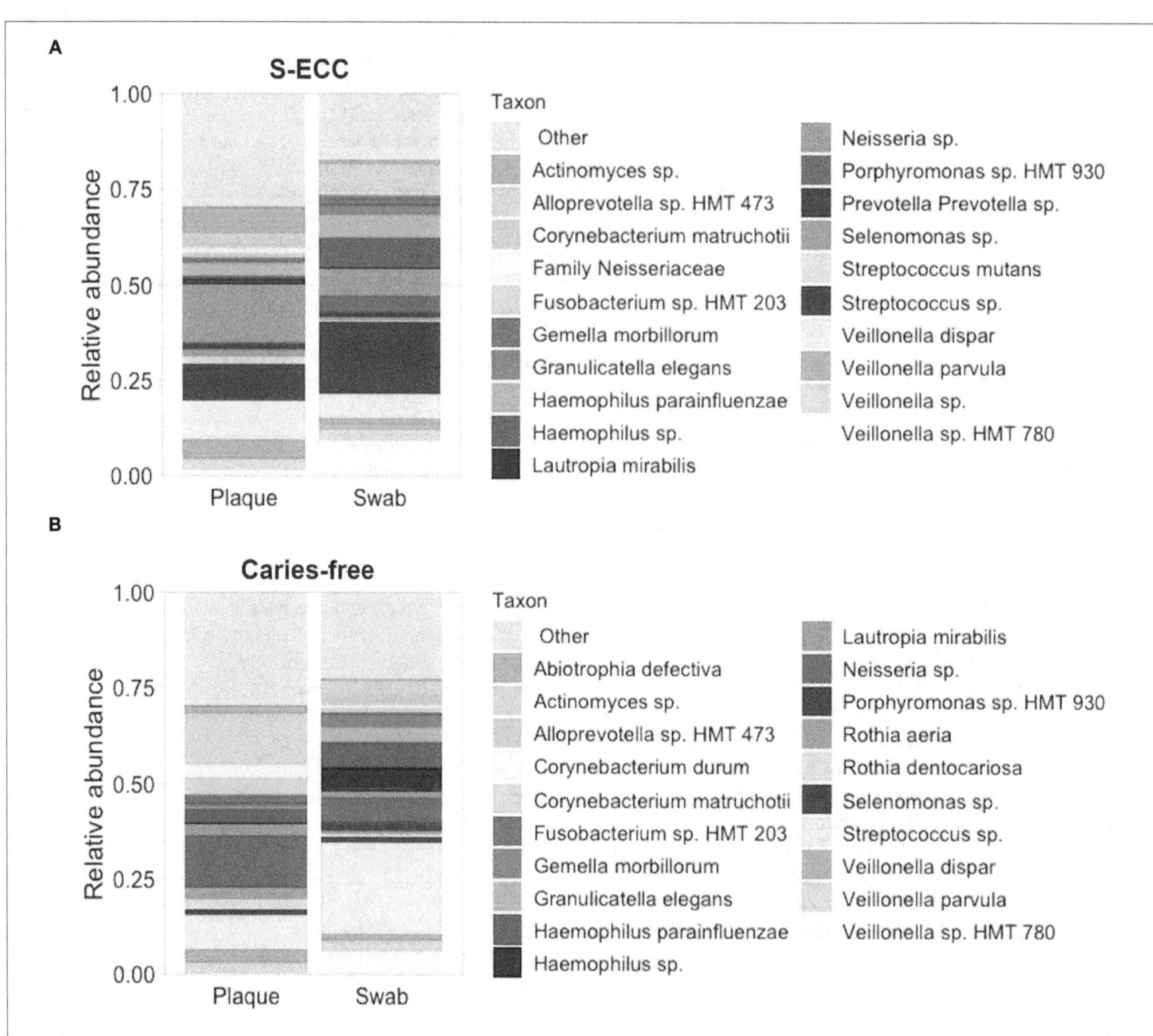

FIGURE 1 | Bacterial taxonomic profiles of dental plaque and oral swab. Relative abundance of the top 20 bacterial taxa in dental plaque and oral swab samples from **(A)** children with S-ECC and **(B)** caries-free children. "Other" indicates the taxa not individually shown. S-ECC, severe early childhood caries.

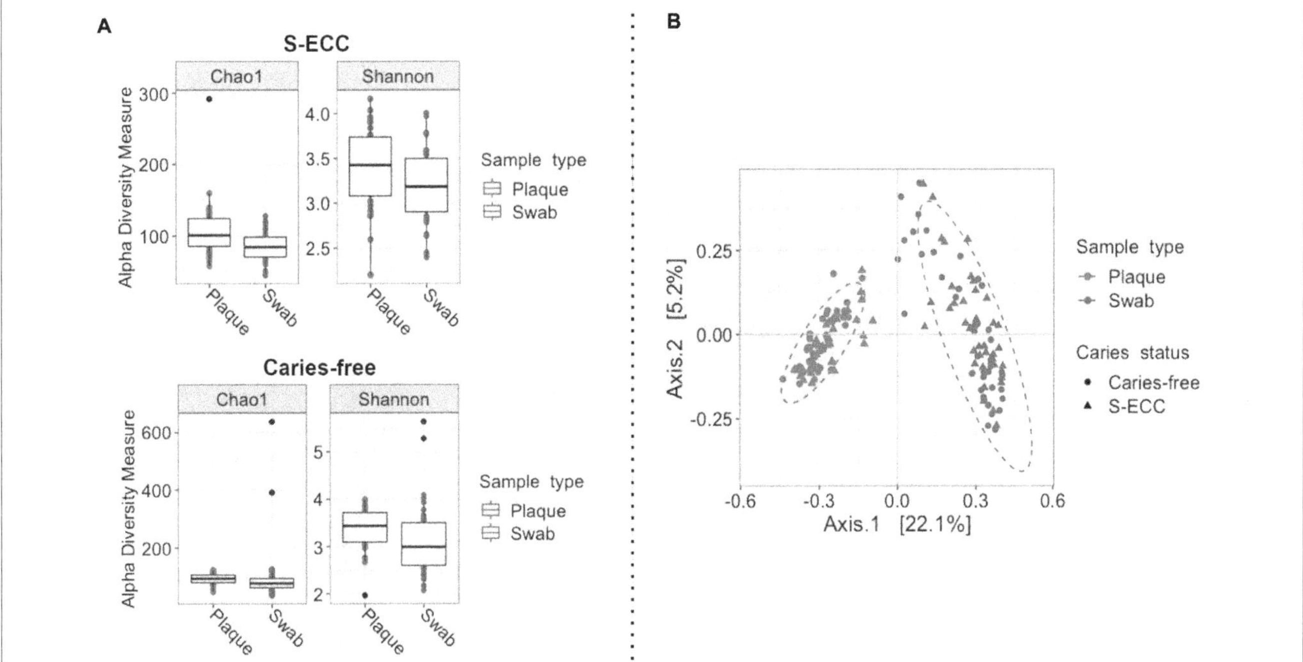

FIGURE 2 | Bacterial diversity of dental plaque and oral swab samples from children with S-ECC and those caries-free. **(A)** For alpha diversity (within-sample) the Shannon and Chao1 diversity and richness measures were calculated according to sample type in both caries-free and S-ECC groups. A significant difference between oral swab and dental plaque alpha diversity and richness was observed in both caries-free and S-ECC groups ($P < 0.05$, paired Wilcoxon test). **(B)** For beta (between-sample) diversity, Bray-Curtis distances were calculated, followed by principal coordinates analysis (PCoA). The plot shows the separation of samples according to sample type (pseudo-F = 40.4, $R^2 = 0.2$, $P = 0.001$, PERMANOVA accounting for the children's caries-status). The ellipses represent a 95% confidence level. S-ECC, severe early childhood caries.

training-test strategy/process was repeated for 30 iterations and the classification performance between caries-free and S-ECC samples were compared by the average of AUROC values from the 30 repeats.

RESULTS

Eighty children who fit the study criteria were recruited and 160 samples (80 dental plaque and 80 oral swabs) were collected. The **Table 1** shows some characteristics of the study participants. Additional information about the participants have been recently published (de Jesus et al., 2020).

Bacterial Community Analysis

After filtering out low quality and chimeric sequences, a total of 8,664,777 16S rRNA reads were obtained, with an average number of 54,154.9 reads per sample (160 samples). A total of 5,421 ASVs were assigned to 141 genera and 320 species. Overall, the most abundant phyla were *Firmicutes* (41.08%) and *Proteobacteria* (27.37%). In oral swabs, *Streptococcus* (overall: 21.81%; S-ECC: 19.22%; Caries-free: 24.41%) was the most abundant genus followed by *Veillonella* (overall: 17.03%; S-ECC: 21.65%; Caries-free: 12.40%) and *Haemophilus* (overall: 13.28%; S-ECC: 13.62%; Caries-free: 12.94%). In dental plaque, *Neisseria* (overall: 16.06%, S-ECC: 15.93%; Caries-free: 16.13%), *Veillonella* (overall: 13.66%; S-ECC: 19.54%; Caries-free: 7.73%), and *Streptococcus* (overall: 11.35%; S-ECC: 12.77%; Caries-free: 9.92%) were the most abundant genera. The taxonomic profile of the dental plaque and oral swab samples are shown in **Figures 1A,B**.

Bacterial alpha diversity (within samples) analysis showed a significant difference between oral swab and dental plaque alpha diversity (Shannon index, S-ECC: $P = 0.0034$; Caries-free: $P = 0.015$) and richness (Chao1 index, S-ECC: $P < 0.001$; Caries-free: $P = 0.025$) in both caries-free and S-ECC groups (**Figure 2A**). Bacterial beta (between-sample) diversity analysis showed a clear separation of samples according to sampling site, oral swab and dental plaque (pseudo-F = 42.71, $R^2 = 0.2$, $P = 0.001$, PERMANOVA accounting for the children's S-ECC status and the paired samples; **Figure 2B**). A significant difference in bacterial community was also observed between the S-ECC and caries-free groups (pseudo-F = 2.85, $R^2 = 0.014$, $P = 0.001$).

Figure 3A shows the relative abundance of the top 20 bacterial species across the subgroups. The differential abundance analysis revealed numerous species that were overabundant in dental plaque or oral swab samples within the S-ECC and caries-free groups (**Figures 3B,C**, adjusted $P < 0.05$, DESeq2). Interestingly, many species were significantly more abundant in dental plaque or oral swab in both S-ECC and caries-free groups. For instance, *Capnocytophaga* sp. oral taxon 326 (S-ECC: −10.83 log2fold change; Caries-free: −4.72 log2fold), *Kingella* sp. oral taxon 012 (S-ECC: −9.52 log2fold change; Caries-free:

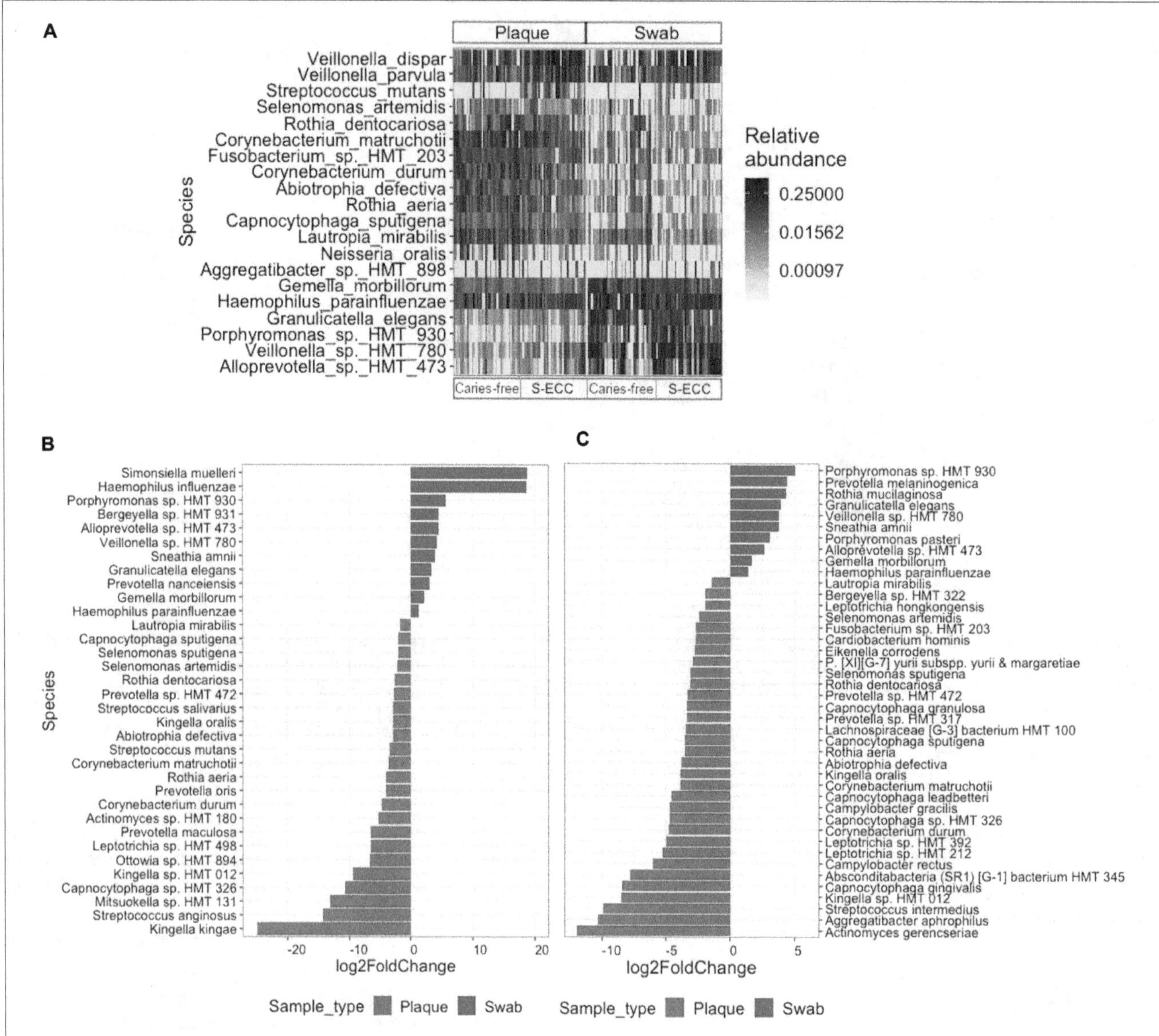

FIGURE 3 | Differential abundance of bacterial species. **(A)** Heatmap showing the relative abundance of the top 20 bacterial species identified in all dental plaque and oral swab samples. **(B,C)** Relative fold change in the abundance of bacterial species in **(B)** samples from children with S-ECC, and **(C)** samples from caries-free children, according to sample type. The differential abundance of the bacterial species was tested using the DESeq2 negative binomial Wald test. **(B,C)** All species listed have an FDR adjusted $P < 0.05$. S-ECC, severe early childhood caries.

−8.57 log2fold change), *Corynebacterium durum* (S-ECC: −4.71 log2fold change; Caries-free: −4.81 log2fold change), *Rothia aeria* (S-ECC: −3.93 log2fold change; Caries-free: −3.56 log2fold change), *Corynebacterium matruchotii (*S-ECC: −3.54 log2fold change; Caries-free: −3.90 log2fold), among others, were more abundant in dental plaque than oral swabs in both caries-free children and those with S-ECC. On the other hand, *Porphyromonas* sp. oral taxon 930 (S-ECC: 5.57 log2fold change; Caries-free: 5.01 log2fold change), *Alloprevotella* sp. oral taxon 473 (S-ECC: 4.35 log2fold change; Caries-free: 2.66 log2fold change*)*, *Veillonella* sp. oral taxon 780 (S-ECC: 4.12 log2fold change; Caries-free: 3.79 log2fold change), *Sneathia amnii (*S-ECC: 3.86 log2fold change; Caries-free: 3.76 log2fold change*)* *Granulicatella elegans* (S-ECC: 3.26 log2fold change; Caries-free: 3.93 log 2fold change), and *Haemophilus parainfluenzae* (S-ECC: 1.26 log2fold change; Caries-free: 1.39 log2fold change) were more abundant in oral swabs in both caries-free and S-ECC groups. In children with S-ECC, the well-known cariogenic bacterium *Streptococcus mutans* was more abundant in dental plaque samples (−3.45 log2fold change, adjusted $P < 0.05$).

Within the oral swab samples, three species were more abundant in S-ECC compared to caries-free: *Veillonella dispar* (2.09 log2fold change), *Prevotella veroralis* (23.33 log2fold change), and *Neisseria bacilliformis* (24.58 log2fold change, adjusted $P < 0.05$, DESeq2). While *Lautropia mirabilis* (−1.41 log2fold change) was significantly more abundant in caries-free

TABLE 2 | Mean relative abundance of the top 20 most abundant fungal taxa.

	S-ECC		Caries-free	
Species	**Plaque**	**Swab**	**Plaque**	**Swab**
*Candida dubliniensis** #	47.76 ± 44.28	13.09 ± 25.16	0.01 ± 0.03	0.00 ± 0.002
Class Agaricomycetes* §	2.52 ± 12.30	11.06 ± 25.85	1.98 ± 6.94	7.21 ± 18.82
*Candida albicans**	9.51 ± 24.79	3.59 ± 14.27	5.16 ± 18.28	1.58 ± 6.65
Blumeria sp. §	3.1 ± 16.65	0.00 ± 0.00	15.08 ± 30.59	0.00 ± 0.00
Family Thelephoraceae*#	2.165 ± 5.35	0.001 ± 0.01	12.85 ± 26.20	1.14 ± 4.07
*Malassezia restricta** § #	0.29 ± 1.03	5.45 ± 18.25	5.55 ± 19.88	0.07 ± 0.38
Candida tropicalis#	3.90 ± 14.90	2.90 ± 9.77	0.00 ± 0.00	0.01 ± 0.04
*Trichosporon asahii** §	0.00 ± 0.00	1.34 ± 8.06	2.99 ± 17.14	0.09 ± 0.56
*Ramicandelaber taiwanensi** §	0.52 ± 1.64	0.09 ± 0.52	3.58 ± 7.00	0.05 ± 0.21
Fusarium sp.* §	0.58 ± 2.46	0.00 ± 0.00	3.01 ± 17.14	0.00 ± 0.00
Meyerozyma guilliermondii§	0.10 ± 0.59	0.00 ± 0.00	3.00 ± 17.14	0.00 ± 0.00
Exophiala radices	0.00 ± 0.00	0.00 ± 0.00	2.65 ± 15.46	0.00 ± 0.00
Candida parapsilosis	0.36 ± 2.16	0.02 ± 0.11	2.204 ± 12.75	0.00 ± 0.00
*Malassezia globosa**	0.00 ± 0.00	2.23 ± 13.41	0.03 ± 0.15	0.00 ± 0.00
Order Malasseziales§	0.27 ± 1.63	0.00 ± 0.00	2.06 ± 11.99	0.00 ± 0.00
*Stereum rugosum**	2.03 ± 12.17	0.00 ± 0.00	0.00 ± 0.00	0.00 ± 0.00
Phylum Rozellomycota§	0.17 ± 0.61	0.10 ± 0.58	1.65 ± 8.99	0.04 ± 0.08
Phylum Chytridiomycota§	0.26 ± 0.93	0.08 ± 0.34	1.24 ± 5.69	0.37 ± 0.71
Phylum Ascomycota§	0.01 ± 0.05	0.03 ± 0.13	0.55 ± 2.19	1.17 ± 5.02
*Wallemia tropicalis**§	0.01 ± 0.07	0.00 ± 0.001	0.001 ± 0.01	0.00 ± 0.00

**Adjusted $P < 0.05$ (DESeq2), dental plaque vs. oral swab in children with S-ECC.*
§ Adjusted $P < 0.05$ (DESeq2), dental plaque vs. oral swab in caries-free children.
#Adjusted $P < 0.05$ (DESeq2), S-ECC vs. caries-free in oral swab samples.
S-ECC, severe early childhood caries.

children's oral swabs (adjusted $P < 0.05$, DESeq2). The differences between the dental plaque microbial composition between children with S-ECC and those caries-free have been previously published (de Jesus et al., 2020). The proportion of bacterial and fungal ASVs assigned to different taxonomic levels are shown in **Supplementary Figure 1**.

Fungal Community Analysis

A total of 8,000,067 filtered ITS1 rRNA reads were obtained, with an average number of reads per sample of 50,000.42 (160 samples). The 622 ASVs where assigned to 63 genera and 59 species. After filtering, ten samples had low reads (<1,000) and were removed from the fungal analysis as well as their respective oral swab or dental plaque pairs, resulting in a total sample size of 140. Differential abundance analysis showed that among the top 20 most abundant fungal taxa, within the S-ECC group, *Stereum rugosum* (−29.03 log2fold change), *Fusarium* sp. (−29.14 log2fold change), *Trichoderma* sp. (−24.79 log2fold change), *Candida albicans* (−10.42 log2fold change), *C. dubliniensis* (−6.04 log2fold change) and others were enriched in dental plaque. While *Trichosporon asahii* (23.97 log2fold change), *Malassezia globosa* (20.36 log2fold change), *M. restricta* (14.9 log2fold change) and others were more abundant in oral swabs. Within the caries-free group, the class Agaricomycetes (13.63 log2 fold change) was more abundant in oral swab, while *Blumeria* sp. (−29.94 log2fold change), *Fusarium* sp. (−23.26 log2fold change), *Wallemia tropicalis* (−22.68 log2fold change), *Malassezia restricta* (−16.44 log2fold change) and others were more abundant in dental plaque. Within the oral swab samples, *Candida dubliniensis* (12.92 log2fold change), *Candida tropicalis* (24.99 log2fold change), and *Malassezia restricta* (24.14 log2fold change) were more abundant in children with S-ECC compared to caries-free controls (**Table 2**, adjusted $P < 0.05$, DESeq2). The results of the differential abundance analysis according to caries status in dental plaque (caries-free vs. S-ECC) have been published previously (de Jesus et al., 2020).

The fungal alpha diversity analysis showed a significant difference in Chao 1 diversity ($P < 0.001$, paired Wilcoxon test) in the caries-free group (**Figure 4A**). Fungal community (β-diversity) analysis also showed a significant difference between dental plaque and oral swab microbiomes (pseudo-F = 5.58, $R^2 = 0.04$, $P = 0.001$, PERMANOVA; **Figure 4B**). The fungal communities of samples from caries-free children and those with S-ECC also showed a significant difference (pseudo-F = 4.17, $R^2 = 0.03$, $P = 0.001$).

Machine Learning Analysis

We first evaluated the model performance using Lasso, Ridge, Elastic Net (Enet), and RandomForest methods to classify S-ECC vs. caries-free. Overall, the Ridge approach with default parameters provided the best classification accuracy while the other three methods provided similar AUROC values (data not shown). Hence, Ridge was the model of choice for further classification.

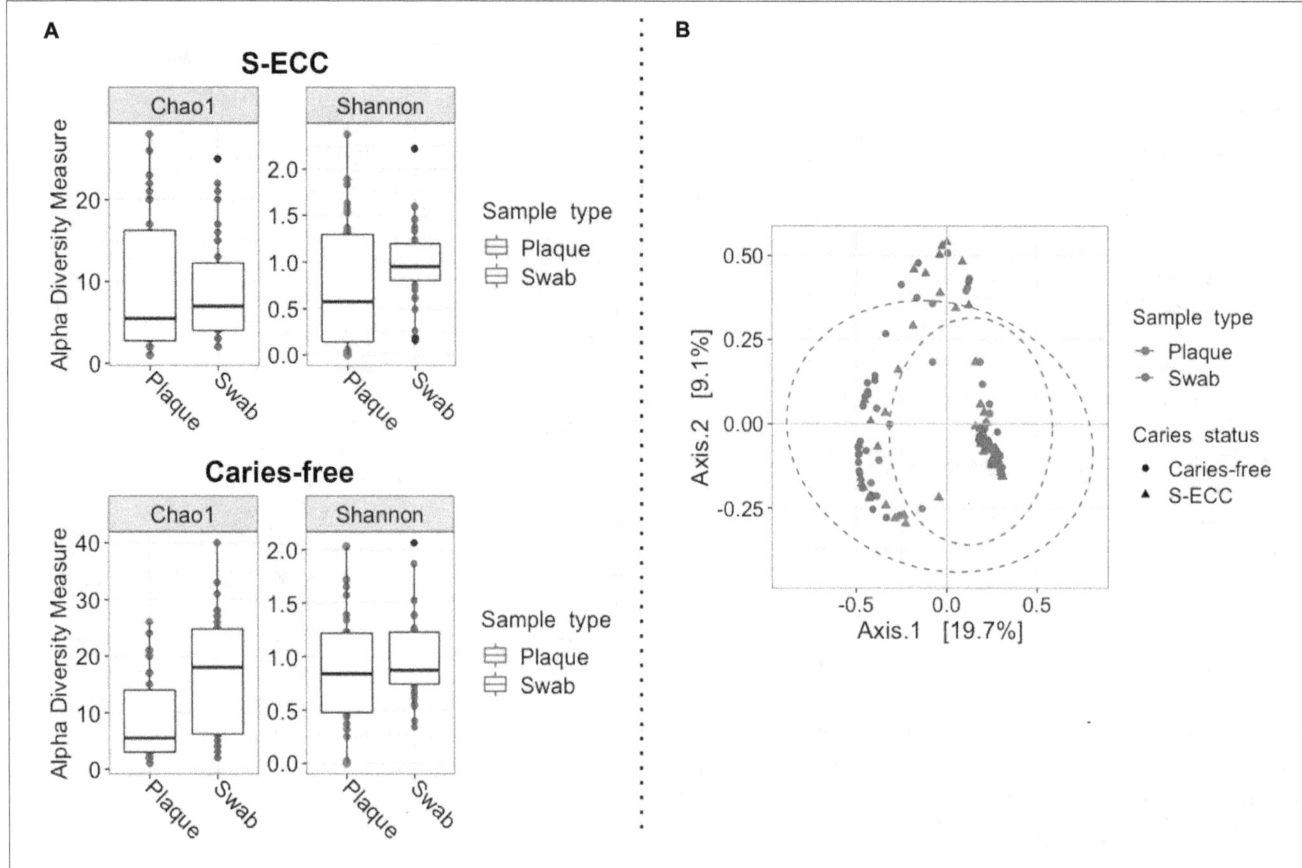

FIGURE 4 | Fungal diversity of dental plaque and oral swab samples. **(A)** For alpha diversity (within-sample) the Shannon and Chao1 diversity and richness measures were calculated according to sample type in both caries-free and S-ECC groups. A significant difference in richness was observed between the sampling sites in the caries-free group ($P < 0.001$, Chao1 index, paired Wilcoxon test). **(B)** For beta (between-sample) diversity, Bray-Curtis distances were calculated, followed by principal coordinates analysis (PCoA, pseudo-F = 11.58, $R^2 = 0.04$, $P = 0.001$, PERMANOVA). The ellipses represent a 95% confidence level. S-ECC, severe early childhood caries.

To evaluate which sampling site, dental plaque or oral swabs, would provide a better classification model for S-ECC vs. caries-free, the samples were grouped according to sampling site. The AUROC values obtained by the Ridge model with bacterial species were 0.92 and 0.91 for dental plaque and oral swab samples, respectively (**Figure 5A**). While, for fungal taxa, the AUROC values were 0.85 and 0.835, respectively (**Figure 5B**). The median relative feature weights used to predict the corresponding models and their ranks are shown in **Figures 5C,D**. Among the most important bacterial features for the S-ECC vs. caries-free classification model are *Gemella morbilorum, Lautropia mirabilis, Actinomyces* oral taxon 525 and *Capnocytophaga* oral taxon 336. While for fungi, *Mycosphaerella tassiana, Betamyces americae meridionalis, Wickerhamiella* sp. and *Cyberlindnera jadinii* were among the most important discriminatory fungal species.

To evaluate if it is possible to differentiate dental plaque samples from oral swab samples based on their bacterial and fungal profiles, both in caries-free and S-ECC groups, the samples were grouped according to caries status. The AUROC values were compared for the models built based on the top 5, 10, 15, 20, and 25 species selected through differential abundance analysis in the training set. For bacteria, in caries-free samples, the maximum AUROC value was 0.80 using 10 species while for S-ECC, the maximum AUROC value was 0.73 with 25 species. For fungi, the maximum AUROC was obtained by 10 species in caries-free samples and 5 in S-ECC samples (**Table 3**). The performance of paired analysis for different number of species is summarized in **Table 3**. It was notable that in site-based classification, in bacteria low number of species provide better classification in caries-free samples. While, for S-ECC samples high number of species are required for improving prediction. For fungi the classification was better with low number of species in both caries-free and S-ECC groups, which might be due to the low alpha diversity in the fungal samples.

DISCUSSION

In this study, first we confirmed that the bacterial and fungal community composition of dental plaque differed significantly from that obtained from oral swabs. Second, we investigated, using machine learning approaches, which sampling site would be the most appropriate to differentiate the oral microbial profile of children with S-ECC and those caries-free. Identifying the

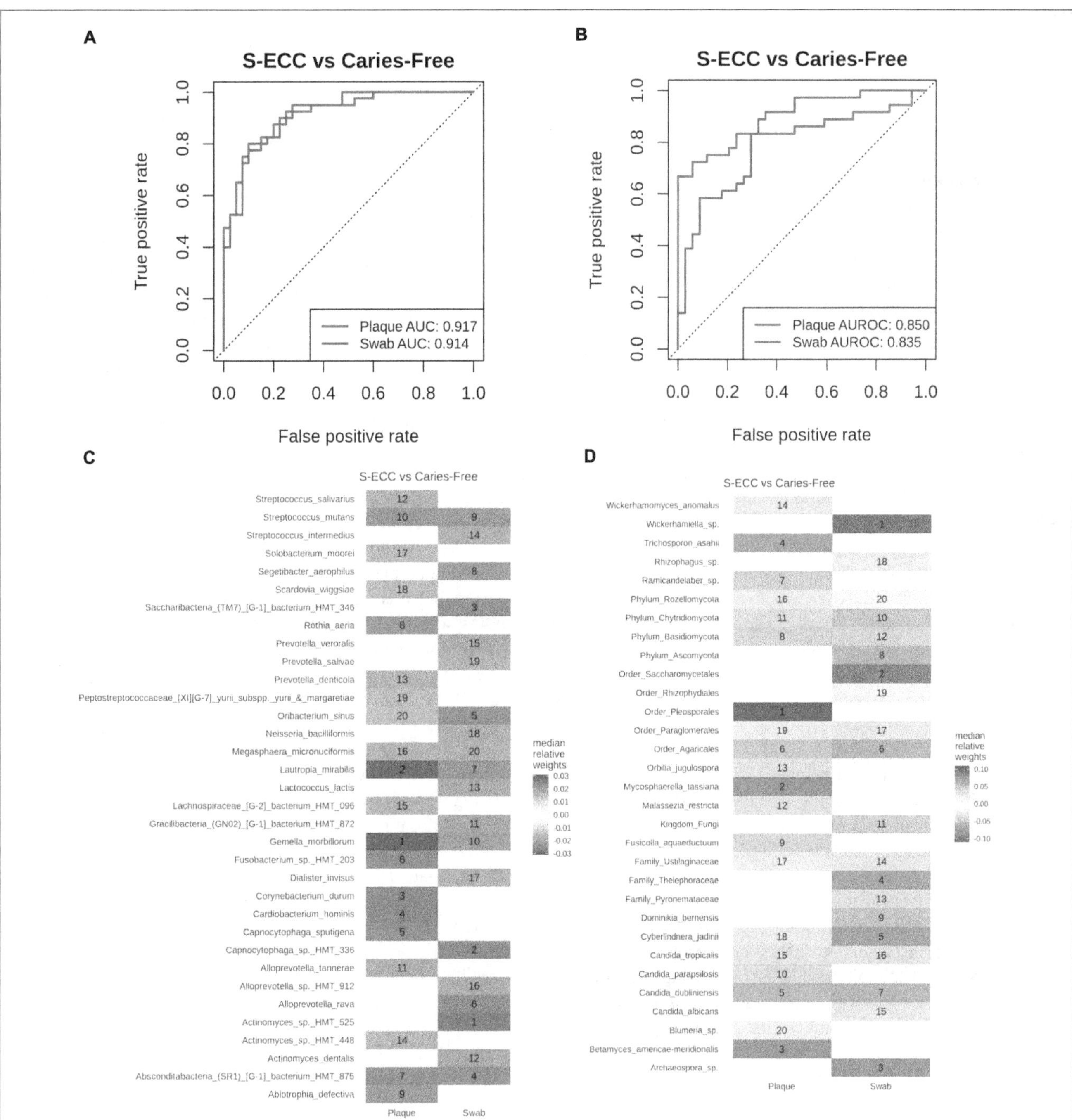

FIGURE 5 | Classification of S-ECC vs. caries-free. **(A,B)** Receiver operating characteristic (ROC) curve representing the cross-validation performance as for the classification of S-ECC and carries-free in **(A)** bacteria and **(B)** fungi using "Ridge" model in Siamcat. The area under the receiver operating characteristic curve (AUROC) represents the sample taken from dental plaques and oral swabs, by red and blue colors, respectively. AUROC values are shown in the bottom-right of the plot. **(C,D)** The relative feature weights used to predict the corresponding model. A maximum of 20 weights in each category were selected to plot on the heatmap and are marked with the ranking of the weights in the heatmap for bacterial **(C)** bacterial and **(D)** fungal taxa. The green color represents the features important in caries-free and brown is for S-ECC.

appropriate type of sample to be used is important to guide future caries association studies. Third, we evaluated whether it could be possible to predict the sampling site (dental plaque vs. oral swab) based on the microbial profile of the samples. Being able to determine the origin of the samples could be useful for the design of future microbiome studies. For instance, if researchers want to collect supragingival plaque, it would be useful to have a way of detecting if during sample collection the supragingival plaque got contaminated with subgingival plaque, as each of those should have unique microbial profiles.

TABLE 3 | Mean AUROC value for plaque vs. swab classification through conditional logistic regression.

	Bacteria		Fungi	
Species	**Caries-free**	**S-ECC**	**Caries-free**	**S-ECC**
5	0.77 ± 0.14	0.67 ± 0.12	0.62 ± 0.17	**0.73 ± 0.15**
10	**0.80 ± 0.13**	0.69 ± 0.15	**0.63 ± 0.18**	0.73 ± 0.16
15	0.73 ± 0.16	0.71 ± 0.17	0.62 ± 0.17	0.69 ± 0.16
20	0.71 ± 0.17	0.72 ± 0.17	0.63 ± 0.19	0.65 ± 0.18
25	0.72 ± 0.16	**0.73 ± 0.17**	0.62 ± 0.17	0.69 ± 0.18

The species column shows the number of species used in the classification and the mean AUROC values are provided with the standard deviation of 30 iterations of the training-test based prediction. The highest AUROC value of each group is bolded.

The oral microbiome is considered highly diverse, compared to other body sites. Although dental plaque, saliva and the buccal mucosa are in close contact, they have diverse microbial communities. The Human Microbiome Project (HMP), for instance, compared the diversity of microbes among five major body areas of 242 healthy individuals and showed that supragingival plaque has higher bacterial alpha diversity compared to the oral mucosa, which agrees with the results reported in the present study (The Human Microbiome Project Consortium, 2012). Hall et al. identified a significant difference between the microbial communities of supragingival plaque, saliva, and tongue samples from health subjects, demonstrating the existence of site-specific oral microbiomes (Hall et al., 2017).

Interestingly, while dental plaque showed increased bacterial alpha diversity compared to oral swabs the fungal alpha diversity showed an opposite pattern, with oral swabs displaying increased fungal alpha diversity. The higher fungal diversity observed in the oral swab may be associated with more fungal DNA of transient colonizers from the environment through mouth breathing and food intake (Xu and Dongari-Bagtzoglou, 2015; Diaz and Dongari-Bagtzoglou, 2021). Furthermore, most oral fungi are present at low biomass and may be difficult to detect in oral samples (Diaz and Dongari-Bagtzoglou, 2021). The above factor may explain why the number of observed fungal ASVs was lower than that of bacteria.

Streptococci was the most abundant bacterial genera in oral swabs, similar to what has been previously reported (Caselli et al., 2020). *Neisseria, Haemophilus* and *Veillonella,* found to be the most abundant in dental plaque or oral swab samples, have also been reported as highly abundant in different oral sites by previous studies (Huse et al., 2012; Caselli et al., 2020). *Streptococcus, Fusobacterium, Gemella,* and *Veillonella* have all been considered core OTUs in different oral sites (Huse et al., 2012; Hall et al., 2017). Here we showed site-specific differences in the abundance of certain species from these genera, with some being significantly more abundant in dental plaque compared to oral swabs or vice-versa. Among children with S-ECC, the known cariogenic bacterium *S. mutans* was significantly enriched in dental plaque samples compared to oral swabs. It also showed to be among the top 10 most important feature for the classification of S-ECC vs. caries-free in both dental plaque and oral swab samples. Other caries associated bacteria such as *Leptotrichia* spp. and *Selenomonas* spp. (Kalpana et al., 2020) were more abundant in dental plaque than oral swab samples from children with S-ECC.

Fungal species from the genera *Candida, Malassezia, Meyerozima,* and *Trichosporon,* were among the most abundant in dental plaque and oral swab, similarly to what has been reported in other studies (Shelburne et al., 2015; Baraniya et al., 2020; Robinson et al., 2020; Diaz and Dongari-Bagtzoglou, 2021). The differential abundance analysis showed a significant difference between *C. dubliniensis* and *C. tropicalis* in the oral swab of caries-free children and children with S-ECC. Those fungal species were also among the top 20 most important features for the classification of S-ECC vs. caries-free in oral swabs. *Candida* spp. are among the most abundant fungal species in the oral cavity and they are associated with different oral diseases (Peters et al., 2017; Diaz et al., 2019). *C. dubliniensis* has only recently been associated with dental caries in children (Al-Ahmad et al., 2016; de Jesus et al., 2020; O'Connell et al., 2020). Here we show that this fungus is not only highly abundant in the dental plaque of children with S-ECC, as previously reported, but it is also enriched in the oral swabs obtained from children with S-ECC compared to those caries-free.

In recent years, machine learning has become a commonly applied approach to early childhood oral health research (Peng et al., 2021). One of the challenges in microbiome data analysis is that the differential analysis methods generally lack the information about predictability. Thus, we used machine learning methods to identify site-specific taxonomic features in dental plaque and oral swabs. The results suggested that both dental plaque and oral swab samples provide a good model for S-ECC vs. caries-free classification. They also suggest that it is possible to differentiate dental plaque from oral swab samples using their microbial profiles. However, site-based classification through fungal species was not optimum in caries-free samples. This could be due to the small number of fungal species that significantly differed in abundance between dental plaque and oral swabs, as observed in the differential abundance analysis.

From our classification results for caries status, it appears that the models using the microbial composition of dental plaque or oral swabs were both able to discriminate between caries-free and S-ECC samples. However, it is important to notice that the species considered to be important for the classification of disease for each sampling site are slightly different. Based on the results from other machine learning models (Lasso, Enet, and RandomForest), we also observed that the choice of the model does not significantly affect the outcome of the analysis (data not shown).

The limitations of this study include, but are not limited to, the lack of information about the socio-economic status of the participants and the convenient sampling used for recruitment, which means that during recruitment the groups were only matched by caries status. As many factors may influence the oral microbial composition, the results of this study may not be generalizable to other populations with different age groups and geographic locations. In this study, an additional enzymatic lysis step was used during DNA extraction from dental plaque samples to disrupt the dental plaque biofilm. Rosenbaum et al. compared the impact of using different DNA extraction methods, including the use of QIAamp DNA Mini Kit (Qiagen) with and without additional enzymatic lysis step, in the oral bacterial (16S rRNA) and fungal (ITS1 rRNA) microbiota. They showed that all tested DNA extraction methods were able to lyse Gram-positive bacterial species. They also reported no significant differences in bacterial and fungal diversity among DNA extraction methods (Rosenbaum et al., 2019). Other studies also found no significant effect of DNA extraction methods in the microbial composition of oral samples (Lim et al., 2017). Therefore, while we do not expect that the additional enzymatic lysis step significantly contributed to the differences observed between the dental plaque and oral swab microbiota, we cannot completely rule out the possible bias associated with the sample preparation on the analyses comparing dental plaque and oral swab microbiomes.

Currently, UNITE is the most commonly used database for taxonomic classification in mycobiome studies of different environments. However, there is an increased concern regarding the lack of taxonomic coverage on the available databases, which creates limitations to studies trying to characterize the human mycobiome (Nilsson, 2016). Here, a high proportion of fungal ASVs (37.14%) could not be classified to a meaningful taxonomic level beyond kingdom. As the reads passed through the quality control process, the observed high number of unclassified ASVs could be a limitation of the database used. Therefore, the construction of a curated ITS database specific for the oral mycobiome, as exists for the oral bacteriome, is urgently needed.

This is a cross-sectional study. Thus, based on our results it is not possible to determine when a significant oral microbial shift from a healthy to a diseased state occurs. Xu et al. performed a longitudinal study where they did a 1-year follow-up of caries-free 3-year-old children (Xu et al., 2018). The authors suggested that prior to any clinical sign of caries, there is a microbial shift that could potentially be used for the diagnosis and prevention of dental caries in young children. Therefore, future longitudinal studies aiming to further characterize the microbial shifts that precede the first clinical signs of dental caries are needed.

In summary, this study characterized the differences in microbial profiles of dental plaque and oral swab samples from children with S-ECC and those caries-free. Importantly, our machine learning results were able to predict the caries-status (S-ECC vs. caries-free) and sampling site (dental plaque vs. oral swab) based on the microbial profile of the samples. In the future, when data from related studies distinguishing oral sampling sites using microbiome profiles are available, we will perform the replication studies to validate our results.

AUTHOR CONTRIBUTIONS

VCJ and PC conceived the study. VCJ, MK, PH, and PC contributed to the design, data analysis, interpretation, and writing of the manuscript. VCJ, BAM, and RJS contributed to data acquisition. KD and RJS contributed to the design, data interpretation, and writing of the manuscript. KD, PH, RJS, and PC contributed to funding acquisition. All authors contributed to the article and approved the submitted version.

ACKNOWLEDGMENTS

We thank the parents/caregivers, participants, and the Misericordia Health Centre.

REFERENCES

1. AAPD (2020). *Policy on Early Childhood Caries (ECC): Classifications, Consequences, and Preventive Strategies." The Reference Manual of Pediatric Dentistry*. Chicago, Ill: American Academy of Pediatric Dentistry, 79–81.
2. Abarenkov, K., Zirk, A., Piirmann, T., Pöhönen, R., Ivanov, F., Nilsson, H. R., et al. (2020a). *"UNITE QIIME Release for Eukaryotes 2." Version 04.02.2020*. London: UNITE Community.
3. Abarenkov, K., Zirk, A., Piirmann, T., Pöhönen, R., Ivanov, F., Nilsson, H. R., et al. (2020b). *"UNITE QIIME Release for Fungi." Version 04.02.2020*. London: UNITE Community.
4. Abarenkov, K., Zirk, A., Piirmann, T., Pöhönen, R., Ivanov, F., Nilsson, H. R., et al. (2020c). *"UNITE QIIME Release for Fungi 2." Version 04.02.2020*. London: UNITE Community.
5. Agnello, M., Marques, J., Cen, L., Mittermuller, B., Huang, A., Chaichanasakul Tran, N., et al. (2017). Microbiome associated with severe caries in Canadian First Nations Children. *J. Dent. Res.* 96, 1378–1385. doi: 10.1177/0022034517718819
6. Al-Ahmad, A., Auschill, T. M., Dakhel, R., Wittmer, A., Pelz, K., Heumann, C., et al. (2016). Prevalence of candida albicans and candida dubliniensis in caries-free and caries-active children in relation to the oral microbiota—a clinical study. *Clin. Oral Investig.* 20, 1963–1971. doi: 10.1007/s00784-015-1696-9
7. Anderson, M. J. (2001). Permutation tests for univariate or multivariate analysis of variance and regression. *Can. J. Fish. Aquat. Sci.* 58, 626–639. doi: 10.1139/f01- 004
8. Andrews, S. (2010). *FastQC: A Quality Control Tool for High Throughput Sequence Data [Online]*. Available online at: http://www.bioinformatics.babraham.ac.uk/ projects/fastqc/ (accessed September 21, 2020).
9. Baraniya, D., Chen, T., Nahar, A., Alakwaa, F., Hill, J., Tellez, M., et al. (2020). Supragingival mycobiome and inter-kingdom interactions in dental caries. *J. Oral Microbiol.* 12:1729305. doi: 10.1080/20002297.2020.1729305
10. Beals, E. W. (1984). Bray-curtis ordination: an effective strategy for analysis of multivariate ecological data. *Adv. Ecol. Res.* 14, 1–55. doi: 10.1016/S0065-2504(08)60168-3
11. Bisanz, J. (2018). *Qiime2R: Importing QIIME2 Artifacts and Associated Data into R Sessions*. San Francisco, CA: GitHub.
12. Bischl, B., Lang, M., Kotthoff, L., Schiffner, J., Richter, J., Studerus, E., et al. (2016). Mlr: machine learning in R. *J. Mach. Learn. Res.* 17, 1–5. doi: 10.11648/j.mlr. 20180301.11
13. Bolyen, E., Rideout, J. R., Dillon, M. R., Bokulich, N. A., Abnet, C. C., Al-Ghalith, G. A., et al. (2019). Reproducible, interactive, scalable and extensible microbiome data science using QIIME 2. *Nat. Biotechnol.* 37, 852–857. doi: 10.1038/s41587-019-0209-9
14. Callahan, B. J., McMurdie, P. J., Rosen, M. J., Han, A. W., Johnson, A. J. A., and Holmes, S. P. (2016). DADA2: high-resolution sample inference from illumina amplicon data. *Nat. Methods* 13, 581–583. doi: 10.1038/nmeth.3869
15. Caselli, E., Fabbri, C., D'Accolti, M., Soffritti, I., Bassi, C., Mazzacane, S., et al. (2020). Defining the oral microbiome by whole-genome sequencing and resistome analysis: the complexity of the healthy picture. *BMC Microbiol.* 20:120. doi: 10.1186/s12866-020-01801-y
16. de Jesus, V. C., Shikder, R., Oryniak, D., Mann, K., Alamri, A., Mittermuller, B., et al. (2020). Sex-based diverse plaque microbiota in children with severe caries. *J. Dent. Res.* 99, 703–712. doi: 10.1177/0022034520908595

17. Depner, M., Taft, D. H., Kirjavainen, P. V., Kalanetra, K. M., Karvonen, A. M., Peschel, S., et al. (2020). Maturation of the gut microbiome during the first year of life contributes to the protective farm effect on childhood asthma. *Nat. Med.* 26, 1766–1775. doi: 10.1038/s41591-020-1095-x
18. Dewhirst, F. E., Chen, T., Izard, J., Paster, B. J., Tanner, A. C. R., Yu, W., et al. (2010). The human oral microbiome. *J. Bacteriol.* 192, 5002–5017.
19. Diaz, P., Hong, B., Dupuy, A., Choquette, L., Thompson, A., Salner, A., et al. (2019). Integrated analysis of clinical and microbiome risk factors associated with the development of oral candidiasis during cancer chemotherapy. *J. Fungi* 5:49. doi: 10.3390/jof5020049
20. Diaz, P. I., and Dongari-Bagtzoglou, A. (2021). Critically appraising the significance of the oral mycobiome. *J. Dent. Res.* 100, 133–140. doi: 10.1177/0022034520956975
21. Fernandes, L. L., Pacheco, V. B., Borges, L., Athwal, H. K., de Paula Eduardo, F., Bezinelli, L., et al. (2020). Saliva in the diagnosis of COVID-19: a review and new research directions. *J. Dent. Res.* 99, 1435–1443. doi: 10.1177/0022034520960070
22. Folayan, M. O., El Tantawi, M., Schroth, R. J., Vukovic, A., Kemoli, A., Gaffar, B., et al. (2020). Associations between early childhood caries, malnutrition and anemia: a global perspective. *BMC Nutr.* 6:16. doi: 10.1186/s40795-020-00340-z Frøslev, T. G., Kjøller, R., Bruun, H. H., Ejrnæs, R., Brunbjerg, A. K., Pietroni, C., et al. (2017). Algorithm for post-clustering curation of DNA amplicon data yields reliable biodiversity estimates. *Nat. Commun.* 8:1188. doi: 10.1038/s41467-017-01312-x
23. Hall, M. W., Singh, N., Ng, K. F., Lam, D. K., Goldberg, M. B., Tenenbaum, H. C., et al. (2017). Inter-personal diversity and temporal dynamics of dental, tongue, and salivary microbiota in the healthy oral cavity. *NPJ Biofilms Microbiomes* 3:2. doi: 10.1038/s41522-016-0011-0
24. Huse, S. M., Ye, Y., Zhou, Y., and Fodor, A. A. (2012). A core human microbiome as viewed through 16S RRNA sequence clusters. *PLoS One* 7:e34242. doi: 10. 1371/journal.pone.0034242
25. Ismail, A., and Sohn, W. (1999). A systematic review of clinical diagnostic criteria of early childhood caries. *J. Public Health Dent.* 59, 171–191. doi: 10.1111/j. 1752-7325.1999.tb03267.x
26. Kalpana, B., Prabhu, P., Bhat, A. H., Senthilkumar, A., Arun, R. P., Asokan, S., et al. (2020). Bacterial diversity and functional analysis of severe early childhood caries and recurrence in India. *Sci. Rep.* 10:21248. doi: 10.1038/s41598-020- 78057-z
27. La Rosa, P. S., Brooks, J. P., Deych, E., Boone, E. L., Edwards, D. J., Wang, Q., et al. (2012). "Hypothesis testing and power calculations for taxonomic-based human microbiome data." *PLoS One* 7:e52078. doi: 10.1371/journal.pone.005 2078
28. Lamont, R. J., Koo, H., and Hajishengallis, G. (2018). The oral microbiota: dynamic communities and host interactions. *Nat. Rev. Microbiol.* 16, 745–759. doi: 10. 1038/s41579-018-0089-x
29. Lim, Y., Totsika, M., Morrison, M., and Punyadeera, C. (2017). The saliva microbiome profiles are minimally affected by collection method or DNA extraction protocols. *Sci. Rep.* 7:8523. doi: 10.1038/s41598-017-07885-3
30. Love, M. I., Huber, W., and Anders, S. (2014). Moderated estimation of fold change and dispersion for RNA-Seq data with DESeq2. *Genome Biol.* 15:550. doi: 10.1186/s13059-014-0550-8
31. Martinsen, E. M. H., Eagan, T. M. L., Leiten, E. O., Haaland, I., Husebø, G. R., Knudsen, K. S., et al. (2021). The pulmonary mycobiome—a study of subjects with and without chronic obstructive pulmonary disease. *PLoS One* 16:e0248967. doi: 10.1371/journal.pone.0248967
32. McMurdie, P. J., and Holmes, S. (2013). Phyloseq: an R package for reproducible interactive analysis and graphics of microbiome census data. *PLoS One* 8:e61217. doi: 10.1371/journal.pone.0061217
33. Nilsson, R. H. (2016). Top 50 most wanted fungi. *MycoKeys* 12, 29–40. O'Connell, L. M., Santos, R., Springer, G., Burne, R. A., Nascimento, M. M., and Richards, V. P. (2020). "Site-specific profiling of the dental mycobiome reveals strong taxonomic shifts during progression of early-childhood caries." *Appl. Environ. Microbiol.* 86, e2825–e2819. doi: 10.1128/AEM.02825-19
34. Paulson, J. N., Stine, O. C., Bravo, H. C., and Pop, M. (2013). Differential abundance analysis for microbial marker-gene surveys. *Nat. Methods* 10, 1200–1202. doi: 10.1038/nmeth.2658
35. Peng, J., Zeng, X., Townsend, J., Liu, G., Huang, Y., and Lin, S. (2021). A machine learning approach to uncovering hidden utilization patterns of early childhood dental care among medicaid-insured children. *Front. Public Health* 8:599187. doi: 10.3389/fpubh.2020.599187
36. Peters, B. A., Wu, J., Hayes, R. B., and Ahn, J. (2017). The oral fungal mycobiome: characteristics and relation to periodontitis in a pilot study. *BMC Microbiol.* 17:157. doi: 10.1186/s12866-017-1064-9
37. Pierce, A., Singh, S., Lee, J., Grant, C., de Jesus, V. C., and Schroth, R. J. (2019). The burden of early childhood caries in canadian children and associated risk factors. *Front. Public Health* 7:328. doi: 10.3389/fpubh.2019.00328
38. Rivers, A. R., Weber, K. C., Gardner, T. G., Liu, S., and Armstrong, S. D. (2018). ITSxpress: software to rapidly trim internally transcribed spacer sequences with quality scores for marker gene analysis. *F1000Res.* 7:1418. doi: 10.12688/ f1000research.15704.1
39. Robinson, S., Peterson, C. B., Sahasrabhojane, P., Ajami, N. J., Shelburne, S. A., Kontoyiannis, D. P., et al. (2020). Observational cohort study of oral mycobiome and inter-kingdom interactions over the course of induction therapy for leukemia. *MSphere* 5, e48–e20. doi: 10.1128/mSphere.00 048-20
40. Rosenbaum, J., Usyk, M., Chen, Z., Zolnik, C. P., Jones, H. E., Waldron, L., et al. (2019). Evaluation of oral cavity DNA extraction methods on bacterial and fungal microbiota. *Sci. Rep.* 9:1531. doi: 10.1038/s41598-018-38 049-6
41. Russell, R. R. (2009). Changing concepts in caries microbiology. *Am. J. Dent.* 22:7. Sapkota, D., Søland, T. M., Galtung, H. K., Sand, L. P., Giannecchini, S., To, K. K. W., et al. (2020). COVID-19 salivary signature: diagnostic and research opportunities. *J. Clin. Pathol.* doi: 10.1136/jclinpath-2020-206834 [Epub ahead of print] .
42. Shelburne, S. A., Ajami, N. J., Chibucos, M. C., Beird, H. C., Tarrand, J., Galloway- Peña, J., et al. (2015). Implementation of a pan-genomic approach to investigate holobiont-infecting microbe interaction: a case report of a leukemic patient with invasive mucormycosis. *PLoS One* 10:e0139851. doi: 10.1371/journal.pone. 0139851
43. Shi, H., and Yin, G. (2015). *R Package: Clogitboost, Version 1.1.* Available online at: https://Cran.r-Project.Org/Web/Packages/Clogitboost/Index.Html (accessed May 3, 2021).
44. Stearns, J. C., Lynch, M. D. J., Senadheera, D. B., Tenenbaum, H. C., Goldberg, M. B., Cvitkovitch, D. G., et al. (2011). Bacterial biogeography of the human digestive tract. *Sci. Rep.* 1:170. doi: 10.1038/srep00170
45. The Human Microbiome Project Consortium (2012). Structure, function and diversity of the healthy human microbiome. *Nature* 486, 207–214. doi: 10.1038/ nature11234
46. Usyk, M., Zolnik, C. P., Patel, H., Levi, M. H., and Burk, R. D. (2017). Novel ITS1 fungal primers for characterization of the mycobiome. *MSphere* 2, e488–e417. doi: 10.1128/mSphere.00488-17
47. Vila, T., Sultan, A. S., Montelongo-Jauregui, D., and Jabra-Rizk, M. A. (2020). Oral candidiasis: a disease of opportunity. *J. Fungi* 6:15. doi: 10.3390/jof601 0015
48. Wickham, H. (2016). *Ggplot2. Use R!.* New York, NY: Springer-Verlag. . Wirbel, J., Pyl, P. T., Kartal, E., Zych, K., Kashani, A., Milanese, A., et al. (2019). Meta-analysis of fecal metagenomes reveals global microbial signatures that are specific for colorectal cancer. *Nat. Med.* 25, 679–689. doi: 10.1038/s41591-019- 0406-6
49. Wirbel, J., Zych, K., Essex, M., Karcher, N., Kartal, E., Salazar, G., et al. (2021). Microbiome meta-analysis and cross-disease comparison enabled by the SIAMCAT machine learning toolbox. *Genome Biol.* 22:93. doi: 10.1186/s13059- 021-02306-1
50. Xu, H., and Dongari-Bagtzoglou, A. (2015). Shaping the oral mycobiota: interactions of opportunistic fungi with oral bacteria and the host. *Curr. Opin. Microbiol.* 26, 65–70. doi: 10.1016/j.mib.2015.06.002
51. Xu, H., Tian, J., Hao, W., Zhang, Q., Zhou, Q., Shi, W., et al. (2018). Oral microbiome shifts from caries-free to caries-affected status in 3-year-old chinese children: a longitudinal study. *Front. Microbiol.* 9:2009. doi: 10.3389/fmicb.2018.02009
52. Xu, H., Zhong, L., Deng, J., Peng, J., Dan, H., Zeng, X., et al. (2020a). High expression of ACE2 receptor of 2019-NCoV on the epithelial cells of oral mucosa. *Int. J. Oral Sci.* 12:8. doi: 10.1038/s41368-020-0 074-x
53. Xu, J., Li, Y., Gan, F., Du, Y., and Yao, Y. (2020b). Salivary glands: potential reservoirs for COVID-19 asymptomatic infection. *J. Dent. Res.* 99, 989–989. doi: 10.1177/002203452091 8518
54. Zhang, Z., Schwartz, S., Wagner, L., and Miller, W. (2000). A greedy algorithm for aligning DNA sequences. *J. Comput. Biol.* 7, 203–214. doi: 10.1089/10665270050081478

7

Evaluating the Effectiveness of Medical–Dental Integration to Close Preventive and Disease Management Care Gaps

David M. Mosen [1*], *Matthew P. Banegas* [1], *John F. Dickerson* [1], *Jeffrey L. Fellows* [1], *Daniel J. Pihlstrom* [2], *Hala M. Kershah* [3], *Jason L. Scott* [1] *and Erin M. Keast* [1]

[1] *Center for Health Research, Kaiser Permanente Northwest, Portland, OR, United States,* [2] *Permanente Dental Associates, Portland, OR, United States,* [3] *Dental Administration, Kaiser Permanente Northwest, Portland, OR, United States*

***Correspondence:**
David M. Mosen
david.m.mosen@kpchr.org

Background: The integration of medical care into the dental setting has been shown to facilitate the closure of care gaps among patients with unmet needs. However, little is known about whether program effectiveness varies depending on whether the care gap is related to preventive care or disease management.

Materials and Methods: We used a matched cohort study design to compare closure of care gaps between patients aged 65+ who received care at a Kaiser Permanente Northwest (KPNW) Medical–Dental Integration (MDI) clinic or a non-MDI dental clinic between June 1, 2018, and December 31, 2019. The KPNW MDI program focuses on closing 12 preventive (e.g., flu vaccines) and 11 disease management care gaps (e.g., HbA1c testing) within the dental setting. Using the multivariable logistic regression, we separately analyzed care gap closure rates (yes vs. no) for patients who were overdue for: (1) preventive services only ($n = 1{,}611$), (2) disease management services only ($n = 538$), or (3) both types of services ($n = 429$), analyzing closure of each care gap type separately. All data were obtained through the electronic health record of KPNW.

Results: The MDI patients had significantly higher odds of closing preventive care gaps (OR = 1.51, 95% CI = 1.30–1.75) and disease management care gaps (OR = 1.65, 95% CI = 1.27–2.15) than the non-MDI patients when they only had care gaps of one type or the other. However, no significant association was found between MDI and care gap closure when patients were overdue for both care gap types.

Conclusions: Patients with care gaps related to either preventive care or disease management who received dental care in an MDI clinic had higher odds of closing these care gaps, but we found no evidence that MDI was helpful for those with both types of care gaps.

Practical Implications: MDI may be an effective model for facilitating the delivery of preventive and disease management services, mainly when patients are overdue for one type of these services. Future research should examine the impact of MDI on long-term health outcomes.

Keywords: integration, Medicare, chronic conditions, preventive, elderly health

INTRODUCTION

Poor oral health, particularly periodontal disease is associated with many common systemic health conditions, including diabetes (1–7), cardiovascular disease (CVD) (7, 8), coronary artery disease (CAD) (9–11), cerebral vascular disease (9, 11–13), hypertension (HTN) (14, 15), cancer (16) and rheumatoid arthritis (RA) (17, 18). Adults aged 65 years and older represent a population at high risk for both and oral and systemic disease, with over 65% having periodontal disease (19, 20) and over 80% having two or more chronic systemic diseases (21, 22).

Previous research has demonstrated that the dental setting can be an ideal setting to promote preventive health for those at risk of developing chronic systemic conditions. For example, Jontell and Glick (23) found that dental healthcare providers can effectively screen and identify patients for serious complications from CVD that they may not be aware of. A systematic review (24) found that screening for dysglycemia in dental clinics was effective in identifying individuals who required triage for further glycemic management.

In a recently published study, we found that a comprehensive medical–dental integration (MDI) program at the Kaiser Permanente Northwest (KPNW) was successful at facilitating the closure of medical care gaps among a population of patients aged 65 years and older who were overdue for either preventive (e.g., flu vaccines) or disease management medical services (e.g., HbA1c testing for persons with diabetes) (25). This research was the first to show that the dental setting can facilitate the provision of recommended evidence-based preventive and disease management medical services for elderly populations (26–28).

Although we found that MDI at KPNW was effective at closing care gaps for preventive and disease management care gaps, there is limited research on whether the effectiveness of MDI on care gaps closure differs by service type: preventive medicine or disease management. For example, MDI is more effective at closing preventive medicine services, such as flu vaccines as opposed to disease management services, such as HbA1c testing for adults with diabetes. Accordingly, the primary objective of this study was to separately examine the association of MDI with the closure of medical care gaps among populations overdue for (1) preventive and/or (2) disease management care gaps. The rationale for conducting this stratified analysis was for program evaluation purposes, namely to understand whether care gaps were closed differently based on the type of medical care gap. Such information can be used for quality improvement purposes to revise and refine the MDI programs.

MATERIALS AND METHODS

The methods for this analysis were presented previously (25). The study population included a retrospective matched cohort analysis of KPNW medical and dental members ($n = 2{,}578$) who received care at any of four MDI clinics of KPNW and those who received care at a non-MDI clinic during the same time period ($n = 2{,}578$; total $n = 5{,}156$). Briefly, we identified all patients who met four inclusion criteria: (1) aged 65 or older; (2) had a dental visit at a KPNW MDI dental clinic between June 1, 2018 and December 31, 2019; (3) had at least one medical care gap at the time of their first (index) dental visit during that time period; and (4) had 12 months of continuous health plan enrollment prior to index dental visit. Using a matching algorithm, we then identified a 1:1 matched sample of patients who met the inclusion criteria except that their index dental visit occurred at one of 13 non-MDI dental clinics during the same time period. Patients from each MDI dental clinic were matched with patients from one of three to four non-MDI dental clinics with a similar total volume of dental staff full-time equivalents (FTEs) and an annual volume of dental visits. Patients were also matched based on sex, care gap type (preventive only, disease management only, or both), age (within 5 years), and index visit date (±60 days). MDI and non-MDI were further propensity-matched based on seven characteristics: Charlson comorbidity index (CCI; 0, 1, 2+); smoking status (yes vs. no); emergency department (ED) utilization in the previous 12 months (any vs. none); hospitalization in previous 12 months (any vs. none); the presence of any of five systemic conditions [diabetes mellitus (DM), RA, CVD, CAD, and HTN; yes vs. no]; periodontal disease status (healthy/early, moderate, and advanced); and a total number of open care gaps at the index visit (continuous).

To assess whether care gap closure varied by service type, we stratified the population into three cohorts based on care gap type(s) at baseline: (1) preventive care gaps only, (2) disease management care gaps only, and (3) both preventive and disease management care gaps. A list of all care gaps and their categories has been described previously (25). Data from the electronic health record (EHR) of KPNW were used for matching and analysis.

The IRB Approval

The protocol for this study was approved by the institutional review board (IRB) within KPNW, who approved a waiver of individual consent for data use (IRB# 00000405 and FWA# 00002344). As this was a "data-only" no-patient contact study, all data storage and analytic practices adhered to the research compliance standards of KPNW.

Setting

The KPNW is a comprehensive healthcare system that currently serves ~605,000 medical members and 250,000 dental members in Oregon and Washington. The KPNW MDI program includes three distinct model types employed in four dental clinics that are in their level of integration (25). The MDI model with the least integration was implemented on June 1st, 2018; the other two models were implemented on August 1st, 2018. Each model is described below.

Least Integration

This model consists of a dental office located in the same building as medical offices (e.g., lab, vision, and nurse treatment center for immunizations) with no medical staff embedded in the dental office. In this model, a dental member assistant (DMA) identifies care gaps at the time of dental visits using the EHR and coordinates closely with other medical departments located within the building to complete the overdue care gaps.

Moderate Integration

In this model, a licensed practice nurse (LPN) is embedded within a stand-alone dental clinic to address care gaps. The LPN can provide immunizations, collect samples for lab-based tests, and provide other basic services [e.g., HbA1c testing, BP screening, and DM foot exams] directly in the dental setting. The LPN also coordinates all other medical services that require offsite referrals (e.g., mammography) or offsite follow-up with primary care (e.g., follow-up regarding abnormal HbA1c results).

Most Integration

This model, implemented in two KPNW locations, consists of co-located medical and dental offices with an embedded LPN within the dental clinic itself. The LPN provides direct services and coordinates with other co-located medical staff to complete additional services. At both clinics following this model, a DMA works closely with the LPN to identify care gaps prior to dental visits. The LPN then provides service to close care gaps that can be directly addressed in the dental setting (e.g., immunizations) and coordinates with other co-located medical departments to address other care gaps after the dental visit (e.g., DM retinopathy screening). The LPN also arranges follow-up care as needed with primary care for care coordination regarding chronic conditions.

Non-MDI dental offices have no embedded medical staff to complete on-site care gap closure or care coordination to complete needed follow-up services. Within the non-MDI clinics, the dental staff uses an EHR-based decision support tool (described below) to remind patients of any care gaps they may have.

Identification of Medical Care Gaps and Outcome Measures

The KPNW dental and medical clinics use an EHR-based program called the panel support tool (PST) to identify patient care gaps. The PST, which has been in use since 2006 (29), uses informatics to track care gaps, patient reminders, and follow-up care (29). The PST lists care gaps based on the current clinical guidelines and evidence for ongoing screening tests and disease management services (26–28).

The primary outcome measure of this study was closure of *all* relevant (1) preventive and (2) disease management medical care gaps present at the index dental visit in each of the three care gap cohorts. For 18 of the 23 measures, care gap closure was assessed at 30 days following the index visit; fecal immunochemical testing, mammography, annual DM exam, retinopathy exam, and smoking cessation were assessed at 60 days following the index visit.

Statistical Analysis

As part of the stratified analysis, we first conducted descriptive analyses of analytic variables to confirm assumptions and as a quality assurance process. In order to assess the performance of our matching algorithm, we calculated standardized differences of demographic and clinical characteristics between MDI and non-MDI patients within each of the three care gap cohorts (**Tables 1.1–1.3**). We used a threshold of $\geq$0.2 to identify variables that are meaningfully different between groups (30); this threshold has been used previously in observational studies (31, 32). Because no differences of 0.2 or higher were found after matching, we did not conduct further adjustment in the stratified regression analysis. Finally, we used three separate logistic regression models to compare rates of closure of care gaps between MDI and non-MDI patients within each of the three care gap cohorts (**Table 2**).

RESULTS

Population Characteristics: Care Gap Cohorts

The preventive care gap cohort included 62.5% (N = 3,222) of the study population, whereas the disease management cohort included 20.9% (N = 1,076) and the combined preventive and disease management gap cohort included 16.6% (N = 858) of the population. Within the three cohorts, patients in the MDI and non-MDI groups were well balanced for care gap type, age, and sex, area deprivation index (ADI) (33) (as a proxy for socioeconomic status), and most clinical and demographic variables after matching (**Tables 1.1–1.3**). Although there was variation between the three cohorts with respect to demographics, comorbidities, systemic conditions, periodontal disease status and open care gaps at baseline, none of these differences exceeded the standard difference $\geq$0.2.

Association Between MDI and Care Gap Closure by Cohort

Table 2 shows the results of the logistic regression analyses testing associations between MDI and care gap closure for each cohort. In the preventive care gap and disease management cohorts, patients seen at MDI clinics had 1.51 the odds of closing all preventive gaps and 1.65 the odds of closing all disease management gaps than patients seen at non-MDI clinics. In the cohort of patients with both types of care gaps, there was no significant association being seen at an MDI clinic and closure of all care gaps.

TABLE 1.1 | Population Characteristics: Preventive Care Gaps Only.

Population characteristics	MDI Clinics $N = 1{,}611$	Non-MDI Clinics $N = 1{,}611$	p-value	Standardized Difference
Baseline gap type				
Preventive alone	1,611 (100.0%)	1,611 (100.0%)	NA	NA
Exact-matched variables				
Age (mean ± S.D.; matched within 5 yrs.)	70.6 ± 5.0	70.8 ± 5.1	0.18	0.05
Sex (exact match)				
Male (vs. female)	580 (36.0%)	580 (36.0%)	1.00	0.00
Propensity-matched variables			0.04	
CCI 0	1,010 (62.7%)	946 (58.7%)		0.04
CCI 1	237 (14.7%)	282 (17.5%)		0.05
CCI 2+	364 (22.6%)	383 (23.8%)		0.02
Current smoker				
Yes (vs. no)	2 (0.1%)	6 (0.4%)	0.16	0.04
ED use in previous 12 months				
Yes (vs. no)	247 (15.3%)	276 (17.1%)	0.17	0.03
Hospitalization in previous 12 months				
Yes (vs. no)	99 (6.1%)	130 (8.1%)	0.03	0.05
Systemic conditions (% yes)				
Diabetes-Mellitus (DM)	166 (10.3%)	179 (11.1%)	0.46	0.02
Rheumatoid Arthritis (RA)	27 (1.7%)	26 (1.6%)	0.89	0.00
Cardiovascular Disease (CVD)	147 (9.1%)	181 (11.2%)	0.05	0.05
Cardiovascular Disease (CAD)	143 (8.9%)	179 (11.1%)	0.03	0.05
Hypertension (HTN)	624 (38.7%)	644 (40.0%)	0.47	0.02
Periodontal disease status			0.87	
Healthy/early	1,273 (79.0%)	1,276 (79.2%)		0.00
Moderate	236 (14.7%)	227 (14.1%)		0.01
Advanced	37 (2.3%)	35 (2.2%)		0.01
Missing	65 (4.0%)	73 (4.5%)		0.02
Total open gaps at index visit (mean ± S.D.)	1.6 ± 0.9	1.6 ± 0.9	0.94	0.00
Non-Propensity matched variables				
SES[b]: Area Deprivation Index (ADI) (Mean ± SD)	4.4 ± 2.4	4.5 ± 2.6	0.33	0.04

$N = 3{,}222$ (62.5% of total population)[a].

[a]*Population includes population of Medicare patients age ≥ 65 with 1+ care gaps at baseline. P-value from t-test for age, count of open gaps at baseline, and ADI state rank; P-value from chi-square for all other variables.*

[b]*SES, socioeconomic status.*

DISCUSSION

This study found that among patients with only preventive or disease management care gaps, receiving care in MDI clinics was associated with significantly greater odds of care gap closure than receiving care at non-MDI clinics. However, there was no significant difference in rates of closure of all care gaps between MDI and non-MDI patients among those with both preventive and disease management care gaps at their index visit. Taken with previously published results by our research team that found the KPNW MDI program was effective at closing care gaps overall (when combining all three care gap cohorts) (25), these findings suggest that the success of the KPNW MDI program may be driven by those who do not have both preventive and disease management care gaps—these cohorts made up over 80% of the eligible population.

This is the first study of which we are aware to examine the association of MDI with the closure of specific types of care gaps. Our findings suggest that MDI is effective at facilitating the use of needed medical services for either preventive or disease management care, suggesting the broad benefits of this approach. This research is consistent with research demonstrating the success of other integration efforts in the dental setting. A study by Jontell and Glick (23) found that oral healthcare professionals can successfully screen and identify patients who are not aware of their risk of developing serious complications from CVD and advise these individuals to seek medical care. Similarly, a recent study (34) found that screening for dysglycemia in dental clinics were effective at identifying high-risk patients who required triage for glycemic management.

The findings from our research have clear program significance. Currently, Medicare does not pay for dental services, except if the care is related to hospitalization. Because

TABLE 1.2 | Population Characteristics: Disease Management Gaps Only.

Population characteristics	MDI Clinics $N = 538$	Non-MDI Clinics $N = 538$	*p*-value	Standardized Difference
Baseline gap type				
Disease management alone	538 (100.0%)	538 (100.0%)	NA	NA
Exact-matched variables				
Age (mean ± S.D.; matched within 5 yrs.)	72.5 ± 5.4	72.6 ± 5.4	0.77	0.02
Sex (exact match)				
Male (vs. female)	285 (53.0%)	285 (53.0%)	1.00	0.00
Propensity-matched variables			0.73	
CCI 0	154 (28.6%)	149 (27.7%)		0.01
CCI 1	122 (22.7%)	133 (24.7%)		0.03
CCI 2+	262 (48.7%)	256 (47.6%)		0.01
Current smoker				
Yes (vs. no)	82 (15.2%)	73 (13.6%)	0.44	0.03
ED use in previous 12 months				
Yes (vs. no)	93 (17.3%)	96 (17.8%)	0.81	0.01
Hospitalization in previous 12 months				
Yes (vs. no)	44 (8.2%)	46 (8.6%)	0.83	0.01
Systemic conditions (% yes)				
Diabetes-Mellitus (DM)	325 (60.4%)	320 (59.5%)	0.76	0.01
Rheumatoid Arthritis (RA)	5 (0.9%)	7 (1.3%)	0.56	0.03
Cardiovascular Disease (CVD)	79 (14.7%)	75 (13.9%)	0.73	0.01
Cardiovascular Disease (CAD)	106 (19.7%)	95 (17.7%)	0.39	0.04
Hypertension (HTN)	429 (79.7%)	419 (77.9%)	0.46	0.02
Periodontal disease status			0.32	
Healthy/early	355 (66.0%)	372 (69.1%)		0.03
Moderate	124 (23.1%)	123 (22.9%)		0.00
Advanced	27 (5.0%)	23 (4.3%)		0.02
Missing	32 (6.0%)	20 (3.7%)		0.07
Total open gaps at index visit (mean ± S.D.)	1.5 ± 0.9	1.4 ± 0.9	0.47	0.04
Non-Propensity matched variables				
SES[b]: Area Deprivation Index (ADI) (Mean ± SD)	4.9 ± 2.2	4.5 ± 2.4	0.01	0.16

N = 1,076 (20.9% of total population)[a].
[a]Population includes population of Medicare patients age ≥ 65 with 1+ care gaps at baseline. P-value from t-test for age, count of open gaps at baseline, and ADI state rank; P-value from chi-square for all other variables.
[b]SES, socioeconomic status.

of the clear benefit in promoting the use of preventive and disease management services among the Medicare population, our results suggest that there may be benefits in the Medicare program offering dental insurance coverage to recipients aged 65 years and over.

We recognize several limitations associated with this analysis. First, all data were collected in one healthcare system, potentially limiting generalizability to other populations. While the KPNW membership reflects the underlying population of the area (29, 35), it has a higher proportion older than age 65 compared to the US population overall, suggesting that more research may be needed to determine if these strategies are equally effective in other populations specifically those who are younger (36). Another limitation is that the retrospective cohort design we used does not allow us to assess causality: other differences between MDI and non-MDI clinics, and patients could account for some of the differences between groups. However, this limitation is reduced due to a robust propensity matching of the samples, which reduced the potential impact of confounders on results.

CONCLUSION AND FUTURE RESEARCH

For about 80% of patients in our study, visiting an MDI clinic was associated with higher odds of closing all care gaps than visiting a non-MDI clinic. For patients overdue for both preventive and disease management of care gaps, we found no significant association between MDI and care gap closure.

Further research is needed to understand why there was no difference in care gap closure between MDI and non-MDI for those with both types of care gaps upon dental visit. Possible factors include more gaps to close at baseline and potentially less adherence among patients with both

TABLE 1.3 | Population Characteristics: Both Gaps.

Population characteristics	MDI Clinics *N* = 429	Non-MDI Clinics *N* = 429	*p*-value	Standardized Difference
Baseline gap type				
Both (Preventive and Management)	429 (100.0%)	429 (100.0%)	NA	NA
Exact-matched variables				
Age (mean ± S.D.; matched within 5 yrs.)	69.8 ± 3.9	70.1 ± 4.1	0.34	0.06
Sex (exact match)				
Male (vs. female)	175 (40.8%)	175 (40.8%)	1.00	0.00
Propensity-matched variables			0.55	
CCI 0	187 (43.6%)	173 (40.3%)		0.04
CCI 1	91 (21.2%)	102 (23.8%)		0.04
CCI 2+	151 (35.2%)	154 (35.9%)		0.01
Current smoker				
Yes (vs. no)	74 (17.2%)	72 (16.8%)	0.86	0.01
ED use in previous 12 months				
Yes (vs. no)	58 (13.5%)	62 (14.5%)	0.69	0.02
Hospitalization in previous 12 months				
Yes (vs. no)	23 (5.4%)	26 (6.1%)	0.66	0.02
Systemic conditions (% yes)				
Diabetes-Mellitus (DM)	216 (50.3%)	220 (51.3%)	0.79	0.01
Rheumatoid Arthritis (RA)	5 (1.2%)	4 (0.9%)	0.74	0.02
Cardiovascular Disease (CVD)	37 (8.6)	48 (11.2%)	0.21	0.06
Cardiovascular Disease (CAD)	60 (14.0%)	53 (12.4%)	0.48	0.03
Hypertension (HTN)	312 (72.7%)	322 (75.1%)	0.44	0.02
Periodontal disease status			0.53	
Healthy/early	289 (67.4%)	288 (67.1%)		0.00
Moderate	91 (21.2%)	80 (18.7%)		0.04
Advanced	18 (4.2%)	20 (4.7%)		0.02
Missing	31 (7.2%)	41 (9.6%)		0.06
Total open gaps at index visit (mean ± S.D.)	3.3 ± 1.4	3.4 ± 1.6	0.42	0.06
Non-propensity matched variables				
SES[b]: Area Deprivation Index (ADI) (Mean ± SD)	5.1 ± 2.5	4.8 ± 2.7	0.20	0.09

N = 858 (16.6% of total population)[a].

[a]Population includes Medicare patients age ≥ 65 with 1+ care gaps at baseline. P-value from t-test for age, count of open gaps at baseline, and ADI state rank; P-value from chi-square for all other variables.

[b]SES, socioeconomic status.

MDI clinics = dental offices with integrated medical and dental services.

TABLE 2 | Logistic Regression Analysis of Medical Care Gap Closure[a], by Care Gap Cohort.

	OR	95 % CI	p-value
Population with Preventive Care Gaps Only (*N* = 3,222)			
MDI Population	1.51	1.30-1.75	<0.0001
Non-MDI Population	1.00	–	–
Population with Disease Management Care Gaps Only (*N* = 1,076)			
MDI Population	1.65	1.27-2.15	0.0002
Non-MDI Population	1.00	—	—
Population with both Preventive and Disease Management Care Gaps (*N* = 858)			
MDI Population	0.94	0.62-1.41	NS
Non-MDI Population	1.00	—	—

[a]Population includes Medicare patients age ≥65 with 1+ care gaps at baseline. All care gap closure assessed at 30 days post index visit, except for FIT testing, mammography, annual DM exam, retinopathy exam, and smoking cessation which was assessed at 60 days post index visit. p-value from Logistic Regression Analysis. NS, not statistically significant at p value < 0.05.

types of care gaps. In addition, future research should directly study the costs and benefits of the MDI model. For health systems and policymakers to evaluate the broader implementation of MDI, it is critical to understand the financial costs and benefits of closing medical-related care gaps in the dental setting, especially for the Medicare population. These could include savings due to improved long-term health outcomes of patients whose care gaps are closed due to MDI.

AUTHOR CONTRIBUTIONS

All authors of the study have met authorship criteria established by the International Committee of Medical Journal Editors statement of Uniform Requirements for Manuscripts submitted to Biomedical Journals. In that regard, all of the co-authors are responsible for the reported research, participated in the concept and design, analysis and interpretation of data, drafting or revising of the manuscript, and have approved the manuscript as submitted.

REFERENCES

1. Kuo LC, Polson AM, Kang T. Associations between periodontal diseases and systemic diseases: a review of the inter-relationships and interactions with diabetes, respiratory diseases, cardiovascular diseases and osteoporosis. *Public Health.* (2008) 122:417–33. doi: 10.1016/j.puhe.2007.07.004
2. Lamster IB, Lalla E, Borgnakke WS, Taylor GW. The relationship between oral health and diabetes mellitus. *J Am Dent Assoc.* (2008) 139:19–24s. doi: 10.14219/jada.archive.2008.0363
3. Skamagas M, Breen TL, LeRoith D. Update on diabetes mellitus: prevention, treatment, and association with oral diseases. *Oral Dis.* (2008) 14:105–14. doi: 10.1111/j.1601-0825.2007.01425.x
4. Taylor GW, Borgnakke WS. Periodontal disease: associations with diabetes, glycemic control and complications. *Oral Dis.* (2008) 14:191–203. doi: 10.1111/j.1601-0825.2008.01442.x
5. Borgnakke WS, Ylostalo PV, Taylor GW, Genco RJ. Effect of periodontal disease on diabetes: systematic review of epidemiologic observational evidence. *J Periodontol.* (2013) 84:S135–52. doi: 10.1111/jcpe.12080
6. Engebretson S, Kocher T. Evidence that periodontal treatment improves diabetes outcomes: a systematic review and meta-analysis. *J Periodontol.* (2013) 84:S153–69. doi: 10.1902/jop.2013.1340017
7. Pihlstrom BL, Michalowicz BS, Johnson NW. Periodontal diseases. *Lancet.* (2005) 366:1809–20. doi: 10.1016/S0140-6736(05)67728-8
8. Dietrich T, Sharma P, Walter C, Weston P, Beck J. The epidemiological evidence behind the association between periodontitis and incident atherosclerotic cardiovascular disease. *J Periodontol.* (2013) 84:S70–84. doi: 10.1902/jop.2013.134008
9. Beck JD, Offenbacher S, Williams R, Gibbs P, Garcia R. Periodontitis: a risk factor for coronary heart disease? *Ann Periodontol.* (1998) 3:127–41. doi: 10.1902/annals.1998.3.1.127
10. Schenkein HA, Loos BG. Inflammatory mechanisms linking periodontal diseases to cardiovascular diseases. *J Periodontol.* (2013) 84:S51–69. doi: 10.1902/jop.2013.134006
11. Beck JD, Moss KL, Morelli T, Offenbacher S. Periodontal profile class is associated with prevalent diabetes, coronary heart disease, stroke, and systemic markers of C-reactive protein and interleukin-6. *J Periodontol.* (2018) 89:157–65. doi: 10.1002/JPER.17-0426
12. Pradeep AR, Hadge P, Arjun Raju P, Shetty SR, Shareef K, Guruprasad CN. Periodontitis as a risk factor for cerebrovascular accident: a case-control study in the Indian population. *J Periodontal Res.* (2010) 45:223–8. doi: 10.1111/j.1600-0765.2009.01220.x
13. Grau AJ, Becher H, Ziegler CM, Lichy C, Buggle F, Kaiser C, et al. Periodontal disease as a risk factor for ischemic stroke. *Stroke.* (2004) 35:496–501. doi: 10.1161/01.STR.0000110789.20526.9D
14. Macedo Paizan ML, Vilela-Martin JF. Is there an association between periodontitis and hypertension? *Curr Cardiol Rev.* (2014) 10:355–61. doi: 10.2174/1573403X10666140416094901
15. Rivas-Tumanyan S, Campos M, Zevallos JC, Joshipura KJ. Periodontal disease, hypertension, and blood pressure among older adults in Puerto Rico. *J Periodontol.* (2013) 84:203–11. doi: 10.1902/jop.2012.110748
16. Linden GJ, Lyons A, Scannapieco FA. Periodontal systemic associations: review of the evidence. *J Periodontol.* (2013) 84:S8–19. doi: 10.1902/jop.2013.1340010
17. Chen HH, Huang N, Chen YM, Chen TJ, Chou P, Lee YL, et al. Association between a history of periodontitis and the risk of rheumatoid arthritis: a nationwide, population-based, case-control study. *Ann Rheum Dis.* (2013) 72:1206–11. doi: 10.1136/annrheumdis-2012-201593
18. Kaur S, White S, Bartold PM. Periodontal disease and rheumatoid arthritis: a systematic review. *J Dent Res.* (2013) 92:399–408. doi: 10.1177/0022034513483142
19. Eke PI, Dye BA, Wei L, Thornton-Evans GO, Genco RJ, CDC Periodontal Disease Surveillance workgroup, et al. Prevalence of periodontitis in adults in the United States: 2009 and 2010. *J Dent Res.* (2012) 91:914–20. doi: 10.1177/0022034512457373
20. Eke PI, Borgnakke WS, Genco RJ. Recent epidemiologic trends in periodontitis in the USA. *Periodontology.* (2020) 82:257–67. doi: 10.1111/prd.12323
21. Lochner KA, Cox CS. Prevalence of multiple chronic conditions among Medicare beneficiaries, United States, (2010). *Prev Chronic Dis.* (2013) 10:E61. doi: 10.5888/pcd10.120137
22. Buttorff C, Ruder T, Bauman M. *Multiple Chronic Conditions in the United States.* Santa Monica, CA: RAND (2017).
23. Jontell M, Glick M. Oral health care professionals' identification of cardiovascular disease risk among patients in private dental offices in Sweden. *J Am Dent Assoc.* (2009) 140:1385–91. doi: 10.14219/jada.archive.2009.0075
24. Glurich I, Bartkowiak B, Berg RL, Acharya A. Screening for dysglycaemia in dental primary care practice settings: systematic review of the evidence. *Int Dent J.* (2018) 68:369–77. doi: 10.1111/idj.12405
25. Mosen DM, Banegas MP, Dickerson JF, Fellows JL, Brooks NB, Pihlstrom DJ, et al. Examining the association of medical-dental integration with closure of medical care gaps among the elderly population. *J Am Dent Assoc.* (2021) 152:302–8. doi: 10.1016/j.adaj.2020.12.010
26. American Diabetes Association. Standards of medical care in diabetes—2014. *Diabetes Care.* (2014) 37(Suppl. 1):S14–80. doi: 10.2337/dc14-S014
27. US Preventive Services Task Force Guides to Clinical Preventive Services. *The Guide to Clinical Preventive Services 2014: Recommendations of the U.S. Preventive Services Task Force.* Rockville, MD: Agency for Healthcare Research and Quality (US) (2014).
28. Arnett DK, Blumenthal RS, Albert MA, Buroker AB, ZD, Hahn EJ, et al. 2019 ACC/AHA guideline on the primary prevention of cardiovascular disease: a report of the American College of Cardiology/American Heart Association Task Force on Clinical Practice Guidelines. *J Am Coll Cardiol.* (2019) 74:e177–232. doi: 10.1016/j.jacc.2019.03.010
29. Livaudais G, Unitan R, Post J. Total panel ownership and the panel support tool- "It's All About the Relationship". *Perm J.* (2006) 10:72–9. doi: 10.7812/TPP/06-002
30. Cohen J. *Statistical Power Analysis for the Behavioral Sciences.* 2nd ed. Hillsdale, NJ: Erlbaum (1988).
31. Austin PC. Balance diagnostics for comparing the distribution of baseline covariates between treatment groups in propensity-score matched samples. *Stat Med.* (2009) 28:3083–107. doi: 10.1002/sim.3697
32. Johnson ES, Dickerson JF, Vollmer WM, Rowley AM, Ritenbaugh C, Deyo RA, et al. The feasibility of matching on a propensity score for acupuncture in a prospective cohort study of patients with chronic pain. *BMC Med Res Methodol.* (2017) 17:42. doi: 10.1186/s12874-017-0318-4
33. Knighton AJ, Savitz L, Belnap T, Stephenson B, VanDerslice J. Introduction of an area deprivation index measuring patient socioeconomic status in an integrated health system: implications for population health. *EGEMS.* (2016) 4:1238. doi: 10.13063/2327-9214.1238
34. Genco RJ, Schifferle RE, Dunford RG, Falkner KL, Hsu WC, Balukjian J. Screening for diabetes mellitus in dental practices: a field trial. *J Am Dent Assoc.* (2014) 145:57–64. doi: 10.14219/jada.2013.7

35. Smith SC Jr., Allen J, Blair SN, Bonow RO, Brass LM, Fonarow GC, et al. AHA/ACC guidelines for secondary prevention for patients with coronary and other atherosclerotic vascular disease: 2006 update: endorsed by the National Heart, Lung, and Blood Institute. *Circulation.* (2006) 113:2363–72. doi: 10.1161/CIRCULATIONAHA.106.174516
36. Vespa J, Armstrong DM, Medina L. *Demographic Turning Points for the United States: Population Projections for 2020 to 2060.* Washington, DC United States Census Bureau (2018). p. 25–1144.

8

Haemophilus pittmaniae and *Leptotrichia* spp. Constitute a Multi-Marker Signature in a Cohort of Human Papillomavirus-Positive Head and Neck Cancer Patients

Jean-Luc C. Mougeot[1], Micaela F. Beckman[1], Holden C. Langdon[1], Rajesh V. Lalla[2], Michael T. Brennan[1] and Farah K. Bahrani Mougeot[1]**

[1] Carolinas Medical Center—Atrium Health, Charlotte, NC, United States, [2] Section of Oral Medicine–University of Connecticut Health, Farmington, CT, United States

***Correspondence:**
Jean-Luc C. Mougeot
jean-luc.mougeot@atriumhealth.org
Farah K. Bahrani Mougeot
farah.mougeot@atriumhealth.org

Objectives: Human papillomavirus (HPV) is a known etiological factor of oropharyngeal head and neck cancer (HNC). HPV positivity and periodontal disease have been associated with higher HNC risk, suggesting a role for oral bacterial species. Our objective was to determine oral microbiome profiles in HNC patients (HPV-positive and HPV-negative) and in healthy controls (HC).

Methods: Saliva samples and swabs of buccal mucosa, supragingival plaque, and tongue were collected from HNC patients (N = 23 patients, n = 92 samples) before cancer therapy. Next-generation sequencing (16S-rRNA gene V3–V4 region) was used to determine bacterial taxa relative abundance (RA). β-Diversities of HNC HPV+ (N = 16 patients, n = 64 samples) and HNC HPV– (N = 7 patients, n = 28 samples) groups were compared using PERMANOVA (pMonte Carlo < 0.05). LEfSe discriminant analysis was performed to identify differentiating taxa (Log LDA > 2.0). RA differences were analyzed by Mann–Whitney U-test (α = 0.05). CombiROC program was used to determine multi-marker bacterial signatures. The Microbial Interaction Network Database (MIND) and LitSuggest online tools were used for complementary analyses.

Results: HNC vs. HC and HNC HPV+ vs. HNC HPV– β-diversities differed significantly (pMonte Carlo < 0.05). *Streptococcus* was the most abundant genus for HNC and HC groups, while *Rothia mucilaginosa* and *Haemophilus parainfluenzae* were the most abundant species in HNC and HC patients, respectively, regardless of antibiotics treatment. LEfSe analysis identified 43 and 44 distinctive species for HNC HPV+ and HNC HPV– groups, respectively. In HNC HPV+ group, 26 periodontal disease-associated species identified by LefSe had a higher average RA compared to HNC HPV– group. The significant species included *Alloprevotella tannerae*, *Fusobacterium periodonticum*, *Haemophilus pittmaniae*, *Lachnoanaerobaulum orale*, and *Leptotrichia* spp. (Mann–Whitney U-test, p < 0.05). Of 43 LEfSe-identified species in HPV+ group, 31 had a higher RA compared to HPV– group (Mann–Whitney U-test,

$p < 0.05$). MIND analysis confirmed interactions between *Haemophilus* and *Leptotrichia* spp., representing a multi-marker signature per CombiROC analysis [area under the curve (AUC) > 0.9]. LitSuggest correctly classified 15 articles relevant to oral microbiome and HPV status.

Conclusion: Oral microbiome profiles of HNC HPV+ and HNC HPV– patients differed significantly regarding periodontal-associated species. Our results suggest that oral bacterial species (e.g., *Leptotrichia* spp.), possessing unique niches and invasive properties, coexist with HPV within HPV-induced oral lesions in HNC patients. Further investigation into host–microbe interactions in HPV-positive HNC patients may shed light into cancer development.

Keywords: head and neck cancer, HPV, oral microbiome, next generation sequencing, *Leptotrichia* spp.

INTRODUCTION

Head and neck cancer (HNC) is the sixth most common cancer worldwide with over 95% comprising squamous cell carcinomas (SCCs) (Jemal et al., 2008; Kumarasamy et al., 2019). Head and neck SCCs are characterized by a locoregional development mainly diagnosed at an advanced stage of the disease, resulting in difficult treatment and eradication of both pre-neoplastic and neoplastic tissue (Carvalho et al., 2005; Ganci et al., 2015). Despite advancements in chemoradiation, ionizing radiation, and surgical resection techniques, HNC has an overall mortality rate of approximately 50% and is characterized by high recurrence rates (Carvalho et al., 2005). While triggers of HNC development have not been fully elucidated, two primary risk factors have been identified, namely, alcohol and tobacco consumptions (Božinović et al., 2019). Most recent studies have identified infection with human papillomavirus (HPV) as a third and more prominent cause of tumor formation (Božinović et al., 2019). HPV-associated SCCs represent the most common HPV-related cancer in the US and are classified by a new staging system for oropharyngeal cancers (National Cancer Institute[1]: van Gysen et al., 2019).

HPV-positive (HPV+) HNC patients are often younger and present with a more advanced cancer stage than HPV-negative (HPV–) HNC patients (Blitzer et al., 2014). It has been reported that the majority of HPV-associated HNCs are caused by HPV16, though more than 220 HPV serotypes have been identified (Tumban, 2019). Two HPV genes, E6 and E7, have been the matter of extensive research due to their role as oncogenes (Yim and Park, 2005). These genes are involved in multiple pathways such as transmembrane signaling, cell cycle regulation, and cell transformation (Yim and Park, 2005). E6 has been shown to promote degradation of tumor suppressor TP53 (Crook et al., 1991), while E7 is able to inhibit retinoblastoma protein (Pal and Kundu, 2020). Aside from E6 and E7, the E5 HPV gene promotes malignancy, has anti-apoptotic effects and plays a role in epidermal growth factor (EGF) receptor-regulated cell proliferation (Venuti et al., 2011).

[1]https://www.cancer.gov/about-cancer/causes-prevention/risk/infectious-agents/hpv-and-cancer

There is a mounting body of evidence that a synergistic interaction between periodontal disease-associated pathogens and HPV exists. Indeed, a case–control study by Tezal et al. (2009) found that HPV+ tumors in 21 patients had a significantly higher alveolar bone loss mean and a fourfold increased risk for HPV+ tumor status for every millimeter of alveolar bone loss caused by periodontal disease.

Overall, without implying a causal effect, a link between oral microbiome dysbiosis and cancer has been suggested by several studies (Kudo et al., 2016; Hayes et al., 2018; Mohammed et al., 2018; Wu et al., 2018; Mougeot et al., 2020). For instance, *Fusobacterium nucleatum* was found overabundant in the oral cavity of patients with colon cancer and lymph node metastasis (Kudo et al., 2016). *F. nucleatum* might initiate oncogenic and proinflammatory responses that stimulate the growth of colon cancer cells (Kudo et al., 2016). Increased levels of blood serum antibodies against the oral bacterial species *Porphyromonas gingivalis* was associated with a twofold higher risk of pancreatic cancer when compared to healthy individuals (Mohammed et al., 2018).

Furthermore, the increased prevalence of *P. gingivalis* and *Aggregatibacter actinomycetemcomitans* was shown to initiate a Toll-like receptor signaling pathway predictive of pancreatic cancer in animal models (Mohammed et al., 2018). Higher levels of firmicutes and bacteroidetes also constitute a potential risk for gastric cancer (Wu et al., 2018). A study by Hayes et al. (2018) suggested an association between the oral microbiome and HNC.

HNC has also been associated with oral cavity diseases such as periodontal disease and dental caries (Michaud et al., 2017; Gasparoni et al., 2021). Periodontitis disrupts the normal oral microbial environment, thereby leading to dysbiosis. Dysbiosis can translate into an abundance shift of opportunistic species, like *P. gingivalis*, which produce several virulence factors resulting in the destruction of periodontal tissues (Rafiei et al., 2017). Chronic periodontitis can result in the release of proinflammatory cytokines from squamous cells, causing inflammation and possible decreased apoptosis (Gholizadeh et al., 2016). In a meta-analysis by Zeng et al. (2013) HNC cancer risk was found to be increased by 2.63-fold in patients with periodontitis.

Using 16S rRNA gene next-generation sequencing and computational approaches, the purpose of this study was to compare microbiome profiles of a limited cohort of HNC patients to those of healthy control subjects, and profiles of HNC HPV+ patients to those of HNC HPV– patients, within the HNC cohort. We also aimed to determine whether bacterial species differentiating HPV+ from HPV– HNC patients are associated with periodontal disease-associated species.

MATERIALS AND METHODS

Patient Recruitment

HNC patients with SCC [N = 30; 8 females, 22 males, age range = 23–75 years (SD = ± 12.02)] were recruited from the OraRad study (U01DE022939) (Brennan et al., 2017; Lalla et al., 2017). OraRad was a multicenter cohort study that collected longitudinal data on radiation-treated HNC patients at 6-month intervals for 2 years. Primary cancer site origin included the base of the tongue, tonsil, neck, tongue, and oral cavity.

Of 30 HNC patients, 23 were clinically classified as HPV+/– into 16 HPV+ and 7 HPV– patients. In addition, healthy control subjects (HC group) (N = 20; age range 24–84, SD = –12.93) were recruited through Atrium Health's Carolinas Medical Center, Charlotte, NC. Of 30 HNC patients, 11 had received antibiotic treatment within 2 weeks of sampling. No HC subject had received antibiotic treatment. The study was approved by the institutional review board, and all participants gave informed consent for the study.

Sample Collection

Saliva (S) samples and swab samples of buccal mucosa (B), supragingival plaque (P), and tongue (T) were collected from HNC patients, pre-cancer treatment at baseline, and from HC subjects. Saliva collection was performed while chewing unsweetened and unflavored gum (The Wrigley Company—Mars, Chicago, IL, United States) for a period of 2 min into a 50-ml conical BD falcon polypropylene centrifuge tube (Corning, Corning, NY, United States).

Buccal mucosal samples were subsequently collected by swabbing both sides of the buccal mucosa for 10 s each. Tongue samples were then obtained by swabbing a 1-cm^2 region on both sides of the mid-dorsal region of the tongue for 5 s. Finally, supragingival plaque samples were obtained by swabbing across the lateral surfaces of all maxillary and mandibular teeth at the junction of the tooth and gingiva. All swab collections were performed using OmniSwabs (GE Life Sciences-Buckinghamshire, United Kingdom).

Bacterial DNA Extraction, Processing, and Sequencing

Bacterial genomic DNA was extracted from oral samples using QIAamp DNA Mini Kit procedure (QIAGEN, Valencia, CA, United States) per manufacturers' instructions. During sample preparation, 50 ng of genomic DNA was used for PCR in which the 16S rRNA gene (V3–V4) region was amplified, followed by purification and processing methods as previously described (Caporaso et al., 2011). Next-generation sequencing was performed using the MiSeq v3 reagent kit and platform (Illumina, Inc., San Diego, CA, United States). To prepare for cluster generation and sequencing, libraries were denatured with NaOH and diluted with a hybridization buffer. Libraries then underwent heat denaturation prior to MiSeq sequencing. Total of 100 ng of each library was pooled together, run on a gel, gel-extracted, and run on a bioanalyzer for quantification. A total concentration of 4 nM of the library was then diluted, and 12 pM of the library was spiked with 20% PhiX. At least 5% PhiX was added as an internal control for low-diversity libraries. Identification of bacterial genera and species was performed using Human Oral Microbe Identification, HOMI*NGS*, which employs a ProbeSeq BLAST program for species/genera identification through recognition of the 16S rRNA gene (V3–V4 region) sequence reads (Caporaso et al., 2011; Mougeot et al., 2016). ProbeSeq loads raw sequence files into a cell array, looping through the array one sequence at a time searching for small sequence strings that 100% match an oligomer (partials are not considered matches). If a match is identified, a counter begins giving counts of the total number of probe-specific "hits." Hits are then accumulated by species/genera and sample.

The sequence reads were matched to 737 ProbeSeq taxon probes, i.e., to species probes (n = 620) or genus probes (n = 117) if not matched to a species probe, or were otherwise recorded as an unmatched read. Matched and unmatched probe count data were provided per taxon per patient as Excel spreadsheets. Species/genus probes containing zeros for all samples were removed from the dataset. Raw abundance data were then transformed into relative abundance (RA) data for further analysis.

Bioinformatic Analysis

α-Diversity

Shannon and Simpson indices were generated using PRIMER$_{v7}$ (PRIMER-E Ltd., Ivybridge, United Kingdom) (Clarke and Gorley, 2006), based on microbiome RA data. RA data of HC subjects (HC group: N = 20) were compared to the RA data of HNC patients including those with antibiotic treatment within 2 weeks of sampling (Grp-All: N = 30). RA data of HC group were also compared to RA data of HNC patients excluding those with antibiotic treatment (Grp-NoAB: N = 19). Subsequently, comparisons of HPV+ vs. HPV– HNC sub-cohorts were performed by including or excluding patients who received antibiotic treatment. Mann–Whitney U-tests were then used to determine significant RA comparisons (α = 0.05) using XLSTAT$_{v2016.02.29253}$ (Data Analysis and Statistical Solution for Microsoft Excel, Addinsoft, Paris, France, 2017).

Permutational Multivariate Analysis of Variance

Patient subgroups used for permutational multivariate analysis of variance (PERMANOVA) included Grp-All (HNC: N = 30; HC: N = 20) and Grp-noAB (HNC: N = 19; HC: N = 20). Sub-analyses were performed based on the multiple sample site combinations "BPST," "BST," and "PST" which provided sufficient power in PRIMER$_{v7}$ program (PRIMER-E Ltd., Ivybridge, United Kingdom) (Clarke and Gorley, 2006) for all

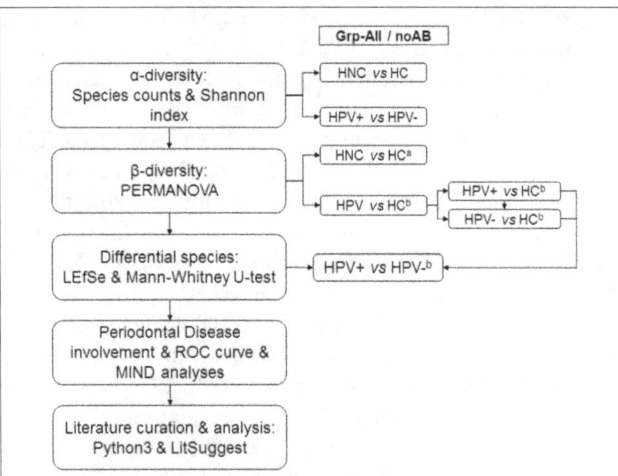

FIGURE 1 | Overall analytical strategy. α-Diversity was calculated for Grp-All HNC vs. HC ($N = 30$; $N = 20$) and HPV+ vs. HPV– ($N = 16$; $N = 7$) and for Grp-noAB HNC vs. HC ($N = 19$; $N = 20$) and HPV+ vs. HPV– ($N = 12$; $N = 3$). Sample sites consisted of different combinations of buccal (B), plaque (P), saliva (S), and tongue (T) samples. β-Diversity was calculated using PERMANOVA by two different analytical designs: (1) [a]Analytical design with "Diagnosis" and "Sample site" as fixed factors and "Antibiotic" as the nested random factor. Comparisons were Grp-All HNC vs. HC and Grp-noAB HNC vs. HC. (2) [b]Analytical design with "HPV status" and "Sample site" as fixed factors and "Antibiotic" as the nested random factor. Grp-All comparisons were as follows: HPV vs. HC ($N = 23$; $N = 20$), HPV+ vs. HC ($N = 16$; $N = 20$), HPV– vs. HC ($N = 7$; $N = 20$), and HPV+ vs. HPV– ($N = 16$; $N = 7$). Grp-noAB comparisons were as follows: HPV vs. HC ($N = 15$; $N = 20$), HPV+ vs. HC ($N = 12$; $N = 20$), HPV– vs. HC ($N = 3$; $N = 20$), and HPV+ vs. HPV– ($N = 12$; $N = 3$). Distinct species were determined using LEfSe and Mann–Whitney *U*-tests for Grp-All and Grp-noAB comparisons of HPV+ vs. HPV– for the sample site combination BPST. Significant LEfSe bacterial species for HPV+ group were investigated for their roles in periodontal disease using conventional methods (PubMed, Google Scholar, etc.). Significant LEfSe HPV+ species using the Mann–Whitney *U*-test were analyzed by using MedCalc ROC curve analysis. Multi-marker combinatorial analysis was completed using CombiROC online tool (http://combiroc.eu/) for the bacterial species identified with MedCalc log(RA + 1) ROC curve AUC of 0.75 or greater ($n = 10$ species). CombiROC utilized raw RA data and log(RA + 1) transformed data. Microbial Interaction Network Database (MIND) online tool was used to identify possible interactions between most significant bacterial species. Python$_{v3.6.2}$ code was used to extract PubMed abstracts matching key words to determine positive and negative training sets and were validated manually. Using NCBI LitSuggest online tool (https://www.ncbi.nlm.nih.gov/research/litsuggest/), 203 PubMed articles were classified to identify articles involving HPV infection in the oral microbiome.

five relevant comparisons (**Figure 1**). Species and genera RA data were square root transformed and converted into Bray–Curtis similarity matrices.

PERMANOVA analyses were performed using a mixed model with unrestricted permutation of raw data, 9,999 permutations, and type III partial sum of squares (Clarke and Gorley, 2006), as previously implemented (Mougeot et al., 2019, 2020). Fixed factors were "Diagnosis" (e.g., HNC vs. HC) and "Sample site" (B, P, S, and T). In this design, the "Antibiotic" treatment (yes or no) variable was used as a random factor nested into "Diagnosis" and "Sample site." Monte Carlo corrected *p*-values ($\alpha = 0.05$) were determined, as appropriate for relatively small sample sizes.

Principal coordinate analysis (PCoA) was completed for the Grp-All: HNC vs. HC BPST sample site combination.

β Diversity Sub-Analyses

Sub-analyses were completed using subsets of Grp-All and Grp-noAB patients, based on $n = 3$ or 4 sample sites per patient (BPST, BST, and PST): HPV+ ($N = 16$) vs. HPV– ($N = 7$) and HPV+ ($N = 12$) vs. HPV– ($N = 3$), respectively. The sample site combinations BPST, BST, and PST and the previously mentioned data transformation were used for PERMANOVAs in PRIMER$_{v7}$ program. Fixed factors used were "HPV status" (positive and negative) and "Sample site" (B, P, S, and T). "Antibiotic" (yes or no) was used as a random factor and nested into "HPV status" and "Sample site." Monte Carlo corrected *p*-values ($\alpha = 0.05$) were determined. PCoA was completed for the Grp-All: HPV+ vs. HPV– BPST sample site combination.

Linear Discriminant Analysis Effect Size

Taxonomy levels were added manually to ProbeSeq derived datasets for Grp-All (HPV+ vs. HPV–) and Grp-noAB (HPV+ vs. HPV–) subsets. The text files were then formatted for linear discriminant analysis (LDA) effect size (LEfSe) using the Galaxy$_{v1.0}$ online tool (Jalili et al., 2020). LEfSe data input consisted of "HPV status" as the option "Class" and "Patient ID" as the option "Subject" (Segata et al., 2011). Data were normalized. Using the "one-against-all" strategy for multi-class analysis, the factorial Kruskal–Wallis test and pairwise Wilcoxon signed-rank test were set at a Monte Carlo significance ($\alpha = 0.05$) to calculate LDA scores. Log LDA scores were set at a threshold > 2.0. Histograms of the differential features (species) were generated, and each species was investigated for its role in periodontal disease.

Receiver-Operating Characteristic Curve Analyses

Conventional Receiver-Operating Characteristic Analysis

Mann–Whitney *U*-tests were completed for LEfSe differential features for HPV+ species probes from Grp-All and Grp-noAB groups. Significant species probes ($\alpha = 0.05$) further underwent receiver-operating characteristic (ROC) curve analysis for Grp-All HPV+ and Grp-noAB HPV+ species probes using the BPST sample combination in MedCalc program (MedCalc Software Ltd, Ostend, Belgium).

RA data were log-transformed with the addition of a pseudo-count [i.e., log(RA + 1)]. Analysis was completed for Grp-All (HPV+; $n = 64$ samples and HPV–; $n = 28$ samples) and Grp-noAB (HPV+; $n = 48$ samples and HPV–; $n = 12$ samples) groups and for each non-zero RA probe in MedCalc program. The area under the curve (AUC) of each probe was calculated, and ROC curves were generated. Significance level was set at $\alpha = 0.05$, and biomarker accuracy was calculated using methods described by Ray et al. (2010).

CombiROC Analysis

ROC curves from MedCalc that had an AUC greater than 0.75 were subjected to combinatorial analysis using CombiROC online tool[2] (Mazzara et al., 2017) based on raw RA data and log(RA + 1) transformed RA data. Using CombiROC, marker profile plots were generated to confirm quality, and the detection threshold was set to 0.001. Using this threshold, combinational analysis was performed which calculated the sensitivity and specificity scores for each marker or combination of markers corresponding to the probability that the microbial data will be positive when HPV is present and the probability that microbial data will be negative when HPV is not present.

A minimum feature filter was set to include at least two markers. Based on a threshold of 10 for sensitivity and 50 for specificity, the best or "gold" combinations of markers were kept, thereby creating optimal multi-marker ROC curves and violin plots. Summary statistics were calculated and recorded for the top two AUC scores of the raw and log(RA + 1) transformed RA data.

Microbial Interaction Network Database Analysis

A microbial interaction network was created to illustrate possible interactions between *Haemophilus* spp. and *Leptotrichia* spp. with other bacterial genera or species, by using Microbial Interaction Network Database ($MIND_{v1.0}$) (Microbial Interaction Network Database, 2019). Default options were selected for human tissue sites, interaction weight, and health or disease conditions.

LitSuggest

An application programming interface was established using the National Center for Biotechnology Information guidelines (National Center for Biotechnology Information, 1988) and $Python_{v3.6.2}$ (van Rossum and Drake, 2009). $Python_{v3.6.2}$ was used to generate classifiers by extracting abstracts from PubMed (1997) through the keywords (i) "oral microbiome" and "HPV" to constitute a positive training set, (ii) "vaginal microbiome" and "HPV" keywords to constitute the negative training set, and (iii) "HPV" and "microbiome" to constitute the test set. Positive and negative training set abstracts were then manually validated. Using the NCBI LitSuggest[3] online tool; a total of 19 positively and 104 negatively classified articles were used to train the model (Allot et al., 2021). Test set classification was then completed using LitSuggest, and full articles were manually verified for relevancy.

RESULTS

The overall analytical strategy is presented in **Figure 1**. Demographics and clinical information of our HNC patient cohort (*N* = 30 patients, sub-cohort of OraRad study) are presented in **Table 1**. Clinical information, including caries and periodontal disease status for OraRad HNC patient cohort, associated with HPV status (*N* = 559 of 572 total patients) has been published elsewhere (Brennan et al., 2021). While no significant differences were noted in age and ethnicity, the male population was over-represented in the HNC patient set in OraRad and this study, as anticipated for oral SCC in general and for HPV-associated oropharyngeal cancers (Fakhry et al., 2018; Mahal et al., 2019). In our sub-cohort, most HPV+ HNC patients had oropharyngeal cancer (e.g., tonsil, base of tongue), whereas most of the HPV– HNC patients had cancer in other sites (**Table 1**).

Abundance, Species Detection, and α-Diversity

Probe count data are provided as **Supplementary Data Files** and can be downloaded from our lab's Github repository[4] (**Supplementary Data Files 1, 2**). Sequencing reads matched 737 total probes (117 genera and 620 species probes) for all samples from HNC and HC groups combined. Comparisons of species and genera detected for HNC vs. HC and HPV+ vs. HPV– are presented in **Supplementary Table 1**. Unmatched reads were removed from RA determinations. For all samples sequencing data, 442 of 620 species probes and 65 of 117 genus probes had at least one matched read. Significant α-diversity differences were identified for Grp-All and Grp-noAB for HNC vs. HC and Grp-noAB HNC vs. HC for the matched sample site combinations BPST, BST, and PST (**Table 2**). *Streptococcus* was the most abundant genus for HNC and HC groups, whereas *Rothia mucilaginosa* and *Haemophilus parainfluenzae* were the most abundant species detected in HNC patients and HC, respectively. Excluding HNC patients treated with antibiotics (Grp-noAB) did not affect these results (data not shown). Overall, the highest and lowest average number of taxa detected per sample were 96.08 and 117.66 for species probes and 24.75 and 26.83 for genus probes (**Supplementary Table 1**).

β-Diversity Analysis

PERMANOVA β-diversity analyses were performed for sample site combinations providing sufficient power based on available oral microbiome data (i.e., BPST, BST, and PST). Significance of β-diversity analyses is presented in **Figure 2**. For the Grp-All comparisons, including HNC HPV+ vs. HNC HPV– comparisons, all but one (i.e., HPV+ vs. HC, BST, pMonte Carlo = 0.261) were significant, regardless of the sample site combinations analyzed. All Grp-noAB comparisons were found significant for "HPV status" and "Sample site." Monte Carlo corrected *p*-values of all comparisons are presented in **Supplementary Table 2**. PCoA plots describing the variations explaining dissimilarity between groups (i.e., HNC vs. HC and HPV+ vs. HPV–) are presented in **Supplementary Figure 1**.

LEfSe Analysis

A total of 44 and 43 species were identified for Grp-All HPV– and HPV+, respectively. A histogram of the differential features is presented in **Figure 3A**. Species of the genera *Actinomyces* and *Leptotrichia* were the most representative of HPV– and HPV+ patient groups, respectively. A total of 52 and 38 species were identified for Grp-noAB HPV– and HPV+, respectively (**Figure 3B**). *Leptotrichia* spp. were the most represented taxa for

[2]http://combiroc.eu

[3]https://www.ncbi.nlm.nih.gov/research/litsuggest

[4]https://github.com/mbeckm01/HPV_HNC.git

TABLE 1 | Patient demographics and clinical characteristics.

	HNC[a]	HC[b]	Combined[c]	HNC HPV+[d]	HNC HPV−[e]	Combined[f]
Patient count (Male/Female)	30 (22/8)	20 (5/15)	50 (27/23)	16 (12/4)	7 (5/2)	23 (17/6)
Antibiotic treatment (Yes/No)	11/19	0/20	11/39	4/12	4/3	8/15
Primary cancer site						
Base of tongue	4		4	4	0	4
Nasopharynx	2		2	1	1	2
Oral cavity	1		1	0	1	1
Oropharynx	1		1	1	0	1
Supraglottis	1		1	0	1	1
Tongue	1		1	0	1	1
Tonsil	8		8	8	0	8
Unknown	5		5	2	3	5
Age:						
Median	55	55	55	54	61	54
Mean	54	52.7	54	54	51	53
Std Dev	12.02	15.29	12.93	6.47	20.29	11.93
Range	23–75	24–84	23–84	40–68	23–75	23–75
Ethnicity count						
M: Caucasian/African American	22/0	5/0	27/0	12/0	5/0	17/0
F: Caucasian/African American	7/1	13/2	20/3	3/1	2/0	5/1
Whole mouth average PD				2.28 (2.03–2.52)	2.09 (1.78–2.40)	2.26 (2.06–2.46)
Whole mouth average CAL				1.74 (1.42–2.07)	1.64 (1.02–2.26)	1.73 (1.46–2.01)
Sample combinations[g]						
BPST	120	80	200	64	28	92
BST	120	72	192	54	30	84
PST	105	69	174	54	21	75
BPS	93	63	156			

[a]*Head and neck cancer (HNC) patient group (primary cancer sites: base of tongue = 4; nasopharynx = 2; oral cavity = 1; oropharynx = 1; supraglottis = 1; tongue = 1; tonsil = 8; unknown = 5).*

[b]*Healthy control (HC) subject group.*

[c]*HNC and HC patient groups combined.*

[d]*HNC human papillomavirus positive (HPV+) patient group (primary cancer sites (N = 16); base of tongue = 4; nasopharynx = 1; oral cavity = 0; oropharynx = 1; supraglottis = 0; tongue = 0; tonsil = 8; unknown = 2).*

[e]*HNC human papillomavirus negative (HPV–) patient group (primary cancer sites (N = 7); base of tongue = 0; nasopharynx = 1; oral cavity = 1; oropharynx = 0; supraglottis = 1; tongue = 1; tonsil = 0; unknown = 3).*

[f]*HNC HPV+ and HPV– patient groups combined.*

[g]*Number of samples for site combinations including B (buccal), P (plaque), S (saliva), and/or T (tongue).*

PD, probing depth; CAL, clinical attachment loss; Std Dev, standard deviation. PD and CAL are shown as the average with 95% confidence intervals in parentheses. Mann–Whitney U-tests comparing whole mouth average PD and whole mouth average CAL separately for HPV+ vs. HPV– patient groups were not found to be significantly different (p > 0.05).

Grp-noAB HPV+ patients, and *Prevotella* spp. were the most represented ones for Grp-noAB HPV– patients. A total of 26 of 43 species in Grp-All HPV+ group (60.5%) and 24 of 38 species in Grp-noAB HPV+ group (63.2%) were recognized for their involvement in periodontal disease by performing manual searches in PubMed (**Supplementary Table 3**).

Receiver-Operating Characteristic Determination

Using the Mann–Whitney *U*-test, 31 of 43 bacterial species in Grp-All HPV+ and 29 of 38 bacterial species in Grp-noAB HPV+ LEfSe were significant ($p < 0.05$) (**Figures 3A,B**). Using MedCalc ROC curve analysis, one species (*Lachnoanaerobaculum sp083*) in Grp-All HPV+ was found not significant. All species in Grp-noAB HPV+ were, however, significant ($p < 0.01$). By minimizing zero inflation, we found 17 of the 31 Grp-All HPV+ species and 16 of the 29 Grp-noAB HPV+ species to be significant (MedCalc Software Ltd, Ostend, Belgium). Minimization of zero inflation is required to optimize ROC analysis for the bacterial species which are more consistently detected across subjects and to increase the "signal-to-noise" ratio for a panel of select candidate bacterial taxa biomarkers. Indeed, *Haemophilus pittmaniae*, *Rumonococcaceae G1* sp. *HOT 075*, and three *Leptotrichia* spp. were determined to be "Excellent" biomarkers in terms of sensitivity, specificity, and accuracy in the Grp-noAB using the log(RA + 1) transformed data with minimized zero inflation (**Supplementary Table 4**). Descriptive statistics of all the species with significant ROC curves are presented in **Supplementary Table 4**. Notably, *Leptotrichia* was the most represented significant genus for both Grp-All and Grp-noAB groups HPV+ vs. HPV– comparisons.

TABLE 2 | α-diversity comparisons: HNC vs. HC and HNC HPV+ vs. HPV–.

Variable[a]	Min[b]	Max[c]	Mean[d]	Std Dev[e]	p-value[f]
Grp-All HNC vs. HC					
BPST					
HNC	42	247	131.65	39.738	**0.045**
HC	53	281	143.5	42.448	
BST					
HNC	42	224	127.87	36.689	**0.004**
HC	72	281	145.96	41.343	
BPS					
HNC	45	247	138.28	42.348	0.378
HC	53	581	143.91	44.884	
PST					
HNC	42	267	135.09	42.93	**0.027**
HC	53	223	146.37	38.401	
Grp-noAB HNC vs. HC					
BPST					
HNC	45	247	131.17	38.434	0.056
HC	53	281	143.5	42448	
BST					
HNC	45	224	139.91	33.5	**0.017**
HC	72	281	145.96	41.343	
BPS					
HNC	45	247	139.55	41.855	0.54
HC	53	281	14.91	44.884	
PST					
HNC	69	267	136.13	42.264	**0.045**
HC	53	223	146.38	38.401	
Grp-All HPV+ vs. HPV–					
BPST					
Negative	42	218	127.25	37.99	0.413
Positive	45	247	133.47	39.39	
BST					
Negative	42	218	119.67	40.014	0.063
Positive	45	214	134.20	34.948	
PST					
Negative	42	218	130.52	40.964	0.483
Positive	69	267	140.30	43.242	
Grp-noAB HPV+ vs. HPV–					
BPST					
Negative	86	177	128.83	28.197	0.919
Positive	45	247	130.17	40.511	
BST					
Negative	86	174	128.08	28.273	0.787
Positive	45	214	130.71	34.437	
PST					
Negative	86	177	133.67	30.332	0.921
Positive	69	267	137.29	45.687	

[a]Sample comparisons from head and neck cancer (HNC) patients with or without human papillomavirus (HPV) and healthy controls (HC) for sample sites buccal (B), plaque (P), saliva (S), and tongue (T) with and without (noAB) antibiotic treatment.
[b]Minimum number of species detected per sample.
[c]Maximum number of species detected per sample.
[d]Mean number of species detected per sample.
[e]Standard deviation of species detected per sample.
[f]Mann–Whitney U-test p-value.
Significant values ($p > 0.05$) are shown in bold. Positive, HPV positive; Negative, HPV negative.

CombiROC and Microbial Interaction Network Database Investigation

From the ROC MedCalc analyses, 10 bacterial species from Grp-All HPV+ group had an AUC of at least 0.75, distinguishing HNC HPV+ from HNC HPV– group (**Supplementary Table 4**). Using RA data in CombiROC program (Mazzara et al., 2017), 24 "gold" combinations were generated out of 2,036 possible combinations containing at least two markers. The best two combinations (greatest AUC) were "Combo XXII" consisting of the microbial species probes *Ruminococcaceae sp075, H. parainfluenzae, H. pittmaniae, Leptotrichia sp212,* and *Leptotrichia sp417* and "Combo XV" consisting of *Ruminococcaceae sp075, H. pittmaniae, Leptotrichia sp212,* and *Leptotrichia sp417* (**Figure 4A**). "Combo XXII" and "Combo XV" had AUCs of 0.941 and 0.928, accuracies of 0.88 and 0.85, and positive predictive values of 0.69 and 0.65, respectively (**Figure 4A**). Using log(RA + 1) data, 46 "gold" combinations were created out of 1,013 possible combinations with the best two combinations of microbial probes being "Combo XLII" and "Combo XXXVI." "Combo XLII" contained a combination of *Gemella sanguinis, H. pittmaniae, Leptotrichia sp212,* and *Ruminococcaceae sp075,* while "Combo XXXVI" contained *TM7 G1 sp352, H. pittmaniae, Leptotrichia sp221, Leptotrichia sp417,* and *Ruminococcaceae sp075* (**Figure 4B**). "Combo XLII" and "Combo XXXVI" had AUCs of 0.943 and 0.938 and positive predictive values of 0.68 and 0.66, respectively. Both of these combinations from log(RA + 1) transformed data had an accuracy of 0.86 (**Figure 4B**). ROC curves, violin plots, and descriptive statistics of each data type are presented in **Figure 4**. Using MIND, *Haemophilus* and *Leptotrichia* were found to have many interactions in common (**Figure 5**).

LitSuggest Performance

From the Python$_{v3.6.2}$ data extraction code, 203 PubMed articles were identified for classification from the model matching the search terms "HPV" and "microbiome." From the classification set of these articles, 36 were determined as positively associated with the search terms "oral microbiome" and "HPV." LitSuggest program found 171 articles negatively classified. Manual validation of the 36 positively associated articles resulted in 21 articles being discarded. A total of 15 remaining articles were correctly determined as positively associated with HPV and the oral microbiome. Of these articles, three were reviews and 12 were research articles evaluating the HPV status in the context of oral tumor and microbiome relationship in SCC patients with oropharynx, including tonsil specifically, as the primary tumor site (**Table 3**).

DISCUSSION

This is the first study to evaluate the microbial differences in HNC HPV+ patients compared to those of healthy individuals and HNC HPV– patients by means of oral samples including saliva, buccal mucosa, supragingival plaque, and tongue swabs using multivariate analysis. We were able to identify 442

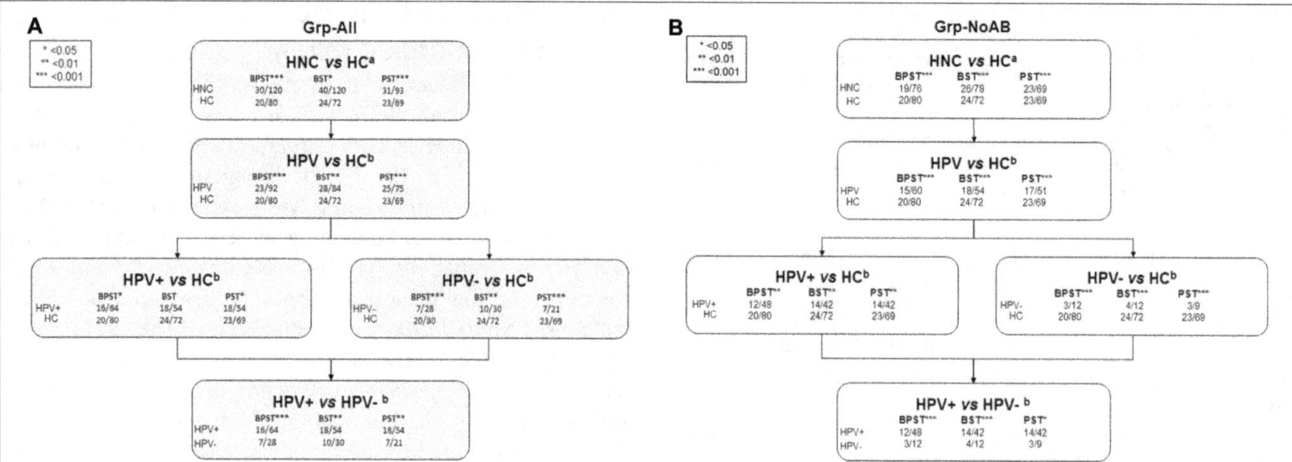

FIGURE 2 | PERMANOVA results comparisons flowchart. **(A)** Grp-All. **(B)** Grp-noAB. β-diversity analyses were performed using PERMANOVA in PRIMER$_{v7}$ software (PRIMER-E Ltd., IvyBridge, United Kingdom) to compare microbial profiles of head and neck cancer (HNC) patients to healthy controls (HC) and to compare microbial profiles of HNC HPV-positive (HPV+) patients to HNC HPV– patients. Sample sites consisted of three to four site combinations of buccal (B), plaque (P), saliva (S), and tongue (T). PERMANOVA analysis was completed using two different analytical designs based on Bray–Curtis similarity matrices determined from square root transformed relative abundance data of 737 probes (620 species and 117 genus probes). Sample site combinations consisted of BPST, BST, and PST for **(A)** Grp-All HNC vs. HC (N = 30; N = 20) and **(B)** Grp-no Antibiotics (Grp-noAB) HNC vs. HC (N = 19; N = 20). [a]For the Grp-All HNC vs. HC comparison, "Diagnosis" was the main fixed factor, and "Sample Site" was the secondary fixed factor. "Antibiotics" was nested into "Diagnosis" and "Sample site" factors as a random variable. Grp-noAB analytical design did not include antibiotics as a factor. [b]For the analytical design considering HPV, "HPV status" and "Sample site" were set as fixed factors and "Antibiotics" as nested as random factor. Grp-noAB analytical design did not include antibiotics as a factor. Level of significance is denoted using an asterisk (*): * < 0.05 = p-value less than 0.05; ** < 0.01 = p-value less than 0.01; *** < 0.001 = p-value less than 0.001.

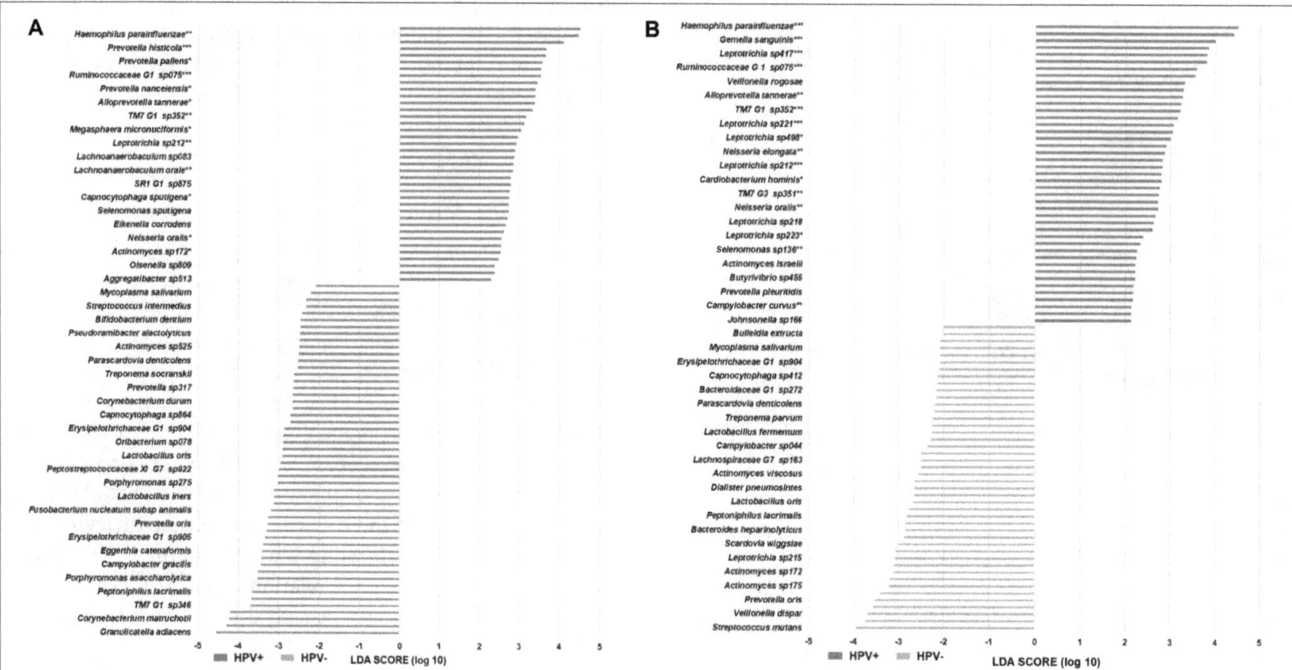

FIGURE 3 | LEfSe histograms of differential features in head and neck cancer patients. **(A)** Grp-All BPST. **(B)** Grp-noAB BPST. Linear discriminant analysis Effect Size (LEfSe) was performed to determine distinct microbiome features in oral samples [stimulated saliva (S) samples and swabs of buccal mucosa (B), supragingival plaque (P), and tongue (T)] of the following: **(A)** Grp-All patient cohort (N = 23) for the head and neck cancer (HNC) HPV-positive (HPV+; N = 16) vs. HPV-negative (HPV–; N = 7) comparisons. **(B)** Grp-noAB patient cohort (N = 15) for HNC HPV+ (N = 12) vs. HPV– (N = 3) that did not receive antibiotics within 2 weeks of sampling. Horizontal histograms depict the discriminant features, i.e., bacterial species, for Grp-All and Grp-noAB potential biomarkers for HPV+ (red) and HPV– (blue). Mann–Whitney U-tests were used to determine significance of HPV+ distinctive species. Level of significance is depicted by an asterisk (*): *p < 0.05; **p < 0.01; ***p < 0.001.

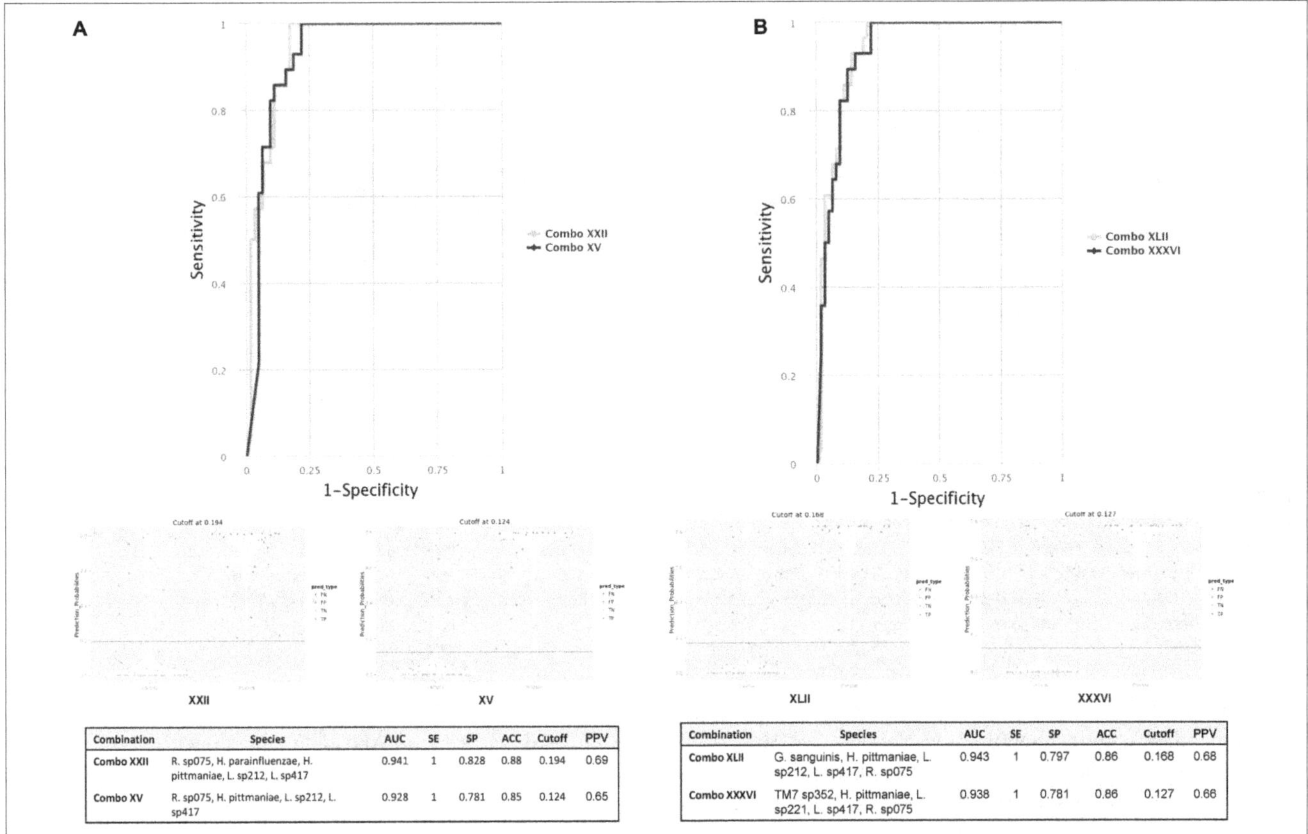

Combination	Species	AUC	SE	SP	ACC	Cutoff	PPV
Combo XXII	R. sp075, H. parainfluenzae, H. pittmaniae, L. sp212, L. sp417	0.941	1	0.828	0.88	0.194	0.69
Combo XV	R. sp075, H. pittmaniae, L. sp212, L. sp417	0.928	1	0.781	0.85	0.124	0.65

Combination	Species	AUC	SE	SP	ACC	Cutoff	PPV
Combo XLII	G. sanguinis, H. pittmaniae, L. sp212, L. sp417, R. sp075	0.943	1	0.797	0.86	0.168	0.68
Combo XXXVI	TM7 sp352, H. pittmaniae, L. sp221, L. sp417, R. sp075	0.938	1	0.781	0.86	0.127	0.66

FIGURE 4 | HNC HPV+ vs. HNC HPV– CombiROC analysis using RA and log(RA + 1) transformed abundance data. **(A)** CombiROC analysis for biomarkers with AUC > 0.75 on RA data. **(B)** CombiROC analysis for biomarkers with AUC > 0.75 on log(RA + 1) data. Significant (α = 0.05) CombiROC program-generated receiver operator characteristic (ROC) curves for **(A)** RA data and **(B)** log(RA + 1) transformed abundance data of candidate microbial biomarkers (AUC > 0.75; *n* = 10 bacterial species) identified *via* MedCalc Software for Grp-All HPV+ vs. HPV– group are shown. **(A)** ROC curves, violin plots, and descriptive statistic summary table for the best two combinations from 10 potential markers using the RA are shown. "Combo XXII" consists of a combination of the markers *Ruminococcaceae sp075*, *Haemophilus parainfluenzae*, *Haemophilis pittmaniae*, *Leptotrichia sp212*, and *Leptotrichia sp417* (ROC curve blue line). "Combo XV" contains markers *Ruminococcaceae sp075*, *H. pittmaniae*, *Leptotrichia sp212*, and *Leptotrichia sp417* (ROC curve black line). **(B)** ROC curves, violin plots, and descriptive statistic summary table for the best two combinations from 10 potential markers using the log(RA + 1) transformed data are shown. "Combo XLII" contains potential markers *Gemella sanguinis*, *H. pittmaniae*, *Leptotrichia sp212*, and *Ruminococcaceae sp075* (ROC curve blue line). "Combo XXXVI" consists of species probes *TM7 G1 sp352*, *H. pittmaniae*, *Leptotrichia sp221*, *Leptotrichia sp417*, and *Ruminococcaceae sp075* (ROC curve black line). Cut-off refers to the optimal value or the highest true positive rate that has the lowest false positive rate. FN, false negative; FP, false positive; TN, true negative; TP, true positive; AUC, area under the curve; SE, sensitivity; SP, specificity; ACC, accuracy; PPV, positive predictive value.

species and 65 genera detected based on HOM*INGS* sequencing data. We confirmed findings from multiple studies indicating that shifts in microbiome profiles which may be defined as "dysbiosis" occur in HNC patients compared to HC subjects (Guerrero-Preston et al., 2016, 2017; Tuominen et al., 2018).

Furthermore, we were able to establish that HNC HPV+ patients have significantly different microbiome than that of HNC HPV– patients (**Supplementary Table 2**). While α-diversity was not significantly different between HNC HPV+ and HNC HPV– patients, α-diversity differed between HNC patients and HC subjects (**Table 2**). Additionally, β-diversity differences were significant for all comparisons in this study except for one out of 30 comparisons (**Supplementary Table 2**). There was a clear separation between the Grp-All HNC patients and HC subjects (**Supplementary Figure 1A**). We were also able to determine that although antibiotic treatment within 2 weeks of sampling is a confounding variable, excluding antibiotic-treated HNC patients did not affect the main results, by comparing the microbiome data of HNC HPV+ patients with the data of HNC HPV– patients (i.e., GrpAll and GrpNoAB) (**Supplementary Table 1**). A visualization of the division of the Grp-All HNC HPV+ vs. HNC HPV– can be seen in **Supplementary Figure 1B.**

Regarding periodontal disease and dental caries status, our sub-cohort is similar to that of the larger OraRad cohort (**Table 1** and Brennan et al., 2021). A study identified by LitSuggest, reviewing findings pertaining to oral HPV infection in relation to periodontitis, suggests periodontal pockets may act as a reservoir for HPV and that oral HPV prevalence may be associated with periodontitis (Shigeishi et al., 2021a). Another recent study characterizing HPV16 DNA prevalence and periodontal disease inflammation in a population of older Japanese women identified an increase of *Prevotella intermedia* and *Porphyromonas* and

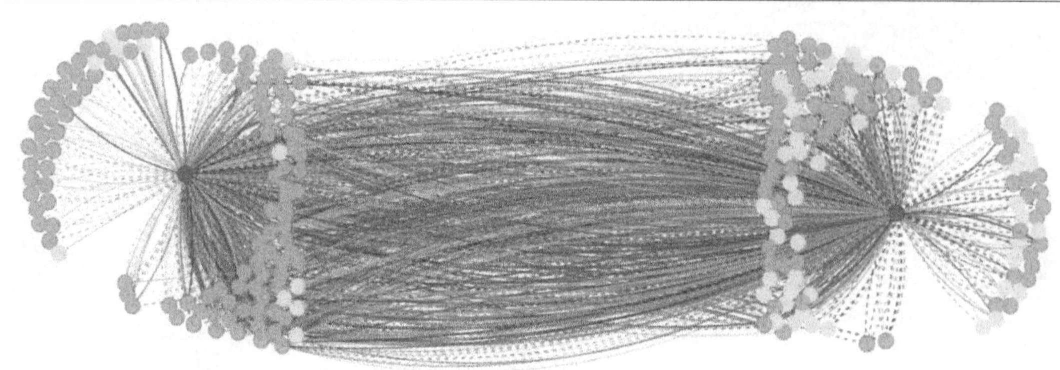

FIGURE 5 | MIND interaction network of *Haemophilus* and *Leptotrichia* spp. Microbial Interaction Network Database (MIND; http://www.microbialnet.org/mind_home.html) results, illustrating a network between *Haemophilus* spp. (left red circle) and *Leptotrichia* spp. (right red circle) by using MIND default options, are presented. Dark green circles depict genera that interact with *Haemophilus* spp./*Leptotrichia* spp., and light green circles depict species that interact with *Haemophilus* spp./*Leptotrichia* spp. The lines between *Haemophilus* spp. and *Leptotrichia* spp. show interactions in common with other genera and species. The different color lines depict the human tissue sites where interactions have been demonstrated in previous studies (MIND; http://www.microbialnet.org/mind_home.html).

a decrease of *Veillonella* and *Prevotella* to be associated with periodontal disease inflammation (Shigeishi et al., 2021b).

Furthermore, a study by Chowdhry et al. (2019) exploring deep-seated infected tissues removed during periodontal flap surgery in chronic periodontitis patients, observed an increased abundance of *Veillonella arula*, *Selenomonas noxia*, *Neisseria oralis*, *P. intermedia*, *Prevotella nigrescens*, and *Capnocytophaga ochracea* in HPV+ samples. Interestingly, in our study we found species of *Capnocytophaga*, *Neisseria*, *Prevotella*, *Selenomonas*, and *Veillonella* spp. to represent distinct taxa for HNC HPV+ patients through LEfSe analysis (**Figure 3**). Species from these genera were also found to be significant using Mann–Whitney *U*-test ($p < 0.05$) (**Figure 3**). While ROC curves were also significant ($p < 0.01$), we determined none of these species to be excellent biomarkers (**Supplementary Table 4**). We agree with Shigeishi et al. (2021b) suggesting that sampling methods of the oral microbiome should be carefully selected for periodontal tissue to ensure detection of HPV DNA directly along with the associated periodontal microbiome.

LEfSe analysis showed 43 bacterial species differentiating Grp-All HNC HPV+ from Grp-All HNC HPV− patients (**Figure 3**). Grp-noAB group analysis confirmed these findings since 24 bacterial species characterizing the HNC HPV+ patients were in common with the species distinctive of Grp-All HNC HPV+ patients (**Figure 3**). *Leptotrichia* spp. were the most prominent and significant species in comparisons performed for both Grp-All and Grp-noAB groups, precluding the possibility that antibiotics alone account for differences between HNC HPV+ and HPV− groups. In addition to LEfSe, Mann–Whitney *U*-tests comparing the RA of HNC HPV+ to HNC HPV− found 5/6 (83%) and 6/6 (100%) *Leptotrichia* spp. for Grp-All and Grp-noAB, respectively, to be significant ($p < 0.05$) (**Figure 3**). For these *Leptotrichia* spp., the RA was found to be greater in samples of HNC HPV+ compared to HNC HPV− patients for Grp-All and Grp-noAB (data not shown). ROC analysis on log(RA + 1) data further confirmed these findings with five Grp-All *Leptotrichia* spp. and six Grp-noAB *Leptotrichia* spp. to have an AUC significantly different from that of 0.5 ($p < 0.01$) (**Supplementary Table 4**). By minimizing zero inflation on log(RA + 1) transformed abundance data for the Grp-noAB group, we determined three *Leptotrichia* spp. (*Leptotrichia sp215*, *sp392*, and *sp417*) to be excellent biomarkers distinguishing HNC HPV+ from HNC HPV− patients, with a sensitivity >95%, a specificity = 100%, and an accuracy >95% (**Supplementary Table 4D**).

A previous study by Bahig et al. (2020) investigating the tumor microenvironment of HPV-associated SCC patients, determined an increased abundance of *Leptotrichia* genus in oral samples at baseline which declined over the course of radiation. This study was positively classified in our LitSuggest analysis (**Table 3**). A study by Oliva et al. (2021) found that *Leptotrichia hofstadii* was abundant in stage III oropharynx cancer, while Zakrzewski et al. (2021) determined *Leptotrichia* genus to be decreased in oropharynx HPV- tumor samples.

Surprisingly, other studies have found *Leptotrichia* spp. to be absent or less abundant at SCC primary tumor sites (Schmidt et al., 2014; Guerrero-Preston et al., 2016, 2017). *Leptotrichia* spp. have also been investigated for their role in periodontal disease (i.e., gingivitis and periodontitis) (**Supplementary Table 3**; Eribe and Olsen, 2017). A systematic review by Pérez-Chaparro et al. (2014) described a study by Griffen et al. (2012) that correlated an increased abundance of *Leptotrichia* genera, *Leptotrichia oral taxon 210*, *Leptotrichia EX103*, and *Leptotrichia IK040* to be associated with deep pockets of patients with periodontal disease. Accordingly, *Leptotrichia* species consist of non-motile facultative anaerobic and anaerobic species mostly present in the oral cavity (Eribe and Olsen, 2017).

We also observed that *H. pittmaniae* had a higher RA in HNC HPV+ than HNC HPV– patients in Grp-All and Grp-noAB (data not shown). This species was identified as a differential feature of HPV+ by LEfSe and was found to have a significant ROC curve using log(RA + 1) data with an AUC of 0.824 (**Figure 3** and **Supplementary Table 4**). Additionally, this species was determined to be an excellent biomarker in the Grp-All and Grp-noAB log(RA + 1) ROC curve analysis with zero inflation minimized as well as a good biomarker when zero inflation was not minimized (**Supplementary Table 3**). *H. pittmaniae* was also

TABLE 3 | LitSuggest positively classified articles (*n* = 15) involving HPV and the oral microbiome in HNC patients.

Year[a]	Author[b]	Purpose of study[c]	Findings[d]	PMID[e]
2021	Gougousis et al., 2021 (review)	Review the significance of biomarkers based on epigenetics and microbiome profile in the diagnosis of HPV-related OSCC.	*Streptococcus salivarius* (+), *Streptococcus gordonii* (+), *Gemella haemolysans*, *Gemella morbillorum* (+), *Johnsonella ignava* (+), and *Streptococcus parasanguinis* (+) highly associated with tumor site. *Gemella adiacens* (+) association with non-tumor site. HPV+ correlation between the genera *Haemophilus* and *Gemella* in oral cavity cancer. *Actinomyces* (+), *Parvimonas* (+), *Selenomonas* (+), and *Prevotella* (+) in OCC compared to OPC. *Corynebacterium* (+) and *Kingella* (+) are associated with decreased risk of oral cancer.	33521000
2021	De Keukeleire et al., 2021 (review)	Knowledge and biomarkers in HNC-SCC.	HPV is a biomarker of HNC-SCC; *Lactobacilli* (+); *Haemophilus* (–); *Neisseria* (–); *Gemellaceae* (–); *Aggregatibacter* (–); *Streptococci* (–); *Fusobacteria* (+); *Fusobacterium nucleatum* (+) associated with lower tumor stage	33916646
2021	De Martin et al., 2021	Characterize microbiome of human palatine tonsil crypts in patients with high-risk HPV-associated tonsil cancer compared to sleep apnea controls.	*Firmicutes* (+); *Actinobacteria* (+); *Veillonella* (+); *Streptococcus* (+); *Prevotella* (+); *Filifactor alocis* and *Prevotella melaninogenica* were distinct features of tonsil cancer	34367729
2021	Oliva et al., 2021	Characterize oral and gut microbiome of HPV+ OSCC patients before and after CRT.	*F. nucleatum* (+), *G. morbillorum* (+), *G. haemolysans* (+), *Leptotrichia hofstadii* (+), *Selenomonas sputigena* (+), and *Selenomonas infelix* (+) in stage III OSCC	33750907
2021	Rajasekaran et al., 2021	Characterize microbiome in patients with HPV-associated early tonsil SCC compared to benign tonsil specimens.	*Burkholderia pseudomallei* was unique to cancer specimens. *Fusobacteria* was identified in HPV-associated OSCC patients in tonsil and lymph node specimens. Negative nodes showed signatures for *Anaplasma phagocytophilum*, *Bacillus subtilis*, *Chlamydia trachomatis*, *Chlamydophila psittaci*, *Lactococcus lactis*, and *Proteus mirabilis*	33905914
2021	Shigeishi et al., 2021a	Characterize HPV16 DNA prevalence and PD inflammation in older Japanese women.	*Prevotella intermedia* (+), *Porphyromonas* (+), *Veillonella* (–), and *Prevotella* (–) in HPV+ periodontal inflammation	33456534
2021	Shigeishi et al., 2021b (review)	Review recent findings of oral HPV infection in relation to periodontitis.	HPV localizes to inflammatory periodontal tissue, and periodontal pockets may act as a reservoir for HPV. Smoking is associated with HPV and periodontitis. Carcinogenic HPV and periodontitis may lead to OCC, but HPV E6/E7 has not been fully investigated in patients with periodontitis. Oral HPV prevalence may be associated with periodontitis.	33728046
2021	Zakrzewski et al., 2021	Compare microbial composition, diversity, and specific bacterial phytotypes between HPV+ and HPV– oropharyngeal tumors using saliva, normal tissue, and tumor tissue.	*Treponema* (+) and *Spirochaetes* (+) were associated with normal tissues of HPV+ patients; *Neisseria*, *Veillonella*, *Fusobacterium*, *P. melaninogenica*, and *Porphyromonas* were associated with HPV status (not significant). *Fusobacteria* (–) in saliva samples (not significant); *Leptotrichia* (–) in HPV-; *Rothia* (–) in HPV+ tumor tissues; *Atopobium* (–) in normal tissue HPV+ patients.	34278648
2020	Bahig et al., 2020	Characterize tumor microenvironment of HPV-associated OSCC with RT +/– cisplatin-based chemotherapy using surface swab of tonsil, base of tongue, and buccal mucosa.	Decreased α-diversity over course of treatment. *Veillonella* (+) and *Leptotrichia* (+) at tumor site. *Actinomyces* (–) and *Leptotrichia* (–) over the course of radiation. *Gemella* (–) and *Streptococcus* (–) between baseline and 1 week and returned to baseline at week 5. *Veillonella* (+) and *Topobium* (+) at week 5.	33367119
2019	Chowdhry et al., 2019	Explore deep-seated infected granulation tissue removed during periodontal flap surgery procedures for residential bacterial species between HPV+ and HPV– chronic periodontitis patients.	Deep-seated granulation tissues showed *Firmicutes* (+), *Proteobacteria* (+), and *Bacteroidetes* (+). *Veillonella arula* (+), *Selenomonas noxia* (+), *Neisseria oralis* (+), *P. intermedia* (+), *Prevotella nigrescens* (+), *Capnocytophaga ochracea* (+) in HPV+ samples. *Prevotella* (+), *Macellibacteroides fermentans* (+), *Porphyromonas endodontalis* (+), *Campylobacter rectus* (+), *Treponema phagedenis* (+) in HPV– samples. *Pseudoxanthomas kaohsiungensis* (+) in females and *Desulfobulbus rhabdoformis* (+) in males.	31111067

(Continued)

TABLE 3 | (Continued)

Year[a]	Author[b]	Purpose of study[c]	Findings[d]	PMID[e]
2018	Lim et al., 2018	Characterize the oral microbiome fluctuation associated with OCC and OSCC compared to healthy controls using oral wash samples.	*Rothia* (–), *Haemophilus* (–), *Corynebacterium* (–), *Paludibacter* (–), *Porphyromonas* (–), *Capnocytophaga* (–) in OCC and OSCC. *Oribacterium* (+) in OCC and OSCC. *Actinomyces* (+), *Parvimonas* (+), *Selenomonas* (+), and *Prevotella* (+) in OCC compared to OSCC. *Haemophilus* (+), *Gemella* (+) with HPV+. *Actinomyces* (+), *Actinobacillus* (+), *Lautropia* (+), *Fusobacterium* (+), *Aggregatibacter* (+) in high-risk individuals. Panel of bacterial species *Rothia*, *Haemophilus*, *Corynebacterium*, *Paludibacter*, *Porphyromonas*, *Oribacterium*, and *Capnocytophaga* showed an area under curve of 0.98, sensitivity of 100%, and specificity of 90%	30123780
2018	Tuominen et al., 2018	Investigate the association between HPV infection and microbiome composition in the placenta, uterine cervix, and mouth in women	*Selenomonas* (+), *TM7* (+), *Megasphaera* (+) with HPV+ in oral samples. *Haemophilus* (+) with HPV– oral samples. Higher richness in HPV+ than HPV– samples.	29955075
2017	Guerrero-Preston et al., 2017	Characterize microbial species in the saliva microbiome and tumor characteristics in HNC-SCC patients.	*Veillonella dispar* (+) in all samples. *S. salivarius* (+), *Streptococcus vestibularis* (+) in HNC-SCC samples. *Lactobacillus* spp. (+), *Parvimonas micra* (+), *Streptococcus mutans* (+), and *F. nucleatum* (+) in salivary HNC-SCC samples. *Fusobacterium periodonticum* (–), *Leptotrichia trevisanii* (–), *L. hofstadii* (–), and *Leptotrichia* (–) in HNC-SCC compared to controls. Lower diversity in HNC-SCC than controls regardless of HPV status. No significant differences when comparing HPV+ to HPV– saliva HNC-SCC samples with control. *F. periodonticum* (+) in saliva from HNC-SCC patients. *Lactobacillus rhamnosus* (+), *Lactobacillus salivarius* (+), *Lactobacillus vaginalis* (+), *Lactobacillus reuteri* (+), *Lactobacillus fermentum* (+), *Lactobacillus johnsonii* (+), *Lactobacillus gasseri* (+) in subset of HNC-SCC samples from Johns Hopkins University. *Lactobacillus* was 710 time higher, and *L. vaginalis* was 52 times higher in HNC-SCC samples compared to controls.	29340028
2017	Wolf et al., 2017	Compare oral salivary microbiome samples of patients with OCC and OSCC vs. healthy controls.	Shannon index found higher diversity in tumor patients but was not significant. Highest LEfSe LDA was from *Proteobacteria*. *Prevotella* (+), *Haemophilus* (+), *Neisseria* (+), *Streptococcus* (+), and *Veillonella* (+) in healthy controls. *Actinomyces* (+), *Schwartzia* (+), *Treponema* (+), and *Selenomonas* (+) in HNC-SCC patients. HPV+ patients demonstrated normal microbiome compared to healthy controls.	28725009
2016	Guerrero-Preston et al., 2016	Compare saliva microbiome from HPV+ and HPV–, OCC, OSCC, and normal cavity epithelium.	*Firmicutes* (+), *Proteobacteria* (+), *Bacteroidetes* (+), *Actinobacteria* (–), and Fusobacteria (–) prior to surgery. At lower levels *Streptococcus* (+), *Prevotella* (+), *Haemophilus* (+), *Lactobacillus* (+), *Veillonella* (+), *Citrobacter* (–), *Kingella* (–) prior to surgery. HNC-SCC patients exhibited lower richness and diversity compared to controls. *Streptococcus*, *Dialister*, and *Veillonella* were able to discriminate tumor from control samples. *Neisseria* (–), *Aggregatibacter* (–), *Haemophilus* (–), and *Leptotrichia* (–) in tumor samples. *Enterobacteriaceae* and *Oribacterium* discriminate OCC from OSCC and normal samples. *Gemellaceae* (+) and *Leuconostoc* (+) only observed in HPV+ samples. α-diversity was reduced post-surgery.	27259999

Using Python$_{v3.6.2}$ program, 203 PubMed articles were retrieved for classification from the model that matched the search terms "HPV" and "microbiome." LitSuggest program determined 36 articles to be positively associated with "HPV" and "oral microbiome." Manual validation of the 36 positively classified articles resulted in 21 articles being discarded. The remaining 15 articles were manually validated as positively classified articles that relate to HNC, HPV, and the oral microbiome.

[a] *Year of publication.*

[b] *First listed author.*

[c] *Purpose or outcomes explored during the study.*

[d] *Findings/results of the study.*

[e] *PubMed ID.*

HPV, human papillomavirus; HNC, head and neck cancer; OSCC, oral squamous cell carcinoma; OCC, oral cavity cancer; OPC, oropharyngeal cancer; SCC, squamous cell carcinoma; CRT, chemoradiotherapy; PD, Parkinson's disease; LDA, linear discriminant analysis; RT, radiotherapy.

included in all four multi-marker ROC combinations including *Leptotrichia* species, suggesting it is a contributor to HPV+ SCC progression (**Figure 4**). *H. pittmaniae* has been suggested as a pathogen possibly responsible for respiratory tract infections in patients with lung diseases (Boucher et al., 2012) but has also been identified at significantly higher levels in male children with active caries (Ortiz et al., 2019). While little is known about *H. pittmaniae* and its role in periodontal disease, the

Haemophilus genus was identified in many positively classified studies per our LitSuggest text mining analysis. In a recent study by De Keukeleire et al. (2021) a decrease in *Haemophilus* was associated with HNC-SCC, confirming findings by Wolf et al. (2017) and Lim et al. (2018). However, studies by Guerrero-Preston et al. (2016) and Gougousis et al. (2021) found the opposite to be true. In our study, we were able to verify findings by Lim et al. (2018) and Tuominen et al. (2018) that an increase in abundance of *Haemophilus* in the oral cavity is associated with HNC-SCC HPV+ samples. Altogether, a microbiome metagenome/metatranscriptome survey focused on *Haemophilus* and *Leptotrichia* at the species and strain levels could provide reliable biomarker signatures with clinical implications for HNC HPV+ patients in the future.

MIND analysis found many microbial interactions between the genera *Leptotrichia* and *Haemophilus* connected through many species and genera (**Figure 5**). These genera have also been shown as two of the nine taxa that facilitate structures in oral plaque and intermingle at the micron scale (Mark Welch et al., 2016). The study by Mark Welch et al. (2016) also suggests that *Corynebacterium* forms long structures with *Streptococcus* and *Porphyromonas* in direct contact. *Streptococcus* creates an environment rich in CO_2, lactate, and acetate, facilitating the contact with *Haemophilus*, *Aggregatibacter*, and *Neisseriaceae* (Mark Welch et al., 2016). With the exception of *Neisseriaceae*, these species are likely essential to aerobic metabolism, allowing *Fusobacterium* and *Leptotrichia* to thrive as key participants in the metabolism of sugars, producing lactic acid (Mark Welch et al., 2016). It is suggested that this metabolism is involved in degradation of oral tissues, possibly leading to dental caries and/or periodontal disease (Eribe and Olsen, 2017).

Text mining used in this study suggests a lack of information involving HPV and the oral microbiome of HNC patients. Of 203 HPV microbiome articles, only 15 were verified as relevant to HPV and the oral microbiome in SCC. Only two studies identified by LitSuggest related oral SCC with HPV and periodontitis (Chowdhry et al., 2019; Shigeishi et al., 2021a). Furthermore, few studies investigated multiple primary tumor sites in SCC patients. Most identified studies in our analysis focused on investigating oropharyngeal SCC (Guerrero-Preston et al., 2016; Wolf et al., 2017; Lim et al., 2018; Bahig et al., 2020; Gougousis et al., 2021; Oliva et al., 2021; Zakrzewski et al., 2021). Only two positively classified articles were found to characterize the microbiome in the tonsil of SCC patients (**Table 3**; De Martin et al., 2021; Rajasekaran et al., 2021). In the future, more studies on HNC-SCC HPV+ patients using larger patient cohorts will be required to determine HNC risk in relation to the oral microbiome and HPV status.

Limitations

While this study was able to show the significance of microbial composition in HNC-SCC HPV+ patients compared to HNC-SCC HPV– patients, we were unable to account for the immune status of the patients. Furthermore, our patient cohort was relatively small, and our design was not optimally balanced due to the various primary cancer sites in our patient cohort. In addition, many factors not addressed in this study may affect HNC progression, such as genetics, oral hygiene practices, and periodontal treatment. However, our main conclusion remains pertinent, in that the species identified as multi-marker combinations, i.e., *H. pittmaniae* and *Leptotrichia* spp., increase in HNC-SCC HPV+ patients regardless of the primary cancer site.

AUTHOR CONTRIBUTIONS

J-LM and FB conceived this microbiome study. MTB and RL had previously established the cited clinical outcomes study "OraRad" and provided clinical insights for this study. J-LM directed the statistical analyses implemented and verified by MFB and HL. MFB, HL, J-LM, and FB contributed to the writing of the manuscript, the overall analysis, and biological interpretation. All authors participated in the revisions of the manuscript and interpretation of the results, gave their final approval, and agreed to be accountable for all aspects of the work.

ACKNOWLEDGMENTS

We are grateful to James Davis, Cynthia Rybczyk, and Jennifer Plascencia for collection of patient samples and the clinical data; Becca Mitchell for providing periodontal status data; Darla Morton for initial steps of sample processing; and Alexis Kokaras for conducting next-generation sequencing and providing the HOM*INGS* ProbeSeq data.

REFERENCES

1. Allot, A., Lee, K., Chen, Q., Luo, L., and Lu, Z. (2021). LitSuggest: a web-based system for literature recommendation and curation using machine learning. *Nucleic Acids Res.* 49, W352–W358. doi: 10.1093/nar/gkab326
2. Bahig, H., Fuller, C. D., Mitra, A., Yoshida-Court, K., Solley, T., Ping Ng, S., et al. (2020). Longitudinal characterization of the tumoral microbiome during radiotherapy in HPV-associated oropharynx cancer. *Clin. Transl. Radiat. Oncol.* 26, 98–103. doi: 10.1016/j.ctro.2020.11.007
3. Blitzer, G. C., Smith, M. A., Harris, S. L., and Kimple, R. J. (2014). Review of the clinical and biologic aspects of human papillomavirus-positive squamous cell carcinomas of the head and neck. *Int. J. Radiat. Oncol. Biol. Phys.* 88, 761–770. doi: 10.1016/j.ijrobp.2013.08.029
4. Boucher, M. B., Bedotto, M., Couderc, C., Gomez, C., Reynaud-Gaubert, M., and Drancourt, M. (2012). *Haemophilus pittmaniae* respiratory infection in a patient with siderosis: a case report. *J. Med. Case Rep.* 6:120. doi: 10.1186/1752- 1947-6-120
5. Božinovic´, K., Sabol, I., Dediol, E., Milutin Gašperov, N., Manojlovic´, S., Vojtechova, Z., et al. (2019). Genome-wide miRNA profiling reinforces the importance of miR-9 in human papillomavirus associated oral and oropharyngeal head and neck cancer. *Sci. Rep.* 9:2306. doi: 10.1038/s41598-019- 38797-z
6. Brennan, M. T., Treister, N. S., Sollecito, T. P., Schmidt, B. L., Patton, L. L., Mohammadi, K., et al. (2017). Dental disease before radiotherapy in patients with head and neck cancer: clinical registry of dental outcomes in head

and neck cancer patients. *J. Am. Dent. Assoc.* 148, 868–877. doi: 10.1016/j.adaj.2017. 09.011

7. Brennan, M. T., Treister, N. S., Sollecito, T. P., Schmidt, B. L., Patton, L. L., Yang, Y., et al. (2021). Epidemiologic factors in patients with advanced head and neck cancer treated with radiation therapy. *Head Neck.* 43, 164–172. doi: 10.1002/hed.26468
8. Caporaso, J. G., Lauber, C. L., Walters, W. A., Berg-Lyons, D., Lozupone, C. A., Turnbaugh, P. J., et al. (2011). Global patterns of 16S rRNA diversity at a depth of millions of sequences per sample. *Proc. Natl. Acad. Sci. U.S.A.* 108(Suppl. 1), 4516–4522. doi: 10.1073/pnas.1000080107
9. Carvalho, A. L., Nishimoto, I. N., Califano, J. A., and Kowalski, L. P. (2005). Trends in incidence and prognosis for head and neck cancer in the United States: a site-specific analysis of the SEER database. *Int. J. Cancer* 114, 806–816. doi: 10.1002/ijc.20740
10. Chowdhry, R., Singh, N., Sahu, D. K., Tripathi, R. K., Mishra, A., Singh, A., et al. (2019). Dysbiosis and variation in predicted functions of the granulation tissue microbiome in HPV positive and negative severe chronic periodontitis. *Biomed. Res. Int.* 2019:8163591. doi: 10.1155/2019/8163591
11. Clarke, K. R., and Gorley, R. N. (2006). *PRIMER v7: User Manual/Tutorial (PRIMER v7).* Plymouth: PRIMER-E, 192.
12. Crook, T., Tidy, J. A., and Vousden, K. H. (1991). Degradation of p53 can be targeted by HPV E6 sequences distinct from those required for p53 binding and trans-activation. *Cell* 67, 547–556. doi: 10.1016/0092-8674(91)90529-8
13. De Keukeleire, S. J., Vermassen, T., Hilgert, E., Creytens, D., Ferdinande, L., and Rottey, S. (2021). Immuno-oncological biomarkers for squamous cell cancer of the head and neck: current state of the art and future perspectives. *Cancers (Basel)* 13:1714. doi: 10.3390/cancers13071714
14. De Martin, A., Lütge, M., Stanossek, Y., Engetschwiler, C., Cupovic, J., Brown, K., et al. (2021). Distinct microbial communities colonize tonsillar squamous cell carcinoma. *Oncoimmunology* 10:1945202. doi: 10.1080/2162402X.2021. 1945202
15. Eribe, E. R. K., and Olsen, I. (2017). *Leptotrichia* species in human infections II.*J. Oral. Microbiol.* 9:1368848. doi: 10.1080/20002297.2017.1368848
16. Fakhry, C., Krapcho, M., Eisele, D. W., and D'Souza, G. (2018). Head and neck squamous cell cancers in the United States are rare and the risk now is higher among white individuals compared with black individuals. *Cancer* 124, 2125–2133. doi: 10.1002/cncr.31322
17. Ganci, F., Sacconi, A., Manciocco, V., Spriano, G., Fontemaggi, G., Carlini, P., et al. (2015). "Radioresistance in head and neck squamous cell carcinoma: possible molecular markers for local recurrence and new putative therapeutic strategies," in *Contemporary Issues in Head and Neck Cancer Management*, ed. L. G. Marcu (London: IntechOpen), 3–34. doi: 10.5772/60081
18. Gasparoni, L. M., Alves, F. A., Holzhausen, M., Pannuti, C. M., and Serpa, M. S. (2021). Periodontitis as a risk factor for head and neck cancer. *Med. Oral. Patol. Oral. Cir. Bucal.* 26, e430–e436. doi: 10.4317/medoral.24270
19. Gholizadeh, P., Eslami, H., Yousefi, M., Asgharzadeh, M., Aghazadeh, M., and Kafil, H. S. (2016). Role of oral microbiome on oral cancers, a review. *Biomed. Pharmacother.* 84, 552–558. doi: 10.1016/j.biopha.2016.09.082
20. Gougousis, S., Mouchtaropoulou, E., Besli, I., Vrochidis, P., Skoumpas, I., and Constantinidis, I. (2021). HPV-related oropharyngeal cancer and biomarkers based on epigenetics and microbiome profile. *Front. Cell Dev. Biol.* 8:625330. doi: 10.3389/fcell.2020.625330
21. Griffen, A. L., Beall, C. J., Campbell, J. H., Firestone, N. D., Kumar, P. S., Yang, Z. K., et al. (2012). Distinct and complex bacterial profiles in human periodontitis and health revealed by 16S pyrosequencing. *ISME J.* 6, 1176–1185. doi: 10.1038/ ismej.2011.191
22. Guerrero-Preston, R., Godoy-Vitorino, F., Jedlicka, A., Rodríguez-Hilario, A., González, H., Bondy, J., et al. (2016). 16S rRNA amplicon sequencing identifies microbiota associated with oral cancer, human papilloma virus infection and surgical treatment. *Oncotarget* 7, 51320–51334. doi: 10.18632/ oncotarget.9710
23. Guerrero-Preston, R., White, J. R., Godoy-Vitorino, F., Rodríguez-Hilario, A., Navarro, K., González, H., et al. (2017). High-resolution microbiome profiling uncovers *Fusobacterium nucleatum*, *Lactobacillus gasseri/johnsonii*, and *Lactobacillus vaginalis* associated to oral and oropharyngeal cancer in saliva from HPV positive and HPV negative patients treated with surgery and chemo-radiation. *Oncotarget* 8, 110931–110948. doi: 10.18632/oncotarget. 20677
24. Hayes, R. B., Ahn, J., Fan, X., Peters, B. A., Ma, Y., Yang, L., et al. (2018). Association of oral microbiome with risk for incident head and neck squamous cell cancer. *JAMA Oncol.* 4, 358–365. doi: 10.1001/jamaoncol.2017.4777
25. Jalili, V., Afgan, E., Gu, Q., Clements, D., Blankenberg, D., Goecks, J., et al. (2020). The Galaxy platform for accessible, reproducible and collaborative biomedical analyses: 2020 update. *Nucleic Acids Res.* 48, W395–W402. doi: 10.1093/nar/ gkaa554
26. Jemal, A., Siegel, R., Ward, E., Hao, Y., Xu, J., Murray, T., et al. (2008). Cancer statistics, 2008. *Cancer J. Clin.* 58, 71–96. doi: 10.3322/CA.2007.0010
27. Kudo, Y., Tada, H., Fujiwara, N., Tada, Y., Tsunematsu, T., Miyake, Y., et al. (2016). Oral environment and cancer. *Genes Environ.* 38:13. doi: 10.1186/ s41021-016- 0042-z
28. Kumarasamy, C., Madhav, M. R., Sabarimurugan, S., Krishnan, S., Baxi, S., Gupta, A., et al. (2019). Prognostic value of miRNAs in head and neck cancers: a comprehensive systematic and meta-analysis. *Cells* 8:772. doi: 10.3390/ cells8080772
29. Lalla, R. V., Treister, N., Sollecito, T., Schmidt, B., Patton, L. L., Mohammadi, K., et al. (2017). Oral complications at 6 months after radiation therapy for head and neck cancer. *Oral Dis.* 23, 1134–1143. doi: 10.1111/odi.12710
30. Lim, Y., Fukuma, N., Totsika, M., Kenny, L., Morrison, M., and Punyadeera, C. (2018). The performance of an oral microbiome biomarker panel in predicting oral cavity and oropharyngeal cancers. *Front. Cell Infect. Microbiol.* 8:267. doi: 10.3389/fcimb.2018.00267
31. Mahal, B. A., Catalano, P. J., Haddad, R. I., Hanna, G. J., Kass, J. I., Schoenfeld, J. D., et al. (2019). Incidence and demographic burden of HPV-associated oropharyngeal head and neck cancers in the United States. *Cancer Epidemiol. Biomark. Prev.* 28, 1660–1667. doi: 10.1158/1055-9965.EPI-19-0038
32. Mark Welch, J. L., Rossetti, B. J., Rieken, C. W., Dewhirst, F. E., and Borisy, G. G. (2016). Biogeography of a human oral microbiome at the micron scale. *Proc. Natl. Acad. Sci. U.S.A.* 113, E791–E800. doi: 10.1073/pnas.1522149113
33. Mazzara, S., Rossi, R. L., Grifantini, R., Donizetti, S., Abrignani, S., and Bombaci, M. (2017). CombiROC: an interactive web tool for selecting accurate marker combinations of omics data. *Sci. Rep.* 7:45477. doi: 10.1038/ srep45477
34. Michaud, D. S., Fu, Z., Shi, J., and Chung, M. (2017). Periodontal disease, tooth loss, and cancer risk. *Epidemiol. Rev.* 39, 49–58. doi: 10.1093/ epirev/mxx006
35. Microbial Interaction Network Database (2019). *THAMBAN G.* Available online at: http://www.microbialnet.org/mind_home.html (accessed September 9, 2021).
36. Mohammed, H., Varoni, E. M., Cochis, A., Cordaro, M., Gallenzi, P., Patini, R., et al. (2018). Oral dysbiosis in pancreatic cancer and liver cirrhosis: a review of the literature. *Biomedicines* 6:115. doi: 10.3390/biomedicines6040115
37. Mougeot, J. C., Beckman, M. F., Langdon, H. C., Brennan, M. T., and Bahrani Mougeot, F. (2020). Oral microbiome signatures in hematological cancers reveal predominance of actinomyces and rothia species. *J. Clin. Med.* 9:4068. doi: 10.3390/jcm9124068
38. Mougeot, J. C., Stevens, C. B., Almon, K. G., Paster, B. J., Lalla, R. V., Brennan, M. T., et al. (2019). Caries-associated oral microbiome in head and neck cancer radiation patients: a longitudinal study. *J. Oral. Microbiol.* 11:1586421. doi: 10.1080/20002297.2019.1586421
39. Mougeot, J. L., Stevens, C. B., Cotton, S. L., Morton, D. S., Krishnan, K., Brennan, M. T., et al. (2016). Concordance of HOMIM and HOMINGS technologies in the microbiome analysis of clinical samples. *J. Oral. Microbiol.* 8:30379. doi: 10.3402/jom.v8.30379
40. National Center for Biotechnology Information (1988). *THAMBAN G.* Available online at: https://www.ncbi.nlm.nih.gov/home/develop/api/ (accessed August 13, 2021).
41. Oliva, M., Schneeberger, P. H. H., Rey, V., Cho, M., Taylor, R., Hansen, A. R., et al. (2021). Transitions in oral and gut microbiome of HPV+ oropharyngeal squamous cell carcinoma following definitive chemoradiotherapy (ROMA LA-OPSCC study). *Br. J. Cancer* 124, 1543–1551. doi: 10.1038/s41416-020-01253-1
42. Ortiz, S., Herrman, E., Lyashenko, C., Purcell, A., Raslan, K., Khor, B., et al. (2019). Sex-specific differences in the salivary microbiome of caries-active children. *J. Oral. Microbiol.* 11:1653124. doi: 10.1080/20002297.2019.1653124
43. Pal, A., and Kundu, R. (2020). Human papillomavirus E6 and E7: the cervical cancer hallmarks and targets for therapy. *Front. Microbiol.* 10:3116. doi: 10. 3389/fmicb.2019.03116I

44. Pérez-Chaparro, P. J., Gonçalves, C., Figueiredo, L. C., Faveri, M., Lobão, E., Tamashiro, N., et al. (2014). Newly identified pathogens associated with periodontitis: a systematic review. *J. Dent. Res.* 93, 846–858. doi: 10.1177/0022034514542468
45. PubMed (1997). *THAMBAN G.* Available online at: https://pubmed.ncbi.nlm.nih.gov/ (accessed August 13, 2021).
46. Rafiei, M., Kiani, F., Sayehmiri, F., Sayehmiri, K., Sheikhi, A., and Zamanian Azodi, M. (2017). Study of Porphyromonas gingivalis in periodontal diseases: a systematic review and meta-analysis. *Med. J. Islam. Repub. Iran.* 31:62. doi: 10.14196/mjiri.31.62
47. Rajasekaran, K., Carey, R. M., Lin, X., Seckar, T. D., Wei, Z., Chorath, K., et al. (2021). The microbiome of HPV-positive tonsil squamous cell carcinoma and neck metastasis. *Oral. Oncol.* 117:105305. doi: 10.1016/j.oraloncology.2021. 105305
48. Ray, P., Le Manach, Y., Riou, B., and Houle, T. T. (2010). Statistical evaluation of a biomarker. *Anesthesiology* 112, 1023–1040. doi: 10.1097/ALN.0b013e3181d47604
49. Schmidt, B. L., Kuczynski, J., Bhattacharya, A., Huey, B., Corby, P. M., Queiroz, E. L., et al. (2014). Changes in abundance of oral microbiota associated with oral cancer. *PLoS One* 9:e98741. doi: 10.1371/journal.pone.0098741
50. Segata, N., Izard, J., Waldron, L., Gevers, D., Miropolsky, L., Garrett, W. S., et al. (2011). Metagenomic biomarker discovery and explanation. *Genome Biol.* 12:R60. doi: 10.1186/gb-2011-12-6-r60
51. Shigeishi, H., Su, C. Y., Kaneyasu, Y., Matsumura, M., Nakamura, M., Ishikawa, M., et al. (2021a). Association of oral HPV16 infection with periodontal inflammation and the oral microbiome in older women. *Exp. Ther. Med.* 21:167. doi: 10.3892/etm.2020.9598
52. Shigeishi, H., Sugiyama, M., and Ohta, K. (2021b). Relationship between the prevalence of oral human papillomavirus DNA and periodontal disease (Review). *Biomed. Rep.* 14:40.
53. Tezal, M., Sullivan Nasca, M., Stoler, D. L., Melendy, T., Hyland, A., Smaldino,P. J., et al. (2009). Chronic periodontitis-human papillomavirus synergy in base of tongue cancers. *Arch. Otolaryngol. Head. Neck Surg.* 135, 391–396. doi: 10.1001/archoto.2009.6
54. Tumban, E. (2019). A current update on human papillomavirus-associated head and neck cancers. *Viruses* 11:922. doi: 10.3390/v11100922
55. Tuominen, H., Rautava, S., Syrjänen, S., Collado, M. C., and Rautava, J. (2018). HPV infection and bacterial microbiota in the placenta, uterine cervix and oral mucosa. *Sci. Rep.* 8:9787. doi: 10.1038/s41598-018-27980-3
56. van Gysen, K., Stevens, M., Guo, L., Jayamanne, D., Veivers, D., Wignall, A., et al. (2019). Validation of the 8th edition UICC/AJCC TNM staging system for HPV associated oropharyngeal cancer patients managed with contemporary chemo-radiotherapy. *BMC Cancer* 19:674. doi: 10.1186/s12885-019- 5894-8
57. van Rossum, G., and Drake, F. L. (2009). *Python 3 Reference Manual.* Scotts Valley, CA: CreateSpace.
58. Venuti, A., Paolini, F., Nasir, L., Corteggio, A., Roperto, S., Campo, M. S., et al. (2011). Papillomavirus E5: the smallest oncoprotein with many functions. *Mol. Cancer* 10:140. doi: 10.1186/1476-4598-10-140
59. Wolf, A., Moissl-Eichinger, C., Perras, A., Koskinen, K., Tomazic, P. V., and Thurnher, D. (2017). The salivary microbiome as an indicator of carcinogenesis in patients with oropharyngeal squamous cell carcinoma: a pilot study. *Sci. Rep.* 7:5867. doi: 10.1038/s41598-017-06361-2
60. Wu, J., Xu, S., Xiang, C., Cao, Q., Li, Q., Huang, J., et al. (2018). Tongue coating microbiota community and risk effect on gastric cancer. *J. Cancer* 9, 4039–4048. doi: 10.7150/jca.25280
61. Yim, E. K., and Park, J. S. (2005). The role of HPV E6 and E7 oncoproteins in HPV-associated cervical carcinogenesis. *Cancer Res. Treat.* 37, 319–324. doi: 10.4143/crt.2005.37.6.319
62. Zakrzewski, M., Gannon, O. M., Panizza, B. J., Saunders, N. A., and Antonsson, A. (2021). Human papillomavirus infection and tumor microenvironment are associated with the microbiota in patients with oropharyngeal cancers-pilot study. *Head Neck* 43, 3324–3330. doi: 10.1002/hed.26821
63. Zeng, X. T., Deng, A. P., Li, C., Xia, L. Y., Niu, Y. M., and Leng, W. D. (2013). Periodontal disease and risk of head and neck cancer: a meta-analysis of observational studies. *PLoS One* 8:e79017. doi: 10.1371/journal.pone.0079017

9

A Framework to Foster Oral Health Literacy and Oral/General Health Integration

Dushanka V. Kleinman[1*†], *Alice M. Horowitz*[2†] *and Kathryn A. Atchison*[3†]

[1] *Department of Epidemiology and Biostatistics, School of Public Health, University of Maryland, College Park, MD, United States,* [2] *Department of Behavioral and Community Health, School of Public Health, University of Maryland, College Park, MD, United States,* [3] *Division of Public Health & Community Dentistry, School of Dentistry, Fielding School of Public Health, University of California, Los Angeles, Los Angeles, CA, United States*

Correspondence:
Dushanka V. Kleinman
dushanka@umd.edu

†These authors have contributed equally to this work

Science and technology advances have led to remarkable progress in understanding, managing, and preventing disease and promoting human health. This phenomenon has created new challenges for health literacy and the integration of oral and general health. We adapted the 2004 Institute of Medicine health literacy framework to highlight the intimate connection between oral health literacy and the successful integration of oral and general health. In doing so we acknowledge the roles of culture and society, educational systems and health systems as overlapping intervention points for effecting change. We believe personal and organizational health literacy not only have the power to meet the challenges of an ever- evolving society and environment, but are essential to achieving oral and general health integration. The new "Oral Health Literacy and Health Integration Framework" recognizes the complexity of efforts needed to achieve an equitable health system that includes oral health, while acknowledging that the partnership of health literacy with integration is critical. The Framework was designed to stimulate systems-thinking and systems-oriented approaches. Its interconnected structure is intended to inspire discussion, drive policy and practice actions and guide research and intervention development.

Keywords: health literacy, organizational health literacy, oral health, oral health literacy, health systems integration, health care services

INTRODUCTION

As a field of study, health literacy, including oral health literacy, grew out of the recognition that the very advances in science and technology that have led to remarkable progress in understanding human health and disease are often lost on the public. Consumers who read health information and patients who leave doctor visits often fail to understand what has been said and what they should do in response. Some of this failure is a result of poor communication by the provider. As the National Academies' Institute of Medicine report noted in 2004, "Nearly half of all American adults—90 million people—have difficulty understanding and acting upon health information" (1). This report highlighted one of the first definitions of health literacy: *The degree to which individuals have the capacity to obtain, process, and understand* basic *health information and services needed to make appropriate health decisions*" (2). Oral health literacy underscores the need to understand basic oral health information in order to make appropriate health decisions, many of which may have overall health implications (3).

In parallel with health literacy has grown a movement to integrate oral and general health in research, education, and clinical care. Their separation, the product of history and tradition, has led many to believe that oral health is less important and outside the realm of general health. But science has long proven otherwise (4–7). Reams of data demonstrate that what happens in the mouth affects, and is affected by, what happens elsewhere in the body. The association between periodontal disease and diabetes was recognized decades ago and the evidence linking oral disease with increased risk for certain cancers, and heart and lung disease is strong (8, 9). Former U.S. Surgeon General C. Everett Koop summed it well saying, "You are not healthy without good oral health" (10).

In this paper we explore the relationship between oral health literacy and oral/general health integration showing that the two are inextricably linked. Achieving oral health literacy enhances the prospects of successful integration and in combination contributes to improved health outcomes, improved quality of care, and cost reductions (3). Together, they work toward reducing health disparities, especially glaring in the health of poor and minority groups, and thus achieving greater health equity. As stated in the Healthy People 2030 overarching goal; *Achieving health and well-being requires eliminating health disparities, achieving health equity, and attaining health literacy* (11).

Our analysis examines factors common to health literacy and integration that, for better or worse, influence them and suggests ways to overcome barriers and move forward. Specifically, we propose that investments in health literacy can open new avenues for advancing progress in developing a stronger health delivery system, improved public health, and enhanced health equity.

A NEW URGENCY

The first decades of the century marked substantive health literacy research and a succession of meetings and publications on health literacy, and oral health literacy in particular. These efforts revealed health literacy associated health outcomes due to personal, provider and health systems factors (1, 12). National action plans and toolkits offered guidance on the interface between health literacy and health outcomes (13, 14). Meanwhile, advocates decried the negative impact on the health of the public and ever-rising costs, due to the lack of understanding of the causes and ways to prevent disease, conflicting and complex health information messages, and poor communication between providers and patients. Then came the year 2020.

The COVID-19 pandemic laid bare the extent of health care inequities in America the limitations in public health infrastructure, and the poor design of our health care delivery systems. An avalanche of information from multiple media platforms created massive confusion from conflicting messages from senior leaders and agencies, conspiracy theories, misinformation, and the lack of a unified national approach (15, 16). In addition, we experienced blatant structural racism, social injustice, and civic unrest. These events continue to cause stress, anxiety, and confusion among the population as a whole and within the health care environment. Specific to oral health, this experience has revealed major oral health inequities, challenged dental care services and the dental care workforce, and revealed the fragmentation in our health care and education systems (17–19). The provision of clear communication to individuals, families, providers, organizations, and jurisdictions was challenged, underscoring the urgency to take action to address the issues. It is clear that improving the health of the U.S. population, which is critical to economic stability and advancement, requires a combination of health practices and policies that emphasize the importance of good health, including oral health, for the entire population.

The groundwork for how next to proceed as society weathers the pandemic storm has been laid out in the earlier events of the decades, mostly under the auspices of the National Academies of Science, Engineering and Medicine's Roundtable on Health Literacy and the Department of Health and Human Services (14, 20). These references include the federal government publications of health priorities and recommendations for each decade, currently ***Healthy People 2030*** (21, 22).

A significant outcome of health literacy research and these national assessments led to changes in the definition of health literacy. The revisions broaden the scope and responsibilities from a focus solely on individuals to a *systems* approach. Healthy People 2030 includes new definitions (**Box 1**) for personal (individual) and organizational health literacy, providing more specificity than the earlier definitions (23).

BOX 1 | New Health Literacy Definitions: Healthy People 2030.

Personal health literacy is the degree to which individuals have the ability, to find, understand, and use information and services to inform health-related decisions and actions for themselves and others.

Organizational health literacy is the degree to which organizations equitably enable individuals to find, understand, and use information and services to inform health-related decisions and actions for themselves and others.

The combination of personal (individual) and organizational health literacy definitions reinforces the need for integration of all health promotion, health care information, and services (both oral and general health). Both definitions highlight the importance of acting on the information to inform health-related decisions and actions, not only for themselves, but also for others. Relevant to integration, the reference to individuals encompasses more than the lay public (individuals, families, communities) and includes health care providers, policy makers, administrators of health and health care programs, and those responsible for developing and disseminating health information. The organizational definition further recognizes the role entities that create health information and those that provide health services play in contributing to health literacy and the importance of their doing so "equitably." This definition also acknowledges that health literacy is dependent on the context (where, when, how, and by and to whom) and serves as the basis for the discussion

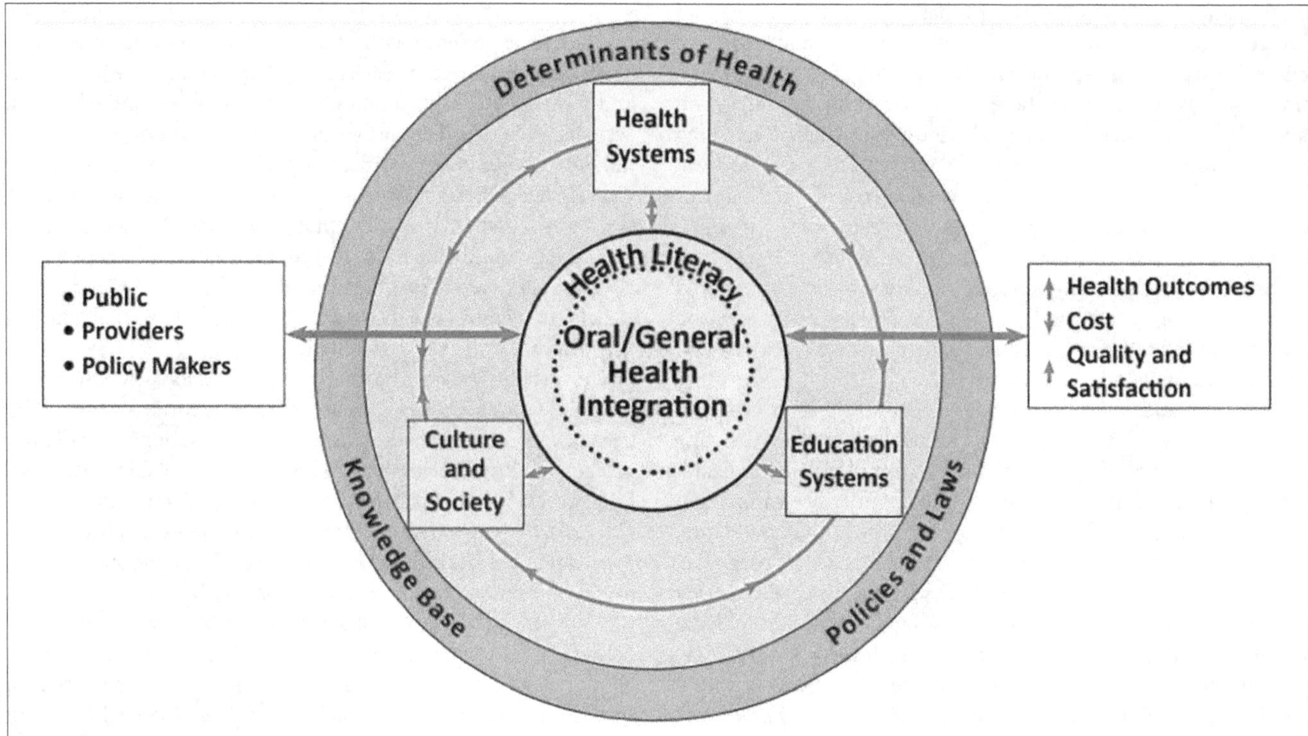

FIGURE 1 | Oral health literacy and health integration framework. Adapted and reproduced with permission from the National Academy of Sciences, Courtesy of the National Academies Press, Washington, DC (24).

in this paper. The new health literacy definitions broaden the imperative for action.

Oral health-related highlights of the pre-pandemic years include activities of the NASEM Roundtable on Health Literacy (Roundtable), which reviewed oral health literacy (25). The 2013 workshop investigated the importance of community support for health literacy, particularly in relation to:

- the health problems of vulnerable populations,
- the role of dental providers in communicating with a diverse patient population, and
- the role of health delivery systems in advancing an understanding of the patient's needs in order to obtain necessary care.

The Roundtable commissioned an environmental scan to assess ways in which health literacy promotes integration of oral health in primary care (26). During a 2018 workshop (27), discussion addressed changes needed in the health system, pointing to:

- the lack of interprofessional collaboration,
- payment systems that minimize prevention, and
- the need for consumer involvement.

TOWARD A HEALTH LITERACY FRAMEWORK TO INFORM INTEGRATION

To discuss the catalytic role of health literacy and health integration, we have selected the health literacy framework presented in the 2004 IOM Report (1) as the foundation. The IOM developed the framework as the organizational principle of the report. It provides a useful visual of "the potential influence on health literacy as individuals interact with educational systems, health systems and cultural, and social factors" at home, work and in the community. It also illustrates that these factors may ultimately contribute to health outcomes and costs. Health literacy sits within a network of systems, culture, and society, each with its own attributes and related legal, social, and ethical issues, which the IOM report refers to as "intervention points." Importantly the IOM report recognized that health systems play a significant role, but that improvements in health literacy must be shared by all sectors.

Our Oral Health Literacy and Health Integration Framework, is designed to recognize the complex factors that contribute to both integration and health literacy and ultimately to health equity (**Figure 1**). The Framework is based on the premise that effective integration of oral and general health is critical, and is enhanced by health literacy. This situation requires a clear understanding of health conditions and needs, care services, community needs and the roles played by individuals, health care providers, and health policy makers.

Health literacy and oral/medical integration are partnered and centrally placed with a permeable membrane between them, emphasizing the interplay. Health literacy is a determinant of health. Limited health literacy by individuals and systems is associated with poor health outcomes, health disparities, reductions in health care quality and increased costs (1, 28, 29).

Equally important, limited health literacy and lack of integration are impediments to achieving health equity. As a determinant of health, health literacy plays a critical role in facilitating:

- the ability of individuals to care for themselves and their families,
- shared decision-making between individuals and their health care providers,
- the ability of providers to communicate in a manner that all patients understand,
- actions that contribute to overall health and well-being,
- health care quality at the community and health care system level, and
- the development and implementation of effective health policies.

Through these roles, health literacy provides an essential foundation for the integration of comprehensive health and health care services, including the integration of oral and medical health care. In contrast, the limited or lack of integration of oral and medical care may contribute to continued poor health literacy within individuals and groups, ultimately resulting in poor population health.

The Framework is nested in a broader environment, including a rapidly evolving knowledge base, emerging health policies and multiple determinants of health. The knowledge base, nurtured by the research community, informs our understanding of health, well-being, and the diseases and conditions that affect the ability of individuals and populations to thrive. Integration is essential in our design and funding of research, from basic through implementation research (30). The knowledge base also informs the development of evidence-based interventions and programs and policies by health systems that support patient health and well-being and prevent harm to the public.

The determinants of health are conditions that affect an individual's or community's ability to thrive. As a determinant of health, health literacy contributes to how individuals manage the conditions of living: their housing, work and social environments, and their engagement in their communities and society at large. These are "non-health care system" determinants and play a major role in lowering or increasing the risk of disease, self-care, and access to health information and care services. Oral health literacy, including the promotion of oral health and access to oral health care contributes positively to the social determinants of health, enabling individuals to meet their basic food and hygiene needs, to be employed, and participate as social beings.

The Framework highlights the role of the public, health care providers, and policy-makers in improving population health and addressing health care inequities. These, and other critical players, such as researchers, educators, and administrators, contribute as individuals in their personal and professional roles and as members of organizations in each of the systems. Intermediate outcomes include improving overall health and well-being, reducing costs, enhancing quality of care, and consumer and provider satisfaction. These outcomes provide feedback into the various systems through the lens of health literacy and oral/general health integration.

Inherent to this Framework are basic questions as to whether the respective health systems, culture, community and society, or the education systems enable or limit integration, and how can health literacy skills and principles contribute to and support integration.

CONDITIONS OF INTEGRATION

Integration and care coordination of oral and general health are dependent upon a complex system of factors (26, 31). For health care, it requires having sufficient knowledge, enabling technologies, and supportive reimbursement mechanisms. The capacity and willingness to integrate and ensure quality of care reflect the level of commitment and agreement among individuals, clinical teams, organizations, and systems. While physical proximity has its benefits, the separation of dental and medical offices, geographically or within the same office building, need not be a deterrent if providers have established a communication system and means for making patient referrals. Even the co-location of providers, such as in a Federally Qualified Health Center housing both dental and medical offices, which allows for personal interactions, would better meet the needs of integrated care with technological enhancements such as interoperable electronic health records. Yet, the foundation for building and sustaining successful integration and care coordination requires a more extensive reach, one that can be enhanced with health literacy.

The interaction of health literacy and integration occurs within and among the larger contexts of culture and society, educational institutions, and health care systems—each of which may, or may not— support integration or promote health literacy.

CULTURE AND SOCIETY

Cultural and societal factors, including communities and neighborhoods, play a large role in determining how individuals identify themselves, the language they speak, the customs or behaviors they follow and their core moral beliefs on what constitutes proper attitudes and behaviors. But they are not static. They are subject to the changes wrought by historical events, developments in art, science and technology, environmental disasters and influences of the media and powerful leaders. The 2004 IOM report recognized the impact of culture and societal factors on individuals, highlighting the importance of ensuring health providers' language and cultural competency in communicating with patients (1). But even in 2004 the report recognized there were multiple challenges to health care information coming from competing sources. These have only grown in the intervening years and with the pandemic have worsened with the addition of misinformation and disinformation, further alarming the public, care providers and policy makers alike.

Achieving health literacy in society today will depend on gaining the trust of a disaffected public and establishing sources of information aligned with the best scientific evidence available. Venues for such resources include libraries, Extension programs, faith and social service groups, and city and county councils.

The perception of dentistry as an outsider contributes to how the public views health providers and services. This perception also affects health care professionals in their development and chosen role. Each specialty has its own traditional culture, norms, language, and how it sees itself (and as other health professionals see it) in relation to the health care system as a whole. This is reflected in where and how professionals practice, how they are reimbursed, and how they interact with other health professionals as well as with the public. For oral health/dental services, these characteristics place oral health care physically and in the minds of the public and policy makers, "outside" the medical care system. This is in addition to legal restrictions imposed by state practice acts that set formal limits on the scope of practice and in this way discourage integration of services among different health care providers. These cultural, societal, and legal factors and perceptions challenge the concept of integration of oral health into overall health and health literacy. On the positive side in support of oral/medical integration, are changes in practice acts and reimbursement for care that are paving the way for new workforce categories (advance practice dental hygienists, dental therapists, community dental health coordinators, and community health workers), and expanded access to oral and medical services. Examples include dental hygienists who practice in medical settings, physician and nurse practitioners who provide fluoride varnish, and dentists who provide vaccines for COVID-19 and triage other conditions. To benefit from these changes and accelerate their implementation, clear communication is needed to describe these changes, why they are important and their impact on health to the public. In turn this can inform the actions of policy makers and health care providers.

EDUCATIONAL SYSTEMS

Educational systems include primary, secondary, and higher education, including health professions education, and non-formal education that is incorporated into programs like Head Start, adult literacy programs and continuing education programs. The link between a student's health and academic outcomes, such as letter grades or test scores is well-established (32). Results from the 2015 national Youth Risk Behavior Survey showed that high school students who earned mostly A's, B's, or C's reported greater use of protective health-related behaviors and significantly lower use of risky behaviors than classmates with D's/F's. National Health Education Standards, currently provide eight comprehensive standards for PreK-12 grades (33). Yet despite national standards, the quality, quantity, and content of health education taught in schools is ultimately decided by state and local entities. The result is that the amount students learn about health in school varies dramatically, and frequently is given short shrift. Further, oral health is often omitted entirely because other health issues such as obesity or sexuality are deemed critical, ignoring the fact that oral health issues play a role in each of those areas (dental caries and sugary diet in obesity and HPV infection in sexuality).

In many ways providing appropriate oral health education for children through their school years is an optimal pathway for achieving oral health literacy. Teaching children about dental caries or teenagers about HPV infections may also increase their parent's oral health literacy. Adult literacy classes may also serve as sources for increasing oral health literacy, focusing on critical topics such as diet, drug use, and association with chronic diseases. Because many adult learners are either foreign born or from disadvantaged homes, they may have a great need for dental treatment and may lack understanding of the U.S. oral health care system, both of which could be covered in the class.

There are similar missed opportunities in health professions education, although progress is being made. In the past decade, more attention has been focused on oral/medical integration and related teaching, spurred by the general movement toward patient-centered care and interprofessional education and practice (34–36). These efforts have resulted in the creation of curricular modules, testing of new education strategies (37–39) and technical assistance toolkits (40, 41). Interprofessional communication is one of the four Interprofessional Education Collaborative (42) competencies, providing a place where health literacy principles and skills can easily be aligned and contribute to enhanced collaboration among health professionals. Health literacy includes communication, but also encompasses the health care delivery environment. This extends beyond the critical patient-provider interaction, and includes factors that guide access to care, care interactions and compliance with treatment, such as clinical information systems and decision support technologies (43). Health professions schools, as institutions, would be ideal sites to incorporate organizational health literacy. Adoption of the attributes of health literate health care organizations could create supportive environments and model how health literacy attributes enhance institutions that provide health care services (20). This exposure during health providers' formative training has the potential for lasting effects upon their graduation.

HEALTH SYSTEMS

Health systems include both public and private health care organizations and programs, third-party payers, health care administrators, employed, or independent private practitioners, plus all the licensing, certification, and accreditation entities as well as medical/dental trade associations. Health systems reflect the "culture of care" and are strongly and inextricably tied to our education systems. The health professions workforce continues to evolve, diversify, and extend into traditional health settings and the emerging knowledge base requires ongoing training and development.

Moving from formal educational settings into health care practice adds new challenges for graduates who may or may not be prepared and oriented to oral/medical integration. While medical and dental schools share similar course work in the first year or two of professional school, few medical schools cover oral tissues and diseases in their curricula or medical residencies. The IPEC competences added skills to non-dental providers to enable interprofessional practice, but there has been little adoption and follow up by physicians, outside of fluoride varnish (44). This means physicians are less likely to refer pregnant patients or diabetic patients for dental care and less likely to urge consumption of tap water to access publicly funded community fluoride programs. Similarly, dentists are less likely to refer their patients for medical care for high blood pressure, diabetes, and HPV vaccines. While all states now reimburse physicians and their staff for oral health counseling and the application of fluoride varnish, there is much more to learn about how the two professions can achieve seamless management of children under the age of 5 (45).

All health care providers contribute to both personal and organizational health literacy, and wherever they practice, their positions place them as front-line communicators and educators to the patients and publics they serve. Provider personal health literacy requires them to be fully capable of finding, understanding, and using information and services to inform health-related decisions, and to communicate the information to their patients, families, and collaborating health providers. Challenges include exponential growth of science findings, evolving changes in evidence-based protocols, the introduction of shared services among providers, and the emerging expansion of the scope of practice. These factors, together with policy changes that reinforce specific new knowledge and practices, such as re-licensure requirements and central monitoring systems, reinforce the importance of personal heath literacy for health providers.

Whether providers are in private practice or employed by health care organizations, they also play a critical role in addressing "organizational health literacy." For providers in hospital systems and health care settings, the relevant oversight accrediting and regulatory agencies provide incentives, such as alignment with The Joint Commission on Accreditation Standards for provider communication and health literacy (46). Dental school accreditation criteria include health literacy as one of the behavioral sciences curriculum elements. It states that "Graduates must be competent in managing a diverse patient population and have the interpersonal and communications skills to function successfully in a multicultural work environment" (47). Dental providers who work in academic institutions need to fulfill both the CODA requirements, and, if interfacing with the medical center, also that of the Joint Commission.

Professional organizations play an important role in providing clinical practice guidelines, techniques to simplify in-office communications, continuing education courses, ethical expectations, and new workforce models for their respective providers and the community. These organizations can also contribute by providing resources on Accreditation, and tools to support health care organizations in addressing provider-patient communication standards in health care settings (46, 48).

CHALLENGES TO MEDICAL AND DENTAL INTEGRATION

The many challenges to oral/medical integration include separate location of practice sites; lack of interoperable patient record systems, separate practice quality review systems, and a lack of common insurance coverage (49). These factors limit coordination and integration of care among health care providers and result in fragmented care for patients. As well, they pose health literacy challenges for patient self-management. In 1999, two-thirds of dentists worked in solo practice; the number in 2019 was 50.3% (50) compared with 15% of physicians (51). The separation of dental practice from the more corporate organization of medical care confuses patients who are accustomed to medical providers who collaborate with their colleagues to manage patients' care, often via referrals within the same health care system and even at the same site. Referrals between dentists and physicians are less common, placing a burden on the patient to manage the communication flow and exchange of patient records between providers (52). A common electronic patient record would facilitate bi-directional communication between practitioners, reducing the patient's burden. It would also facilitate the management of chronic conditions, such as obesity, diabetes, and others associated with common risk factors such as diet, smoking, alcohol use, the environment, and access to health care (53). Currently, several initiatives and health systems such as Marshfield Clinic Health System, HealthPartners, Kaiser Permanente, Apple Tree Dental and others, are addressing these challenges (26, 54–56).

Larger Links

Connecting a private dental practice to a larger health system such as an accountable care organization could introduce provider communication quality measures, such as measuring the extent to which the doctor listens carefully to patients, and explains things in a way patients can understand (57). Training physicians on The Joint Council of Accreditation's "What did the doctor say? Improving Health Literacy to Protect Patient Safety" (58) offers a roadmap for how dental education curricula could incorporate health literacy principles to improve safety and quality in next generation dental practitioners. These organizational standards help hospitals, ambulatory care facilities, and behavioral health facilities achieve a higher quality of care and patient safety. The provision of educational materials to medical practices on the Universal Precautions Health Literacy Toolkit, and the importance of adopting the National Standards for Culturally and Linguistically Appropriate Services (CLAS) can facilitate patient understanding of care instructions (59).

Separate Insurance

The lack of a common insurance system to handle medical and dental coverage is a point of serious confusion for even the most health literate consumers. Preventive messages from physicians rarely include the association with dental diseases, such as caries, which continues to be the condition representing the highest global burden of disease (60). This missed opportunity increases the challenge for people with lower health literacy to learn about the connection between the mouth and body, and to recognize the need for daily prevention and regular dental visits. Recent studies have demonstrated that medical organizations can reduce overall health care costs (predominantly hospital costs) for people with chronic medical conditions, such as diabetes by covering the cost of periodontal cleanings (61, 62). This approach provides an opportunity for enhanced education.

Workforce and Beyond

The report of the Primary Care Collaborative for 2021 provides a timely snapshot of the current state of innovations in oral health and primary care integration. A call to action recommends expanding oral health coverage and access, aligning oral health and primary care with new payment models, and enhancing the health workforce (31). Each of the integration challenges and their solutions have clear health literacy implications. Implementing the proposed "health literate care model" as described by Koh et al. could provide additional support and reinforce oral/medical integration practices (43). This approach could foster the anticipated health care transformation toward a greater prevention orientation, population health focus, and primary and social care-based systems (63).

CONCLUDING COMMENTS

The long-recognized need for oral and general health care integration has grown. Achieving such integration is complex and difficult, requiring a long-term commitment and coordinated efforts. Work to achieve integration has resulted in progress in some areas but remains challenging in others, necessitating a call for new and different approaches. A coordinated, sustained, multilevel approach that includes health literacy is needed. Along with investments in science assessments of policies and laws and their impact on the determinants of health are needed as well as implementation of quality improvement methods for clinical and public health services and systems.

The Oral Health Literacy and Health Integration Framework provides an interconnected structure to inspire discussion, drive policy and practice actions, and guide future research and intervention. We adapted the 2004 IOM health literacy framework (1), adding oral and general health integration, with an accompanying rationale for partnering health literacy and integration. The power of both personal and organizational health literacy efforts provides a strong foundation for an ever-changing and evolving society and environment. We propose that using the lens of the public we serve, health care providers we support, and policy-makers we inform adds an important dimension to foster systems thinking.

The Framework was developed to acknowledge the complexity of efforts needed to achieve an equitable health system that includes oral health, highlights the critical partnering role of health literacy, and stimulates systems thinking and systems-oriented approaches. Stroh's description of when the value of systems thinking is most effective suits the current stage and problems of integrating oral and general health. As Stroh [(64) p. 23–24] wrote, incorporating systems thinking into a broader systems approach is especially effective when:

- "A problem is chronic and has defied people's best intentions to solve it.
- Diverse stakeholders find it difficult to align their efforts despite shared intentions.
- They (diverse stakeholders) try to optimize their part of the system without understanding their impact on the whole.
- Stakeholders' short-term efforts might actually undermine the intent to solve the problem.
- People are working on a large number of disparate initiatives at the same time.
- Promoting particular solutions (such as best practices) comes at the expense of engaging in continuous learning."

An essential part of the systems thinking process involves taking the time to explore the direct and indirect contributing factors and to identify intended and unintended consequences. It also requires a continuous quality improvement and engagement approach.

Next steps involve testing the use of the Oral Health Literacy and Health Integration Framework as a tool to help with our collective work and impact. An initial phase may include mapping existing oral and general health integration efforts and noting the degree to which they include health literacy. The activity clusters could be used to identify advances, reveal knowledge gaps and inform collaborative efforts. Ultimately, we should strive for a common agenda with mutually reinforcing activities, shared measurement, and continuous communication.

AUTHOR CONTRIBUTIONS

All authors listed have made a substantial, direct and intellectual contribution to the work, and approved it for publication.

ACKNOWLEDGMENTS

We acknowledge the substantial editing contribution of Joan Wilentz.

REFERENCES

1. IOM, Kindig DA, Panzer AM, Nielsen LB. (editors) (2004). *Health Literacy: A Prescription to End Confusion*. Washington, DC: The National Academies Press.
2. Ratzan SC, Parker RM. Introduction. In: Selden CR, Zorn M, Ratzan SC, Parker RM, editors. *National Library of Medicine Current Bibliographies in Medicine: Health Literacy*. Bethesda, MD: National Institutes of Health, U.S. Department of Health and Human Services (2000).
3. Horowitz AM, Kleinman DV, Atchison KA, Weintraub JA, Rozier RG. The evolving role of health literacy in improving oral health. *Stud Health Technol. Inform.* (2020) 25:95–114. doi: 10.3233/SHTI200025
4. USDHHS. U. S. Department of Health and Human Services. *Oral Health in America: A Report of the Surgeon*. General Rockville, MD: U.S. Department of Health and Human Services, National Institute of Dental and Craniofacial Research, National Institutes of Health (2000). Available online at: https://www.nidcr.nih.gov/sites/default/files/2017-10/hck1ocv.%40 (accessed May 19, 2021).

5. USDHHS. *National Call to Action to Promote Oral Health*. Rockville, MD: U.S. Department of Health and Human Services, Public Health Service, National Institutes of Health, National Institute of Dental and Craniofacial Research. NIH Publication No. 03-5303 (2003).
6. IOM. *Advancing Oral Health in America*. Washington, DC: The National Academies Press (2011).
7. Institute of Medicine and NRC National Research Council. *Improving Access to Oral Health Care for Vulnerable and Underserved Populations*. Washington, DC: The National Academies Press (2011).
8. Beck JD, Papapanou PN, Philips KH, Offenbacher S. Periodontal medicine: 100 years of progress. *J Dent Res*. (2019) 98:1053–62. doi: 10.1177/0022034519846113
9. Baeza M, Morales A, Cisterna C, Cavalla F, Jara G, Isamitt Y, et al. Effect of periodontal treatment in patients with periodontitis and diabetes: systematic review and meta-analysis. *J Appl Oral Sci*. (2020) 28:e20190248. doi: 10.1590/1678-7757-2019-0248
10. Koop CE. *Oral Health 2000*. Second National Consortium Advance Program, 2 (1993).
11. USDHHS. USDHHS Office of Disease Prevention and Health Promotion (ODPHP). *Healthy People 2030 Framework*. (2021). Available online at: https://health.gov/healthypeople/about/healthy-people-2030-framework (accessed May 8, 2021).
12. Koh HK, Berwick DM, Clancy CM, Baur C, Brach. C., Harris LM, et al. New federal policy initiatives to boost health literacy can help the nation move beyond the cycle of costly 'crisis care.' *Health Aff*. (2012) 31:434–43. doi: 10.1377/hlthaff.2011.1169
13. USDHHS. *AHRQ Health Literacy Universal Precautions Toolkit, Second Edition*. AHRQ Publication No. 15-0023-ERockville F, MD. Agency for Healthcare Research and Quality, U.S. Department of Health and Human Services (2015). Available online at: https://www.ahrq.gov/sites/default/files/publications/files/healthlittoolkit2_3.pdf (accessed May 8, 2021).
14. USDHHS ODPHP. *National Action Plan to Improve Health Literacy*. Washington, DC (2010). Available online at: https://health.gov/sites/default/files/2019-09/Health_Literacy_Action_Plan.pdf (accessed May 8, 2021).
15. World Health Organization (WHO) (2020). *Risk Communication and Community Engagement Readiness and Response to Coronavirus Disease (COVID-19)*. (2020). Available online at file:///C:/WHO-2019-nCoV-RCCE-2020.2-eng.pdf (accessed on May 13, 2021).
16. Airhihenbuwa CO, Iwelunmor J, Manodowafa D, Ford CL, Oni T, Agyemang C, et al. Culture matters in communicating the global response to COVID-19. *Prev Chronic Dis*. (2020) 17:200–45. doi: 10.5888/pcd17.200245
17. Zachary B, Weintraub JA. Oral health and COVID-19: increasing the need for prevention and access. *Prev Chronic Dis*. (2020) 17:E82. doi: 10.5888/pcd17.200266
18. The Gerontological Society of America Webinar (2021). The Gerontological Society of America (GSA) *Webinar Pandemic Driven Disruptions in Oral Health*. (2021). Available online at: geron_org/images/gsa/documents/Pandemic_Driven_Disruptions_in_Oral_Health.pdf (accessed May 12, 2021).
19. Weintraub JA, Quinonez RB, Smith AJ, Kraszeski MM, Rankin MS, Matthews NS. Responding to a pandemic. *JADA*. (2020) 151:P825–34. doi: 10.1016/j.adaj.2000.08
20. Brach C, Keller D, Hernandez LM, Bauer C, Parker R, Dreyer B, et al. *Ten Attributes of Health Literate Health Care Organizations*. Washington, DC: Institute of Medicine; Discussion Paper (2012). Available online at: https://nam.edu/wp-content/uploads/2015/06/BPH_Ten_HLit_Attributes.pdf (accessed May 8, 2021).
21. USDHHS ODPHP. *Health Literacy in Healthy People*. Health.gov. (2030). Available online at: https://health.gov/our-work/healthy-people/healthy-people-2030/health-literacy-healthy-people-2030 (accessed May 8, 2021).
22. USDHHS Oral Health Strategic Framework (2014–2017) Oral Health Coordinating Committee (2014). *HHS Oral Health Strategic Framework 2014–2017*. Available online at: https://www.hrsa.gov/sites/default/files/oralhealth/oralhealthframework.pdf (accessed May 8, 2021).
23. Santana S, Brach C, Harris L, Ochiai E, Blakey C, Bevington F, et al. Updating health literacy for healthy people 2030: defining its importance for a new decade in public health. *J Public Health Manag Pract*. (2021). doi: 10.1097/PHH.0000000000001324. [Epub ahead of print].
24. Institute of Medicine. *Health Literacy: A Prescription to End Confusion*. Washington, DC: Courtesy of the National Academies Press (2004).
25. IOM. *Oral Health Literacy: Workshop Summary*. Washington, DC: The National Academies Press (2013).
26. Atchison KA, Rozier RG, Weintraub JA. *Integrating Oral Health, Primary Care, and Health Literacy: Considerations for Health Professional Practice, Education, and Policy*. Commissioned by the Roundtable on Health Literacy, Health and Medicine Division, the National Academies of Sciences, Engineering, and Medicine, the Paper is found by clicking the button at this website (2017). Available online at: https://www.nationalacademies.org/our-work/integrating-dental-and-general-health-through-health-literacy-practices-a-workshop
27. National Academies of Sciences Engineering and Medicine. *Integrating Oral and General Health Through Health Literacy Practices: Proceedings of a Workshop*. Washington, DC: The National Academies Press (2019).
28. Institute of Medicine, Adams K, Corrigan JM. (editors). *Priority Areas for National Action: Transforming Health Care Quality*. Washington, DC: The National Academies Press (2003).
29. Vernon JA, Trujillo A, Rosenbaum S, DeBuono B. *Low Health Literacy: Implications for National Health Policy*. Washington, DC: Department of Health Policy, School of Public Health and Health Services, The George Washington University (2007). Available online at: https://publichealth.gwu.edu/departments/healthpolicy/CHPR/downloads/LowHealthLiteracyReport10_4_07.pdf (accessed May 10, 2021).
30. Somerman M, Mouradian WE. Integrating oral and systemic health: innovations in transdisciplinary science, health care and policy. *Front Dent Med*. (2020) 1:599214. doi: 10.3389/fdmed.2020.599214
31. Primary Care Collaborative. *Innovations in Oral Health and Primary Care Integration: Alignment with the Shared Principles of Primary Care*. (2021). Available online at: https://www.pcpcc.org/resource/OHPCintegrationreport (accessed May 8, 2021).
32. Rasberry CN, Tiu GF, Kann L, McManus T, Michael SL, Merlo CL, et al. Health-related behaviors and academic achievement among high school students-United States, 2015. *MMWR Morb. Mortal Wkly. Rep*. (2017) 66:921–7. doi: 10.15585/mmwr.mm6635a1
33. Birch DA, Goekler S, Auld EM, Lohrmann DK, Lyde A. Quality assurance in teaching K–12 health education: paving a new path forward. *Health Promot. Pract*. (2019) 20:845–57. doi: 10.1177/1524839919868167
34. CIPCOH. *Center for the Integration of Primary Care and Oral Health*. Harvard School of Dental Medicine (2021). Available online at: https://cipcoh.hsdm.harvard.edu/ (accessed May 8, 2021).
35. NIIOH. *National Interprofessional Initiative on Oral Health (NIIOH)*. (2021). Available online at: https://www.niioh.org/content/about-us (accessed on May 8, 2021).
36. Oral Health Nursing Education and Practice. Available online at: http://ohnep.org/ (accessed May 8, 2021).
37. Haber J, Hartnett E, Cipolina J, Allen K, Crowe R, Roitman J, et al. Attaining interprofessional competencies by connecting oral health to overall health. *J Dent Educ*. (2020) 85:504–12. doi: 10.1002/jdd.12490
38. Ferullo A, Silk H, Savageau JA. Teaching oral health in U.S. medical schools: results of a national survey. *Acad Med*. (2011) 86:226–30. doi: 10.1097/ACM.0b013e3182045a51
39. STFM. *Society of Teachers of Family Medicine (STFM) Group on Oral Health*. (2005). Smiles for Life Oral Health. Available online at: http://www.smilesforlifeoralhealth.org/ (accessed May 8, 2021).
40. USDHHS Health Resources Services Administration (HRSA) HIV/AIDS Bureau, 2019. *Integration of Oral Health and Primary Care Technical Assistance Toolkit*. (2019). Available online at: https://targethiv.org/sites/default/files/file-upload/resources/hab-oral-health-integration-toolkit_july%202019.pdf (accessed at May 8, 2021).
41. Qualis Health. *Safety Net Medical Home Initiative. Implementation Guide Supplement*. Organized, Evidence-based care: Oral health integration (2016). Available online at: https://www.qualishealth.org/sites/default/files/Guide-Oral-Health-Integration.pdf (accessed on: May 8, 2021).

42. Interprofessional Education Collaborative. *Core competencies for Interprofessional Collaborative Practice: 2016 Update*. Washington, DC: Interprofessional Education Collaborative (2016). Available online at: https://ipec.memberclicks.net/assets/2016-Update.pdf (accessed May 8, 2021).
43. Koh HK, Brach C, Harris LM, Parchman ML. A proposed "Health Literate Care Model" would constitute a systems approach to improving patients' engagement in care. *Health Aff.* (2013) 32:357–67. doi: 10.1377/hlthaff.2012.1205
44. Sams LD, Rozier RG, Wilder RS, Quinonez RB. Adoption and implementation of policies to support preventive dentistry initiatives for physicians: a national survey of medicaid programs. *AJPH.* (2013) 103:e83–90. doi: 10.2105/AJPH.2012.301138
45. Kranz AM, Rozier RG, Stein BD, Dick AW. Do oral health services in medical offices replace pediatric dental visits? *J Dent Res.* (2020) 99:891–7. doi: 10.1177/0022034520916161
46. Cordero T. The Joint Commission. *Helping Organizations Address Health Literacy.* (2018). Avaialble online at: https://www.jointcommission.org/resources/news-and-multimedia/blogs/dateline-tjc/2018/11/helping-organizations-address-health-literacy/ (accessed 2, 2021).
47. Commission on Dental Accreditation. *Accreditation Standards for Dental Education Programs.* (2019). Available at: https://www.ada.org/\sim/media/CODA/Files/predoc_standards.pdf?la=en (accessed May 8, 2021).
48. American Dental Association, Public Programs. *Health Literacy.* (2021). Available online at: https://www.ada.org/en/public-programs/health-literacy-in-dentistry (accessed May 24, 2021).
49. Norwood CW, Maxey HL, Randolph C, Gano L, Kochbar K. Administrative challenges to the integration of oral health with primary care. *J Ambulatory Care Manage.* (2017) 40:204–13. doi: 10.1097/JAC.0000000000000151
50. ADA News. *Dentists' Practice Ownership Decreasing.* Chicago, IL (2018). Available online at: https//ada.org/en/publications/ada-news/2018-archive/april/dentists-practice-ownership-decreasing (accessed May 24, 2021).
51. Kane CK. Updated data on physician practice arrangements: for the first time, fewer physicians are owners than employees. American Medical Association (2018). Available online at: https://www.ama-assn.org/system/files/2019-07/prp-fewer-owners-benchmark-survey-2018.pdf (accessed May 19, 2021).
52. Atchison KA, Rozier RG, Weintraub JA. *Integration of Oral Health and Primary Care: Communication, Coordination, and Referral.* NAM Perspectives. Discussion Paper, National Academy of Medicine, Washington, DC (2018).
53. Sheiham A, Watt RG. The common risk factor approach: a rational basis for promoting oral health. *Community Dent Oral Epidemiol.* (2000) 28:399–406. doi: 10.1034/j.1600-0528.2000.028006399.x
54. Atchison K, Weintraub J, Rozier R. Bridging the dental-medical divide: case studies integrating oral health care and primary health care. *J Am Dental Assoc.* (2018) 149:850–8. doi: 10.1016/j.adaj.2018.05.030
55. Helgeson M. Economic models for prevention: making a system work for patients. *BMC Oral Health.* (2015) 15(Suppl 1):S11. doi: 10.1186/1472-6831-15-S1-S11
56. MacNeil, RL, Hilario, H, Ryan, MM, Glurich I, Nycz GR, Acharya A, et al. The case for integrated oral and primary medical health care delivery: marshfield clinic health system. *J Dent Educ.* (2020) 84:924–31. doi: 10.1002/jdd.12289
57. Press Ganey Associates (2018). Available online at: https://helpandtraining.pressganey.com/documents/hcahps_communication_guidelines.pdf (accessed March 7, 2021).
58. The Joint Commission. *"What Did the Doctor Say?" Improving Health Literacy to Protect Patient Safety.* Oakbrook Terrace, IL: The Joint Commission (2007).
59. USDHHS, Office of Minority Health. *National Standards for Culturally and Linguistically Appropriate Services (CLAS) in Health and Health Care (n.d.).* Available online at: https://minorityhealth.hhs.gov/omh/browse.aspx?lvl=1&lvlid=6 (accessed August 22, 2021).
60. Marcenes W, Kassebaum NJ, Bernabé E., Flaxman A, Naghavi M, Lopez A, et al. Global burden of oral conditions in 1990-2010: a systematic analysis. *J Dent Res.* (2013) 92:592–7. doi: 10.1177/0022034513490168
61. Nasseh K, Vujicic M, Glick M. The Relationship between periodontal interventions and healthcare costs and utilization. Evidence from an integrated dental, medical, and pharmacy commercial claims database. *Health Econ.* (2017) 26:519–27. doi: 10.1002/hec.3316
62. Jeffcoat MK, Jeffcoat RL, Gladowski PA, Bramson JB, Blum JJ, et al. Impact of periodontal therapy on general health: evidence from insurance data for five systemic conditions. *Am J Prev Med.* (2014) 47:166–74. doi: 10.1016/j.amepre.2014.04.001
63. Zimlichman E, Nicklin W, Aggarwal R, Bates DW. *Health care 2030: The coming transformation.* NEJM Catalyst Innovation in Care Delivery. Available online at: https://catalyst.nejm.org/doi/full/10.1056/CAT.20.0569 (accessed May 11, 2021).
64. Stroh DP. *Systems Thinking for Social Change.* Vermont: Chelsea Green Publishing (2015).

10

Characterization of Oral *Enterobacteriaceae* Prevalence and Resistance Profile in Chronic Kidney Disease Patients Undergoing Peritoneal Dialysis

*Carolina F. F. A. Costa[1,2], Ana Merino-Ribas[2,3], Catarina Ferreira[4], Carla Campos[5], Nádia Silva[6], Luciano Pereira[2,6], Andreia Garcia[2], Álvaro Azevedo[7,8], Raquel B. R. Mesquita[4], António O. S. S. Rangel[4], Célia M. Manaia[4] and Benedita Sampaio-Maia[2,7]**

[1]Instituto de Ciências Biomédicas Abel Salazar, Universidade do Porto, Porto, Portugal, [2]Nephrology & Infectious Diseases R&D Group, INEB – Instituto de Engenharia Biomédica, i3S – Instituto de Investigação e Inovação em Saúde, Universidade do Porto, Porto, Portugal, [3]Nephrology Department, Hospital Universitari Doctor Josep Trueta, Girona, Spain, [4]Universidade Católica Portuguesa, CBQF - Centro de Biotecnologia e Química Fina – Laboratório Associado, Escola Superior de Biotecnologia, Porto, Portugal, [5]Instituto Português de Oncologia do Porto Francisco Gentil (IPO), Porto, Portugal, [6]Nephrology Department, Centro Hospitalar Universitário de São João, Porto, Portugal, [7]Faculdade de Medicina Dentária, Universidade do Porto, Porto, Portugal, [8]Laboratório para a Investigação Integrativa e Translacional em Saúde Populacional (ITR), Porto, Portugal

***Correspondence:**
Benedita Sampaio-Maia
bmaia@fmd.up.pt

Chronic Kidney Disease (CKD) is a growing public-health concern worldwide. Patients exhibit compromised immunity and are more prone to infection than other populations. Therefore, oral colonization by clinically relevant members of the *Enterobacteriaceae* family, major agents of both nosocomial and dialysis-associated infections with frequent prevalence of antibiotic resistances, may constitute a serious risk. Thus, this study aimed to assess the occurrence of clinically relevant enterobacteria and their antibiotic resistance profiles in the oral cavity of CKD patients undergoing peritoneal dialysis (CKD-PD) and compare it to healthy controls. Saliva samples from all the participants were cultured on MacConkey Agar and evaluated regarding the levels of urea, ammonia, and pH. Bacterial isolates were identified and characterized for antibiotic resistance phenotype and genotype. The results showed that CKD-PD patients exhibited significantly higher salivary pH, urea, and ammonia levels than controls, that was accompanied by higher prevalence and diversity of oral enterobacteria. Out of all the species isolated, only the prevalence of *Raoultella ornithinolytica* varied significantly between groups, colonizing the oral cavity of approximately 30% of CKD-PD patients while absent from controls. Antibiotic resistance phenotyping revealed mostly putative intrinsic resistance phenotypes (to amoxicillin, ticarcillin, and cephalothin), and resistance to sulfamethoxazole (~43% of isolates) and streptomycin (~17%). However, all isolates were resistant to at least one of the antibiotics tested and multidrug resistance isolates were only found in CKD-PD group (31,6%). Mobile genetic elements and resistance genes were detected in isolates of the species *Raoultella ornithinolytica*, *Klebsiella pneumoniae*, *Klebsiella oxytoca*, *Escherichia coli*, and *Enterobacter asburiae*, mostly originated from CKD-PD patients. PD-related infection history revealed that *Enterobacteriaceae* were responsible for ~8% of peritonitis and ~16% of exit-site infections episodes in CKD-PD patients, although no association was found to oral enterobacteria colonization at the time of sampling. The results suggest that the CKD-induced alterations of the oral milieu might promote a dysbiosis of the commensal oral microbiome, namely the proliferation of clinically relevant *Enterobacteriaceae* potentially harboring acquired antibiotic resistance genes. This study highlights the importance of the oral cavity as a reservoir for pathobionts and antibiotic resistances in CKD patients undergoing peritoneal dialysis.

Keywords: chronic kidney disease, oral microbiome, oral dysbiosis, peritoneal dialysis, *Enterobacteriaceae*, *Raoultella ornithinolytica*, antibiotic resistance

INTRODUCTION

Chronic kidney disease (CKD) is an increasing global health issue, defined as decreased kidney function shown by a glomerular filtration rate of less than 60 ml/min/1.73 m^2, or markers of kidney damage, or both, for a duration of at least 3 months (Webster et al., 2017; Benjamin and Lappin, 2021). CKD is commonly progressive and when patients reach end-stage renal disease, they may require renal replacement therapies, such as hemodialysis, peritoneal dialysis (PD) or kidney transplantation (Murdeshwar and Anjum, 2021). CKD patients exhibit increased mortality and morbidity, especially associated with cardiovascular events (Webster et al., 2017; Benjamin and Lappin, 2021).

The decrease in kidney function leads to the accumulation of substances in the body that in normal conditions would be eliminated in the urine (Lisowska-Myjak, 2014). These substances, known as uremic toxins, build up inside the organism and cause alterations in various body sites, including the oral cavity, with higher levels of urea, ammonia and pH being commonly detected in the saliva of CKD patients (Gupta et al., 2015; Simões-Silva et al., 2017). These changes are thought to be major selective factors responsible for altering the oral microbiome, which has shown significant association with CKD status (Simões-Silva et al., 2017, 2018; Hu et al., 2018).

On the other hand, it has been hypothesized that the oral microbiome may contribute in some extent to the progression of CKD. Three mechanisms have been proposed that link oral infection, especially periodontitis, to secondary systemic effects (Li et al., 2000; Simões-Silva et al., 2018). These include the generalized spread of infection from the oral cavity as a result of transient bacteremia; generalized injury resulting from circulating toxins of oral microbial origin; and systemic inflammation as a result of immunological activation induced by oral microorganisms (Li et al., 2000; Simões-Silva et al., 2018).

Among other complications, the accumulation of uremic toxins in the body leads to a chronic inflammatory status which can cause the suppression of lymphocytes and cell-mediated immunity, making CKD patients more prone to infections than other populations (Gupta et al., 2015). In fact, infectious episodes persist as the main weakness of PD programs, with peritonitis and exit-site/tunnel infections remaining as the most common and relevant concerns for these patients (Mujais, 2006; Liakopoulos et al., 2017). While Gram-positive agents (mainly *Staphylococcus* spp. and *Streptococcus* spp.) are responsible for the majority of infections, Gram-negative bacteria (mainly *Pseudomonas* spp. and members of the family *Enterobacteriaceae*) are more likely to provoke more severe infections with poor outcomes (Li and Chow, 2011; Liakopoulos et al., 2017).

The *Enterobacteriaceae* family is of particular relevance in end-stage renal disease patients. Aside from being recognized agents of nosocomial infections, *Enterobacteriaceae* are responsible for 10 to 12% of all peritoneal dialysis-associated peritonitis, constituting a significant risk for patients on PD programs (Jain and Blake, 2006; Szeto et al., 2006). Regarding the oral microbiome, enterobacteria are frequent inhabitants of periodontal pockets (Gonçalves et al., 2007), potentially contributing to generalized inflammation and disease progression in these patients. Furthermore, *Enterobacteriaceae* are critical level pathogens regarding antibiotic resistance phenotypes. The mechanisms of antibiotic resistance in these bacteria may be intrinsic due to the presence of features encoded by chromosomal genes related with functions such as antibiotic inactivating enzymes and non-enzymatic paths (efflux pumps, permeability or target modifications) that are observed in all or most of the members of a given bacterial species (Ruppé et al., 2015). In contrast, acquired antibiotic resistance is due to gene mutation or, more frequently, to incorporation of genes received through mobile genetic elements, such as plasmids or phages that often harbor genes encoding ß-lactamases, aminoglycosides modifying enzymes, or non-enzymatic mechanisms (Cox and Wright, 2013).

Antimicrobial resistant enterobacteria are quite prevalent in CKD patients and are the cause of serious drug-resistant infectious episodes (Wang et al., 2019). Probably because of frequent hospitalizations and frequent need for antibiotic therapy, patients with CKD tend to have more infections by drug resistant bacteria than people with normal kidney function (Fysaraki et al., 2013; Salloum et al., 2020). In 2014, outpatient hemodialysis facilities in the United States reported that, out of the isolates identified as agents of bloodstream infections and exit-site-related infections, 17.8% of *Escherichia coli* and 14.6% of *Klebsiella* spp. isolates were resistant to cephalosporins and 4.8% of *Enterobacter* spp. isolates were resistant to carbapenems (Nguyen et al., 2017). In another study conducted in a hemodialysis unit in a hospital in Algeria, 100% of *K. pneumoniae* isolates associated with catheter-related infections produced extended spectrum beta-lactamase and were resistant to at least gentamicin (Sahli et al., 2017). Regarding peritoneal dialysis, in PD patients who developed dialysis-associated peritonitis between 2002 and 2011, 54.3% of Enterobacteriaceae isolates were resistant to third-generation cephalosporins and 76.1% were resistant to fluoroquinolones (ciprofloxacin), and all of them produced extended spectrum beta-lactamase (Prasad et al., 2014). This data shows that a large percentage of enterobacteria responsible for dialysis-related infections in CKD patients also exhibit resistance to one or more antibiotic drugs.

Taking into consideration the above mentioned, this work aimed to assess the prevalence and antibiotic resistance profile of clinically relevant enterobacteria in the oral cavity of CKD patients undergoing PD.

MATERIALS AND METHODS

Participant Recruitment

Chronic kidney disease patients undergoing peritoneal dialysis (CKD-PD, $n = 44$) followed at the outpatient clinic of the Nephrology Department of Centro Hospitalar Universitário de São João were invited to participate in this study. Exclusion criteria for this group included inability to give informed consent, pregnancy, recent history of infection (less than 3 months), recent history of antibiotic therapy (less than 3 months), and severe acute illness. Samples were collected according to patient attendance to the clinic over a period of 4 months. Relevant clinical and demographic information was gathered for each individual through a semi-structured interview and by reviewing the patient's computerized clinical reports. The occurrence of PD-related infectious episodes associated with species from the *Enterobacteriaceae* family was retrieved from clinical records from the date of entrance in the PD program until the moment of oral sample collection.

The control group was recruited from the student body of the Faculdade de Medicina Dentária da Universidade do Porto ($n = 37$). Relevant clinical and demographic information was gathered through a semi-structured interview. Exclusion criteria for the control group included inability to give informed consent, pregnancy, recent history of infection (less than 3 months), recent history of antibiotic therapy (less than 3 months), and compromised oral health (occurrence of gum disease, such as gingivitis or periodontitis, and a caries index including decayed, missing or filled teeth superior to 5). Controls had no history of chronic or systemic diseases (such as diabetes, hypertension, obesity, allergies, autoimmune diseases, etc.), no history of genetic disorders, no history of renal disease, and had not been diagnosed for any other health condition.

The protocols for the study were approved by both the Ethics Committee for Health of Centro Hospitalar Universitário de São João (approval number 200/18) and the Ethics Committee for Health of Faculdade de Medicina Dentária da Universidade do Porto (approval number 12/2019) and followed the 1964 Helsinki declaration and its later amendments; all recruited participants gave their written informed consent.

Sample Collection

Unstimulated whole saliva was collected *via* the spitting method (Navazesh, 1993) into sterile containers, at least 1 h after eating or tooth brushing. Prior to the collection, the subjects did a water mouthwash to minimize typical dry-mouth sensation and to clean the oral cavity. Saliva collection began after swallowing the residual saliva present in the mouth and allowing newly produced saliva to accumulate. Part of the saliva samples (~1 ml) were stored at −20°C until biochemical analysis and the remaining volume was kept refrigerated for microbiological evaluation.

Saliva Biochemical Analysis

The biochemical analysis was carried out using a sequential injection analysis system with potentiometric detection for the determination of urea and ammonia in saliva samples as previously described (Thepchuay et al., 2020), and the pH was measured using pH strips (5.0–8.0, Duotest, Germany and 1–14, Merck, Germany).

Oral Microbiota Isolation and Identification

Up to 2 h after collection, refrigerated saliva samples were serially diluted with sterile 0.9% NaCl solution and were plated in triplicate in MacConkey Agar (VWR Chemicals BDH, Belgium). This culture medium was used in order to target non-fastidious non-strict anaerobic Gram-negative species. After aerobic incubation at 37°C for 48 h, the total number of colonies was counted and the results were expressed in colony-forming units per mL of saliva (CFU/ml).

From each saliva sample, all colonies with distinct appearances were reisolated in the same medium, which resulted in the selection of 2 to 3 isolates per individual saliva sample. Additionally, urease production was tested by incubating colonies on Urea Broth (Panreac, Spain) at 37°C for 24 h. Isolates were then stored in Brain Heart Infusion broth (BHI; Biolab Zrt., Hungary) supplemented with 10% glycerol at −80°C and were later identified by matrix-assisted laser desorption/ionization–time-of-flight mass spectrometry (MALDI-TOF MS, Bruker MALDI Biotyper).

The MALDI-TOF MS analysis was conducted directly from fresh (<24 h) bacterial colonies according to manufacturer's instructions. When necessary, formic acid 70% was added to samples to improve identification. Only isolates which obtained an identification score value equal or higher than 2.0, corresponding to probable identification to species level, were considered properly identified.

Antibiotic Resistance Phenotype and Genotype

Antibiotic resistance phenotype was determined using the Kirby–Bauer disk-diffusion method to test the following antibiotics: amoxicillin (AML, 25 μg), gentamycin (GEN, 10 μg),

TABLE 1 | CKD-PD patients' clinical information, including etiology of CKD, residual renal function, blood pressure, time on PD, and PD-related infection history.

	CKD-PD patients
Etiology of CKD (%)	
Diabetic nephropathy	25.0%
Hepatorenal polycystic disease	20.5%
Glomerular disease	13.7%
Urologic (nephrectomy, neoplasia, chronic PNC)	9.1%
Chronic interstitial nephritis	4.5%
Nephroangiosclerosis	2.3%
Vasculitis	2.3%
Unknown	22.7%
Residual renal function (mL/min)	5.9 ± 4.0
Blood pressure (mmHg)	
Systolic	140 ± 18
Diastolic	80 ± 10
PD vintage (months)	31.7 ± 30.2
Infection history[a] (%)	
Peritonitis	27.3%
By *Enterobacteriaceae*	2.3%
Exit-site infections	45.5%
By *Enterobacteriaceae*	9.1%

Results are shown in prevalence (%) or mean ± SD. [a]Prevalence of infections refers to PD patients that had at least one infection episode from the date of entrance in the PD program until the moment of oral sample collection. CKD, chronic kidney disease; PD, peritoneal dialysis; CKD-PD, chronic kidney disease patients undergoing peritoneal dialysis.

TABLE 2 | Demographic information and biochemical salivary parameters of healthy controls and CKD-PD patients.

	Controls	CKD-PD patients	*p* value
Age (years)	19.7 ± 1.2	55.9 ± 11.0	<0.001
Sex (male %)	18.9%	65.9%	<0.001
Saliva Biochemistry			
pH	6.7 ± 0.3	8.1 ± 0.8	<0.001
Urea (mg/dL)	20.4 ± 14.2	85.2 ± 46.2	<0.001
Ammonia (mg/dL)	16.1 ± 12.8	63.6 ± 38.1	<0.001

Results are shown in prevalence (%) or mean ± SD. CKD-PD, chronic kidney disease patients undergoing peritoneal dialysis.

ciprofloxacin (CIP, 5 μg), sulfamethoxazole/trimethoprim (SXT, 1.25/23.75 μg), tetracycline (TET, 30 μg), cephalothin (CP, 30 μg), meropenem (MEM, 10 μg), ceftazidime (CAZ, 30 μg), ticarcillin (TIC, 75 μg), colistin (CT, 50 μg), sulfamethoxazole (SUL, 25 μg) and streptomycin (STR, 10 μg; Oxoid™, Hampshire, UK). Assays were conducted as recommended for *Enterobacteriaceae* (CLSI, 2017). As a quality control, *Escherichia coli* strain ATCC 25922 was included in all assays.

PCR-based gene screening (primers and PCR conditions described in **Supplementary Table S1**) used DNA extracts obtained from fresh pure cultures: bacterial colonies were resuspended in 50 μl of nuclease-free water and heated for 10 min at 95°C; subsequently, the mixture was refrigerated on ice for 5 min and centrifuged at 14 000 rpm for 5 min for sedimentation of cell debris; the supernatant was used as template for PCR reactions (Wiedmann-al-Ahmad et al., 1994). PCR gel electrophoresis pictures are presented in **Supplementary Figures S1–S9**. The screened genetic determinants included resistance determinants to β-lactams (*bla*$_{TEM}$, *bla*$_{CTX\text{-}M}$, *bla*$_{OXA}$ and *bla*$_{SHV}$), sulfonamides (*sul1*) and quinolones (*qnrS*), and mobile genetic elements related with genetic recombination and gene acquisition, plasmid replicon types (incF, incHI1 and incHI2), representative of incompatibility groups circulating among *Enterobacteriaceae*, and class 1 integron integrase (*intI1*).

Data Analysis

All data analysis was carried out using IBM SPSS Statistics for Windows, Version 23.0 (IBM Corp, NY, United States). When appropriate, the chi-square independence test was used to analyze hypotheses regarding the categorical variables, using continuity correction for 2×2 Tables. T-test for independent samples was used for the continuous variables, using Levene's test for equal variances. In order to evaluate potential confounders like age and sex, binary logistic regression (Enter method) was applied for the presence of *Raoultella ornithinolytica* as dependent variable and the type of participant as another covariate with bootstrapping technique with 95% of confidence. A significance level of 0.05 was considered.

RESULTS

Clinical Characterization of CKD-PD Patients

Clinical information relating to the CKD-PD patients is included in **Table 1**. The most prevalent etiology of CKD was diabetic nephropathy and, at the time of sampling, the average time on PD therapy was 32 months, ranging from 2 months up to 12.4 years. Regarding salivary biochemical parameters, pH, urea, and ammonia levels were all significantly higher in CKD-PD patients compared to healthy controls (**Table 2**).

Oral *Enterobacteriaceae* Prevalence

CKD-PD patients exhibited significantly higher microbial counts and *Enterobacteriaceae* prevalence (**Table 3**). *Enterobacteriaceae* diversity was also higher in CKD-PD patients, with only three species being isolated from healthy controls while seven species (two in common with the controls and an additional five) were isolated from the study group, from a total of eight isolated species (**Table 3**). Six of the total eight species tested positive for urease production (excluding *Escherichia coli* and *Klebsiella aerogenes*; **Table 3**). Out of all *Enterobacteriaceae* species identified, only *Raoultella ornithinolytica* exhibited significantly higher prevalence in CKD-PD patients, being absent from the oral cavity of healthy controls.

Because controls and CKD patients vary significantly in terms of age and gender, binary logistic regression was applied for the presence of *Raoultella ornithinolytica* as dependent variable containing three independent variables: sex, age and type of participants. The full model with bootstrapping technique

TABLE 3 | Bacterial counts in MacConkey Agar and prevalence of participants colonized by urease producing (*) and non-producing *Enterobacteriaceae* species.

	Controls	CKD-PD patients	*P* value
Counts, CFU/ml	$8.8\times10^3 \pm 1.5\times10^4$	$3.1\times10^4 \pm 4.9\times10^4$	0.008
Enterobacteriaceae prevalence, %	10.8%	43.2%	0.003
*Raoultella ornithinolytica**	0%	29.5%	0.001
*Klebsiella oxytoca**	0%	2.3%	>0.999
*Klebsiella pneumoniae**	5.4%	2.3%	0.878
Klebsiella aerogenes	0%	2.3%	>0.999
*Enterobacter asburiae**	2.7%	4.5%	>0.999
Escherichia coli	2.7%	0%	0.930
*Citrobacter koseri**	0%	2.3%	>0.999
*Citrobacter freundii**	0%	2.3%	>0.999

*Results are shown in prevalence (%) or mean ± SD. *Species that tested positive for urease production. CKD-PD, chronic kidney disease patients undergoing peritoneal dialysis.*

TABLE 4 | Total number of PD-related infection episodes, including peritonitis and exit-site infections (ESI), and the infectious agent identified.

Infectious agent	PD-related infection episodes (n = 50)	
	Peritonitis ($n = 13$)	ESI ($n = 37$)
Others	12 (92.3%)	31 (83.8%)
Enterobacteria	1 (7.7%)	6 (16.2%)
Klebsiella pneumoniae	0	2 (5.4%)
Klebsiella oxytoca	1 (7.7%)	0
Enterobacter spp.	0	3 (8.1%)
Escherichia coli	0	1 (2.7%)

PD, Peritoneal dialysis.

containing all predictors was statically significant (χ^2 (3, N = 81) = 18.041, $p < 0.001$). According to the bootstrapping technique, only the type of participants (controls or CKD) made a unique statistically significant contribution ($p < 0.001$) in the model (CKD patients' coefficient, B = 20.299; CI95% = 17.675; 22.954). On the other hand, statistical significance was not attained for sex nor age, respectively ($p = 0.760$) and ($p = 0.956$).

Enterobacteriaceae-Related Infection History

During the complete period of PD therapy, around one quarter of the studied population had at least one peritonitis and around half of the patients had at least one ESI (**Table 1**). When one looks to the total number of infectious episodes (**Table 4**), *Enterobacteriaceae* were responsible for 7.7% of all peritonitis and for 16.2% of all ESI episodes, and the identified infectious agents include the genera *Klebsiella*, *Enterobacter* and *Escherichia*. No association was found between previous *Enterobacteriaceae* infectious agents and the oral enterobacteria colonization of the CKD-PD patients at the time of sampling.

Antibiotic Resistance Profiling

Enterobacteriaceae isolates ($n = 23$) obtained from different individuals exhibited mainly intrinsic antibiotic resistance phenotypes (CLSI, 2017; EUCAST, 2020; **Supplementary Table S2**). Specifically, resistance to amoxicillin (in all isolates of *Klebsiella* spp., one isolate of *Citrobacter freundii*, 2 out of 3 isolates of *Enterobacter* spp., and 12 out of 14 isolates from *R. ornithinolytica*), resistance to ticarcillin (2 out of 3 isolates of *Klebsiella* spp. and in 10 out of 14 isolates from *R. ornithinolytica*), and resistance to cephalothin (in all isolates of *Enterobacter* spp.) were observed. In addition to intrinsic antibiotic resistance, sulfamethoxazole (in *Enterobacter asburiae*, *Escherichia coli*, *Klebsiella pneumoniae*, and *Raoultella ornithinolytica* isolates), and streptomycin (in *Enterobacter asburiae* and *Raoultella ornithinolytica* isolates) resistances were also observed. Only 6 isolates (2 isolates of *Enterobacter asburiae* and 4 of *Raoultella ornithinolytica*) exhibited multidrug resistance, all of them originated from CKD-PD patients. These results are depicted in **Supplementary Table S2**. Overall, out of the 23 *Enterobacteriaceae* isolates, about 83% were resistant to amoxicillin, 52% showed resistance to ticarcillin, 43% to sulfamethoxazole, 35% to ciprofloxacin and 17% to streptomycin. 100% of the isolates were resistant to at least one of the antibiotics tested. The percentage of sensitivity to the studied antibiotics is presented in **Supplementary Figure S10**.

Among the genes screened, neither the antibiotic resistance genes bla_{TEM}, bla_{OXA} and *qnrS*, nor the plasmid replicon types incHI1 and incHI2 were detected. The other genetic determinants were observed in one *Escherichia coli* isolate from a healthy control (*sul1*); in 2 of the 3 *Enterobacter asburiae* isolates from CKD-PD patients and controls (*sul1*, $n = 1$ and *sul1* and *intI1*, $n = 1$); in the *Klebsiella oxytoca* isolate from a CKD-PD patient ($bla_{CTX\text{-}M}$, normally associated with the plasmid replicon type incF); in 2 isolates of *Klebsiella pneumoniae* from controls (bla_{SHV}, $n = 2$, probably intrinsic in this species, and *sul1*, $n = 1$); and in 4 of the 14 *Raoultella ornithinolytica* isolates from CKD-PD patients (*sul1* and *intI1*, $n = 3$ and *intI1*, $n = 1$). These results are depicted in **Supplementary Table S2**. Overall, the bla_{SHV} gene alone or with *sul1* and $bla_{CTX\text{-}M}$ with replicon type incF were detected in 4.3% of isolates. The *sul1* gene alone was found in 8.7% of isolates and *sul1* with *intI1* were found in 17.4% of isolates. None of the tested genes were detected in approximately 57% of isolates. The prevalence of these genetic elements is presented in **Supplementary Figure S11**.

DISCUSSION

Overall, our results show that the accumulation of uremic toxins in patients with advanced CKD and the consequent changes in the oral milieu (such as the increase in salivary urea, ammonia and pH) may indeed act as selecting factors on the oral microbiome, leading to an oral dysbiosis with proliferation of pathobionts in the oral cavity. In fact, 6 of the 8 species identified in **Table 3** tested positive for urease production. Thus, it was observed that more urease-producing species were found in the oral cavity of CKD patients in comparison to the oral cavity of healthy controls, which is expected to be due to the previously reported adaptation of the microbiome to the altered conditions of the oral milieu, evidenced in **Table 2** (Hu et al., 2018; Rysz et al., 2021).

The increased prevalence of *Enterobacteriaceae* spp. is significantly relevant in CKD patients. While enterobacteria are only occasionally detected in the oral cavity of healthy individuals, colonization is much more prevalent in immunocompromised patients, people who come in contact with hospital environments frequently, and people suffering from hyposalivation, oral lesions, and systemic disease, a scenario that fits CKD patients (Peleg and Hooper, 2010; Posse et al., 2017). Perhaps, all these reasons also contributed to the higher prevalence of *Enterobacteriaceae* in the oral microbiota of our CKD patients as well as to the fact that *Enterobacteriaceae* were responsible for approximately 8% of the peritoneal dialysis-associated peritonitis and 16% of exit-site infections in our group of patients, highlighting the clinical relevance of our results.

The increased prevalence of *Raoultella ornithinolytica* in CKD patients undergoing PD is a particularly significant finding. Formerly classified as *Klebsiella ornithinolytica*, *R. ornithinolytica*, a histamine-producing aquatic-commensal enterobacteria, is a virulent pathogen of community-acquired and emerging nosocomial infections, particularly associated with invasive procedures (Seng et al., 2016; Hajjar et al., 2018, 2020). *R. ornithinolytica* is able to occasionally survive in human saliva and a case report has pointed it as a cause of primary peritonitis in humans (Sibanda, 2014; Seng et al., 2016), thus aggravating the risk of its presence in the oral cavity of patients undergoing peritoneal dialysis. Regarding the oral microbiome, the high rate of colonization by *Raoultella ornithinolytica* is a very interesting finding in itself, since this species is still not described in the Human Oral Microbiome Database.[1]

Although no association was found between previous *Enterobacteriaceae* infectious agents in the group of CKD patients and oral colonization by enterobacteria at the time of sampling, the difficulty in the identification of *R. ornithinolytica* and common misidentification as belonging to the *Klebsiella* genus should be considered, as a misidentification of the infectious agent is a possibility (Ponce-Alonso et al., 2016). Additionally, the hypothesis of an oral-peritoneal association regarding infection cannot be discarded without further studies, especially when all the *Enterobacteriaceae*-related infectious episodes reported in these patients occurred at least 1 year prior to the collection of the samples used in this study.

It is important to note that all the species identified in this study are clinically relevant and constitute potential cause of infection, with many being associated with PD-related infections (Barraclough et al., 2009; Li and Chow, 2011). Although contamination concerns for patients undergoing peritoneal dialysis typically tend to focus on contamination from external origins, the oral microbiome may be a major source of contamination both through external and internal routes (Li and Chow, 2011; Smith and Nehring, 2021). Bacteria inhabiting the oral cavity can translocate into the bloodstream as a result from routine daily activities, such as tooth brushing or invasive dental procedures, becoming opportunistic infectious agents in distant body sites such as the peritoneum (Smith and Nehring, 2021). In fact, the risk associated with the presence of pathogenic bacteria in the oral-nasal cavities of CKD patients is already recognized, which is why these patients are frequently screened for nasal carriage of *Staphylococcus aureus* as a way to prevent infection and the efficacy of prophylactic intranasal antibiotics for the treatment of confirmed nasal carriage of *S. aureus* has been tested in several prospective studies (Grothe et al., 2014; Li et al., 2016). Furthermore, the presence of these bacteria in the oral cavity can stimulate the immune system and contribute to the inflammatory state in CKD, which then leads to cardiovascular events, the main cause of death in these patients (Li et al., 2000; Webster et al., 2017; Höfer et al., 2021).

The oral cavity has also recently been highlighted as a potential reservoir of antibiotic resistance genes (Roberts and Mullany, 2010; Jiang et al., 2018; de Sousa Moreira Almeida et al., 2020). Resistance against amoxicillin was observed in 83% of isolates, although in these cases it is possibly intrinsic (Cox and Wright, 2013). However, putative acquired genetic elements related with antibiotic resistance were observed in 10 out of 23 oral isolates, 3 from healthy individuals (*sul1* in *Escherichia coli* and bla_{SHV} in *Klebsiella pneumoniae*) and 7 from CKD patients (*sul1*, *intI1*, $bla_{CTX\text{-}M}$ and incF in *Enterobacter asburiae*, *Raoultella ornithinolytica* and *Klebsiella oxytoca*). Curiously, the 5 isolates harboring the gene *intI1* and the one exhibiting the high mobile replicon type incF and $bla_{CTX\text{-}M}$ genes all originated from CKD patients. These observations raise the interest to investigate the vulnerability of some population groups to be colonized by bacteria harboring acquired antibiotic resistance genes and mobile genetic elements (de Sousa Moreira Almeida et al., 2020). Overall, regarding the resistance phenotype, 100% of the *Enterobacteriaceae* isolates were resistant to at least one of the antibiotics tested and only 6 isolates, all originating from CKD-PD patients, exhibited multidrug resistance. Genetic elements related to resistance were also detected in approximately 43% of isolates. Antibiotic-resistant enterobacteria are known agents of dialysis-associated infections in CKD patients, frequently originating serious life-threatening complications (Wang et al., 2019). Therefore, it is important to keep screening isolates from CKD patients for antimicrobial resistances, in order to plan efficient therapeutic interventions in case of infection.

[1]http://www.homd.org/

Our study presents several strengths and some limitations. The fact that the control and CKD groups differ in age and gender may constitute a limitation of our study, although a binary logistic regression was applied using the prevalence of *Raoultella ornithinolytica* (the only member of the *Enterobacteriaceae* family with a significantly different prevalence between groups) as the dependent variable and sex, age, and type of participants as independent variables, confirming that only the type of participants (controls or CKD-PD) made a unique statistically significant contribution. Moreover, though ideally the groups should display similar demographic characteristics, several studies have reported that the oral microbiome does not suffer significant alterations throughout adulthood, with no significant differences being reported by gender or age groups (adults and young adults) at species level. Alterations in the healthy oral microbiota are only significant before adulthood or after the age of 65–70 years-old (Crielaard et al., 2011; Belstrøm et al., 2014; Lira-Junior et al., 2018; Verma et al., 2021). As so, the healthy young adults constituting the control group in this study are nevertheless representative of healthy reference values. Regarding methodology, although MALDI-TOF MS is a universally used method that has been routinely used in clinical microbiology (He et al., 2010; Tsuchida et al., 2020) and is considered extremely adequate for the identification of enterobacteria (Richter et al., 2013), it presents some limitations, as is the example of the inability to differentiate *Escherichia coli* from *Shigella* species (Devanga Ragupathi et al., 2017).

When one looks to the study strengths, firstly, it highlights how the uremic state in CKD can cause a dysbiosis of the oral microbiome and lead to a proliferation of enterobacteria, which are clinically relevant pathogens for patients on PD programs. Additionally, the identification of *Raoultella ornithinolytica* as a colonizer of the oral cavity is of extreme importance. The isolation of *R. ornithinolytica* from saliva samples has been reported before in the literature (Heggendorn et al., 2013; Derafshi et al., 2017), but never in such a high prevalence as in this study and never as an oral colonizer of CKD patients. It is important to keep in mind that this is an emerging species both in terms of infectious episodes in humans and in terms of resistance to antibiotic agents (Seng et al., 2016; Hajjar et al., 2020), two factors that make *R. ornithinolytica* a clinically relevant cause of concern, not only to CKD patients, but to the general population. The profiling of *Enterobacteriaceae* isolates in terms of antibiotic resistance, both regarding resistance phenotypes and the presence of genetic elements, is another strong point of this paper. As mentioned before, antibiotic-resistant enterobacteria are responsible for a significant percentage of infections in CKD patients (Prasad et al., 2014; Nguyen et al., 2017; Sahli et al., 2017; Wang et al., 2019), which makes their screening crucial for the clinical follow-up of said patients, given it can provide information for efficient antibiotic prescription in case of infection. Of note that infections are a major problem in peritoneal dialysis programs, leading to patients' deaths or exclusion from peritoneal dialysis programs (Li et al., 2016). Therefore, the search of predisposing factors that lead to peritonitis and catheter-related infections in CKD-PD patients is of outmost importance. Finally, our study also contributes to the profiling of antibiotic resistance genes in the oral microbiome. In recent years, the oral cavity has been highlighted as a reservoir for resistance genes (de Sousa Moreira Almeida et al., 2020) and the profiling of these genes provides extremely relevant information for dentistry and the treatment of oral infections.

CONCLUSION

Our results suggest that the accumulation of uremic toxins in CKD patients induces alterations in the oral milieu, which, in turn, exert selective pressure on the oral microbiome, leading to its dysbiosis with significantly increased prevalence of urease-producing enterobacteria, specifically of *Raoultella ornithinolytica*, an opportunistic enterobacteria. Antibiotic resistance phenotyping revealed mostly intrinsic resistances, although resistances to sulfamethoxazole and streptomycin were also detected. Multidrug resistance was exclusively found in CKD-PD patients isolates. These results, together with the detection of acquired antibiotic resistance genes, alert to the possibility of the oral microbiota as a potential reservoir of resistance genes.

Enterobacteriaceae are known opportunistic pathogens of CKD patients, and this CKD-induced oral dysbiosis can potentially lead to an increase of resistant infectious and inflammatory episodes, contributing, in turn, to the progression of the disease and to its mortality rate. For all these reasons, studying the oral microbiome and its associated resistome and comprehend its role in infection episodes and in the progression of systemic diseases is of extreme relevance to ensure the health and well-being of CKD patients undergoing peritoneal dialysis.

AUTHOR CONTRIBUTIONS

RM, AR, and BS-M contributed to conception and design of the study. CC, AM-R, CC, NS, LP, CF and AG contributed to data acquisition. CC, AM-R, CC, CF, RM, AR, CM and BS-M contributed to data analysis and interpretation. CC, CF, AA, RM, AR, CM and BS-M performed the statistical analysis. CC wrote the first draft of the manuscript. All authors contributed to manuscript revision, read, and approved the submitted version.

FUNDING

This work is a result of the project POCI-01-0145-FEDER-029777, co-financed by Competitiveness and Internationalisation Operational Programme (POCI), under the PORTUGAL 2020 Partnership Agreement, through the European Regional Development Fund (ERDF) and through national funds by the FCT – Fundação para a Ciência e a Tecnologia. CC fellowship was supported by FCT/MCTES scholarship with the reference 2020.08540.BD. This work and CF were financially supported by FEDER through project "Assessing the risks associated with environmental antibiotic resistant bacteria: propagation and transmission to humans" (PTDC/CTA-AMB/28196/2017) - Programa Operacional Competitividade e Internacionalização, and by National Funds from FCT - Fundação para a Ciência e a Tecnologia and was hosted by CBQF through FCT project UIDB/50016/2020.

ACKNOWLEDGMENTS

We would like to thank the kind participants in our study.

REFERENCES

1. Barraclough, K., Hawley, C. M., McDonald, S. P., Brown, F. G., Rosman, J. B., Wiggins, K. J., et al. (2009). *Corynebacterium peritonitis* in Australian peritoneal dialysis patients: predictors, treatment and outcomes in 82 cases. *Nephrol. Dial. Transplant.* 24, 3834–3839. doi: 10.1093/ndt/gfp322
2. Belstrøm, D., Holmstrup, P., Nielsen, C. H., Kirkby, N., Twetman, S., Heitmann, B. L., et al. (2014). Bacterial profiles of saliva in relation to diet, lifestyle factors, and socioeconomic status. *J. Oral Microbiol.* 6:23609. doi: 10.3402/jom.v6.23609
3. Benjamin, O., and Lappin, S. L. (2021). "End-stage renal disease," in *StatPearls [Internet]* (Treasure Island (FL): StatPearls Publishing).
4. CLSI (2017). Performance Standards for Antimicrobial Susceptibility Testing. *27th Edn.* Wayne, PA: Clinical and Laboratory Standards Institute.
5. Cox, G., and Wright, G. D. (2013). Intrinsic antibiotic resistance: mechanisms, origins, challenges and solutions. *Int. J. Med. Microbiol.* 303, 287–292. doi: 10.1016/j.ijmm.2013.02.009
6. Crielaard, W., Zaura, E., Schuller, A. A., Huse, S. M., Montijn, R. C., and Keijser, B. J. F. (2011). Exploring the oral microbiota of children at various developmental stages of their dentition in the relation to their oral health. *BMC Med. Genet.* 4:22. doi: 10.1186/1755-8794-4-22
7. de Sousa Moreira Almeida, V., Azevedo, J., Leal, H. F., de Queiroz, A. T. L., da Silva Filho, H. P., and Reis, J. N. (2020). Bacterial diversity and prevalence of antibiotic resistance genes in the oral microbiome. *PLoS One* 15:e0239664. doi: 10.1371/journal.pone.0239664
8. Derafshi, R., Bazargani, A., Ghapanchi, J., Izadi, Y., and Khorshidi, H. (2017). Isolation and identification of nonoral pathogenic bacteria in the oral cavity of patients with removable dentures. *J. Int. Soc. Prev. Commun. Dent.* 7, 197–201. doi: 10.4103/jispcd.JISPCD_90_17
9. Devanga Ragupathi, N. K., Muthuirulandi Sethuvel, D. P., Inbanathan, F. Y., and Veeraraghavan, B. (2017). Accurate differentiation of *Escherichia coli* and *Shigella* serogroups: challenges and strategies. *New Microbes New Infect.* 21, 58–62. doi: 10.1016/j.nmni.2017.09.003
10. EUCAST (2020). Intrinsic Resistance and Unusual Phenotypes, version 3.2. Available at: https://www.eucast.org/fileadmin/src/media/PDFs/EUCAST_files/ Expert_Rules/2020/Intrinsic_Resistance_and_Unusual_Phenotypes_Tables_ v3.2_20200225.pdf
11. Fysaraki, M., Samonis, G., Valachis, A., Daphnis, E., Karageorgopoulos, D. E., Falagas, M. E., et al. (2013). Incidence, clinical, microbiological features and outcome of bloodstream infections in patients undergoing hemodialysis. *Int. J. Med. Sci.* 10, 1632–1638. doi: 10.7150/ijms.6710
12. Gonçalves, M. O., Coutinho-Filho, W. P., Pimenta, F. P., Pereira, G. A., Pereira, J. A. A., Mattos-Guaraldi, A. L., et al. (2007). Periodontal disease as reservoir for multi-resistant and hydrolytic enterobacterial species. *Lett. Appl. Microbiol.* 44, 488–494. doi: 10.1111/j.1472-765X.2007.02111.x
13. Grothe, C., Taminato, M., Belasco, A., Sesso, R., and Barbosa, D. (2014). Screening and treatment for *Staphylococcus aureus* in patients undergoing hemodialysis: A systematic review and meta-analysis. *BMC Nephrol.* 15:202. doi: 10.1186/1471-2369-15-202
14. Gupta, M., Gupta, M., and Abhishek, (2015). Oral conditions in renal disorders and treatment considerations – A review for pediatric dentist. *Saudi Dent. J.* 27, 113–119. doi: 10.1016/j.sdentj.2014.11.014
15. Hajjar, R., Ambaraghassi, G., Sebajang, H., Schwenter, F., and Su, S. H. (2020). *Raoultella ornithinolytica*: emergence and resistance. *Infect. Drug. Resist.* 13, 1091–1104. doi: 10.2147/IDR.S191387
16. Hajjar, R., Schwenter, F., Su, S.-H., Gasse, M.-C., and Sebajang, H. (2018). Community-acquired infection to *Raoultella ornithinolytica* presenting as appendicitis and shock in a healthy individual. *J. Surg. Case Rep.* 2018:rjy097. doi: 10.1093/jscr/rjy097
17. He, Y., Li, H., Lu, X., Stratton, C. W., and Tang, Y.-W. (2010). Mass spectrometry biotyper system identifies enteric bacterial pathogens directly from colonies grown on selective stool culture media. *J. Clin. Microbiol.* 48, 3888–3892. doi: 10.1128/JCM.01290-10
18. Heggendorn, F. L., Gonçalves, L. S., Dias, E. P., Silva Junior, A., Galvão, M. M., and Lutterbach, M. T. (2013). Detection of sulphate-reducing bacteria in human saliva. *Acta Odontol. Scand.* 71, 1458–1463. doi: 10.3109/00016357.2013.770163
19. Höfer, K., Turnowsky, A., Ehren, R., Taylan, C., Plum, G., Witte, H., et al. (2021). The impact of a needs-oriented dental prophylaxis program on bacteremia after toothbrushing and systemic inflammation in children, adolescents, and young adults with chronic kidney disease. *Pediatr. Nephrol.* doi: 10.1007/s00467-021-05153-1
20. Hu, J., Iragavarapu, S., Nadkarni, G. N., Huang, R., Erazo, M., Bao, X., et al. (2018). Location-specific oral microbiome possesses features associated with CKD. *Kidney Int. Rep* 3, 193–204. doi: 10.1016/j.ekir.2017.08.018
21. Jain, A. K., and Blake, P. G. (2006). Non-pseudomonas gram-negative peritonitis. *Kidney Int.* 69, 1107–1109. doi: 10.1038/sj.ki.5000257
22. Jiang, S., Zeng, J., Zhou, X., and Li, Y. (2018). Drug resistance and gene transfer mechanisms in respiratory/oral bacteria. *J. Dent. Res.* 97, 1092–1099. doi: 10.1177/0022034518782659
23. Li, P. K.-T., and Chow, K. M. (2011). Infectious complications in dialysis – epidemiology and outcomes. *Nat. Rev. Nephrol.* 8, 77–88. doi: 10.1038/nrneph.2011.194
24. Li, X., Kolltveit, K. M., Tronstad, L., and Olsen, I. (2000). Systemic diseases caused by oral infection. *Clin. Microbiol. Rev.* 13, 547–558. doi: 10.1128/CMR.13.4.547
25. Li, P. K.-T., Szeto, C. C., Piraino, B., de Arteaga, J., Fan, S., Figueiredo, A. E., et al. (2016). ISPD peritonitis recommendations: 2016 update on prevention and treatment. *Perit. Dial. Int.* 36, 481–508. doi: 10.3747/pdi.2016. 00078
26. Liakopoulos, V., Nikitidou, O., Kalathas, T., Roumeliotis, S., Salmas, M., and Eleftheriadis, T. (2017). Peritoneal dialysis-related infections recommendations: 2016 update. What is new? *Int. Urol. Nephrol.* 49, 2177–2184. doi: 10.1007/ s11255-017-1632-9
27. Lira-Junior, R., Åkerman, S., Klinge, B., Boström, E. A., and Gustafsson, A. (2018). Salivary microbial profiles in relation to age, periodontal, and systemic diseases. *PLoS One* 13:e0189374. doi: 10.1371/journal.pone.0189374
28. Lisowska-Myjak, B. (2014). Uremic toxins and their effects on multiple organ systems. *Nephron Clin. Pract.* 128, 303–311. doi: 10.1159/000369817
29. Mujais, S. (2006). Microbiology and outcomes of peritonitis in North America. *Kidney Int.* 70, 55–62. doi: 10.1038/sj.ki.5001916
30. Murdeshwar, H. N., and Anjum, F. (2021). "Hemodialysis," in *StatPearls [Internet]* (Treasure Island (FL): StatPearls Publishing).
31. Navazesh, M. (1993). Methods for collecting saliva. *Ann. N. Y. Acad. Sci.* 694, 72–77. doi: 10.1111/j.1749-6632.1993.tb18343.x
32. Nguyen, D. B., Shugart, A., Lines, C., Shah, A. B., Edwards, J., Pollock, D., et al. (2017). National healthcare safety network (NHSN) dialysis event surveillance report for 2014. *Clin. J. Am. Soc. Nephrol.* 12, 1139–1146. doi: 10.2215/CJN.11411116
33. Peleg, A. Y., and Hooper, D. C. (2010). Hospital-acquired infections due to gram-negative bacteria. *N. Engl. J. Med.* 362, 1804–1813. doi: 10.1056/NEJMra0904124
34. Ponce-Alonso, M., Rodríguez-Rojas, L., del Campo, R., Cantón, R., and Morosini, M. I. (2016). Comparison of different methods for identification of species of the genus *Raoultella*: report of 11 cases of *Raoultella* causing bacteraemia and literature review. *Clin. Microbiol. Infect.* 22, 252–257. doi: 10.1016/j.cmi.2015.10.035
35. Posse, J. L., Dios, P. D., and Scully, C. (2017). "Systemic bacteria transmissible by kissing," in *Saliva Protection and Transmissible Diseases* (London, U.K: Elsevier Inc.), 29–51.
36. Prasad, K. N., Singh, K., Rizwan, A., Mishra, P., Tiwari, D., Prasad, N., et al. (2014). Microbiology and outcomes of peritonitis in northern India. *Perit. Dial. Int.* 34, 188–194. doi: 10.3747/pdi.2012.00233
37. Richter, S. S., Sercia, L., Branda, J. A., Burnham, C. A., Bythrow, M., Ferraro, M. J., et al. (2013). Identification of *Enterobacteriaceae* by matrix-assisted

laser desorption/ionization time-of-flight mass spectrometry using the VITEK MS system. *Eur. J. Clin. Microbiol. Infect. Dis.* 32, 1571–1578. doi: 10.1007/ s10096-013-1912-y

38. Roberts, A. P., and Mullany, P. (2010). Oral biofilms: A reservoir of transferable, bacterial, antimicrobial resistance. *Expert Rev. Anti-Infect. Ther.* 8, 1441–1450. doi: 10.1586/eri.10.106

39. Ruppé, É., Woerther, P.-L., and Barbier, F. (2015). Mechanisms of antimicrobial resistance in gram-negative bacilli. *Ann. Intensive Care* 5, 61. doi: 10.1186/ s13613-015-0061-0

40. Rysz, J., Franczyk, B., Ławiński, J., Olszewski, R., Ciałkowska-Rysz, A., and Gluba-Brzózka, A. (2021). The impact of CKD on uremic toxins and gut microbiota. *Toxins* 13, 252. doi: 10.3390/toxins13040252

41. Sahli, F., Feidjel, R., and Laalaoui, R. (2017). Hemodialysis catheter-related infection: rates, risk factors and pathogens. *J. Infect. Public Health* 10, 403–408. doi: 10.1016/j.jiph.2016.06.008

42. Salloum, S., Tawk, M., and Tayyara, L. (2020). Bacterial resistance to antibiotics and associated factors in two hospital centers in Lebanon from January 2017 to June 2017. *Infect. Prev. Pract.* 2:100043. doi: 10.1016/j.infpip.2020. 100043

43. Seng, P., Boushab, B. M., Romain, F., Gouriet, F., Bruder, N., Martin, C., et al. (2016). Emerging role of *Raoultella ornithinolytica* in human infections: a series of cases and review of the literature. *Int. J. Infect. Dis.* 45, 65–71. doi: 10.1016/j.ijid.2016.02.014

44. Sibanda, M. (2014). Primary peritonitis caused by *Raoultella ornithinolytica* in a 53-year-old man. *JMM Case Rep.* 1. doi: 10.1099/jmmcr.0.002634

45. Simões-Silva, L., Ferreira, S., Santos-Araujo, C., Tabaio, M., Pestana, M., Soares-Silva, I., et al. (2018). Oral colonization of *staphylococcus* species in a peritoneal dialysis population: A possible reservoir for PD-related infections? *Can. J. Infect. Dis. Med. Microbiol.* 2018:5789094. doi: 10.1155/2018/5789094

46. Simões-Silva, L., Silva, S., Santos-Araujo, C., Sousa, J., Pestana, M., Araujo, R., et al. (2017). Oral yeast colonization and fungal infections in peritoneal dialysis patients: A pilot study. *Can. J. Infect. Dis. Med. Microbiol.* 2017:4846363. doi: 10.1155/2017/4846363

47. Smith, D. A., and Nehring, S. M. (2021). "Bacteremia," in *StatPearls [Internet]* (Treasure Island (FL): StatPearls Publishing).

48. Szeto, C. C., Chow, V. C., Chow, K. M., Lai, R. W., Chung, K. Y., Leung, C. B., et al. (2006). *Enterobacteriaceae* peritonitis complicating peritoneal dialysis: a review of 210 consecutive cases. *Kidney Int.* 69, 1245–1252. doi: 10.1038/ sj.ki.5000037

49. Thepchuay, Y., Costa, C. F. F. A., Mesquita, R. B. R., Sampaio-Maia, B., Nacapricha, D., and Rangel, A. O. S. S. (2020). Flow-based method for the determination of biomarkers urea and ammoniacal nitrogen in saliva. *Bioanalysis* 12, 455–465. doi: 10.4155/bio-2020-0036

50. Tsuchida, S., Umemura, H., and Nakayama, T. (2020). Current status of matrix- assisted laser desorption/ionization–time-of-flight mass spectrometry (MALDI- TOF MS) in clinical diagnostic microbiology. *Molecules* 25:4775. doi: 10.3390/ molecules25204775

51. Verma, D., Srivastava, A., Garg, P. K., Akhter, Y., Dubey, A. K., Mishra, S., et al. (2021). Taxonomic profiling and functional characterization of the healthy human oral bacterial microbiome from the north Indian urban sub-population. *Arch. Microbiol.* 203, 927–939. doi: 10.1007/s00203-020-02084-7 Wang, T. Z., Kodiyanplakkal, R. P. L., and Calfee, D. P. (2019). Antimicrobial resistance in nephrology. *Nat. Rev. Nephrol.* 15, 463–481. doi: 10.1038/ s41581-019-0150-7

52. Webster, A. C., Nagler, E. V., Morton, R. L., and Masson, P. (2017). Chronic kidney disease. *Lancet* 389, 1238–1252. doi: 10.1016/S0140-6736(16)32064-5 Wiedmann-al-Ahmad, M., Tichy, H. V., and Schön, G. (1994). Characterization of Acinetobacter type strains and isolates obtained from wastewater treatment plants by PCR fingerprinting. *Appl. Environ. Microbiol.* 60, 4066–4071. doi: 10.1128/aem.60.11.4066-4071.1994

11

Periodontitis is Associated with Risk of Conventional Stent Restenosis

Raphael Osugue[1], *Nidia C. Castro dos Santos*[1,2], *Cassia F. Araujo*[1], *Flavio X. de Almeida*[2], *Magda Feres*[2] *and Mauro P. Santamaria*[1*]

[1] *Division of Periodontics, Institute of Science and Technology, UNESP - São Paulo State University, São José dos Campos, Brazil,* [2] *Dental Research Division, Guarulhos University, Guarulhos, Brazil*

Correspondence:
Mauro P. Santamaria
mauro.santamaria@unesp.br

Objectives: Percutaneous coronary angioplasty with stent implantation has been established as the main form of treatment of atherosclerosis. However, 16 to 44% of patients may evolve with stent restenosis. Periodontitis is an inflammatory condition associated with bacterial infection, that may lead to periodontal tissue destruction and tooth loss. This study aimed to evaluate the association between stent restenosis and periodontitis.

Materials and Methods: Coronary angiography exams presenting stent imaging with and without restenosis were analyzed. Patients meeting the inclusion and exclusion criteria were selected and allocated in 2 groups: case (restenosis) and control (without restenosis). We evaluated if systemic and periodontal variables were predictors of restenosis (primary outcome) using a multivariable stepwise logistic regression. Additionally, we compared clinical and periodontal conditions between the control and case groups (secondary outcomes) using Chi-square test and ANOVA test.

Results: Data from 49 patients (case $n = 15$; control $n = 34$) were analyzed. The results showed that stages III and IV periodontitis and lack of physical activity were significant predictors of stent restenosis (OR 5.82 and 5.98, respectively). Comparisons regarding the diagnosis of periodontal conditions between control and case groups did not present significant differences in the incidence of periodontitis and alveolar bone loss.

Conclusion: Stages III and IV periodontitis increased the incidence of stent restenosis. These findings suggest that advanced stages of periodontal disease might lead to the occurrence of negative outcomes after coronary angioplasty with stent placement.

Keywords: atherosclerosis, cardiovascular disease, stent restenosis, periodontitis, inflammation

INTRODUCTION

Atherosclerosis is a progressive fibroproliferative chronic systemic inflammatory process that affects the intima layer of the middle and large vessels, culminating in the formation of atherosclerotic plaque. Its etiology is multifactorial with dyslipidemia, systemic arterial hypertension, diabetes, smoking, and the genetic hereditary component as the main risk factors for the development of atherosclerosis and coronary artery disease (CAD) (1). These factors increase the permeability of the intima to plasma lipoproteins in the subendothelial space, which when oxidized by macrophages become foam cells that are the main component of fatty striae. These immunogenic components stimulate the migration and proliferation of smooth muscle cells from the middle to the intimal layer to produce extracellular matrix that will form part of the fibrous cap of the atherosclerotic plaque (2, 3).

In the last three decades, interventional cardiology has established itself as the main form of myocardial revascularization in the treatment of coronary artery disease. Despite advances in procedural techniques and materials, about 16 to 44% of patients eventually evolve into an event called stent restenosis (4, 5). Restenosis is the onset of new obstruction >50% in the segment previously treated with stent (6) and occurs between the second and sixth month (7, 8) up to the 8 months after implantation of a conventional stent (9). Clinically it may manifest with the return of signs and/or symptoms of myocardial ischemia, associated with angiographic confirmation of new obstruction of the stent. This is the most commonly used concept and is based on vascular physiology studies where from this degree of obstruction we can observe impairment of the coronary flow reserve (10, 11).

Periodontal diseases are inflammatory diseases associated with bacterial infection (12). The initial clinical presentation is gingivitis, which perpetuates the infectious-inflammatory process over the years. In susceptible individuals, gingivitis may be modified by multiple host response genes and, in combination with lifestyle and environmental factors, can culminate in the destructive form of periodontal disease, namely periodontitis (13). Periodontitis is considered a worldwide health problem (14) that over the years has demanded global health policies and programs that can assist in its prevention and treatment (15). It is a highly prevalent disease, with its moderate form affecting 50% and a severe form affecting 5 to 15% of the global adult population (16). Since it was suggested that periodontitis could decrease life expectancy (17), much has been researched on the influence of this disease on quality of life and systemic health of individuals, including cardiovascular disease (18, 19), pregnancy complications (20), neurological diseases (21, 22) and diabetes (23, 24).

Host-microbe interaction in the periodontium can initiate or even aggravate atherosclerotic processes through the activation of innate immunity, bacteremia, and direct involvement of cytokines and inflammatory proteins of oral microbiota (25–27). The association between atherosclerosis and periodontal diseases has already been corroborated in both acute coronary disease and acute myocardial infarction (28, 29), indicating the presence of periodontal diseases as a factor of clinical decompensation of coronary atherosclerosis (30). Despite this, we do not know whether the chronic inflammatory process triggered by periodontal diseases can interfere with the long-term outcome of patients undergoing coronary angioplasty with a consequent episode of restenosis. Whether periodontal diseases, due to their chronic systemic inflammatory state, would be contributing to an increase in restenosis rates of conventional stents is not defined in the literature. Besides that, it is not routine in the clinical practice of interventional cardiologists to consider the oral health status before performing surgical coronary angioplasty. To date, there are no studies evaluating the possible relationship between conventional stent restenosis and periodontal diseases. Therefore, the aim of the present study is to evaluate the association between stent restenosis and periodontitis.

MATERIALS AND METHODS

Experimental Design

This was an observational, retrospective, case-control, population-based study designed to evaluate the association between conventional stent restenosis and periodontal diseases. This study was approved by the human subjects ethics board of UNESP (CAAE: 60607916.9.0000.0077) and was conducted in accordance with the Helsinki Declaration of 1975, as revised in 2013.

Study Population and Inclusion and Exclusion Criteria

Data from coronary angiography examinations performed at Pio XII Hospital (São José dos Campos, SP, Brazil) from January 4th, 2016 to February 28th, 2018 were analyzed. The study population consisted of patients who underwent coronary angiography at the referred hospital during the established period. Detailed medical records were obtained. Volunteers who fulfilled the inclusion criteria were invited to participate in the study. Inclusion criteria were prior coronary angioplasty with conventional stent implantation; aged ≥40. Exclusion criteria were: edentulism; diabetes mellitus with glycated hemoglobin (HbA1c) levels >7.0%; pharmacological stent implantation; restenosis in stents implanted over the previous 2 years. Informed consent was provided by each volunteer after a thorough explanation of the nature, risks, and benefits of the clinical investigations.

Allocation

Patients were allocated into two groups according to the criteria below:

- Case Group: Patients who underwent coronary angiography examination of stent with restenosis, whose stent implantation occurred within 2 years.
- Control Group: Patients who presented coronary angiography with stent image without restenosis regardless of the implantation period.

Cardiovascular Evaluation

For the screening and selection of candidates for both study groups, the reports previously made by interventional cardiologists at the Pio XII Hospital were used. For the definition of angiographic restenosis in coronary angiography reports, the Interventional Cardiology societies criteria were used. These criteria are based on studies of vascular physiology, in which the impairment of coronary flow reserve can be observed considering the degree of obstruction, and consists of the presence of >70% from the lesion in the stent-treated segment (within the stent and within 5 mm beyond the stent) (4). Restenosis was classified using the Guideline Reference for Percutaneous Coronary Intervention by the American Heart Association (31, 32). This classification is based on the geographic distribution of intimal hyperplasia in reference to the implanted stent. Peripheral blood was collected to evaluate HbA1c levels and lipid profile. Anthropometric measures including weight and height were recorded. Body mass index (BMI) was calculated as the weight divided by the square of height (kg/m^2).

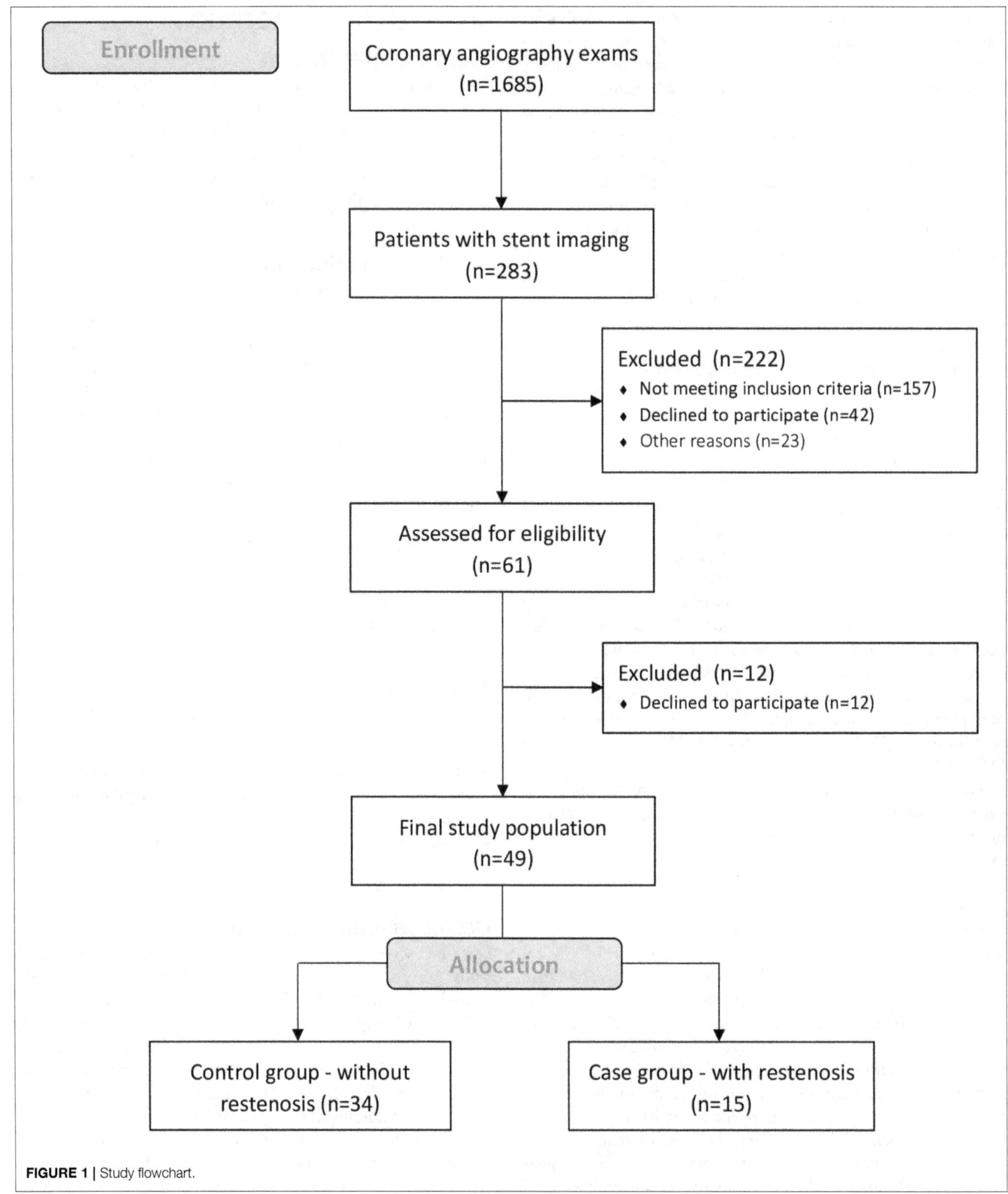

FIGURE 1 | Study flowchart.

Periodontal Evaluation

All patients were scheduled for a periodontal evaluation at the Department of Periodontology at the Institute of Science and Technology, São Paulo State University–Unesp (São José dos Campos, SP, Brazil). In this session, a throughout periodontal examination was performed by two trained and calibrated periodontists (CFA and NCCS). The examiners participated in a calibration exercise in which PD and CAL of 10 patients were measured twice within a 24-h interval. These measurements were subjected to an intraclass correction test. The agreement for the variables was >90%.

The evaluated parameters were: (1) Probing depth (PD); (2) Clinical attachment level (CAL); (3) Gingival recession (GR); (4) Bleeding on probing (BoP); (5) Supragingival biofilm accumulation (Pl) (33). All clinical measures were assessed using a manual probe (University of North Carolina Probe PCPUNC-BR 15, Hu-Friedy).

The presence or absence of periodontal diseases, the diagnosis, and classification of the diseases, the quantification of the extent and severity of the diseases, and the estimated duration of the diseases were determined (34, 35).

Alveolar Bone Loss Analysis

Panoramic radiographs were obtained by a radiologist and evaluated by a trained examiner. The examiner was blind to the status of each group of participants. The severity of alveolar bone loss was measured as a percentage of bone loss in the interproximal sites of each tooth (36). Each site was assigned a score from 1 through 4 according to alveolar bone (1: 0 to 24%; 2: 25 to 49%; 3: 50 to 74%; 4: 75 to 100%). We defined a mean bone loss score ≤2 as mild to moderate periodontal bone loss and score >2 as severe alveolar bone loss.

Statistical Analysis

Data were recorded as mean and standard deviation, median with quartiles or percentage according to the different variables analyzed. Normal distribution was tested by Shapiro-Wilk. For the comparison of quantitative variables, the mean and standard deviation were used. For percentages, Chi-square test (χ^2) was used for qualitative variables. ANOVA test was used to compare groups for mean age and BMI. A multivariable stepwise logistic regression was performed to verify if there is a relationship between restenosis (dependent variable) and independent variables. All data analyses were performed using IBM SPSS, Minitab, and Excel Office. A significance level of 0.05 (5%) was defined for this study, and all confidence intervals throughout the study were constructed with 95% statistical confidence.

TABLE 1 | Socioeconomic and clinical characteristics for control and case groups.

Variables	Control group (n = 34)	Case group (n = 15)	P-value
Gender (male)	24 (70%)[A]	13 (86%)[A]	0.228
Age (years)	60.60±8.00[A]	59.10±8.50[A]	0.542
BMI (kg/m^2)	27.91±3.50[A]	27.12±3.46[A]	0.495
Arterial hypertension	31 (96%)[A]	12 (85%)[A]	0.158
Diabetes mellitus	8 (23%)[A]	5 (33%)[A]	0.474
Dyslipidemia	27 (84%)[A]	12 (86%)[A]	0.907
CAD	16 (50%)[A]	9 (64%)[A]	0.371
Smoker	7 (22%)[A]	2 (14 %)[A]	0.550
Former smoker	9 (28%)[A]	9 (64%)[B]	0.021
Obesity	9 (28%)[A]	3 (21%)[A]	0.634
Brushing	30 (96%)[A]	14 (100%)[A]	0.497

BMI, body mass index; CAD, coronary artery disease.
Different uppercase indicates statistically significant differences between groups. Age and BMI were compared using one-way ANOVA. Intergroup percentages were compared using Chi-square test (χ^2).

TABLE 2 | Stepwise logistic regression considering restenosis as an outcome variable for all volunteers (n = 49).

	Restenosis		
	OR	95% C.I.	P-value
Periodontitis			
No	1.0		
Stages III and IV	5.82	1.35–25.07	0.018
Physical activity			
Yes	1.0		
No	5.98	1.07–33.62	0.042

Covariables included are periodontitis, diabetes, obesity, smoking, physical activity, age, gender, number of teeth, and alveolar bone loss.
Nagelkerke R^2 = 0.248.

RESULTS

A total of 1,685 coronary angiography examinations performed during the period from January 4th, 2016 to February 28th, 2018 were analyzed. At the end of volunteer selection, 61 patients were eligible. Of these, 49 patients accepted to participate in the study and underwent periodontal evaluation (**Figure 1**). **Table 1** presents sociodemographic characteristics of the control group (n = 34) and the case group (n = 15). There was no statistical difference between most of the variables analyzed, except for previous smoking history (**Table 1**).

A binary logistic regression was performed to determine if demographic, systemic, and periodontal variables were predictors of restenosis. "Stages III and IV periodontitis" and "No regular physical activity" were significant predictors when restenosis was a dependent outcome variable (OR 5.82 and 5.98, respectively). Other stages of periodontitis, controlled diabetes, obesity, current smoking, age, gender, number of teeth, and severe alveolar bone loss were not statistically significant (**Table 2**).

We evaluated the groups according to the frequency of different diagnoses and classifications of periodontal diseases. There was a higher percentage of gingivitis and Stages I and II periodontitis when the control group was compared to the case group. On the other hand, Stages III and IV periodontitis presented higher percentages in the case group than

TABLE 3 | Incidence of periodontal diseases for the control and case groups.

Variables	Control group		Case group		*P*-value
	n	%	*n*	%	
Gingivitis	8	23.5	2	13.3	0.414
Stage I periodontitis	5	14.7	1	6.7	0.466
Stage II periodontitis	10	29.5	3	20.0	0.492
Stage III periodontitis	5	14.7	5	33.3	0.111
Stage IV periodontitis	6	17.6	4	26.7	0.470

Chi-square test (χ^2) was used to compare the frequency of periodontal diseases between groups ($p < 0.05$).

in the control group. Despite these differences, no statistical significance was observed ($p > 0.05$) (**Table 3**).

For the comparison of alveolar bone loss scores between groups, the case group presented 4 (36%) patients with alveolar bone loss score ≤ 2, while 7 (63%) patients presented score >2. In the control group, we observed that 11 (38%) patients presented score ≤ 2, and 18 (62%) patients presented score >2. No statistical significance was observed in the intergroup comparison.

DISCUSSION

Stages III and IV periodontitis increased the risk of chances for stent restenosis. These results suggest that periodontitis is an important factor to be considered in the clinical cardiological evaluation routine before and after coronary angioplasty interventions.

Growing evidence suggests a link between periodontitis and cardiovascular disease, especially regarding the risk factors shared between these conditions. In this study population, all patients presented atherosclerosis and had already received conventional stent implantation treatment. Thus, the high prevalence of periodontal disease found in our study population is justified, confirming the same results found in a previous study (37). Besides having common risk factors, a mechanism linking the two diseases has been elucidated in a recent longitudinal study. Van Dyke et al. (38) evaluated the F-fluorodeoxyglucose positron emission tomography/computed tomography of 304 individuals, quantifying periodontal and arterial inflammation. The authors showed that periodontitis is associated with arterial inflammation and that periodontitis predicted subsequent major adverse cardiovascular events (38). These findings corroborate the main results of our study, which underscore the hypothesis that periodontitis could influence the occurrence and treatment of CAD.

In addition to periodontitis, we observed that physical activity was associated with a lower restenosis rate. It is well-documented that physical activity helps to control many cardiovascular risk factors (39). In patients with stable CAD, the measurement of C-reactive protein (CRP) may be useful as an independent marker to assess the likelihood of recurrent events, including death, myocardial infarction, or stent restenosis (40), and physical activity in this type of patient is a factor that in itself reduces inflammatory markers such as CRP (41). Thus, the regular practice of physical activity could contribute as a protective factor for restenosis by reducing inflammation.

Risk factors associated with the development of periodontitis comprise local, systemic, and genetic factors, including smoking, diabetes, and possibly obesity (42). Contributions for cardiovascular disease are also multifactorial, which encompass ethnicity, age, family history of CAD, dyslipidemia, hypertension, smoking, obesity, and diabetes. Hence, there are many potentially important confounders for the association between periodontitis and atherosclerotic disease (19). The presence of confounding factors is a relevant limitation aspect of several observational studies (43). In the present study, we assessed if there was an association between risk factors shared by the two diseases and restenosis, but no significant results were observed.

Although diabetes mellitus is considered a risk factor that increases the likelihood of restenosis, patients with controlled diabetes (HbA1c <7.0%) do not present high restenosis rates after conventional stent implantation (44, 45). For this reason, patients with controlled diabetes were included in this study. As expected, controlled diabetes was not associated with an increased risk for restenosis in this study. One of the exclusion criteria was the presence of pharmacological stents, for the use of pharmacological stents alters the physiology of the stent endothelialization phenomenon by inhibiting the cell cycle in different stages, thus delaying the stent phenomenon of cell migration and proliferation (46). Despite the benefits of pharmacological stents observed in large randomized controlled clinical trials, the use of drug-eluting stenting implies longer dual anti-aggregation therapy, thereby increasing the risk of bleeding (47) and decreasing the cost-effectiveness of the procedure (48).

The findings of this study demonstrate that periodontitis is an important predictor of stent restenosis. Nevertheless, this result should be interpreted with caution. The main limitation of this study is the small sample size. Of the 1,685 coronary angiography examinations, 1,402 patients did not present stent imaging, which resulted in 283 possible volunteers for the study. Then, volunteer selection was particularly difficult for the exclusion criterion "edentulism," which was highly prevalent in the analyzed population. Possibly, most individuals presenting edentulism had lost their teeth due to periodontitis previously to this study. Thus, the number of observed events (restenosis) was modest (15 patients). The main strength of the present study is that periodontal diseases were evaluated as possible predictors for stent restenosis for the first time. This hypothesis was mechanistically plausible and demonstrated to be clinically relevant in this population. Additionally, evaluating the association between periodontal diseases and negative outcomes after cardiological interventions help to increase the awareness of the relevance of periodontal evaluation and treatment in patients with atherosclerosis.

Stages III and IV periodontitis is associated with the incidence of stent restenosis. These findings suggest that advanced stages of periodontal disease might lead to the occurrence of negative outcomes after coronary angioplasty with stent placement.

AUTHOR CONTRIBUTIONS

RO: conception and design, selection of volunteers, and interpretation of data. NC: data acquisition, analysis, interpretation of data, and drafting article. CA: data acquisition and interpretation of data. FA: interpretation of data. MF: interpretation of data and drafting article. MS: conception and design, direction and implementation, interpretation, and drafting article. All authors contributed to the article and approved the submitted version.

REFERENCES

1. Yahagi K, Kolodgie FD, Otsuka F, Finn A V, Davis HR, Joner M, et al. Pathophysiology of native coronary, vein graft, and in-stent atherosclerosis. *Nat Rev Cardiol.* (2016) 13:79–98. doi: 10.1038/nrcardio.2015.164
2. Ross R, Glomset JA. The pathogenesis of atherosclerosis (first of two parts). *N Engl J Med.* (1976) 295:369–77. doi: 10.1056/NEJM197608122950707
3. Otsuka F, Kramer MC, Woudstra P, Yahagi K, Ladich E, Finn A V, et al. Natural progression of atherosclerosis from pathologic intimal thickening to late fibroatheroma in human coronary arteries: a pathology study. *Atherosclerosis.* (2015) 241:772–82. doi: 10.1016/j.atherosclerosis.2015.05.011
4. Weintraub WS, Ghazzal ZM, Douglas JS, Liberman HA, Morris DC, Cohen CL, et al. Long-term clinical follow-up in patients with angiographic restudy after successful angioplasty. *Circulation.* (1993) 87:831–40. doi: 10.1161/01.CIR.87.3.831
5. Gershlick A, Brack MJ, More RS, Syndercombe-Court D, Balcon R. Angiographic restenosis after angioplasty: comparison of definitions and correlation with clinical outcome. *Coron Artery Dis.* (1993) 4: 73–81.
6. Roubin GS, King SB, Douglas JS. Restenosis after percutaneous transluminal coronary angioplasty: the Emory University Hospital experience. *Am J Cardiol.* (1987) 60:39B–43B. doi: 10.1016/0002-9149(87) 90482-6
7. Serruys PW, Luijten HE, Beatt KJ, Geuskens R, de Feyter PJ, van den Brand M, et al. Incidence of restenosis after successful coronary angioplasty: a time-related phenomenon. A quantitative angiographic study in 342 consecutive patients at 1, 2, 3, and 4 months. *Circulation.* (1988) 77:361–71. doi: 10.1161/01.CIR.77.2.361
8. Nobuyoshi M, Kimura T, Nosaka H, Mioka S, Ueno K, Yokoi H, et al. Restenosis after successful percutaneous transluminal coronary angioplasty: serial angiographic follow-up of 229 patients. *J Am Coll Cardiol.* (1988) 12:616–23. doi: 10.1016/S0735-1097(88)80046-9
9. Gruentzig AR, King SB, Schlumpf M, Siegenthaler W. Long-term follow-up after percutaneous transluminal coronary angioplasty. The early Zurich experience. *N Engl J Med.* (1987) 316:1127–32. doi: 10.1056/NEJM198704303161805
10. Holmes DR, Schwartz RS, Webster MW. Coronary restenosis: what have we learned from angiography? *J Am Coll Cardiol.* (1991) 17(6 Suppl B):14B–22B. doi: 10.1016/0735-1097(91)90934-2
11. Kuntz RE, Baim DS. Defining coronary restenosis. Newer clinical and angiographic paradigms. *Circulation.* (1993) 88:1310–23. doi: 10.1161/01.CIR.88.3.1310
12. Page RC, Kornman KS. The pathogenesis of human periodontitis: an introduction. *Periodontol.* (1997) 14:9–11. doi: 10.1111/j.1600-0757.1997.tb00189.x
13. Bartold PM, Van Dyke TE. Periodontitis : a host-mediated disruption of microbial homeostasis. Unlearning learned concepts. *Periodontology.* (2013) 62:203–17. doi: 10.1111/j.1600-0757.2012.00450.x
14. Armitage GC, Research S ienc. TC of the AA of P. Diagnosis of periodontal diseases. *J Periodontol.* (2003) 74:1237–47. doi: 10.1902/jop.2003.74.8.1237
15. Petersen PE, Ogawa H. Strengthening the prevention of periodontal disease: the WHO approach. *J Periodontol.* (2005) 76:2187–93. doi: 10.1902/jop.2005.76.12.2187
16. Holtfreter B, Albandar JM, Dietrich T, Dye BA, Eaton KA, Eke PI, et al. Standards for reporting chronic periodontitis prevalence and severity in epidemiologic studies: proposed standards from the Joint EU/USA Periodontal Epidemiology Working Group. *J Clin Periodontol.* (2015) 42:407–12. doi: 10.1111/jcpe.12392
17. Buset SL, Walter C, Friedmann A, Weiger R, Borgnakke WS, Zitzmann NU. Are periodontal diseases really silent? A systematic review of their effect on quality of life. *J Clin Periodontol.* (2016) 43:333–44. doi: 10.1111/jcpe.12517
18. Dietrich T. Age-dependent associations between chronic periodontitis/edentulism and risk of coronary heart disease. *Bone.* (2008) 23:1–7. doi: 10.1161/CIRCULATIONAHA.107.711507
19. Tonetti MS, Van Dyke TE. Periodontitis and atherosclerotic cardiovascular disease: consensus report of the Joint EFP/AAP Workshop on Periodontitis and Systemic Diseases. *J Clin Periodontol.* (2013) 40(Suppl. 14):24–9. doi: 10.1111/jcpe.12089
20. Armitage GC. Bi-directional relationship between pregnancy and periodontal disease. *Periodontol.* (2013) 61:160–76. doi: 10.1111/j.1600-0757.2011.00396.x
21. Hellvard A, Ryder MI, Hasturk H, Walker GD, Benedyk M, Lee A, et al. Porphyromonas gingivalis in Alzheimer's disease brains: evidence for disease causation and treatment with small-molecule inhibitors. *Sci Adv.* (2019) 5:eaau3333. doi: 10.1126/sciadv.aau3333
22. Gil-Montoya JA, Sanchez-Lara I, Carnero-Pardo C, Fornieles F, Montes J, Vilchez R, et al. is periodontitis a risk factor for cognitive impairment and dementia? A case-control study. *J Periodontol.* (2015) 86:244–53. doi: 10.1902/jop.2014.140340
23. Taylor GW. Bidirectional interrelationships between diabetes and periodontal diseases: an epidemiologic perspective. *Ann Periodontol.* (2001) 6:99–112. doi: 10.1902/annals.2001.6.1.99
24. Casanova L, Hughes FJ, Preshaw PM. Diabetes and periodontal disease: a two-way relationship. *Br Dent J.* (2014) 217:433–7. doi: 10.1038/sj.bdj.2014.907
25. Schenkein HA, Loos BG. Inflammatory mechanisms linking periodontal diseases to cardiovascular diseases. *J Clin Periodontol.* (2013) 40(Suppl. 14). doi: 10.1111/jcpe.12060
26. Flores MF, Montenegro MM, Furtado M V, Polanczyk CA, Rosing CK, Haas AN. Periodontal status affects C-reactive protein and lipids in patients with stable heart disease from a tertiary care cardiovascular clinic. *J Periodontol.* (2014) 85:545–53. doi: 10.1902/jop.2013.130255
27. Reyes L, Herrera D, Kozarov E, Roldan S, Progulske-Fox A. Periodontal bacterial invasion and infection: contribution to atherosclerotic pathology. *J Clin Periodontol.* (2013) 40:S30–50. doi: 10.1111/jcpe.12079
28. Widén C, Holmer H, Coleman M, Tudor M, Ohlsson O, Sättlin S, et al. Systemic inflammatory impact of periodontitis on acute coronary syndrome. *J Clin Periodontol.* (2016) 9:713–9. doi: 10.1111/jcpe.12540
29. Sidhu RK. Association between acute myocardial infarction and periodontitis: a review of the literature. *J Int Acad Periodontol.* (2016) 18:23–33.
30. Vedin O, Hagstrom E, Gallup D, Neely ML, Stewart R, Koenig W, et al. Periodontal disease in patients with chronic coronary heart disease: prevalence and association with cardiovascular risk factors. *Eur J Prev Cardiol.* (2015) 22:771–8. doi: 10.1177/2047487314530660
31. Mehran R, Dangas G, Abizaid AS, Mintz GS, Lansky AJ, Satler LF, et al. Angiographic patterns of in-stent restenosis: classification and implications for long-term outcome. *Circulation.* (1999) 100:1872–8. doi: 10.1161/01.CIR.100.18.1872
32. Levine GN, Bates ER, Blankenship JC, Bailey SR, Bittl JA, Cercek B, et al. 2011 ACCF/AHA/SCAI Guideline for Percutaneous Coronary Intervention: a report of the American College of Cardiology Foundation/American Heart Association task force on practice guidelines and the society for cardiovascular angiography and interventions. *Circulation.* (2011). 124:e574–651. doi: 10.1161/CIR.0b013e31823a5596
33. Ainamo J, Bay I. Problems and proposals for recording gingivitis and plaque. *Int Dent J.* (1975) 25:229–35.
34. Caton J, Armitage G, Berglundh T, Chapple ILC, Jepsen S, Kornman K, et al. A new classification scheme for periodontal and peri-implant diseases and conditions – Introduction and key changes from the 1999 classification. *J Clin Periodontol.* (2018) 45:S1–8. doi: 10.1111/jcpe.12935
35. Papapanou PN, Sanz M, Buduneli N, Dietrich T, Feres M, Fine DH, et al. Periodontitis: consensus report of workgroup 2 of the 2017 World Workshop

on the classification of periodontal and peri-implant diseases and conditions. *J Clin Periodontol.* (2018) 45:S162–70. doi: 10.1111/jcpe.12946

36. Schei O, Waerhaug J, Lovdal A, Arno A. Alveolar bone loss as related to oral hygiene and age. *J periodontol.* (1959) 30:7–16. doi: 10.1902/jop.1959.30.1.7
37. Accarini R, Godoy MF. Periodontal disease as a potential risk factor for acute coronary syndromes. *Arq Bras Cardiol.* (2007) 88:539–43. doi: 10.1590/s0066-782x2006001800007
38. Van Dyke TE, Kholy K El, Ishai A, Takx RAP, Mezue K, Abohashem SM, et al. Inflammation of the periodontium associates with risk of future cardiovascular events. *J Periodontol.* (2021) 92:348–58. doi: 10.1002/JPER.19-0441
39. Milani R V., Lavie CJ, Mehra MR. Reduction in C-reactive protein through cardiac rehabilitation and exercise training. *J Am Coll Cardiol.* (2004) 43:1056–61. doi: 10.1016/j.jacc.2003.10.041
40. Pearson TA, Mensah GA, Alexander RW, Anderson JL, Cannon RO, Criqui M, et al. Markers of inflammation and cardiovascular disease: application to clinical and public health practice: a statement for healthcare professionals from the centers for disease control and prevention and the American Heart Association. *Circulation.* (2003) 107:499–511. doi: 10.1161/01.CIR.0000052939.59093.45
41. Rahimi K, Secknus MA, Adam M, Hayerizadeh BF, Fiedler M, Thiery J, et al. Correlation of exercise capacity with high-sensitive C-reactive protein in patients with stable coronary artery disease. *Am Heart J.* (2005) 150:1282–9. doi: 10.1016/j.ahj.2005.01.006
42. Borrell LN, Papapanou PN. Analytical epidemiology of periodontitis. *J Clin Periodontol.* (2005) 32(Suppl. 6):132–58. doi: 10.1111/j.1600-051X.2005.00799.x
43. Hyman J. The importance of assessing confounding and effect modification in research involving periodontal disease and systemic diseases. *J Clin Periodontol.* (2006) 33:102–3. doi: 10.1111/j.1600-051X.2005.00881.x
44. Corpus RA, George PB, House JA, Dixon SR, Ajluni SC, Devlin WH, et al. Optimal glycemic control is associated with a lower rate of target vessel revascularization in treated type II diabetic patients undergoing elective percutaneous coronary intervention. *J Am Coll Cardiol.* (2004) 43:8–14. doi: 10.1016/j.jacc.2003.06.019
45. Kassaian SE, Goodarzynejad H, Boroumand MA, Salarifar M, Masoudkabir F, Mohajeri-Tehrani MR, et al. Glycosylated hemoglobin (HbA1c) levels and clinical outcomes in diabetic patients following coronary artery stenting. *Cardiovasc Diabetol.* (2012) 11:82. doi: 10.1186/1475-2840-11-82
46. Morice M-C, Serruys PW, Souza JE. A randomized comparison of a Sirolimus-eluting stent with a standard stent for coronary revascularization. *N Engl J Med.* (2002) 346:1773–80. doi: 10.1056/NEJMoa012843
47. Yeh RW, Normand SLT, Wolf RE, Jones PG, Ho KKL, Cohen DJ, et al. Predicting the restenosis benefit of drug-eluting versus bare metal stents in percutaneous coronary intervention. *Circulation.* (2011) 124:1557–64. doi: 10.1161/CIRCULATIONAHA.111.045229
48. Amin AP, Spertus JA, Cohen DJ, Chhatriwalla A, Kennedy KF, Vilain K, et al. Use of drug-eluting stents as a function of predicted benefit. *Arch Intern Med.* (2012) 172:1145–52. doi: 10.1001/archinternmed.2012.3093

12

Oral Microbiome Dysbiosis is Associated with Symptoms Severity and Local Immune/Inflammatory Response in COVID-19 Patients

Irene Soffritti[1†], Maria D'Accolti[1†], Chiara Fabbri[2], Angela Passaro[3], Roberto Manfredini[4], Giovanni Zuliani[3], Marco Libanore[5], Maurizio Franchi[2], Carlo Contini[6] and Elisabetta Caselli[1]*

[1] Section of Microbiology, CIAS Research Center and LTTA, Department of Chemical and Pharmaceutical Sciences, University of Ferrara, Ferrara, Italy, [2] Section of Dentistry, Department of Biomedical and Specialty Surgical Sciences, University of Ferrara, Ferrara, Italy, [3] Unit of Internal Medicine, Department of Translational Medicine, University of Ferrara, Ferrara, Italy, [4] Medical Clinic Unit, Department of Medical Sciences, University of Ferrara, Ferrara, Italy, [5] Unit of Infectious Diseases, University Hospital of Ferrara, Ferrara, Italy, [6] Section of Infectious Diseases and Dermatology, Department of Medical Sciences, University of Ferrara, Ferrara, Italy

***Correspondence:**
Elisabetta Caselli
csb@unife.it

† These authors have contributed equally to this work

The human oral microbiome (HOM) is the second largest microbial community after the gut and can impact the onset and progression of several localized and systemic diseases, including those of viral origin, especially for viruses entering the body via the oropharynx. However, this important aspect has not been clarified for the new pandemic human coronavirus SARS-CoV-2, causing COVID-19 disease, despite it being one of the many respiratory viruses having the oropharynx as the primary site of replication. In particular, no data are available about the non-bacterial components of the HOM (fungi, viruses), which instead has been shown to be crucial for other diseases. Consistent with this, this study aimed to define the HOM in COVID-19 patients, to evidence any association between its profile and the clinical disease. Seventy-five oral rinse samples were analyzed by Whole Genome Sequencing (WGS) to simultaneously identify oral bacteria, fungi, and viruses. To correlate the HOM profile with local virus replication, the SARS-CoV-2 amount in the oral cavity was quantified by digital droplet PCR. Moreover, local inflammation and secretory immune response were also assessed, respectively by measuring the local release of pro-inflammatory cytokines (L-6, IL-17, TNFα, and GM-CSF) and the production of secretory immunoglobulins A (sIgA). The results showed the presence of oral dysbiosis in COVID-19 patients compared to matched controls, with significantly decreased alpha-diversity value and lower species richness in COVID-19 subjects. Notably, oral dysbiosis correlated with symptom severity ($p = 0.006$), and increased local inflammation ($p < 0.01$). In parallel, a decreased mucosal sIgA response was observed in more severely symptomatic patients ($p = 0.02$), suggesting that local immune response is important in the early control of virus infection and that its correct development is influenced by the HOM profile. In conclusion, the data presented here suggest that the HOM profile may be important in defining the individual susceptibility to SARS-CoV-2 infection, facilitating inflammation and virus replication, or rather, inducing a protective IgA response. Although it is not possible to determine whether the alteration in the microbial community is the cause or effect of the SARS-CoV-2 replication, these parameters may be considered as markers for personalized therapy and vaccine development.

Keywords: oral microbiome, COVID-19, symptom severity, inflammatory cytokines, secretory IgA

INTRODUCTION

The human oral microbiome (HOM) is the second largest and complex microbial community after that of the gut in the human body (Wade, 2013; Caselli et al., 2020a). HOM dysbiosis is often associated with periodontal inflammation and has been reportedly associated with several local and systemic disease conditions (Baghbani et al., 2020; Caselli et al., 2020a), including those sustained by viral infections (Cagna et al., 2019; Baghbani et al., 2020). Indeed, the role of HOM in the establishment of the infection of many viruses entering the body via the oropharynx has been reportedly recognized (Baghbani et al., 2020). The microbial component of a eubiotic HOM can inhibit pathogen colonization by competitive exclusion and/or by empowering the immune response (Wilks et al., 2013). There is evidence that crucial mutual interactions occur between viruses and the microbiome (Wilks and Golovkina, 2012) and that the microbiome can regulate and is in turn regulated by viruses via different mechanisms (Li et al., 2019). Respiratory viruses spread by aerosol transmission encounter oral and upper respiratory microbiota and are modulated in their ability to establish infection and able to induce changes in the resident microbiota (Li et al., 2019). The microbiota can produce antiviral compounds (defensins) against several viruses, including respiratory or oral viruses such as adenoviruses, herpesviruses, papillomaviruses, orthomyxoviruses, and coronaviruses (Pfeiffer and Sonnenburg, 2011). On the other hand, viruses can alter the microbiota, favoring dysbiosis and disease progression (Lynch, 2014).

The new pandemic human coronavirus SARS-CoV-2, causing COVID-19 disease, is a respiratory virus that uses the oropharynx as the primary site of replication, but the potential impact of HOM in the development of infection is still not elucidated. In particular, no data are available about the non-bacterial components of the HOM (fungi, viruses), which have been shown crucial for other diseases. Concerning the current pandemics by SARS-CoV-2, the presence of gingival inflammation/periodontitis has been associated with a 3.5-fold increased risk of admission to intensive care units (ICU), a 4.5-fold greater risk of assisted ventilation, and a consistent impressive 8.81-fold higher risk of death in COVID-19 patients, independently from other concomitant risk factors (Marouf et al., 2021).

The novel human Severe Acute Respiratory Syndrome Coronavirus type (SARS-CoV-2) is a single strand RNA virus belonging to the *Coronaviridae* family, β-coronavirus genus (Contini et al., 2020), which has spread worldwide. The associated disease, Corona Virus Disease 2019 (COVID-19), is currently reported by the World Health Organization (WHO) to have caused about 120 million cases with >2.6 million deaths (World Health Organization [WHO], 2021). In Italy, to date over 3.2 million cases have been reported, with other 102,000 deaths. The disease is characterized by the involvement of the lower respiratory tract, often accompanied by elevated blood levels of inflammatory cytokines/chemokines, the so-called "cytokine storm" (de la Rica et al., 2020; Jose and Manuel, 2020), by ageusia and/or hyposmia (Contini et al., 2020; Li et al., 2020; Prasad et al., 2020), and neurological and enteric symptoms in severely symptomatic patients (Contini et al., 2020; Gupta et al., 2020).

An extraordinarily high number of studies were published the last year, yet the mechanisms underlying virus proliferation in the primary site of infection and understanding of how the virus can become more invasive at the site of entry is still unclear, even though this could shed important light on the very first phases of the infection. It is recognized that SARS-CoV-2 enters the body mainly via the oropharynx, where it finds epithelial cells expressing the ACE2 and TMPRSS2 virus receptors (Herrera et al., 2020), and the virus has been detected in saliva (Henrique Braz-Silva et al., 2020; To et al., 2020). Thus, the resident oral microbiome may influence the ability of SARS-CoV-2 to take root and establish the infection. Similar to what is reported for other viruses affecting the oral and respiratory tract, the virus-host interplay in this site may define the vulnerability of the infected subject and the subsequent development of the disease or rather the early control of virus infection and prevention of severe disease. Like other microbial communities in the body, the oral microbiome can represent a protective barrier against exogenous pathogens (Zaura et al., 2009; Wade, 2013; He et al., 2015; Deo and Deshmukh, 2019) and it contributes to the lung microbiome, thus potentially affecting also the microbial environment in the lungs (Bassis et al., 2015). The oral microbiome can contribute to regulating mucosal immunity and inflammation, which might affect pathogenic potential directly or indirectly (Belkaid and Hand, 2014; Lamont et al., 2018).

Although there is potential interest in understanding these networks in SARS-CoV-2 infection, no information is yet available about the microbiome profile in COVID-19 patients, except for a two as yet unpublished reports describing the bacterial component of the oral microbiome by NGS (Iebba et al., 2020; Ward et al., 2021). However, several reports have evidenced that the non-bacterial components of the microbiome can be very important in defining individual susceptibility to diseases besides bacteria (the mycome and virome), thus the use of Whole

Genome Sequencing (WGS) technology may be more useful in elucidating the microbial environment potentially impacting on SARS-CoV-2 infecting ability.

The present work aimed to characterize, for the first time, the oral microbiome of COVID-19 patients by WGS, comparing its profile to controls, and simultaneously evaluating the presence of inflammatory cytokines and local IgA immune response, to better understand the features of the oral environment that could potentially support SARS-CoV-2 infection and related disease, and to identify eventual markers for the risk of developing a severe infection.

MATERIALS AND METHODS

Ethics Statement

Recruitment of study participants was performed according to the protocol approved by the Ethics Committee Area Vasta Emilia Centro della Regione Emilia-Romagna (CE-AVEC): approval document no. 408/2020/Oss/UniFe, approved on April 21, 2020.

Design of the Study

A cross-sectional observational study was performed to characterize the oral microbiome and local response in COVID-19 patients compared to non-COVID-19 subjects. All participants were recruited from the University Hospital of Ferrara, in the COVID-19 and the non-COVID Infectious ward, respectively. Study participants were recruited in the period April to July 2020. Each study participant was recruited after signing informed consent. Clinical and epidemiological data were collected from the clinicians of the enrolled ward. The study was registered and published prospectively in the ISRCTN International Registry (study n° ISRCTN87832712; doi: 10.1186/ISRCTN87832712).

Study Participants

All study participants were recruited among the hospitalized patients of the University Hospital of Ferrara. Inclusion criteria were: age >18 years, written consent to participate in the study, and molecular diagnosis of SARS-CoV-2 infection (for COVID-19 group only). Exclusion criteria included: pregnancy, breastfeeding, uncooperative patient (inability to perform oral rinse to collect samples), lack of written agreement. COVID-19 patients were stratified into four categories based on symptoms: asymptomatic (1, no symptoms), paucisymptomatic (2, aspecific flu-like symptoms), symptomatic (3, including specific respiratory symptoms), severely symptomatic (4, needing ventilation). The control group consisted of SARS-CoV-2-negative subjects affected by non-respiratory diseases. The number of study participants was decided based on the subjects hosted at the University Hospital of Ferrara in the study period.

Clinical Specimens

Oral rinse samples were collected in 5 mL of sterile phosphate-buffered saline (PBS), as previously described (Caselli et al., 2020a). The specimens were immediately inactivated with 0.1% SDS, refrigerated (2–8°C), and processed within 4 h. Briefly, all samples were vortexed and centrifuged at 15,000 × g for 10 min at 4°C to divide the corpuscular part from the supernatant, which were immediately frozen in liquid nitrogen and kept at −80°C until use.

Nucleic Acid Extraction From Clinical Specimens

Total nucleic acids (DNA and RNA) were extracted from the pellets by using the Maxwell CSC platform equipped with the HT Viral TNA Kit (Promega, Milan, Italy), following the manufacturer's instructions (Comar et al., 2019). Extracted total nucleic acids (TNAs) were checked and quantified by nanodrop spectrophotometric (Thermo Fisher Scientific, Milan, Italy) reading at 260/280 nm. The amplificability of extracted DNA was checked by PCR amplification of human, bacterial, and fungal genes. Namely, human β-actin, bacterial 16S rRNA gene (pan bacterial PCR, *panB*), and mycetes ITS gene (pan fungal PCR, *panF*) were respectively, analyzed, as previously described (Borghi et al., 2016; Caselli et al., 2016, 2018).

Library Preparation and Sequencing

Extracted TNA (100 ng) were retrotranscribed and analyzed by WGS by the NGS Service of the University of Ferrara (Department of Morphology, Surgery and Experimental Medicine, University of Ferrara), who carried out library preparation, sequencing, and taxonomic analysis. Briefly, WGS libraries were prepared using NEBNext® Fast DNA Fragmentation and Library Prep Kit for Ion Torrent TM (Thermo Fisher Scientific, Milan, Italy), following the manufacturer's protocol. Samples were then sequenced by using the Ion Gene Studio S5 System (Thermo Fisher Scientific, Milan, Italy). Low-quality sequence data removal was performed directly on the Ion S5 GeneStudio sequencer, as part of in-built processing. Briefly, the Torrent Suite software (Thermo Fisher Scientific, Milan, Italy), installed in the sequencer, automatically clips adapter sequences and trims low-quality bases from the 3′ end of each read. Reads with quality less than Q20 were also discarded. Additionally, PRINSEQ open source application (Schmieder and Edwards, 2011) was used to remove reads with lengths of less than 100 nucleotides. The taxonomic assignment has been performed using Kraken2 (Pubmed ID: 24580807) and a database consisting of archaea, bacteria, fungi, protozoa, and viruses. Raw sequencing data and bioinformatics analyses have been deposited in the European Nucleotide Archive (ENA) website (accession number PRJEB42999).

SARS-CoV-2 Detection and Quantification

Extracted TNA (100 ng) was used for SARS-CoV-2 detection and quantification by droplet digital PCR (ddPCR), by using the SARS-CoV-2 ddPCR Kit (Bio-Rad Laboratories, Milan, Italy). Briefly, three targets are analyzed in each sample by FAM and HEX labeled probes, targeting SARS-CoV-2 N1 and N2 genes, and human RPP30 gene, this last was used as a control and to normalize the virus counts. The assay sensitivity was between

0.260 copies/μl to 0.351 copies/μl, respectively, for the genetic markers N1 and N2.

IgA Analysis

The presence of anti-SARS-CoV-2 secretory IgA (sIgA) in the oral samples was evaluated by a CE-IVD ELISA assay designed to detect IgA directed against the virus S1 protein (Euroimmun, Lubeck, Germany). The test was previously reported to have high specificity/sensitivity for IgA detection in serum/plasma samples (>95%) and ocular fluids (Caselli et al., 2020b). For oral rinse analysis, the samples were diluted 1:5 in saline, allowing optimal detection of IgA and differentiation between positive samples and controls, as detected in preliminary assays. Each sample was assessed in triplicate. Sample positivity was expressed following the manufacturer's instruction, as the ratio (R) between the absorbance ($OD_{450\ nm}$) value detected in samples and that detected in the calibrator sample provided by the manufacturer. Samples were considered negative if R values were < 0.8, weakly positive with R values comprised between 0.8 and 1.1, and strongly positive with $R \geq 1.1$.

Cytokines Analysis

Oral specimens were analyzed for the presence of pro-inflammatory cytokines, by using ELISA assays specifically detecting and quantitating the following cytokines: IL-6, IL-17, TNFα, and GM-CSF (Thermo Fisher Scientific, Life-Technologies, Milan, Italy).

Statistical Analyses

Statistical analyses were performed with Agilent GeneSpring GX v11.5 software (Agilent Technologies, Santa Clara, CA, United States) and R (R 2019, R Core Team, available as free software at https://www.r-project.org/). Microbiome data were expressed as the relative abundance of each taxonomic unit at the genus or species level. The null hypothesis was tested by the Kruskal–Wallis test. Pairwise *post hoc* analysis was performed by the non-parametric Dunn test which includes correction for multiple comparisons. A Chi-square test was used to assess gender distribution significance. Alpha-diversity obtained by measuring the Shannon H' diversity index was used to describe the microbiome diversity between clinical samples. ELISA results were analyzed by Student's t-test. Linear regression and correlation analyses (Spearman r correlation coefficient) were conducted to evaluate the correlation between patients' clinical parameters (a non-continuous discrete variable), and continuous variables including microbiome profile, immune and inflammation responses. A p-value ≤ 0.05 was considered significant.

RESULTS

Patients' Characteristics

Seventy-five eligible subjects, including 39 COVID-19 patients and 36 controls, were enrolled in the study. COVID-19 patients included 20 males (51.3%) and 19 females (48.7%), with a mean age of 71.1 ± 18.4 years (range 25–99). Oral rinses were collected from COVID-19 patients at 0–43 days since the first SARS-CoV-2-positive nasopharyngeal swab. At the time of sample collection, 11/39 (28.2%) COVID-19 patients were asymptomatic, 7/39 (17.9%) presented mild symptoms, 21/39 (55.3%) were symptomatic, with 2 of them (2/39, 5.1%) showing severe respiratory symptoms requiring ventilation. All recruited COVID-19 patients received hydroxychloroquine and azithromycin on hospitalization (Gautret et al., 2020). The control group consisted of SARS-CoV-2-negative subjects admitted for non-respiratory diseases at the non-COVID Infectious Disease ward, and included 22 males and 14 females (respectively, 61% and 39% of the group), with a mean age of 66.5 ± 18.8 years (range 20–94). The characteristics of study participants are reported in **Table 1**. No statistical differences were evidenced between COVID-19 and control group with regard to age (Kruskal–Wallis test; $p = 0.27$, n.s.) and gender (Chi-square test; $\chi^2 = 0.734$, $p = 0.39$, n.s.). Similarly, no statistically significant differences were evidenced between COVID-19 disease sub-groups (asymptomatic, pauci-symptomatic, and symptomatic) regarding age (Kruskal–Wallis test; $p = 0.21$, n.s.) or gender distribution (Chi-square test; $\chi^2 = 0.256$, $p = 0.88$, n.s.).

SARS-CoV-2 Load in COVID-19 Patients

Although all the enrolled COVID-19 patients were confirmed to be SARS-CoV-2 positive at hospital admission by the routine molecular test performed on nasopharyngeal swab by the Hospital microbiology laboratory, we wanted to assess the presence of SARS-CoV-2 in the oral cavity of all the enrolled subjects at the time of oral rinse withdrawal. The oral rinse samples were analyzed by digital droplet PCR (ddPCR), able to detect and quantify the virus genomes, contrarily to the routinely used diagnostic assays (Falzone et al., 2020; Suo et al., 2020). While the results confirmed the absence of positivity in the control group, in the COVID-19 group both positive and negative oral rinse specimens were observed, as summarized in **Figure 1**. Quantitative analysis showed that 16/39 subjects harbored a high load of SARS-CoV-2 (from 101 to 3,963 genome copies in 20 μl of the amplified sample), 17/39 had lower but detectable amounts of virus (from 3 to 100 genome copies in 20 μl), whereas 6/39 patients did not display any detectable virus copy in the oral cavity at the time of oral withdrawal (<3 copies in 20 μl). It is noteworthy that the virus load detected in the oral cavity correlated with symptom severity (Spearman $r = 0.774$; 95% CI 0.608–0.875) ($p < 0.0001$), defining specific subpopulations of COVID-19 patients.

Oral Microbiome in COVID-19 Patients

Whole Genome Sequencing analysis of the oral microbiome evidenced significant differences in the profiles of the COVID-19 compared to controls. Alpha-diversity values were lower in COVID-19 patients vs. controls ($p = 0.01$) (**Figure 2A**). Interestingly, the comparison between severely symptomatic COVID-19 subgroups and controls revealed the most significant differences (**Figure 2B**), with an inverse correlation between alpha-diversity value and symptoms (Spearman $r = -0.431$, 95% CI $-0.666/-0.120$,

TABLE 1 | Characteristics of COVID-19 and control study participants.

Subject n°	Control group		COVID-19 group				Age/gender distribution
	Gender	**Age**	**Gender**	**Age**	**Days after NPS**	**COVID-19 symptoms (*)**	
1	F	74	M	76	13	3	***Age:***
2	M	72	F	72	4	3	**CTR:** 66.5 ± 18.8 years
3	M	73	F	56	0	1	**COVID-19:** 71.1 ± 18.4 years
4	F	86	M	49	3	1	**CTR vs. COVID-19:** $p = 0.27$, n.s.
5	F	38	F	49	6	2	
6	F	66	M	99	6	2	
7	F	67	F	80	18	4	
8	F	40	F	73	16	3	
9	M	53	F	68	2	1	
10	M	42	F	33	18	2	
11	M	75	F	51	2	2	
12	F	86	M	76	4	3	
13	M	60	M	82	8	3	
14	M	59	F	87	29	1	
15	M	83	M	47	6	1	
16	M	86	F	91	18	3	
17	F	86	M	89	5	3	
18	M	71	F	94	16	3	***Gender:***
19	M	88	M	94	20	2	**CTR:** 22/36 males (61%)
20	M	84	M	80	15	3	**COVID-19:** 20/39 males (51.3%)
21	F	88	M	85	18	3	**CTR vs. COVID-19:** $p = 0.39$, n.s.
22	F	86	F	83	7	3	
23	M	20	M	25	10	3	
24	F	94	F	78	18	4	
25	F	46	F	83	49	3	
26	F	76	F	45	17	3	
27	M	50	M	82	1	1	
29	M	51	F	82	2	1	
30	M	53	M	59	0	2	
31	M	45	M	45	43	1	
32	M	70	M	57	5	3	
33	F	85	F	86	4	3	
34	M	49	F	48	3	2	
35	M	67	M	90	11	3	
36	M	49	F	70	0	1	
37	M	76	M	81	51	1	
38	–	–	M	87	23	3	
39	–	–	M	78	11	1	
	–	–	M	63	18	3	

(*) Symptom score was: 1, asymptomatic; 2, paucisymptomatic; 3, symptomatic; 4, severely symptomatic.
NPS, nasopharyngeal swab.
Age and gender distribution significance were assessed, respectively, by Kruskal–Wallis and Chi-square tests.

$p = 0.006$). The decrease of alpha diversity was higher in male compared to female patients (**Figure 2C**), which paralleled symptoms severity.

The microbiome profile appeared profoundly altered in COVID-19 patients compared to controls (**Figure 3**). In particular, the relative abundance of the bacterial genera *Streptococcus, Veillonella, Prevotella, Lactobacillus, Capnocytophaga, Porphyromonas, Abiotrophia, Aggregatibacter, Atopobium* was increased in COVID-19 compared to controls, whereas *Rothia, Haemophilus, Parvimonas, Fusobacterium*, and *Gemella* spp. were decreased (**Figure 3A**). Notably, *Enterococcus* and *Enterobacter* genera were exclusively present in COVID-19 patients, and not detectable in control subjects. At the species level (**Figure 3B**), COVID-19 patients had decreased amounts of *Haemophilus parainfluenzae* and *parahaemolyticus, Gemella morbillorum* and *sanguinis, Parvimonas micra*, and

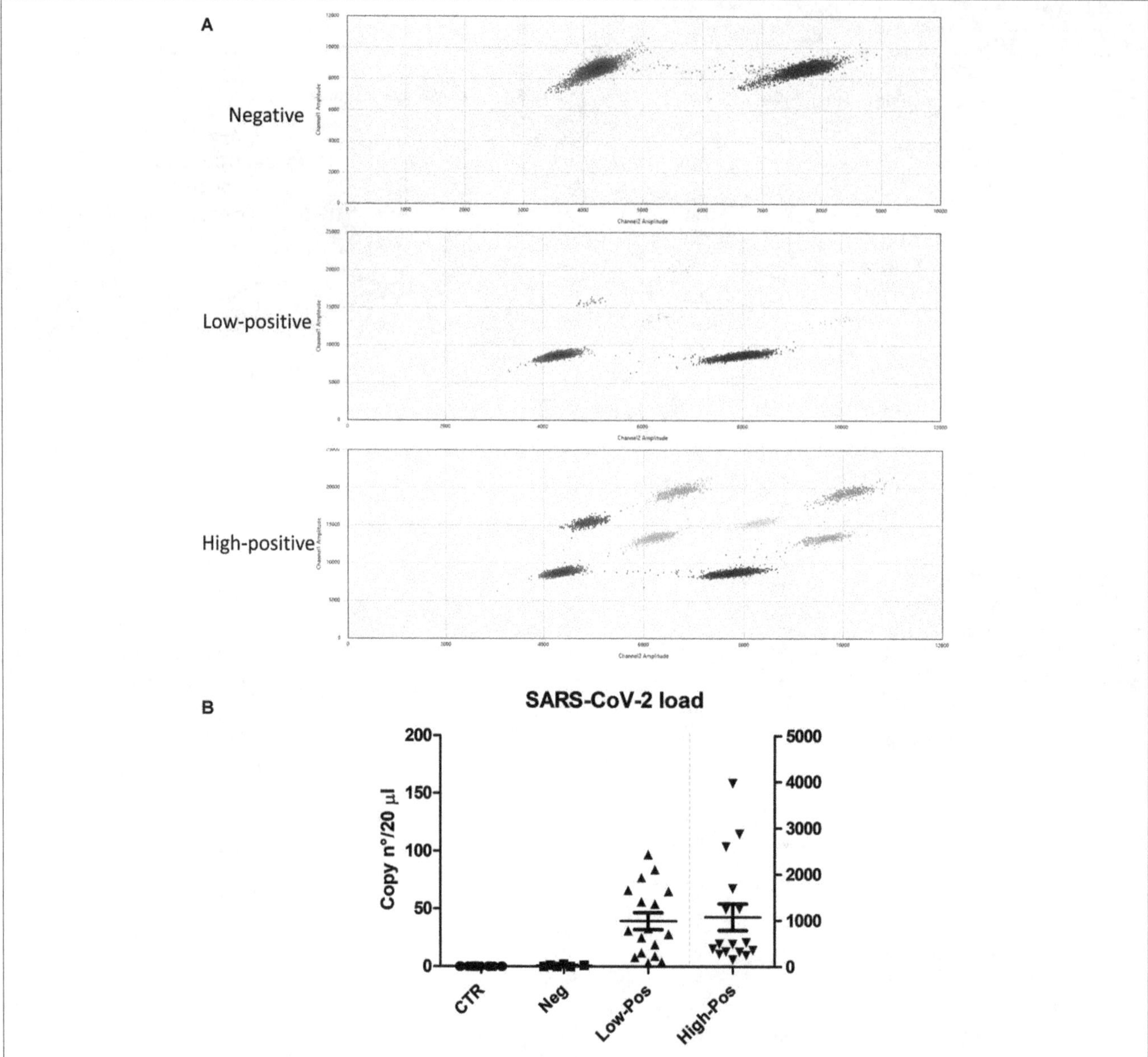

FIGURE 1 | SARS-CoV-2 load in control and COVID-19 subjects, as measured by ddPCR. **(A)** Graphical representation of the values detected by the use of three different molecular probes: negative samples, only the clouds corresponding to the housekeeping control genes are detectable (gray and purple clouds); low- and high-positive samples, the clouds corresponding to the virus genes are detectable and counted (positives to individual FAM probes: gray, red, and yellow; positives to individual HEX probes: purple, blue, and pink; double positives to FAM/HEX probes: beige and orange). **(B)** Virus load, expressed as genome copy number per analyzed sample (20 µl of extracted nucleic acid); left *y* axis refers to control, negative and low-positive values, whereas right *y* axis refers to high-positive COVID-19 subjects. Mean value ± SEM is also reported.

Neisseria subflava, whereas *Neisseria mucosa*, *Veillonella parvula*, *Lactobacillus fermentum*, *Enterococcus faecalis*, *Atopobium parvulum*, *Acinetobacter baumannii* were increased. Notably, many species of periodontopathogenic bacteria (*Prevotella melaninogenica*, *jejuni*, *denticola*, and *oris*; *Eikenella corrodens*; *Capnocytophaga sputigena* and *gingivalis*; and *Aggregatibacter aphrophilus*) were significantly increased in COVID-19 compared to control subjects. **Figure 4** summarizes the taxa significantly altered in COVID-19 patients compared to controls, with significance values.

It is of note that high differences were observed relative to the fungal component of the oral microbiome (**Figure 5**). Contrary to the decreased richness of the bacterial component, the fungal fraction of the oral microbiome was increased in COVID-19 patients compared to controls, both as total normalized counts and as species richness. In detail, while the oral mycobiome of controls was essentially constituted by *Candida* and *Saccharomyces* spp. (47% and 52% of relative abundance, respectively), in COVID-19 patients *Aspergillus*, *Nakaseomyces*, and *Malassezia* spp. were detectable at a fair

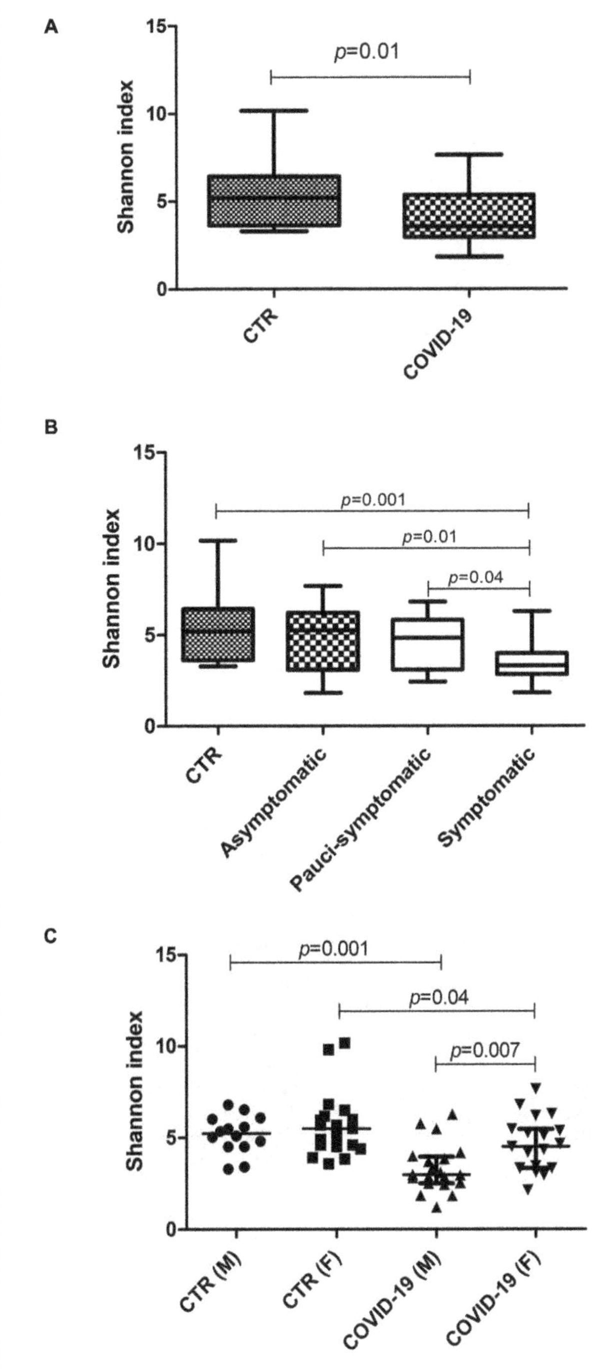

FIGURE 2 | Alpha-diversity values in the oral microbiomes of control and COVID-19 subjects. **(A)** Comparison between control and COVID-19 patients, expressed as median and range values. **(B)** Comparison between controls and COVID-19 asymptomatic, pauci-symptomatic, and symptomatic subjects; median and range values are shown. **(C)** Comparison between genders (M, male; F, female) in the control and COVID-19 groups; median values with interquartile range are shown for each group.

by *Candida* and *Saccharomyces* spp. (47 and 52% of relative abundance, respectively), in COVID-19 patients *Aspergillus*, *Nakaseomyces*, and *Malassezia* spp. were detectable at a fair level, with respective relative abundance values of 4%, 3%, and <1%. The species *Candida albicans*, *Saccharomyces cerevisiae*, *Aspergillus fumigatus*, and *Malassezia restricta* were identified.

Interestingly, the oral virome also appeared more abundant in COVID-19 patients compared to controls (**Figure 6**). While viruses represented 0.07% of the microbial community in controls, their relative abundance increased to 1.12% in COVID-19 patients. *Lymphocryptovirus* and *Simplexvirus* genera of the Herpesviridae family were detected both in COVID-19 and control subjects. However, Epstein Barr virus (EBV) resulted reactivated in 11/39 COVID-19 patients and in only 2/36 controls. Moreover, Herpes simplex virus type 1 (HSV-1) and four bacteriophages targeted, respectively, toward *Staphylococcus* (Staphylococcus phage ROSA), *Streptococcus* (Streptococcus phage EJ-1 and phage PH10), and *Lactobacillus* (Lactobacillus phage phiadh), were also increased in COVID-19 patients compared to controls.

Oral IgA Response in COVID-19 Patients

To assess the development of a mucosal immune response against SARS-CoV-2 in the oral cavity, oral secretory IgA was searched and quantified by specific ELISA in the oral rinse samples of COVID-19 patients and controls. A mucosal IgA response was detected in 25/39 (64.1%) COVID-19 patients and no controls (p = 0.0008). Interestingly, the extent of mucosal response was different among the symptom subgroups of patients (**Figure 7**). In fact, 10/39 patients (25.6%) exhibited a very high concentration of sIgA (R > 2.0), whereas 15/39 patients (38.5%) had intermediate values (0.8 < R < 2.0), and 14/39 (35.9%) showed the presence of a barely detectable (R~0.8 threshold value) or no sIgA response. Of note, 6/10 COVID-19 patients displaying high oral sIgA titer were asymptomatic/paucisymptomatic, evidencing a trend toward an inverse correlation between the salivary sIgA concentration and symptom severity (Spearman r−0.355; 95% CI −0.600 to 0.047; p = 0.02).

Oral Cytokines in COVID-19 Patients

Since the so-called "cytokine storm" is a hallmark of severe COVID-19 disease, we investigated the release of pro-inflammatory cytokines in the oral cavity. Namely, the four main cytokines/chemokines detected in the blood of COVID-19 patients were analyzed: IL-6, IL-17, TNFα, and GM-CSF. The results showed that both IL-6 (p = 0.005) and IL-17 (p = 0.02) were significantly higher in COVID-19 oral samples than in controls (**Figure 8**). TNFα and GM-CSF were also more concentrated in COVID-19 patients compared to controls, but the differences were not statistically significant. However, the differences became significant by comparing COVID-19 symptomatic subgroup with controls (TNFα p = 0.005; GM-CSF p = 0.002), highlighting that more inflammation was detectable in the subjects undergoing a more severe course of the disease.

Inflammation also correlated with the oral microbiome dysbiosis, being more pronounced in subjects with a more evident decrease of alpha-diversity and species richness (p < 0.01).

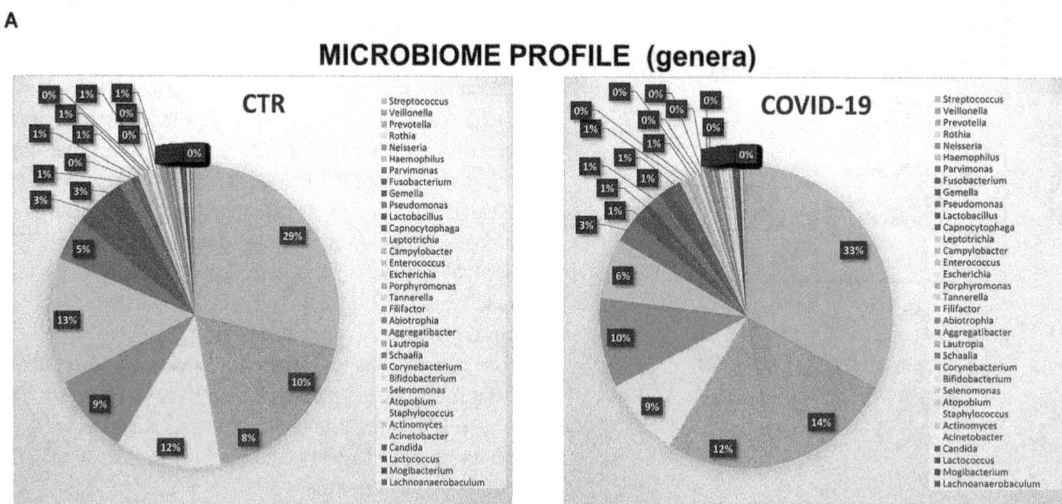

B

MICROBIOME PROFILE (species)

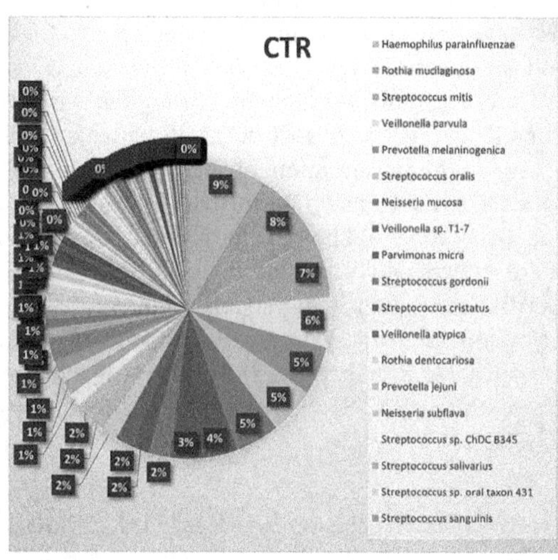

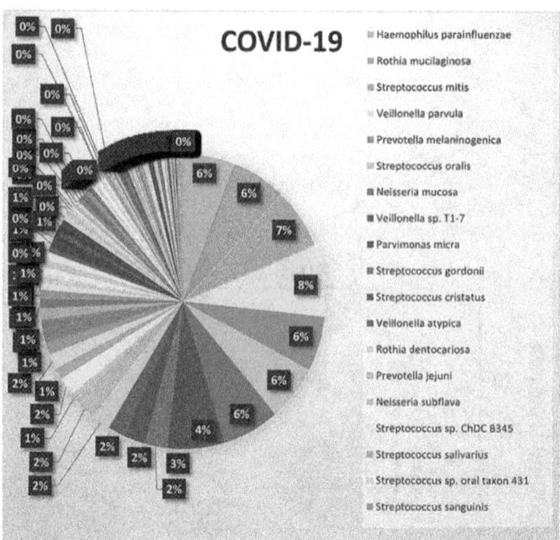

FIGURE 3 | Relative abundance and distribution of microorganisms in the oral cavity of control (CTR) and COVID-19 subjects. **(A)** Percentage distribution of most detected microbial genera. **(B)** Percentage distribution of most detected microbial species.

DISCUSSION

Recent reports have shed light on the role of the microbiome in several diseases, including those of viral origin, suggesting that the commensal microbiota may potentially favor or hamper viral infections. However, most studies consider the gut microbiome, neglecting the role of an oral one. In addition, most if not all studies discuss only bacterial microbiota, whereas fungi and viruses are also important components of the commensal microbiota. Concerning SARS-CoV-2 infection, COVID-19 patients have been reported to harbor oral pathogenic bacteria (such as cariogenic or periodontopathic pathogens) (Bao et al., 2020; Patel and Sampson, 2020; Xiang et al., 2020). Oral dysbiosis might favor the establishment of SARS-CoV-2 infection through different mechanisms, as known for other respiratory viruses, including alteration of the respiratory epithelium, promotion of adhesion of respiratory pathogens, and increase of local inflammation (Baghbani et al., 2020). Despite such suggestions, the profile of the HOM is currently still not clarified, especially in the non-bacterial components, rendering it difficult to understand whether the HOM dysbiosis may be considered a risk factor for COVID-19 development (Patel and Sampson, 2020). Two recent preprints reported on the bacterial profile of HOM in COVID-19 patients, suggesting relationships between some bacteria and SARS-CoV-2 infection (Iebba et al., 2020; Ward et al., 2021). However, to date, no studies have

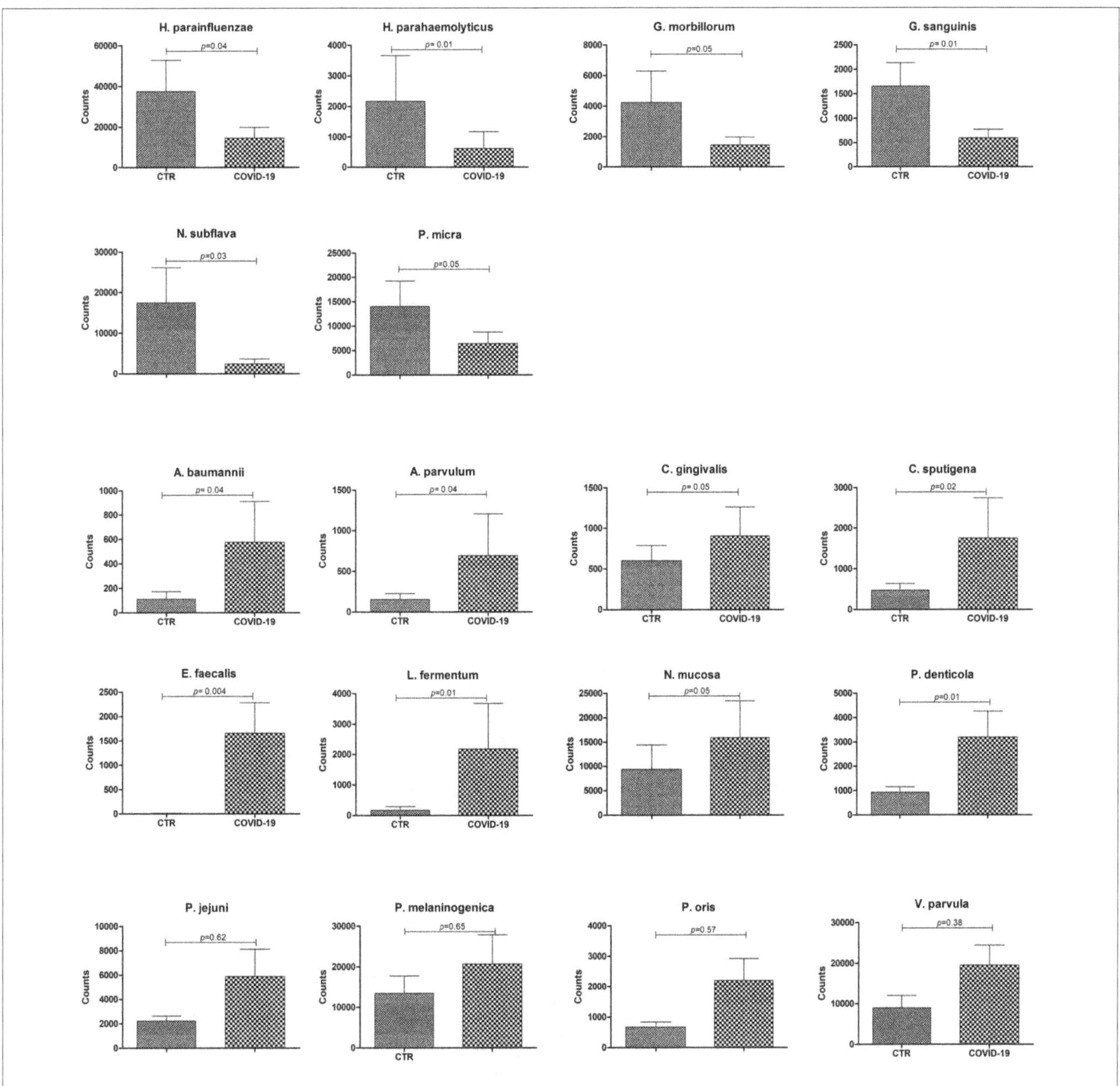

FIGURE 4 | Significantly altered taxa in control (CTR) and COVID-19 subjects. The results are expressed as normalized counts ± SEM values. Significance *p*-values for each comparison are also displayed.

completely addressed HOM profiling, including fungal and viral components.

Thus, our study aimed to characterize by metagenomics (WGS deep sequencing) the oral microbiome of COVID-19, to get a comprehensive view of its bacterial, fungal, and viral components.

The results showed very significant differences in the HOM composition between COVID-19 and control subjects, highlighting a decrease in the alpha-diversity and bacterial species richness in COVID-19 patients compared to controls, and a significant correlation between such decrease and symptom severity ($p = 0.006$). These data are in line with previous observations highlighting a decrease in the alpha variety and species richness upon HCV, HIV, and influenza infection (Sun et al., 2016; Inoue et al., 2018), with a parallel increase of pro-inflammatory cytokines like IL-6, TNFα, and IL-1β (Yildiz et al., 2018; Ramos-Sevillano et al., 2019).

Our results also showed an increase in the relative abundance of genera associated with poor oral hygiene and periodontitis in COVID-19 patients (*Prevotella, Lactobacillus, Capnocytophaga, Porphyromonas, Abiotrophia, Aggregatibacter,* and *Atopobium*), suggesting an association between those bacteria and SARS-CoV-2 infection, similar to that reported for other respiratory viruses (Andrews et al., 2012; Wang et al., 2016). The exclusive

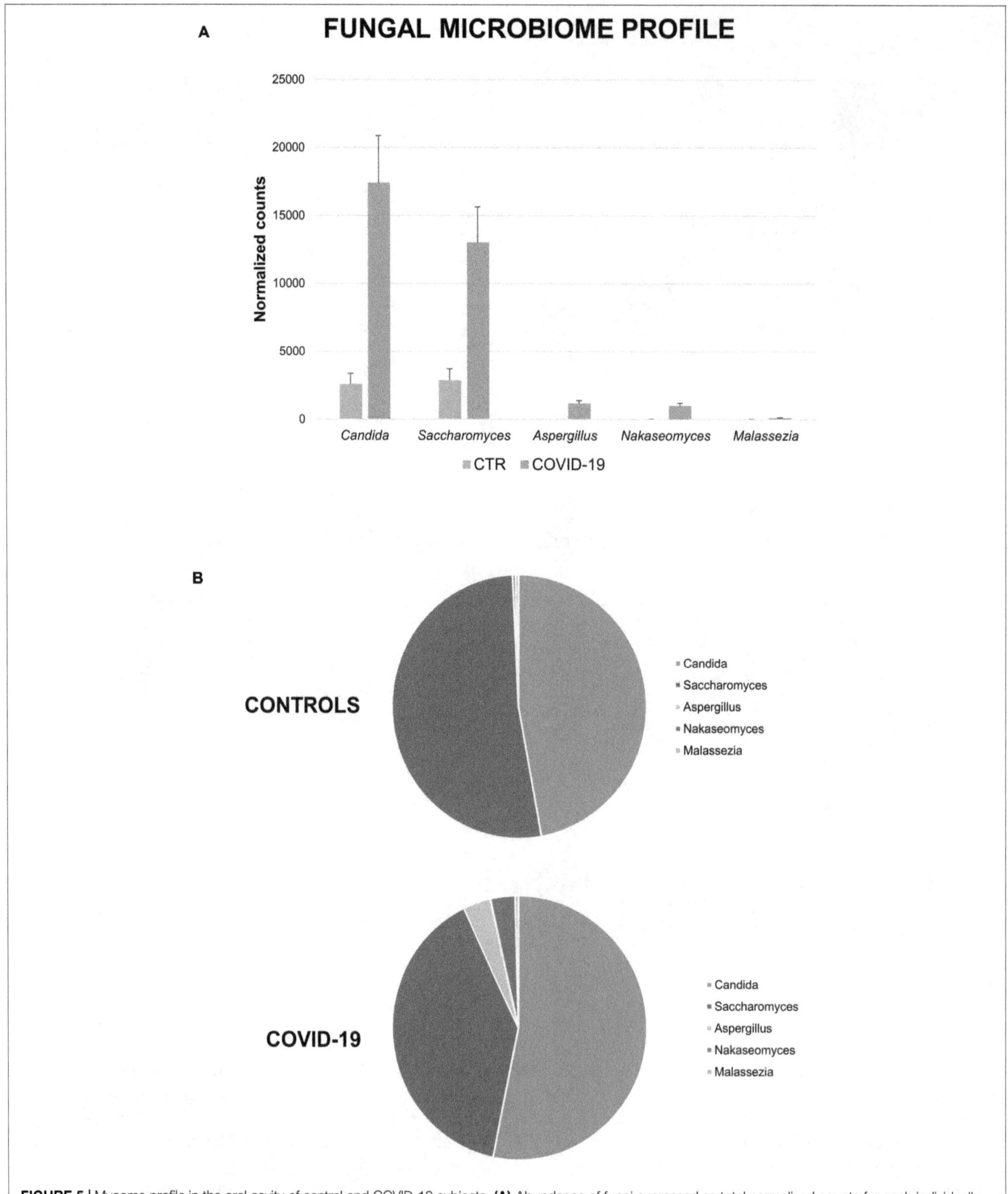

FIGURE 5 | Mycome profile in the oral cavity of control and COVID-19 subjects. **(A)** Abundance of fungi expressed as total normalized counts for each individually detected mycetes. **(B)** Percentage distribution of the fungal genera in controls and COVID-19 patients.

presence of *Enterococcus* and *Enterobacter* genera in COVID-19 patients suggests that they might be a microbial marker of susceptibility for SARS-CoV-2 infection. Even more interesting, fungi were instead more abundant in COVID-19 patients than in controls, with some genera (*Aspergillus*, *Nakaseomyces*, and *Malassezia*) only detectable in COVID-19 subjects, besides the

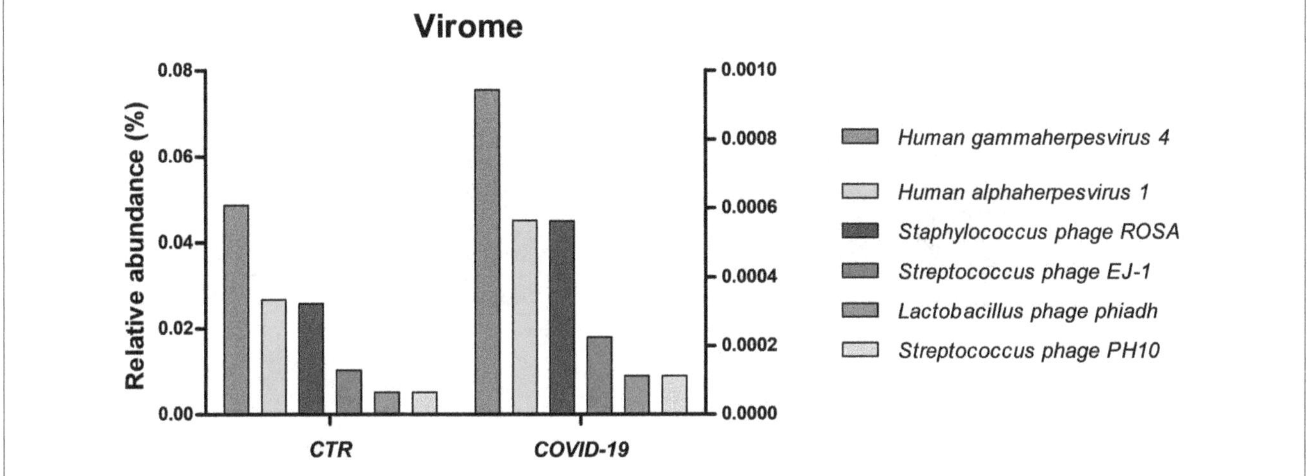

FIGURE 6 | Virome profile in the oral cavity of control (CTR) and COVID-19 subjects. The results are expressed as relative abundance (%). Left *y* axis refers to Human gammaherpesvirus 4 and Human alphaherpesvirus 1 (green bars), whereas right *y* axis refers to the amount of the four detected bacteriophage (orange-red bars).

more common *Candida* and *Saccharomyces* genera. In this regard, significant differences in fungal community with a higher richness of fungal species were detected in HIV-infected compared to uninfected individuals (Mukherjee et al., 2014) and in HBV/HCV symptomatic patients, where the diversity of intestinal fungi was positively associated with disease progression (Chen et al., 2011). Oral mycetes may be increased in the mouth because of bacterial alterations, ultimately favoring SARS-CoV-2 infection, due to the increased inflammation originated by fungi enzymatic and catabolic/toxic activity in the mouth (Chen X. et al., 2020). Beyond the potential mechanisms underlying the cooperation between SARS-CoV-2 and fungi, the results suggest that it could be important to consider this component of HOM in the management of virus infection.

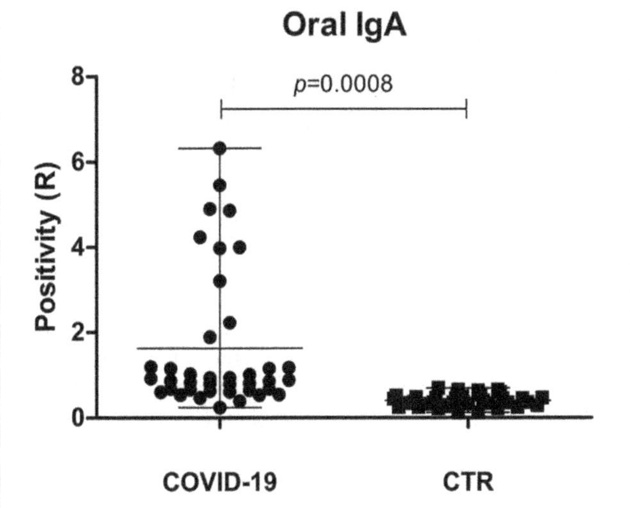

FIGURE 7 | Mucosal sIgA response in the oral cavity of COVID-19 and control (CTR) subjects. The positivity is expressed as the ratio (R) between the value detected in the sample and the threshold control value, following manufacturer's instructions; mean value with range is also shown.

Another non-bacterial HOM component that was augmented in COVID-19 patients was the viral one (from 0.07 to 1.12% of the total microbiome). HSV-1 and EBV herpesviruses were most present, and EBV coinfection was evidenced in about 30% of COVID-19 patients compared to only 5% of controls. In this regard, the HOM dysbiosis may have facilitated the activation/reactivation of oral viruses, and in turn, the high presence of herpesviruses infection/reactivation may further impair proper immune control (Jasinski-Bergner et al., 2020), thus potentially contributing to worse efficiency of the immune response against SARS-CoV-2. Consistent with this, EBV infection was detected in COVID-19 patients, associated with increased risk of severe COVID-19 symptoms and fatal outcome (Roncati et al., 2020; Chen et al., 2021), and correlated increased levels of IL-6 (Lehner et al., 2020). Similarly, alpha-herpesvirus (HSV-1, VZV) reactivation was observed, impacting the prognosis of COVID-19 patients (Le Balc'h et al., 2020; Hernandez et al., 2021). Thus, the presence of Herpesviridae infections in the oral cavity and their direct consequences deserve further investigation.

In parallel with the HOM profile, our work also characterized the local inflammatory and immune response as critical parameters to understand the evolution of the SARS-CoV-2 infection at the primary site of entry.

A hallmark of disease severity in COVID-19 is the uncontrolled inflammatory response, with the detection of IL-6, IL-17, TNFα, and GM-CSF at the serum/blood level (Chen G. et al., 2020; Mehta et al., 2020; Parra-Medina et al., 2020), the so-called "cytokine storm." Here we showed a significant increase of those cytokines in the oral cavity of COVID-19 patients, indicating the development of inflammation right at the entry site of the virus. It is noteworthy that the level of oral inflammation paralleled the symptom severity, pointing to the importance of oral conditions for the subsequent systemization of virus infection and inflammation cascade.

A still unanswered point in COVID-19 progression regards the development and role of the local immune response against

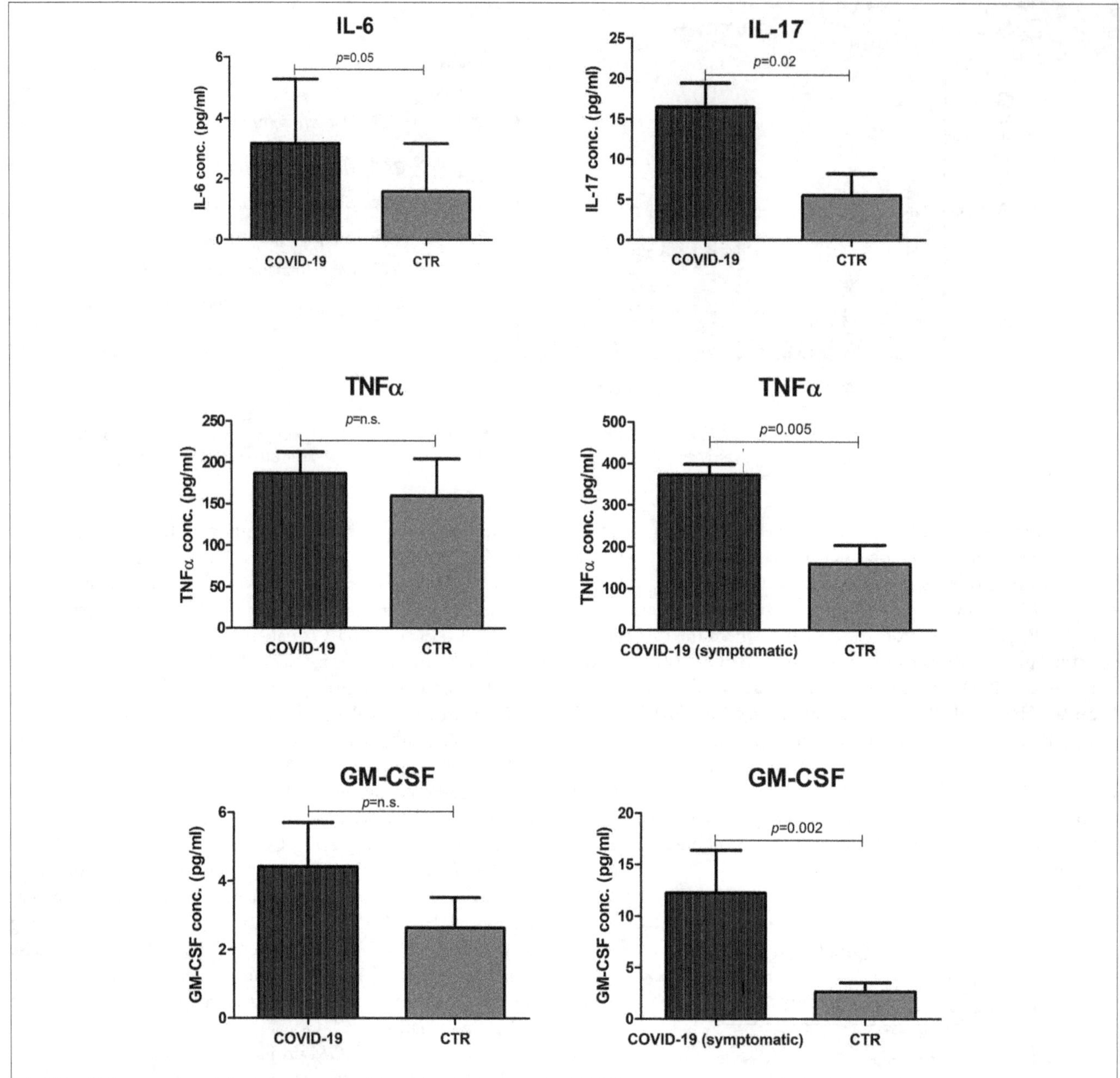

FIGURE 8 | Presence of pro-inflammatory cytokines/chemokines in the oral cavity of COVID-19 patients and controls (CTR). The results are expressed as the mean values ± SEM of the concentration (pg/ml) for each indicated cytokine.

SARS-CoV-2. Mucosal sIgA has long been known to be crucial in controlling viruses that enter the body via mucosal surfaces (Yan et al., 2002); sIgA were indeed found in the ocular fluid of at least 40% of COVID-19 patients (Caselli et al., 2020b), and microbiome composition is reportedly known to interact with and influence IgA response, in different anatomical niches including the nares (Salk et al., 2016; Grosserichter-Wagener et al., 2019; Pabst and Slack, 2020). Here, we demonstrate anti-SARS-CoV-2 sIgA in the oral cavity and that they are significantly more abundant in asymptomatic/paucisymptomatic COVID-19 patients ($p = 0.02$), suggesting that sIgA may be important in controlling virus penetration in the body.

The main limitation of our study is the number of enrolled subjects, who represented all the eligible subjects hosted at the enrolled center. The enrollment of a higher number of subjects, ideally in a multi-center study, may confirm the generalizability of the study results. A higher number of subjects would also enable us to stratify patients for age, thus providing a direct comparison of more homogeneous microbial populations, as the microbiome composition is dependent on the subject's age (Bourgeois et al., 2017; Caselli et al., 2020a). The relatively low number of recruited patients in our study also did not enable us to evidence a high statistically significant correlation between sIgA production and protection from severe COVID-19. Thus, studying a higher number of patients may be of importance to ascertain this point, especially in developing effective prevention strategies and vaccines.

Overall, the data presented here suggest a correlation between HOM dysbiosis and individual susceptibility to SARS-CoV-2 severe infection, indicating an interplay between HOM profile (including mycobiome and virome), inflammation, and mucosal IgA response. If HOM alteration is the cause or effect of severe COVID-19, it is not currently possible to distinguish, because the presence of SARS-CoV-2 in the oral cavity may impact microbiome dysbiosis (Xiang et al., 2020; de Oliveira et al., 2021). On the other hand, connections between oral dysbiosis and post-viral complications have been reported, suggesting that improving oral health may reduce the risk of complications from COVID-19 (Sampson et al., 2020), thus supporting the hypothesis of a role of dysbiosis in the virus-induced disease. Toward this direction, recent studies reported that SARS-CoV-2 load can be reduced by the use of chlorhexidine mouthwashes (Yoon et al., 2020), supporting the use of antiseptics against coronavirus infection (Koch-Heier et al., 2021; Mateos Moreno et al., 2021), and clinical studies are developing accordingly (Carrouel et al., 2020) and hopefully will help to clarify this aspect.

These findings may be important in defining markers useful to predict the development of symptomatic COVID-19, and open new therapeutic opportunities addressed to balance HOM and inflammation to prevent the development of severe symptoms. In this direction, IL-6 inhibitors have been reported to reduce the odds of COVID-19 mortality (Sinha et al., 2021), and specific probiotic administration has been proposed to balance microbiome dysbiosis and prevent the development of virus-induced respiratory diseases (Wang et al., 2016) and may represent a possible intervention in COVID-19 patients.

AUTHOR CONTRIBUTIONS

IS and MD'A analyzed the samples. CF and MF contributed to the design of the study, protocol for oral sampling, and interpretation of data. AP provided COVID-19 clinical samples and patient data. RM and GZ provided COVID-19 clinical samples and interpretation of clinical data. ML and CC provided control clinical samples. CC contributed to writing the manuscript. EC designed the study, elaborated the results, and wrote the manuscript. All authors read and approved the final manuscript.

ACKNOWLEDGMENTS

The authors thank the team of the Medical Clinic Unit (Head: RM), Internal Medicine Unit (Head: GZ), and Infectious Disease Unit (Head: CC) for their assistance and technical support: Benedetta Boari, Gloria Brombo, Eleonora Capatti, Andrea Cutini, Edoardo Dalla Nora, Andrea D'Amuri, Gloria Ferrocci, Alfredo De Giorgi, Francesca Di Vece, Fabio Fabbian, Laura Fornasari, Christian Molino, Elisa Misurati, Michele Polastri, Tommaso Romagnoli, Giovanni Battista Vigna, Alessandro Bella, Stefania Bonazzi, Beatrice Bonsi, Paola Chessa, Angela Colangiulo, Daniele Deplano, Valeria Fortunato, Enrico Giorgini, Salvatore Greco, Patrizia Guasti, Gaetano Lo Coco, Mariarosaria Lopreiato, Francesco Luciani, Chiara Mancino, Lisa Marabini, Sara Morrone, Chiara Pazzaglini, Dario Pedrini, Chiara Pistolesi, Ugo Politti, Federica Ristè, Rossella Roversi, Alessandro Scopa, Chiara Marina Semprini, Ruana Tiseo, Daniela Tortola, Grazia Vestita, Alessandra Violi, Aurora Bonazza, Altea Gallerani, and Martina Maritati.

REFERENCES

1. Andrews, T., Thompson, M., Buckley, D. I., Heneghan, C., Deyo, R., Redmond, N., et al. (2012). Interventions to influence consulting and antibiotic use for acute respiratory tract infections in children: a systematic review and meta-analysis. *PLoS One* 7:e30334. doi: 10.1371/journal.pone.0030334
2. Baghbani, T., Nikzad, H., Azadbakht, J., Izadpanah, F., and Haddad Kashani, H. (2020). Dual and mutual interaction between microbiota and viral infections: a possible treat for COVID-19. *Microb. Cell Fact.* 19:217. doi: 10.1186/s12934- 020-01483-1
3. Bao, L., Zhang, C., Dong, J., Zhao, L., Li, Y., and Sun, J. (2020). Oral microbiome and SARS-CoV-2: beware of lung co- infection. *Front. Microbiol.* 11:1840. doi: 10.3389/fmicb.2020.01 840
4. Bassis, C. M., Erb-Downward, J. R., Dickson, R. P., Freeman, C. M., Schmidt, T. M., Young, V. B., et al. (2015). Analysis of the upper respiratory tract microbiotas as the source of the lung and gastric microbiotas in healthy individuals. *mBio* 6:e00037-15. doi: 10.1128/mBio.00037-15
5. Belkaid, Y., and Hand, T. W. (2014). Role of the microbiota in immunity and inflammation. *Cell* 157, 121–141. doi: 10.1016/j.cell.2014.03.011
6. Borghi, A., D'Accolti, M., Rizzo, R., Virgili, A., Di Luca, D., Corazza, M., et al. (2016). High prevalence of specific KIR types in patients with HHV-8 positive cutaneous vascular lesions: a possible predisposing factor? *Arch. Dermatol. Res.* 308, 373–377. doi: 10.1007/s00403-016-1643-x
7. Bourgeois, D., David, A., Inquimbert, C., Tramini, P., Molinari, N., and Carrouel, F. (2017). Quantification of carious pathogens in the interdental microbiota of young caries-free adults. *PLoS One* 12:e0185804. doi: 10.1371/ journal.pone. 0185804
8. Cagna, D. R., Donovan, T. E., McKee, J. R., Eichmiller, F., Metz, J. E., Albouy, J. P., et al. (2019). Annual review of selected scientific literature: a report of the committee on scientific investigation of the american academy of restorative dentistry. *J. Prosthet. Dent.* 122, 198–269. doi: 10.1016/j.prosdent.2019.05.010
9. Carrouel, F., Viennot, S., Valette, M., Cohen, J. M., Dussart, C., and Bourgeois, D. (2020). Salivary and nasal detection of the SARS-CoV-2 virus after antiviral mouthrinses (BBCovid): a structured summary of a study protocol for a randomised controlled trial. *Trials* 21:906. doi: 10.1186/s13063-020-04846-6
10. Caselli, E., Brusaferro, S., Coccagna, M., Arnoldo, L., Berloco, F., Antonioli, P., et al. (2018). Reducing healthcare-associated infections incidence by a probiotic- based sanitation system: a multicentre, prospective, intervention study. *PLoS One* 13:e0199616. doi: 10.1371/journal.pone.0199616
11. Caselli, E., D'Accolti, M., Vandini, A., Lanzoni, L., Camerada, M. T., Coccagna, M., et al. (2016). Impact of a probiotic-based cleaning intervention on the microbiota ecosystem of the hospital surfaces: focus on the resistome remodulation. *PLoS One* 11:e0148857. doi: 10.1371/journal.pone.0148857
12. Caselli, E., Fabbri, C., D'Accolti, M., Soffritti, I., Bassi, C., Mazzacane, S., et al. (2020a). Defining the oral microbiome by whole-genome sequencing and resistome analysis: the complexity of the healthy picture. *BMC Microbiol.* 20:120. doi: 10.1186/s12866-020-01801-y
13. Caselli, E., Soffritti, I., Lamberti, G., D'Accolti, M., Franco, F., Demaria, D., et al. (2020b). Anti-SARS-Cov-2 IgA response in tears of COVID-19 patients. *Biology* 9:374. doi: 10.3390/biology9110374
14. Chen, G., Wu, D., Guo, W., Cao, Y., Huang, D., Wang, H., et al. (2020). Clinical and immunological features of severe and moderate coronavirus disease 2019. *J. Clin. Invest.* 130, 2620–2629. doi: 10.1172/JCI137244

15. Chen, T., Song, J., Liu, H., Zheng, H., and Chen, C. (2021). Positive Epstein-Barr virus detection in corona virus disease 2019 (COVID-19) patients. *Lancet Resp. Med.* [Epub ahead of print]. doi: 10.2139/ssrn.3555268
16. Chen, X., Liao, B., Cheng, L., Peng, X., Xu, X., Li, Y., et al. (2020). The microbial coinfection in COVID-19. *Appl. Microbiol. Biotechnol.* 104, 7777–7785. doi: 10.1007/s00253-020-10814-6
17. Chen, Y., Chen, Z., Guo, R., Chen, N., Lu, H., Huang, S., et al. (2011). Correlation between gastrointestinal fungi and varying degrees of chronic hepatitis B virus infection. *Diagn. Microbiol. Infect. Dis.* 70, 492–498. doi: 10.1016/j. diagmicrobio.2010.04.005
18. Comar, M., D'Accolti, M., Cason, C., Soffritti, I., Campisciano, G., Lanzoni, L., et al. (2019). Introduction of NGS in environmental surveillance for healthcare-associated infection control. *Microorganisms* 7:708. doi: 10.3390/ microorganisms7120708
19. Contini, C., Caselli, E., Martini, F., Maritati, M., Torreggiani, E., Seraceni, S., et al. (2020). COVID-19 is a multifaceted challenging pandemic which needs urgent public health interventions. *Microorganisms* 8:1228. doi: 10.3390/ microorganisms8081228
20. de la Rica, R., Borges, M., and Gonzalez-Freire, M. (2020). COVID-19: in the eye of the cytokine storm. *Front. Immunol.* 11:558898. doi: 10.3389/ fimmu.2020. 558898
21. de Oliveira, G. L. V., Oliveira, C. N. S., Pinzan, C. F., de Salis, L. V. V., and Cardoso, C. R. B. (2021). Microbiota modulation of the gut-lung axis in COVID-19. *Front. Immunol.* 12:635471. doi: 10.3389/fimmu.2021.635471
22. Deo, P. N., and Deshmukh, R. (2019). Oral microbiome: unveiling the fundamentals. *J. Oral Maxillofac. Pathol.* 23, 122–128. doi: 10.4103/jomfp. JOMFP_304_18
23. Falzone, L., Musso, N., Gattuso, G., Bongiorno, D., Palermo, C. I., Scalia, G., et al. (2020). Sensitivity assessment of droplet digital PCR for SARS-CoV-2 detection. *Int. J. Mol. Med.* 46, 957–964. doi: 10.3892/ijmm.2020.4673
24. Gautret, P., Lagier, J. C., Parola, P., Hoang, V. T., Meddeb, L., Mailhe, M., et al. (2020). Hydroxychloroquine and azithromycin as a treatment of COVID-19: results of an open-label non-randomized clinical trial. *Int. J. Antimicrob. Agents* 56:105949. doi: 10.1016/j.ijantimicag.2020.105949
25. Grosserichter-Wagener, C., Radjabzadeh, D., van der Weide, H., Smit, K. N., Kraaij, R., Hays, J. P., et al. (2019). Differences in systemic IgA reactivity and circulating Th subsets in healthy volunteers with specific microbiota enterotypes. *Front. Immunol.* 10:341. doi: 10.3389/fimmu.2019.00341
26. Gupta, A., Madhavan, M. V., Sehgal, K., Nair, N., Mahajan, S., Sehrawat, T. S., et al. (2020). Extrapulmonary manifestations of COVID-19. *Nat. Med.* 26, 1017–1032. doi: 10.1038/s41591-020-0968-3
27. He, J., Li, Y., Cao, Y., Xue, J., and Zhou, X. (2015). The oral microbiome diversity and its relation to human diseases. *Folia Microbiol.* 60, 69–80. doi: 10.1007/ s12223-014-0342-2
28. Henrique Braz-Silva, P., Pallos, D., Giannecchini, S., and To, K. K. (2020). SARS- CoV-2: what can saliva tell us?. *Oral Dis.* 27(Suppl. 3), 746–747. doi: 10.1111/ odi.13365
29. Hernandez, J. M., Singam, H., Babu, A., Aslam, S., and Lakshmi, S. (2021). SARS-CoV-2 infection (COVID-19) and herpes simplex virus-1 conjunctivitis: concurrent viral infections or a cause-effect result? *Cureus* 13:e12592. doi: 10. 7759/cureus.12592
30. Herrera, D., Serrano, J., Roldan, S., and Sanz, M. (2020). Is the oral cavity relevant in SARS-CoV-2 pandemic? *Clin. Oral Investig.* 24, 2925–2930. doi: 10.1007/ s00784-020-03413-2
31. Iebba, V., Zanotta, N., Campisciano, G., Zerbato, V., Di Bella, S., Cason, C., et al. (2020). Profiling of oral microbiota and cytokines in COVID-19 patients. *bioRxiv* [Preprint]. doi: 10.1101/2020.12.13.422589
32. Inoue, T., Nakayama, J., Moriya, K., Kawaratani, H., Momoda, R., Ito, K., et al. (2018). Gut dysbiosis associated with hepatitis C virus infection. *Clin. Infect. Dis.* 67, 869–877. doi: 10.1093/cid/ciy205
33. Jasinski-Bergner, S., Mandelboim, O., and Seliger, B. (2020). Molecular mechanisms of human herpes viruses inferring with host immune surveillance. *J. Immunother. Cancer* 8:841. doi: 10.1136/jitc-2020-000841
34. Jose, R. J., and Manuel, A. (2020). COVID-19 cytokine storm: the interplay between inflammation and coagulation. *Lancet Respir. Med.* 8, e46–e47. doi: 10.1016/ S2213-2600(20)30216-2
35. Koch-Heier, J., Hoffmann, H., Schindler, M., Lussi, A., and Planz, O. (2021). Inactivation of SARS-CoV-2 through treatment with the mouth rinsing solutions ViruProX((R)) and BacterX((R)) Pro. *Microorganisms* 9:e030521. doi: 10.3390/microorganisms9030521
36. Lamont, R. J., Koo, H., and Hajishengallis, G. (2018). The oral microbiota: dynamic communities and host interactions. *Nat. Rev. Microbiol.* 16, 745–759. doi: 10. 1038/s41579-018-0089-x
37. Le Balc'h, P., Pinceaux, K., Pronier, C., Seguin, P., Tadie, J. M., and Reizine, F. (2020). Herpes simplex virus and cytomegalovirus reactivations among severe COVID-19 patients. *Crit. Care* 24:530. doi: 10.1186/s13054-020-03252-3
38. Lehner, G. F., Klein, S. J., Zoller, H., Peer, A., Bellmann, R., and Joannidis, M. (2020). Correlation of interleukin-6 with Epstein-Barr virus levels in COVID- 19. *Crit. Care* 24:657. doi: 10.1186/s13054-020-03384-6
39. Li, J., Gong, X., Wang, Z., Chen, R., Li, T., Zeng, D., et al. (2020). Clinical features of familial clustering in patients infected with 2019 novel coronavirus in Wuhan, China. *Virus Res.* 286:198043. doi: 10.1016/j.virusres.2020.198 043
40. Li, N., Ma, W. T., Pang, M., Fan, Q. L., and Hua, J. L. (2019). The commensal microbiota and viral infection: a comprehensive review. *Front. Immunol.* 10:1551. doi: 10.3389/fimmu.2019.01551
41. Lynch, S. V. (2014). Viruses and microbiome alterations. *Ann. Am. Thorac. Soc.* 11(Suppl. 1), S57–S60. doi: 10.1513/AnnalsATS.201306-158MG
42. Marouf, N., Cai, W., Said, K. N., Daas, H., Diab, H., Chinta, V. R., et al. (2021). Association between periodontitis and severity of COVID-19 infection: a case- control study. *J. Clin. Periodontol.* 48, 483–491. doi: 10.1111/jcpe.13435
43. Mateos Moreno, M. V., Obrador, A. M., Marquez, V. A., and Ferrer Garcia, M. D. (2021). Oral antiseptics against coronavirus: in vitro and clinical evidence. *J. Hosp. Infect.* 113, 30–43. doi: 10.1016/j.jhin.2021.04.004
44. Mehta, P., McAuley, D. F., Brown, M., Sanchez, E., Tattersall, R. S., Manson, J. J., et al. (2020). COVID-19: consider cytokine storm syndromes and immunosuppression. *Lancet* 395, 1033–1034. doi: 10.1016/S0140-6736(20) 30628-0
45. Mukherjee, P. K., Chandra, J., Retuerto, M., Sikaroodi, M., Brown, R. E., Jurevic, R., et al. (2014). Oral mycobiome analysis of HIV-infected patients: identification of Pichia as an antagonist of opportunistic fungi. *PLoS Pathog.* 10:e1003996. doi: 10.1371/journal.ppat.1003996
46. Pabst, O., and Slack, E. (2020). IgA and the intestinal microbiota: the importance of being specific. *Mucosal Immunol.* 13, 12–21. doi: 10.1038/ s41385-019-0227-4
47. Parra-Medina, R., Herrera, S., and Mejia, J. (2020). Comments to: a systematic review of pathological findings in COVID-19: a pathophysiological timeline and possible mechanisms of disease progression. *Mod. Pathol.* [Epub ahead of print]. doi: 10.1038/s41379-020-0631-z
48. Patel, J., and Sampson, V. (2020). The role of oral bacteria in COVID-19. *Lancet Microbe* 1:e105. doi: 10.1016/S2666-5247(20)30057-4
49. Pfeiffer, J. K., and Sonnenburg, J. L. (2011). The intestinal microbiota and viral susceptibility. *Front. Microbiol.* 2:92. doi: 10.3389/fmicb.2011.00 092
50. Prasad, N., Gopalakrishnan, N., Sahay, M., Gupta, A., Agarwal, S. K., and Nephrology, C. (2020). Epidemiology, genomic structure, the molecular mechanism of injury, diagnosis and clinical manifestations of coronavirus infection: an overview. *Indian J. Nephrol.* 30, 143–154. doi: 10.4103/ijn.IJN_191_20
51. Ramos-Sevillano, E., Wade, W. G., Mann, A., Gilbert, A., Lambkin-Williams, R., Killingley, B., et al. (2019). The effect of influenza virus on the human oropharyngeal microbiome. *Clin. Infect. Dis.* 68, 1993–2002. doi: 10.1093/cid/ ciy821
52. Roncati, L., Lusenti, B., Nasillo, V., and Manenti, A. (2020). Fatal SARS-CoV-2 coinfection in course of EBV-associated lymphoproliferative disease. *Ann. Hematol.* 99, 1945–1946. doi: 10.1007/s00277-020-04098-z
53. Salk, H. M., Simon, W. L., Lambert, N. D., Kennedy, R. B., Grill, D. E., Kabat, B. F., et al. (2016). Taxa of the nasal microbiome are associated with influenza-specific IgA response to live attenuated influenza vaccine. *PLoS One* 11:e0162803. doi: 10.1371/journal.pone.0162803
54. Sampson, V., Kamona, N., and Sampson, A. (2020). Could there be a link between oral hygiene and the severity of SARS-CoV-2 infections? *Br. Dent. J.* 228, 971–975. doi: 10.1038/s41415-020-1747-8
55. Schmieder, R., and Edwards, R. (2011). Quality control and preprocessing of metagenomic datasets. *Bioinformatics* 27, 863–864. doi: 10.1093/bioin formatics/btr026
56. Sinha, P., Jafarzadeh, S. R., Assoumou, S. A., Bielick, C. G., Carpenter, B., Garg, S., et al. (2021). The effect of IL-6 inhibitors on mortality among hospitalized COVID-19 patients: a multicenter Study. *J. Infect. Dis.* 223, 581–588. doi: 10. 1093/infdis/jiaa717

57. Sun, Y., Ma, Y., Lin, P., Tang, Y. W., Yang, L., Shen, Y., et al. (2016). Fecal bacterial microbiome diversity in chronic HIV-infected patients in China. *Emerg. Microbes Infect.* 5:e31. doi: 10.1038/emi.2016.25

58. Suo, T., Liu, X., Feng, J., Guo, M., Hu, W., Guo, D., et al. (2020). ddPCR: a more accurate tool for SARS-CoV-2 detection in low viral load specimens. *Emerg. Microbes Infect.* 9, 1259–1268. doi: 10.1080/22221751.2020.1772 678

59. To, K. K., Tsang, O. T., Yip, C. C., Chan, K. H., Wu, T. C., Chan, J. M., et al. (2020). Consistent detection of 2019 novel coronavirus in saliva. *Clin. Infect. Dis.* 71, 841–843. doi: 10.1093/cid/ciaa149

60. Wade, W. G. (2013). The oral microbiome in health and disease. *Pharmacol. Res.* 69, 137–143. doi: 10.1016/j.phrs.2012.11.006

61. Wang, Y., Li, X., Ge, T., Xiao, Y., Liao, Y., Cui, Y., et al. (2016). Probiotics for prevention and treatment of respiratory tract infections in children: a systematic review and meta-analysis of randomized controlled trials. *Medicine* 95:e4509. doi: 10.1097/MD.0000000000004509

62. Ward, D. V., Bhattarai, S., Rojas-Correa, M., Purkayastha, A., Holler, D., Da Qu, M., et al. (2021). The intestinal and oral microbiomes are robust predictors of covid-19 severity the main predictor of COVID-19-related fatality. *medRxiv* [Preprint]. doi: 10.1101/2021.01.05.20249061

63. Wilks, J., Beilinson, H., and Golovkina, T. V. (2013). Dual role of commensal bacteria in viral infections. *Immunol. Rev.* 255, 222–229. doi: 10.1111/imr. 12097

64. Wilks, J., and Golovkina, T. (2012). Influence of microbiota on viral infections. *PLoS Pathog.* 8:e1002681. doi: 10.1371/journal.ppat.1002681

65. World Health Organization [WHO] (2021). *WHO Coronavirus Disease (COVID-19) Dashboard.* Geneva: World Health Organisation.

66. Xiang, Z., Koo, H., Chen, Q., Zhou, X., Liu, Y., and Simon-Soro, A. (2020). Potential implications of SARS-CoV-2 oral infection in the host microbiota. *J. Oral Microbiol.* 13:1853451. doi: 10.1080/20002297.2020.1853451

67. Yan, H., Lamm, M. E., Bjorling, E., and Huang, Y. T. (2002). Multiple functions of immunoglobulin A in mucosal defense against viruses: an in vitro measles virus model. *J. Virol.* 76, 10972–10979. doi: 10.1128/jvi.76.21.10972-10979.2002

68. Yildiz, S., Mazel-Sanchez, B., Kandasamy, M., Manicassamy, B., and Schmolke, M. (2018). Influenza A virus infection impacts systemic microbiota dynamics and causes quantitative enteric dysbiosis. *Microbiome* 6:9. doi: 10.1186/s40168-017- 0386-z

69. Yoon, J. G., Yoon, J., Song, J. Y., Yoon, S. Y., Lim, C. S., Seong, H., et al. (2020). Clinical significance of a high SARS-CoV-2 viral load in the saliva. *J. Korean Med. Sci.* 35:e195. doi: 10.3346/jkms.2020.35.e195

70. Zaura, E., Keijser, B. J., Huse, S. M., and Crielaard, W. (2009). Defining the healthy "core microbiome" of oral microbial communities. *BMC Microbiol.* 9:259. doi: 10.1186/1471-2180-9-259

13

A Multi-Disciplinary Review on the Aerobiology of COVID-19 in Dental Settings

Darya Dabiri[1*], *Samuel Richard Conti*[2], *Niloufar Sadoughi Pour*[3], *Andrew Chong*[4], *Shaahin Dadjoo*[5], *Donya Dabiri*[1], *Carol Wiese*[1], *Joyce Badal*[6], *Margaret Arleen Hoogland*[7], *Heather Raquel Conti*[2], *Travis Roger Taylor*[8], *George Choueiri*[3] and *Omid Amili*[3]

[1] Department of Dentistry, Division of Pediatric Dentistry, University of Toledo, Toledo, OH, United States, [2] Department of Biological Sciences, University of Toledo, Toledo, OH, United States, [3] Department of Mechanical, Industrial and Manufacturing Engineering (MIME), University of Toledo, Toledo, OH, United States, [4] Department of Cariology, Restorative Sciences & Endodontics, University of Michigan, Ann Arbor, MI, United States, [5] Department of Orthodontics and Dentofacial Orthopedics, The Eastman Institute for Oral Health, University of Rochester, Rochester, NY, United States, [6] Department of Medicine, University of Toledo, Toledo, OH, United States, [7] Mulford Health Sciences Library, University of Toledo, Toledo, OH, United States, [8] Department of Medical Microbiology and Immunology, University of Toledo, Toledo, OH, United States

***Correspondence:**
Darya Dabiri
darya.dabiri@utoledo.edu*

The COVID-19 pandemic pushed dental health officials around the world to reassess and adjust their existing healthcare practices. As studies on controlled COVID-19 transmission remain challenging, this review focuses on particles that can carry the virus and relevant approaches to mitigate the risk of pathogen transmission in dental offices. This review gives an overview of particles generated in clinical settings and how size influences their distribution, concentration, and generation route. A wide array of pertinent particle characterization and counting methods are reviewed, along with their working range, reliability, and limitations. This is followed by a focus on the effectiveness of personal protective equipment (PPE) and face shields in protecting patients and dentists from aerosols. Direct studies on severe acute respiratory syndrome coronavirus 2 (SARS-CoV-2) are still limited, but the literature supports the use of masks as an important and effective non-pharmaceutical preventive measure that could reduce the risk of contracting a respiratory infection by up to 20%. In addition to discussing about PPE used by most dental care professionals, this review describes other ways by which dental offices can protect patients and dental office personnel, which includes modification of the existing room design, dental equipment, and heating, ventilation, and air conditioning (HVAC) system. More affordable modifications include positioning a high-efficiency particulate air (HEPA) unit within proximity of the patient's chair or using ultraviolet germicidal irradiation in conjunction with ventilation. Additionally, portable fans could be used to direct airflow in one direction, first through the staff working areas and then through the patient treatment areas, which could decrease the number of airborne particles in dental offices. This review concludes that there is a need for greater awareness amongst dental practitioners about the relationship between particle dynamics and clinical dentistry, and additional research is needed to fill the broad gaps of knowledge in this field.

Keywords: COVID-19, particle measurement, bioaerosol, dental procedures, particle topography

INTRODUCTION

Severe acute respiratory syndrome coronavirus 2 (SARS-CoV-2), which is the causative virus of coronavirus disease-2019 (COVID-19), presents challenges greater than that posed by seasonal influenza ($R_0 \sim 1.2$), Middle East respiratory syndrome (MERS) ($R_0 \sim 1.4$), or severe acute respiratory syndrome (SARS) ($R_0 \sim 3$) due to its high reproductive number ($R_0 = 1.4$–3.9) (1–3). The most recent global assessment of R_0 for COVID-19 is 4.08. This high reproductive number contributed to the unprecedented global spread of SARS-CoV-2 (4).

According to a scientific brief published by the WHO on March 29, 2020, the primary transmission mode of SARS-CoV-2 is through respiratory droplets and contact routes (i.e., oral secretions) with a diameter >5 μm (5, 6). These droplets enter the air through speaking, coughing, and sneezing by individuals in close contact with each other (5–8). Short-range inhalation of aerosols can be a route of COVID-19 transmission as with many respiratory pathogens (9). Oral cavity is another important site for SARS-CoV-2 infection (10). The most reported mode of pathogen spread is through respiratory droplets. Individuals that are pre-symptomatic or asymptomatic do not significantly cough or sneeze, yet are responsible for more than 50% of COVID-19 transmission (11), and hence it is important to study the effect of particles expired through normal breathing and oral cavity secretions (10, 12).

Dental practices across the globe closed down for non-emergency dental care during peak COVID-19 periods because of the higher risk of virus transmission during dental appointment due to the close proximity of patient–provider and the use of modern dental tools, such as high-speed handpieces, ultrasonic scalers, air turbines, and air-water syringes, in the presence of contaminated salivary secretions (5, 10, 13–15). It is important to note that dental professionals demonstrated high compliance (72.8%) to CDC guidelines during the COVID-19 pandemic, which has led to very low cases of COVID-19 transmission in dental settings (16). In this review, the authors present studies focused on the transport of particles, the various methods of characterizing the particles, bioaerosols in dentistry, and finally recommendations for reducing the transmission of potentially virus-laden droplets generated during routine dental treatments.

PARTICLES

To better understand the modifications that could be adopted by dental offices to minimize transmission of SARS-CoV-2, the team elaborates on the definition of particle and droplet, transmission of particles *via* bioaerosols, and the natural production and dissemination of aerosols produced during cleaning or treatment at a dental office.

Definitions of Particle and Droplet

In dental settings, particles are generated from patient–provider interactions, dental equipment, and dental procedures. Our review defines droplets as water-based with a mean diameter >5 μm. Aerosols (or airborne nuclei) are defined as liquid or solid particles typically <5 μm in diameter. Particulate matters (PMs) are arguably interchangeable with aerosols and typically refer to solid (or liquid) particles in the size range of sub-micron to 10 μm. Particle concentration refers to the count (or particle mass) per unit volume, e.g., count/m^3 (or μg/L).

Size influences the behavior and trajectory of droplets and aerosols/particles. Within a 1 m radius, droplets larger than 50 μm display ballistic or jet-like movements. Intermediate size droplets can either fall on the surface or can stay in the air and travel approximately 2 m before settling down. Smaller droplets and aerosols are the least impacted by gravity and can stay airborne for long durations. For example, a dust particle with a diameter of 10 μm falls 1 m in air at rest in ~5.5 min, whereas a 1 μm particle takes over 9 h to travel the same distance. Owing to air currents, such small particles may spread throughout the room, especially after the volatile liquid in the droplet dries out (17).

Bioaerosols Production and the Influencing Factors

Human lungs inspire approximately 0.5–0.75 L per breath during rest. Air expelled through nasal respiration produces an exit velocity of ~0.5 m/s, whereas the exit velocity while speaking with a normal volume and pace exhibits ~0.3 m/s. In contrast, during periodic coughing, the exit velocity dramatically increases to 4–5 m/s (18). Direct observations of human sneezing and coughing reveal that these airflows consist of initially hot and moist turbulence followed by cool and buoyant clouds containing droplets of varying sizes. A single cough may expel ~700 particles as compared with a sneeze that may produce over 40,000 particles (19). In this regard, most of the particles and droplets produced from a sneeze are relatively large and may be easily blocked by the use of a simple mask. In addition to coughing and sneezing, speaking can generate droplets of size ranging from 20 to 500 μm (5). However, the estimated concentration of droplets per cough is 2.4–5.2 cm^{-3}, which is significantly more than that of speech, 0.004–0.223 cm^{-3} (20).

In addition to particle size, environmental factors such as temperature and relative humidity influence the potency and distribution of infectious respiratory droplets and particles. For example, a 100 μm droplet will evaporate in approximately 10 s after expulsion while a 1 μm droplet will evaporate within 0.001 s (19). Increased air temperature, however, leads to an immediate decrease in particles post expulsion. By contrast, however, in an environment of elevated humidity, these numbers increase. Regardless of humidity or temperature, particles or droplets with a diameter of <0.1 μm evaporate almost immediately or cannot contain enough viral material to be infectious (9).

Viruses can be transmitted *via* droplets produced by sneezing and coughing, with diameters varying in the range of 0.1 μm-0.9 mm (21). Once an individual begins coughing, the duration and position of the mouth influence the area covered by the expelled droplets, which can degrade into categories of smaller size (9). Viral, fungal, and bacterial particles react in different ways depending on changes in temperature or humidity of the environment. The maximum stability of influenza occurs at 20–40% humidity and has a minimum stability at 50% humidity (22). Studies have suggested that SARS-CoV-2 exhibits similar survival curves in response to increases in temperature and humidity (23). With respect to coronaviruses at room temperature, they remain viable on surfaces for up to 9 days (24). At temperatures >30°C, the survival of these viruses decreases dramatically (24).

Bioaerosols in the Practice of Dentistry

Dissemination of Microorganisms

Dissemination of microorganisms in dental operatories can occur directly, by contact with bacteria on the surfaces of dental instruments and dental providers, or indirectly, *via* splatter of droplets larger than 100 μm in diameter or by particles <100 μm in diameter suspended in air (25). Most dental bioaerosol studies have investigated bacterial colonies on the surfaces of dental instruments as the main pathogen. The potential for disease transmission of airborne bacteria (e.g., tuberculosis), viruses (e.g., measles and SARS), and bloodborne viruses, which can become aerosolized by blood splatter *via* high-speed handpieces used in dentistry and orthodontics, is not known (26–28). COVID-19 transmission is primarily through respiratory droplets and less likely through fomite transmission (29). The two most notable sources of droplet and aerosol generation in dental settings are procedures involving air turbine handpieces and ultrasonic instruments.

Air Turbine Handpieces

Studies have demonstrated that air turbine handpieces atomize 20 times more bacteria when compared to air spray. This production of bioaerosols is equivalent to the concentration produced by biological motions such as sneezing (30). A prophylactic hygiene handpiece with a pumice cup and pumice is often used for cleaning teeth. This common dental procedure produces a volume of aerosolized bacteria comparable to that resulting from a cough (31). *Tubercle bacilli* were found in droplet scatterings generated by dental air turbine handpieces within a range of 6 inches to over 4 feet from the patient's mouth (26). This distance is larger than the distance between providers and patients, indicating a working dentist/assistant will undoubtedly be affected (30).

Ultrasonic Instruments

Ultrasonic instruments also produce significant amounts of aerosols and the vibration of the tip generates significant amounts of heat. Water is used to cool the instrument, which results in the generation of significant splatter. When mixed with saliva and plaque from the oral cavity, aerosolized splatter from ultrasonic instruments has the potential to become highly infectious and a major risk factor for disease transmission (31). Moreover, ultrasonic instrumentation can transmit 100,000 microbes/ft^3 with aerosolization of up to 6 ft (32). In the absence of a favorable air current, microbes can survive for a period ranging from 35 min to 17 h. Using microbiological analysis, significantly higher bacterial counts were detected after scaling treatments, with the presence of Staphylococcus and Streptococcus species being the most notable (26). Results also showed high numbers of colony forming units (CFUs) and identified strictly oral anaerobes on all microbial plates from both groups, which meant that a significant amount of contamination occurred during ultrasonic scaling (26).

METHODS OF CHARACTERIZING BIOAEROSOLS

Aerosolized particles can be classified into three categories: natural (e.g., fog, dust, and mist), anthropogenic (e.g., air pollution and smoke), and biological (e.g., bioaerosols) which are primarily released by humans and animals. These particles are carried through natural and anthropogenic means (33, 34). Bioaerosols contain both volatile and non-volatile material and their behavior and transmissibility depend on their size. Smaller bioaerosol particles penetrate more easily and go farther into the respiratory tract, which means they are more likely to transmit diseases compared to the larger particles (19).

Over the years, researchers have developed a variety of instruments to assist with particle sizing and classification. A broad list of instruments used in bioaerosol particle counting and sizing is presented in **Table 1**, and a summary of measured particle size distributions is shown in **Figure 1**. More recently, researchers have started using machine learning to analyze SARS-CoV-2 infected particles (44).

RECOMMENDATIONS TO MINIMIZE COVID-19 TRANSMISSION IN DENTAL SETTINGS

Patient/Staff as Source of Particle

Although there are differences in aerodynamic behavior and properties between droplets and particles, both provide mechanisms for transmitting pathogenic microorganisms between patient and dental personnel. Human interactions (speaking, sneezing, and coughing), even without any symptom, can be a source of respiratory pathogen transmission in an indoor setting (5, 20), such as in dental offices. Dental providers working with high-speed handpieces have routine exposure to bodily fluids including respiratory particles and oral secretions (10, 34). Ultrasonic scalers, air turbines, three-in-one syringes, and air-water syringes are also significant contributors to bioaerosol generation (31).

Personal Protective Equipment

Personal protective equipment (PPE) is an important mitigation strategy (45). Global sources for producing PPE continue to be insufficient due to a large number of COVID-19 cases, misinformation, panic buying, and stockpiling (6). It is imperative to revisit the current and developing PPE options with respect to their efficacy. The WHO has listed the following PPEs as necessary for healthcare workers: medical masks, N95 respirators, filtering facepiece respirators-2 (FFP2) standard or equivalent, gowns, gloves, aprons, and eye protection (goggles or face shields) (6). A recent study on COVID-19 prevalence among dentists, while adhering to

TABLE 1 | Experimental methods used for particle count and characterization.

Method	Description	Select bioaerosol studies and comments
Aerodynamic particle sizer (APS)	Uses the principle of inertia to size particles. Particles pass between two laser beams and the scattered light is collected on a photodetector. By measuring the time delay between pulses generated as particles pass through the laser beams, the velocity and diameter of particles are measured.	Morawska et al. (35): studied particle concentration and size distribution near the mouth for a range of breath exercises. Voiced activities produced higher particle concentrations than whispered ones which indicated particles were produced by the vibrating vocal cords. Whispered counting and breathing produced similar amount of particles.
Andersen cascade impactors (ACI)	Also known as cascade sampler impactors. Used to measure the size distribution of non-volatile aerosolized particles (36). A suction pump is used to draw air through a series of 6-8 stages which are used to separate different particle sizes.	Two types can be found; one for viable particles (meaning viruses and bacteria which can be grown on a series of Petri dishes) and the other for non-viable particles.
Droplet deposition analysis (DDA)	Uses optical or electron microscopes to measure the size of deposited droplets on a surface by using a substrate which preserves traces of the deposited droplets.	Duguid (37): measured the droplet size of sneezing, coughing, and speaking. Found similar size distribution for all activities, but smaller droplets much more frequent in sneezing. 95% of droplets were between 2 and 100 μm. Most common are in the range of 4-8 μm (38).
Interferometric Mie imaging (IMI) and particle image velocimetry (PIV)	An out-of-focus imaging technique of particles illuminated by a laser light sheet (39). It may be used simultaneously with particle image/tracking velocimetry (PIV/PTV) to measure instantaneous velocity fields.	VanSciver et al. (40): measured cough velocity of 29 healthy subjects within the range of 1.5 and 28.8 m/s. Chao et al. (20): studied 11 human subjects and measured the size distribution and velocity of droplets during speaking and coughing using IMI APS and PIV. Found the mean diameter of particles was 13.5 and 16 μm and velocity was 11.7 and 3.1 m/s for coughing and speaking respectively. Zhu et al. (41): studied transport properties of the saliva droplets of coughing in an indoor environment by using both PIV and numerical methods. The initial coughing velocity was estimated between 6 and 22 m/s with an average velocity of 11.2 m/s and the impacted area was 2 m or larger.
Laser diffraction (LD)	Utilizes the light scattering principle to measure the distribution of particle size by determining the unique variations in the intensity of light scattered as a laser beam travels through a scattered particulate sample. Large particles scatter light at small angles and vice versa. The angular light intensity data is then evaluated to assess the size of the particles responsible for producing such scattering patterns.	Zayas et al. (21): used laser diffraction to measure voluntary cough aerosols of 45 healthy non-smokers and found a size range of 0.1-900 μm of which 97% of droplets were found to be less than 1 μm.
Optical particle counters (OPC)	Works on the concept of light scattering from illuminated particles. Two types are generally found: LED and laser-based counters; the first is better for counting larger particles, while the latter is better for smaller particles.	Papineni and Rosenthal (42): measured exhaled droplets from mouth breathing, nose breathing, coughing, and talking. They also used an analytical transmission electron microscope (analytical TEM) and found particle sizes with the OPC in the range of 0.3-2.5 μm and with the analytical TEM in the range of 0.4-7.6 μm. Edwards et al. (43): measured expired air particle count and size and reported the size range of droplets between 0.085 μm and >0.5 μm with a mode between 0.15 and 0.2 μm.
Spray droplet size analyzer (SDSA)	A laser diffraction-based droplet sizer that can detect aerosols and particles between 0.1-2,000 μm.	Lindsley et al. (22): measured the concentration of aerosols from a cough aerosol simulator. A major peak in aerosol concentrations was measured in the size range of 3-10 μm.

the listed PPEs, indicated a very low percentage of only 0.9% (16). While combinations of PPE are recommended, the effectiveness of specific PPE at preventing SARS-CoV-2 infection has not been quantified. Determining the effectiveness of PPE is complicated due to the limited controlled human infection studies. "Silent spreaders" may expose healthcare workers at work and elsewhere if basic non-pharmaceutical interventions are not universally adopted and enforced (46, 47). In the absence of PPE measures, historical data from similarly transmitted respiratory diseases, such as tuberculosis in dental settings showed a transmission of 10%, which was more than double the reported data from the National Health and Nutrition Examination Survey (NHANES) in the year 2000 (48).

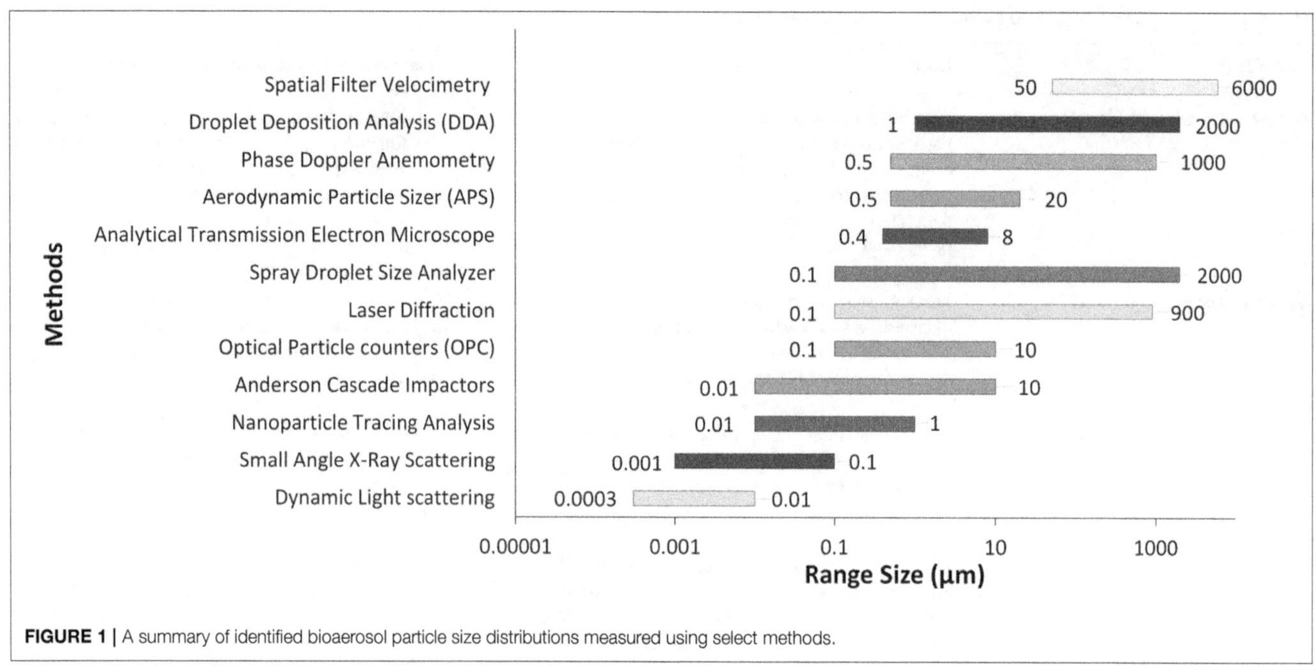

FIGURE 1 | A summary of identified bioaerosol particle size distributions measured using select methods.

Face Shields

Most harmful particles are generated during the initial part of a cough (49). Healthcare providers working at a distance of 46 cm from an infected patient may inhale 0.9% of these harmful particles. Wearing a face shield can reduce the inhalation of aerosols by 96% and surface contamination by 97% for droplets with a volume median diameter (VMD) of 8.5 μm. However, for smaller droplets with a VMD of 3.4 μm, the reduction rates are lower with 68 and 76% for aerosols and surface contamination, respectively (45). Face shields may reduce the inhalation of large harmful aerosol particles for a short time. However, smaller particles remain in the air for longer periods and could bypass the face shield. These particles pose inhalation risks for healthcare providers and patients (50).

Face Masks

A study conducted on 47 human subjects with influenza showed that the average cough profiles had a volume of 4.16 L with a peak flow rate of 11.1 L/s (22). A mask designed to suppress droplets at this volume and flow rate could be an effective inhibitor for smaller cough volumes and lesser peak flow rates (18). A different study reported that each patient suffering from influenza released ~38 pL of particles in the size range of <10 μm. After being diagnosed and receiving treatment, the study participants released ~26 pL of particles per cough. Droplets become infectious when they encounter the mucous membranes, e.g., oral and nasal cavities of the body (51). Studies on influenza-related diseases support the use of surgical masks for effective reduction of infection (47). Using masks in crowded places could reduce the risk of contracting influenza-like respiratory infections by 20% (52). Masks made of foam, cloth, or paper are less effective at filtering bacterial aerosols (50).

Masks vs. Respirators

According to the CDC, the N95 FFP can block at least 95% of 0.3 μm particles. Most research pertaining to the efficacy of face masks has been done by quantifying the number of respiratory viruses in exhaled breaths of participants with acute respiratory virus illness (17). Surgical masks can effectively reduce the emission of influenza-laden respiratory droplets but not particles (53). When subjects cough while wearing a surgical mask or N95, the dispersion of forward moving viral aerosol particles decreases but the lateral dispersion patterns of particles increases (54). N95s and surgical masks offer similar levels of protection against viral infection of respiratory diseases in non-aerosol producing environments (55).

Equipment as Source of Particles (Room Design/Equipment Modification)

Dental buildings can contain high levels of circulating bioaerosols. Air-conditioning and ventilation systems in these settings should be maintained on a regular basis to minimize recirculation of contaminants (56). Cooling towers, air-conditioning, and mechanical ventilation systems are known sources of *Legionella pneumophila* (57). The risks to dentists, patients, and others who are routinely exposed to bioaerosols remain unclear, prompting the need for further research (14).

Office or Clinic Design

Multiple actions can be taken to decrease the transmission of infectious particles in healthcare settings. Electronic-based patient triages and check-ins, automatic doors, motion-sensing lights, and hand-sanitizer dispensers reduce the physical interface among patients, physicians, and interior surfaces. The use of thermal imaging to screen for elevated body temperatures ensures a safe distance between ingress patients and office staff while shortening the initial screening process. Since dental procedures generate mists and aerosols, local exhaust ventilation should be positioned with consideration of the aerosol flow direction as well as the location of the physician and the patient (9, 58–61).

Heating, Ventilation, and Air Conditioning System Design

Dental offices are advised to use a systems-based approach with engineering controls to minimize cross contamination. For example, fans could be used to direct the airflow first through the staff working areas and then through the patient treatment areas, thereby reducing workplace risks involving airborne particles or droplets (62). Positioning of patients in front of each other should be avoided whenever possible (9). Operatories should be oriented parallel to the direction of airflow, which will assist in directing the flow of airborne contaminants (62).

The CDC also recommends positioning the heads of patients away from pedestrian corridors and closer to the back wall and return air vents (9, 63). Several studies have evaluated the characteristics of plumes generated by exhaled droplets and noted that a top exhaust system is more efficient than the traditional air conditioning systems (64). Ultraviolet (UV) germicidal irradiation, including UV-C at 254 nm, in conjunction with ventilation is emerging as a cost-effective tool for reducing viral aerosols (52, 65, 66). In the design of future dental offices, the designation of negative-pressure isolation rooms, antechambers, and 24/7 HVAC systems could improve aerobiological controls (63).

Interior Design

It is important to consider an interior design that prompts safe conduct of ordinary activities. Visual signage is a good option to communicate instructions clearly to the general public. For example, clear marking of risk zones with visual aids or creating visual cues for specific activities raises awareness and allows policies to be followed easily (58). Additionally, creating signage that indicates "clean" areas around donning rooms and PPE carts can establish easy-to-follow protocols. Efficient and regimented routines create less interaction and reduce cross-contamination. The efficacy of visual signage is increased if supplemented with an office culture based on safety and education. Additionally, anti-bacterial surface coatings reduce healthcare-associated infections (HAIs) by 36% while also decreasing CFUs and clinically relevant pathogens by ~59–75% (67). Other design initiatives worth considering are sanitizing stations, maintaining social distancing whenever possible in the reception and treatment rooms, and dedicated PPE recycling bins in each room (58).

CONCLUSIONS

Respiratory droplets are the primary mode of SARS-CoV-2 transmission. Human and simulated studies have demonstrated that sneezing and high-volume coughs in patients pose a significant risk for viral transmission. Environmental conditions effect the potency of viruses shed from human coughing and sneezing as well as dental procedures. SARS-CoV-2 reacts inversely to temperature and humidity, which are factors that can be controlled in a closed dental setting. One of the biggest concerns for dental providers is the working proximity to potentially active SARS-CoV-2 sources, as intermediate size (10–50 μm) droplets can travel as far as 2 m away from the source. Furthermore, these droplets are easily disseminated by air currents. Surgical masks and respirators appear to provide significant protection against viral particle transmission from infected individuals, although the risk is not completely eliminated. While we highlighted various methods used to study the size and distribution of airborne droplets and particles, these methods for the most part do not measure the viral load and more specialized tools need to be developed. Implementing some of the recommendations we proposed and a greater awareness amongst dental practitioners about the relationship between particle dynamics and clinical dentistry, can help improve safety in dental practice. Finally, while this review provides a broad overview of past and current studies related to pathogen and particle transmission in dental settings, there is a clear gap in our understanding of how dental practices specifically affect the transmission of SARS-CoV-2; therefore, much more research is needed in this area. This knowledge is imperative to addressing the current crisis, and those that might be faced in the future.

AUTHOR CONTRIBUTIONS

All authors gave their final approval and agreed to be accountable for all aspects of the work.

ACKNOWLEDGMENTS

The authors thank the National Institutes of Health (grant number: X01 DE030405-01) for the partial financial support for this article through the National Dental PBRN collaborative group funding U19-DE-028717 and U01-DE-028727. The authors thank Mohammad Reza D. Jahanshahi, Armon Jahanshahi, Dr. Michael Nedley, Dr. Mel Krajden, Dr. Yvonne Kapila, and Dr. Daniel Clauw for their expertise and guidance.

REFERENCES

1. Coburn BJ, Wagner BG, Blower S. Modeling influenza epidemics and pandemics: insights into the future of swine flu (h1n1). *BMC Med.* (2009) 7:30. doi: 10.1186/1741-7015-7-30
2. Yin Y, Wunderink RG. Mers, sars and other coronaviruses as causes of pneumonia. *Respirology.* (2018) 23:130–7. doi: 10.1111/resp.13196
3. Wang J, Pan L, Tang S, Ji JS, Shi X. Mask use during covid-19: a risk adjusted strategy. *Environ Pollut.* (2020) 266:115099. doi: 10.1016/j.envpol.2020.115099
4. Yu CJ, Wang ZX, Xu Y, Hu MX, Chen K, Qin G. Assessment of basic reproductive number for covid-19 at global level: a meta-analysis. *Medicine.* (2021) 100:e25837. doi: 10.1097/MD.0000000000025837

5. Bax A, Bax CE, Stadnytskyi V, Anfinrud P. Sars-cov-2 transmission via speech-generated respiratory droplets. *Lancet Infect Dis.* (2021) 21:318. doi: 10.1016/S1473-3099(20)30726-X
6. *Modes of Transmission of Virus Causing Covid-19: Implications for IPC Precaution Recommendations: Scientific Brief.* Geneva: World Health Organization (2020).
7. Peng X, Xu X, Li Y, Cheng L, Zhou X, Ren B. Transmission routes of 2019-ncov and controls in dental practice. *Int J Oral Sci.* (2020) 12:9. doi: 10.1038/s41368-020-0075-9
8. Sun P, Lu X, Xu C, Sun W, Pan B. Understanding of covid-19 based on current evidence. *J Med Virol.* (2020) 92:548–51. doi: 10.1002/jmv.25722
9. *Covid-19 Overview and Infection Prevention and Control Priorities in Non-US Healthcare Settings.* Atlanta, GA: Centers for Disease Control and Prevention (2021).
10. Huang N, Pérez P, Kato T, Mikami Y, Okuda K, Gilmore RC, et al. Sars-cov-2 infection of the oral cavity and saliva. *Nat Med.* (2021) 27:892–903. doi: 10.1038/s41591-021-01296-8
11. Johansson MA, Quandelacy TM, Kada S, Prasad PV, Steele M, Brooks JT, et al. Sars-cov-2 transmission from people without covid-19 symptoms. *JAMA Netw Open.* (2021) 4:e2035057. doi: 10.1001/jamanetworkopen.2020.35057
12. Scheuch G. Breathing is enough: for the spread of influenza virus and sars-cov-2 by breathing only. *J Aerosol Med Pulm Drug Deliv.* (2020) 33:230–4. doi: 10.1089/jamp.2020.1616
13. Ather A, Patel B, Ruparel NB, Diogenes A, Hargreaves KM. Coronavirus disease 19 (covid-19): implications for clinical dental care. *J Endod.* (2020) 46:584–95. doi: 10.1016/j.joen.2020.03.008
14. Bahador M, Alfirdous RA, Alquria TA, Griffin IL, Tordik PA, Martinho FC. *Aerosols generated during endodontic treatment: a special concern during the coronavirus disease 2019 pandemic. J Endod.* (2021) 47:732-9. doi: 10.1016/j.joen.2021.01.009
15. Caprioglio A, Pizzetti GB, Zecca PA, Fastuca R, Maino G, Nanda R. Management of orthodontic emergencies during 2019-ncov. *Prog Orthod.* (2020) 21:10. doi: 10.1186/s40510-020-00310-y
16. Estrich CG, Mikkelsen M, Morrissey R, Geisinger ML, Ioannidou E, Vujicic M, et al. Estimating covid-19 prevalence and infection control practices among us dentists. *J Am Dent Assoc.* (2020) 151:815–24. doi: 10.1016/j.adaj.2020.09.005
17. *Interim Guidance on Planning for the Use of Surgical Masks and Respirators in Health Care Settings During an Influenza Pandemic.* Atlanta, GA: Centers for Disease Control and Prevention (2006).
18. Kähler CJ, Hain R. Fundamental protective mechanisms of face masks against droplet infections. *J Aerosol Sci.* (2020) 148:105617. doi: 10.1016/j.jaerosci.2020.105617
19. Fernstrom A, Goldblatt M. Aerobiology and its role in the transmission of infectious diseases. *J Pathog.* (2013) 2013:493960. doi: 10.1155/2013/493960
20. Chao CYH, Wan MP, Morawska L, Johnson GR, Ristovski ZD, Hargreaves M, et al. Characterization of expiration air jets and droplet size distributions immediately at the mouth opening. *J Aerosol Sci.* (2009) 40:122–33. doi: 10.1016/j.jaerosci.2008.10.003
21. Zayas G, Chiang MC, Wong E, MacDonald F, Lange CF, Senthilselvan A, et al. Cough aerosol in healthy participants: fundamental knowledge to optimize droplet-spread infectious respiratory disease management. *BMC Pulm Med.* (2012) 12:11. doi: 10.1186/1471-2466-12-11
22. Lindsley WG, Reynolds JS, Szalajda JV, Noti JD, Beezhold DH. A cough aerosol simulator for the study of disease transmission by human cough-generated aerosols. *Aerosol Sci Technol.* (2013) 47:937–44. doi: 10.1080/02786826.2013.803019
23. van Doremalen N, Bushmaker T, Morris DH, Holbrook MG, Gamble A, Williamson BN, et al. Aerosol and surface stability of sars-cov-2 as compared with sars-cov-1. *N Engl J Med.* (2020) 382:1564–7. doi: 10.1056/NEJMc2004973
24. Kampf G, Todt D, Pfaender S, Steinmann E. Persistence of coronaviruses on inanimate surfaces and their inactivation with biocidal agents. *J Hosp Infect.* (2020) 104:246–51. doi: 10.1016/j.jhin.2020.01.022
25. Miller RL, Micik RE, Abel C, Ryge G. Studies on dental aerobiology. II. Microbial splatter discharged from the oral cavity of dental patients. *J Dent Res.* (1971) 50:621–5. doi: 10.1177/00220345710500031701
26. Belting CM, Haberfelde GC, Juhl LK. Spread of organisms from dental air rotor. *J Am Dent Assoc.* (1964) 68:648–51. doi: 10.14219/jada.archive.1964.0145
27. Bennett AM, Fulford MR, Walker JT, Bradshaw DJ, Martin MV, Marsh PD. Microbial aerosols in general dental practice. *Br Dent J.* (2000) 189:664–7. doi: 10.1038/sj.bdj.4800859
28. Harrel SK, Molinari J. Aerosols and splatter in dentistry: a brief review of the literature and infection control implications. *J Am Dent Assoc.* (2004) 135:429–37. doi: 10.14219/jada.archive.2004.0207
29. CDC. *Science Brief: Sars-Cov-2 and Surface (fomite) Transmission for Indoor Community Environments.* CDC (2021). Available online at: https://www.cdc.gov/coronavirus/2019-ncov/more/science-and-research/surface-transmission.html
30. Pelzner RB, Kempler D, Stark MM, Barkin PR, Graham DA. Laser evaluation of handpiece contamination. *J Dent Res.* (1977) 56:1629–34. doi: 10.1177/00220345770560123601
31. Micik RE, Miller RL, Mazzarella MA, Ryge G. Studies on dental aerobiology. I. Bacterial aerosols generated during dental procedures. *J Dent Res.* (1969) 48:49–56. doi: 10.1177/00220345690480012401
32. Nejatidanesh F, Khosravi Z, Goroohi H, Badrian H, Savabi O. Risk of contamination of different areas of dentist's face during dental practices. *Int J Prev Med.* (2013) 4:611–5.
33. Asadi S, Bouvier N, Wexler AS, Ristenpart WD. The coronavirus pandemic and aerosols: does covid-19 transmit via expiratory particles? *Aerosol Sci Technol.* (2020) 0:1–4. doi: 10.1080/02786826.2020.1749229
34. Ge ZY, Yang LM, Xia JJ, Fu XH, Zhang YZ. Possible aerosol transmission of covid-19 and special precautions in dentistry. *J Zhejiang Univ Sci B.* (2020) 21:361–8. doi: 10.1631/jzus.B2010010
35. Morawska L, Johnson G, Ristovski Z, Hargreaves M, Mengersen K, Corbett S, et al. Size distribution and sites of origin of droplets expelled from the human respiratory tract during expiratory activities. *J Aerosol Sci.* (2009) 40:256–69. doi: 10.1016/j.jaerosci.2008.11.002
36. Andersen AA. New sampler for the collection, sizing, and enumeration of viable airborne particles. *J Bacteriol.* (1958) 76:471–84. doi: 10.1128/jb.76.5.471-484.1958
37. Duguid JP. The size and the duration of air-carriage of respiratory droplets and droplet-nuclei. *J Hyg.* (1946) 44:471–9. doi: 10.1017/S0022172400019288
38. Kohli R, Mittal KL. *Developments in Surface Contamination and Cleaning: Detection, Characterization, and Analysis of Contaminants.* Oxford: Elsevier Inc (2012).
39. Ragucci R, Cavaliere A, Massoli P. Drop sizing by laser light scattering exploiting intensity angular oscillation in the mie regime. *Particle Particle Systems Characterization.* (1990) 7:221-5. doi: 10.1002/ppsc.19900070136
40. VanSciver M, Miller S, Hertzberg J. Particle image velocimetry of human cough. *Aerosol Sci Technol.* (2011) 45:415–22. doi: 10.1080/02786826.2010.542785
41. Zhu S, Kato S, Yang J-H. Study on transport characteristics of saliva droplets produced by coughing in a calm indoor environment. *Build Environ.* (2006) 41:1691–702. doi: 10.1016/j.buildenv.2005.06.024
42. Papineni RS, Rosenthal FS. The size distribution of droplets in the exhaled breath of healthy human subjects. *J Aerosol Med.* (1997) 10:105–16. doi: 10.1089/jam.1997.10.105
43. Edwards DA, Man JC, Brand P, Katstra JP, Sommerer K, Stone HA, et al. Inhaling to mitigate exhaled bioaerosols. *Proc Natl Acad Sci USA.* (2004) 101:17383–8. doi: 10.1073/pnas.0408159101
44. Nemati M, Ansary J, Nemati N. Machine-learning approaches in covid-19 survival analysis and discharge-time likelihood prediction using clinical data. *Patterns.* (2020) 1:100074. doi: 10.1016/j.patter.2020.100074
45. Bouadma L, Barbier F, Biard L, Esposito-Farèse M, Le Corre B, Macrez A, et al. Personal decision-making criteria related to seasonal and pandemic a(h1n1) influenza-vaccination acceptance among french healthcare workers. *PLoS ONE.* (2012) 7:e38646. doi: 10.1371/journal.pone.0038646
46. Froum SH, Froum SJ. Incidence of covid-19 virus transmission in three dental offices: A 6-month retrospective study. *Int J Periodontics Restorative Dent.* (2020) 40:853–9. doi: 10.11607/prd.5455
47. Jefferson T, Del Mar C, Dooley L, Ferroni E, Al-Ansary LA, Bawazeer GA, et al. Physical interventions to interrupt or reduce the spread of respiratory viruses: systematic review. *BMJ.* (2009) 339:b3675. doi: 10.1136/bmj.b3675

48. Merte JL, Kroll CM, Collins AS, Melnick AL. An epidemiologic investigation of occupational transmission of mycobacterium tuberculosis infection to dental health care personnel: infection prevention and control implications. *J Am Dent Assoc.* (2014) 145:464–71. doi: 10.14219/jada.2013.52
49. Day JB, Jones BM, Afshari AA, Frazer DG, Goldsmith W. Temporal characteristics of aerosol generation during a voluntary cough. A67 airway function and aerosols in children, adults and mice. *Am Thorac Soc.* (2010). A2183. doi: 10.1164/ajrccm-conference.2010.181.1_MeetingAbstracts.A2183
50. Balachandar S, Zaleski S, Soldati A, Ahmadi G, Bourouiba L. Host-to-host airborne transmission as a multiphase flow problem for science-based social distance guidelines. *Int J Multiphase Flow.* (2020) 132:103439. doi: 10.1016/j.ijmultiphaseflow.2020.103439
51. Harris C, Carson G, Baillie JK, Horby P, Nair H. An evidence-based framework for priority clinical research questions for covid-19. *J Glob Health.* (2020) 10:011001. doi: 10.7189/jogh.10.011001
52. Barasheed O, Alfelali M, Mushta S, Bokhary H, Alshehri J, Attar AA, et al. Uptake and effectiveness of facemask against respiratory infections at mass gatherings: a systematic review. *Int J Infect Dis.* (2016) 47:105–11. doi: 10.1016/j.ijid.2016.03.023
53. Leung NHL, Chu DKW, Shiu EYC, Chan KH, McDevitt JJ, Hau BJP, et al. Respiratory virus shedding in exhaled breath and efficacy of face masks. *Nat Med.* (2020) 26:676–80. doi: 10.1038/s41591-020-0843-2
54. Bartoszko JJ, Farooqi MAM, Alhazzani W, Loeb M. Medical masks vs n95 respirators for preventing covid-19 in healthcare workers: a systematic review and meta-analysis of randomized trials. *Influenza Other Respir Viruses.* (2020) 14:365–73. doi: 10.1111/irv.12745
55. Noti JD, Lindsley WG, Blachere FM, Cao G, Kashon ML, Thewlis RE, et al. Detection of infectious influenza virus in cough aerosols generated in a simulated patient examination room. *Clin Infect Dis.* (2012) 54:1569–77. doi: 10.1093/cid/cis237
56. Leggat PA, Kedjarune U. Bacterial aerosols in the dental clinic: a review. *Int Dent J.* (2001) 51:39–44. doi: 10.1002/j.1875-595X.2001.tb00816.x
57. Zemouri C, de Soet H, Crielaard W, Laheij A. A scoping review on bio-aerosols in healthcare and the dental environment. *PLoS ONE.* (2017) 12:e0178007. doi: 10.1371/journal.pone.0178007
58. *Ashrae Position Document on Infectious Aerosols.* Atlanta, GA: American Society for Heating, Ventilating and Air-Conditioning Engineers (2020).
59. Novoselac A, Siegel JA. Impact of placement of portable air cleaning devices in multizone residential environments. *Build Environ.* (2009) 44:2348–56. doi: 10.1016/j.buildenv.2009.03.023
60. Qian H, Zheng X. Ventilation control for airborne transmission of human exhaled bio-aerosols in buildings. *J Thorac Dis.* (2018) 10(Suppl 19):S2295–304. doi: 10.21037/jtd.2018.01.24
61. Yang J, Sekhar C, Wai DCK, Raphael B. Computational fluid dynamics study and evaluation of different personalized exhaust devices. *HVACandR Res.* (2013) 19:934–46. doi: 10.1080/10789669.2013.826066
62. Olmedo I, Nielsen PV, Ruiz de Adana M, Jensen RL, Grzelecki P. Distribution of exhaled contaminants and personal exposure in a room using three different air distribution strategies. *Indoor Air.* (2012) 22:64–76. doi: 10.1111/j.1600-0668.2011.00736.x
63. Kurnitski J, Boerstra A, Franchimon F, Mazzarella L, Hogeling J, Hovorka F. How to Operate and Use Building Services in Order to Prevent the Spread of the Coronavirus Disease (covid-19) Virus (sars-cov-2) in Workplaces. REHVA European Federation of Heating, Ventilation and Air Conditioning Association (2020). Available online at: https://www.rehva.eu/fileadmin/user_upload/REHVA_COVID-19_guidance_document_V4_23112020.pdf
64. *Dentistry Workers and Employers.* Washington, DC: Department of Labor - Occupational Safety and Health Administration (2020).
65. Bedell K, Buchaklian AH, Perlman S. Efficacy of an automated multiple emitter whole-room ultraviolet-c disinfection system against coronaviruses MHV and mers-cov. *Infect Control Hosp Epidemiol.* (2016) 37:598–9. doi: 10.1017/ice.2015.348
66. Walker CM, Ko G. Effect of ultraviolet germicidal irradiation on viral aerosols. *Environ Sci Technol.* (2007) 41:5460–5. doi: 10.1021/es070056u
67. Ellingson KD, Pogreba-Brown K, Gerba CP, Elliott SP. Impact of a novel antimicrobial surface coating on health care-associated infections and environmental bioburden at 2 urban hospitals. *Clin Infect Dis.* (2020) 71:1807–13. doi: 10.1093/cid/ciz1077

14

Human Microbiota in Esophageal Adenocarcinoma: Pathogenesis, Diagnosis, Prognosis and Therapeutic Implications

Wanyue Dan[1,2†], Lihua Peng[1†], Bin Yan[1], Zhengpeng Li[1] and Fei Pan[1]*

[1] *Department of Gastroenterology and Hepatology, The First Medical Center, Chinese PLA General Hospital, Beijing, China,*
[2] *Medical School of Nankai University, Tianjin, China*

Correspondence:
Fei Pan
panfei@plagh.org

†These authors have contributed equally to this work and share first authorship

Esophageal adenocarcinoma (EAC) is one of the main subtypes of esophageal cancer. The incidence rate of EAC increased progressively while the 5-year relative survival rates were poor in the past two decades. The mechanism of EAC has been studied extensively in relation to genetic factors, but less so with respect to human microbiota. Currently, researches about the relationship between EAC and the human microbiota is a newly emerging field of study. Herein, we present the current state of knowledge linking human microbiota to esophageal adenocarcinoma and its precursor lesion—gastroesophageal reflux disease and Barrett's esophagus. There are specific human bacterial alternations in the process of esophageal carcinogenesis. And bacterial dysbiosis plays an important role in the process of esophageal carcinogenesis *via* inflammation, microbial metabolism and genotoxicity. Based on the human microbiota alternation in the EAC cascade, it provides potential microbiome-based clinical application. This review is focused on novel targets in prevention, diagnosis, prognosis, and therapy for esophageal adenocarcinoma.

Keywords: microbiota, esophageal adenocarcinoma, Barrett's esophagus, gastroesophageal reflux disease, microbial therapy

INTRODUCTION

Esophageal cancer (EC) is the seventh most common cancer with an estimated 604, 000 new cases worldwide in 2020. It is also the sixth leading cause of cancer death with an estimated 544,000 deaths in 2020 (Sung et al., 2021). The age-standardized 5-year net survival of the EC patients was in the range of 10–30% between 2010 and 2014, except in Japan and Korea. In many countries, the age-standardized 5-year net survival trends increased by 6–10% from 2000 to 2014 (Allemani et al., 2018). Tackling the global burden of the EC is one of the major challenges in this century.

There are two main distinctive histological subtypes that account for more than 95% of EC, esophageal adenocarcinoma (EAC) and esophageal squamous cell carcinoma (ESCC). Generally, ESCC occurs in the upper two-thirds of the esophagus, whereas EAC typically occurs in the lower third of the esophagus (Arnold et al., 2020). In recent decades, the incidence rate of EAC in the United States has increased to 7.2 per 100,000 populations, while the incidence rate of ESCC has been sharply decreasing (Simard et al., 2012). From 1999 to 2008, the incidence rate of EAC showed an increasing trend in all races, except for American Indian or Alaska native, whose average annual percent change was −0.1. Although increased progressively during 1992 through 2007, 5-year relative survival rates for EAC were poor (Simard et al., 2012). Gastroesophageal reflux disease (GERD) and obesity have been identified as strong risk factors for EAC. Tobacco smoking and alcohol consumption might facilitate EAC development. In contrast, weight loss, estrogens, dietary fiber, and vegetable intake might protect against its development (Coleman et al., 2018). These risk factors provided clues for the primary prevention of EAC, thus public health interventions to modify them are advisable (Lagergren and Lagergren, 2013; Thrumurthy et al., 2019). Our knowledge of the human microbiota has expanded exponentially with the development of novel molecular methods, especially metagenome sequencing. Much of the current literature on cancer pays particular attention to the human microbiota (Plottel and Blaser, 2011). Accumulating evidence suggests that human microbiota contributes to colorectal cancer, gastric cancer, liver cancer, lung cancer and breast cancer (Schwabe and Jobin, 2013). Besides, the human microbiota is widely regarded as a potential co-factor for the development of EAC and its precursor Barrett's esophagus (BE) (Peters et al., 2017; Quante et al., 2018).

Herein, we present the current state of knowledge linking human microbiota to esophageal adenocarcinoma, with a primary focus on its potential clinical applications.

HUMAN MICROBIOTA

The human genetic makeup is virtually identical. Different from the human genome, the metagenome of the human microbiome shows greater variability (Lloyd-Price et al., 2016). The human microbiota is a highly individual, complex, and dynamic community in each healthy individual (Consortium, 2012; Gilbert et al., 2018). There are 10–100 trillion symbiotic microorganisms and 500–1000 species of bacteria in the human body, whereas the number of sub-species could be far more (Turnbaugh et al., 2007). Even in the same person, it will be extraordinarily different from before. Besides, there are diverse archaea, fungi, and viruses colonizing in the human body, although the current understanding of them remains limited. The digestive tract is the largest microbial habitat in the human body, which has the largest number of microbes and the most kind of species (Gupta et al., 2017). The gastrointestinal microbiota has three main ways of colonization: in the epithelial mucosa, in digest particles, and suspension solution (Dominguez-Bello et al., 2019). Investigators have been devoted to identifying the core microbiota, which is characterized by a group genera of being found in all populations regardless of their geographical location, ethnic background or residence. A population-level analysis reported a 14-genera core microbiota (*Lachnospiraceae*, *Ruminococcaceae*, *Bacteroides*, *Faecalibacterium*, *Blautia*, *Roseburia*, *Erysipelotrichaceae*, *Coprococcus*, *Dorea*, *Clostridiaceae*, *Hyphomicrobiaceae*, *Clostridiales*, *Veillonellaceae*, *Clostridium* XIVa) by assessing human fecal samples (Falony et al., 2016).

Given the well-established carcinogenesis that *Helicobacter pylori* had in gastric cancer and human papillomavirus had in cervical cancer, human microbiota was starting to be considered as a key factor that influences both human health and disease in the past decade (Bashan et al., 2016). Along with the deep-going of the research, in addition to special pathogens, the imbalance of normal microbiota can also cause diseases, such as allergy and psoriasis. Studies in colon cancer animal models have revealed evidence for tumor-promoting effects of the microbiota dysbiosis. There is a significant decrease in the number of tumors with the treatment of wide-spectrum antibiotics (Schwabe and Jobin, 2013). In addition, microbial diversity is associated with disease status. It is well established that type 2 diabetes and inflammatory bowel disease have low intestinal microbial diversity, as well as cervical intraepithelial neoplasia and bacterial vaginosis have high vaginal microbial diversity (Fredricks et al., 2005; Consortium, 2012; Qin et al., 2012; Mitra et al., 2015; Proctor, 2019). The mechanisms by which the human microbiota is involved in carcinogenesis primarily includes inflammation, immunity, metabolism, genomic integration, and genotoxicity (Scott et al., 2019). As an example, Gram-negative bacteria could acquire carcinogenic ability by producing genotoxin (He et al., 2019). Consequently, Microbiome Wide Association Studies, including DNA sequencing, metabolomics, proteomics, and computation, are providing potential microbiome-based screening tools, diagnostic markers, and adjuvant therapies (Kåhrström et al., 2016). It links microbial community structure and metabolites with disease status, which will lead clinical researches to a new field in the future.

HUMAN MICROBIOTA ALTERNATION IN THE ESOPHAGEAL ADENOCARCINOMA CASCADE

Esophageal Dysbiosis in the Esophageal Adenocarcinoma Cascade

Unlike the oral cavity, stomach, or intestine, the esophagus has its unique microbiota. A total of 41 genera belonging to six phyla of bacteria colonizing in the normal distal esophageal were identified (Pei et al., 2004). Six phyla consisted of *Firmicutes*, *Bacteroides*, *Actinobacteria*, *Proteobacteria*, *Fusobacteria*, and TM7. And top five genera were *Streptococcus*, *Prevotella*, *Veillonella*, *Rothia*, and *Megasphaera*. Furthermore, shotgun sequencing identified that there were not only abundant bacteria but also a relatively low abundance of viruses and eukaryotes in the esophagus, such as betaherpesvirus 7 and *Candida glabrata* (Deshpande et al., 2018). The esophageal microbiota is classified mainly into three main community types, and it has been proved significant differences across the three types. Among them, the predominant genus is *Streptococcus* in type 2 and it is *Prevotella* in type 3. Type 1 is an intermediate type between type 1 and type 2, which is composed of not only *Streptococcus* and *Prevotella*, but also increased abundances of *Haemophilus* and *Rothia* (Deshpande et al., 2018). Although there is no statistical difference in the total amount of microbial DNA among normal esophagus, reflux esophagitis (RE), and BE, the microbial communities are different among them. By detecting bacterial populations of the distal esophagus, the percentage of Bacteroidetes in the normal esophagus, RE, and BE increased successively, but the percentage of Proteobacteria was detected successively (Liu et al., 2013). The normal esophageal mucosa had higher levels of Gram-positive *Firmicutes* and *Actinobacteria* compared to RE, BE, and EAC (Zhou et al., 2020). The microbe composition of esophagus samples including low-grade dysplasia (LGD), high-grade dysplasia (HGD), EAC, and healthy controls, were analyzed by 16S DNA sequencing. The top five different microbial taxa in abundance at the phylum level were *Firmicutes, Proteobacteria, Bacteroidetes, Actinobacteria*, and *Fusobacteria*. Compared with controls, phylum *Planctomycetes* and genus *Balneola* were decreased across disease groups, especially in HGD and EAC. And phylum *Crenarchaeota* was similarly decreased (Peter et al., 2020). The influence of age, host genetics and disease status on the esophageal microbiome has been identified. In support of these findings, a prospective study showed age was positively associated with the relative abundance of *Streptococcus* and negatively associated with relative abundance of *Prevotella melaninogenica* by using amplicon sequencing from 106 subjects. Deshpande et al. (2018) (Elliott et al., 2017) demonstrated a connection between host genetics and the composition of the esophageal microbiome with the help of MicrobiomeGWAS. Although the disease did not affect the global taxonomic composition of the esophageal microbiome, increasing Gram-negative bacteria taxa were found in esophageal carcinogenesis, which was only appearing in the disease states (Deshpande et al., 2018).

In order to avoid the interference of microorganisms in other parts of the digestive tract, investigators put forward various methods. At earlier stages of research on esophageal microbial colonization, esophageal biopsy and aspiration specimen measurement were applied in analyzing esophageal microbial composition. By Yang's preliminary statistics of previous cultivation-independent studies on esophageal microbiota, the number of bacterial species detected by biopsy samples ranged from 7 to 166 (Yang et al., 2014). And they found enrichment of *Streptococcus* on esophageal microbiota. In another research, a total of 18 species were isolated from normal esophageal mucosa, while only three genera were detected in esophageal aspirate specimens, including *Lactobacilli, Streptococci*, and yeasts (Macfarlane et al., 2007). For patients with Barrett's esophagus, the highest relative proportions were *Anaerococcus, Streptococcus*, and *Alloicoccus* in the esophagus, while the highest relative proportions were *Fusobacterium, Prevotella*, and *Dialister* in the uvula (Okereke et al., 2019). Recently, the microbial communities of EAC samples were examined by means of Cytosponge. EAC tissues had decreased microbial diversity, including a reduction of Gram-positive taxa (*Granulicatella, Atopobium, Actinomyces*, and *Solobacterium*) as well as Gram-negative taxa (*Veillonella, Megasphaera*, and *Campylobacter*) compared with healthy controls (Elliott et al., 2017). These studies confirmed that decreased microbial diversity and altered microbial composition may play a significant role in the EAC cascade.

Oral Dysbiosis in the Esophageal Adenocarcinoma Cascade

The oral cavity is the initial part of the digestive tract. It consists of oral lips, cheek, palate, teeth, tongue, and salivary gland. Microorganisms inhabit the available surface of oral cavity, such as the surfaces of teeth, tongue and mucosal membranes (Lamont et al., 2018). Thus, polymicrobial communities which inhabit the oral cavity have unique biogeography. The Human Microbiome Project (HMP) collected the specimens of 15 to 18 body sites from over 200 individuals. Seven of body sites were taken from the mouth including buccal mucosa, keratinized attached gingiva, hard palate, saliva, tongue and two surfaces along with the tooth. Segata et al. (2012) analyzed sub-gingival plaques, supra-gingival plaques, stool and oral specimens from the HMP. They demonstrated that the microbial communities of the tongue are similar to saliva and the microbial communities of buccal mucosa are similar to keratinized attached gingiva and hard palate, while the microbial communities of sub-gingival and supra-gingival plaque were distinct from others. The site-specialist hypothesis for oral microbiota was proposed that there was a prime habitat for oral microbiota where most of oral microorganisms grew and divided (Mark Welch et al., 2019). Besides, microbial compositions in the oral cavity and esophagus are similar but essentially different (**Figure 1**). Dong et al. (2018) collected oral samples from saliva, tongue dorsum and supragingival plaque, as well as esophageal samples from upper, middle and lower of the esophagus. There were 594 genera subjected to 29 phyla in the esophagus and 365 genera subjected to 29 phyla in the oral cavity. Both of them detected high relative abundances of bacteria, including *Streptococcus, Neisseria, Prevotella, Actinobacillus*, and *Veillonella*. The predominant genus in the esophagus was *Streptococcus*, while the predominant genus in the oral cavity was *Neisseria*.

It is well-established that oral microbiota has a close association with many oral diseases, such as periodontitis, tooth reduction, dental caries. In addition to these diseases, oral microbiota alteration has been suggested to play an important role in diabetes, rheumatoid arthritis, chronic obstructive pulmonary diseases, cardiovascular diseases, and cancer (Gupta et al., 2017; Bourgeois et al., 2019b; Sun et al., 2020; Tuominen and Rautava, 2021). In particular, the relative abundance of *Porphyromonas gingivalis* in patients with digestive tract cancer (tongue/pharyngeal cancer, EC, gastric cancer, colorectal cancer) was higher than that in healthy controls (Kageyama et al., 2019). Other studies have reported the relationship between oral microbiota and EAC. On the one hand, a prospective study showed that a history of periodontal disease and tooth loss was associated with a 43% and 59% increased risk of EAC over 22–28 years of follow-up (Lo et al., 2021). On the other hand, the salivary bacterial diversity was significantly higher in EC patients than that in healthy controls (Kageyama et al., 2019). And a case–control study in China showed a significant shift in oral microbiota between the EC patients

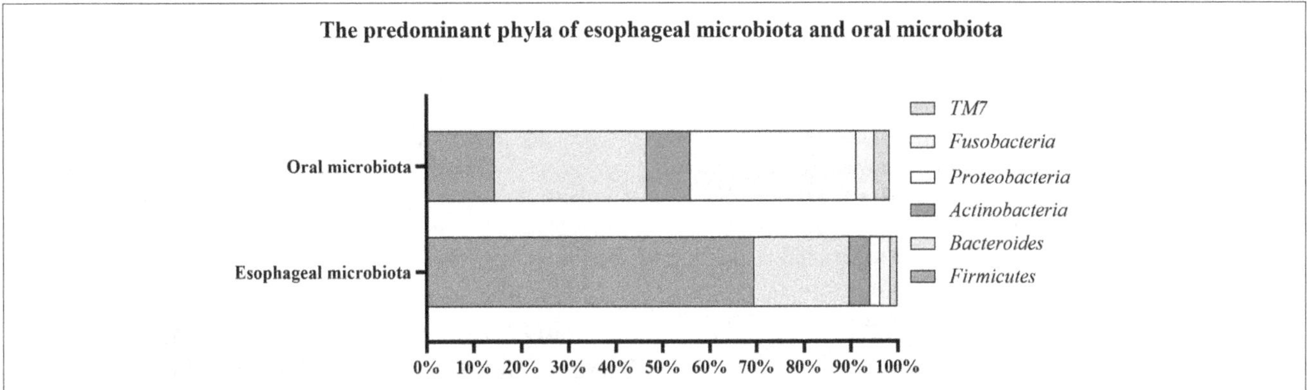

FIGURE 1 | The predominant phyla of esophageal microbiota and oral microbiota. The top six most abundant phyla of esophageal microbiota consisted of *Firmicutes* (69.60%), *Bacteroides* (20.20%), *Actinobacteria* (4.30%), *Proteobacteria* (2.20%), *Fusobacteria* (2.20%), *TM7* (1.40%); And the top six most abundant phyla of oral microbiota consisted of *Proteobacteria* (35.34%), *Bacteroides* (32.20%), *Firmicutes* (14.48%), *Actinobacteria* (9.26%), *Fusobacteria* (3.76%), *TM7* (3.25%).

and the healthy participants. By detecting salivary microbial communities, EC patients had a higher relative abundance of phylum *Firmicutes*, class *Negativicutes*, order *Selenomonadales*, family *Veillonellaceae*, and genus *Prevotella*, and a lower relative abundance of phylum *Proteobacteria*, class *Betaproteobacteria*, order *Neisseriales*, family *Neisseriaceae*, and genus *Neisseria* in contrast with healthy individuals (Zhao et al., 2020). Moreover, another research showed that BE patients had a higher relative abundance of *Firmicutes* and a lower relative abundance of Proteobacteria in saliva compared to patients without BE (Snider et al., 2018), which was in accordance with the EC patients. All of these researches support a link between oral microbiota and EAC development.

HUMAN MICROBIOTA IN ESOPHAGEAL ADENOCARCINOMA

Determination of the variation in human microbiota between health and disease is crucial to understanding the biases that occur in disease. There were many studies of the esophageal microbiota alteration in EAC. One prior case-control study found altered microbial communities in esophageal carcinogenesis, notably increases in *Proteobacteria* and reductions in *Firmicutes*. Besides, two families, *Verrucomicrobiaceae* and *Enterobacteriaceae*, became increasingly in HGD and EAC (Snider et al., 2019). Similarly, Zaidi and colleagues found a high prevalence of *Escherichia coli* in EAC and BE patients, while it was lacking in the tumor adjacent normal epithelium. All these indicated that the shift toward *Enterobacteriaceae* in esophageal carcinogenesis was not accidental. According to the research of the esophageal microbiome, there is a reduction of *Streptococcus* and an increase of *Prevotella* in EAC compared with healthy controls (Lopetuso et al., 2020). Zhou and colleagues discovered a unique esophageal microbiota in EAC subjects. Compared with normal esophageal, there were abundant *Proteobacteria* and *Firmicutes*, mostly like *Staphylococcus aureus*, *Streptococcus infantis*, *Moryella* sp. and *Lactobacillus salivarius*, and rare *Actinobacteria* (*Rothia mucilaginosa*) in the EAC esophageal microbiota (Zhou et al., 2020). Most of them were lactic acid-producing bacteria. As is well established, sustained high lactate level could promote angiogenesis, immune escape, cell migration and metastasis, thus supporting the tumorigenesis and progression (San-Millán and Brooks, 2017). The authors proposed that increased lactic acid-producing bacteria in the esophageal may work as one of the factors contributing to the development of the EAC. Additionally, there is a high prevalence of *Candida albicans* and *Candida glabrata* in more than half of the human EAC samples (Zaidi et al., 2016), which suggests the existence of fungal microbiota in the esophagus.

Esophageal adenocarcinoma has been studied extensively in relation to the esophageal microbiota, but relatively insufficiency so with respect to microbiota at other sites of the human body. A prospective study examined the relationship between EAC and oral microbiota. In mouthwash samples, there was a high amount of *Tannerella forsythia*, *Actinomyces cardiffensis*, *Veillonella* oral taxon 917, and *Selenomonas* oral taxon 134 was associated with higher EAC risk, whereas a low amount of *Prevotella nanceiensis*, *Corynebacterium durum*, *Streptococcus pneumoniae*, *Lachnoanaerobaculum umeaense*, *Solobacterium moorei*, *Oribacterium parvum*, *Neisseria flavescens*, *Neisseria sicca*, and *Haemophilus* oral taxon 908 was associated with lower EAC risk (Peters et al., 2017). If these results turn out to characterize the shift with the progression of EAC, rather than simply correlative, they demonstrate potential prevention *via* protecting against microbial exposure.

HUMAN MICROBIOTA IN GASTROESOPHAGEAL REFLUX DISEASE AND BARRETT'S ESOPHAGUS

Gastroesophageal reflux disease was regarded as a risk factor for EAC and BE was established as the precursor lesion of EAC. It is of momentous significance to clarify the human microbiota of GERD and BE for the EAC researches. An early study by Yang in 2009 found the potential link between alterations in the human distal esophageal microbiome and reflux-related disorders. The bacterial communities of 34 patients were checked after biopsies of the distal esophagus by 16S rRNA gene sequencing. The authors classified the human esophageal microbiome into two types according to the results of gene analysis. The type I esophageal microbiome was more relevant to the normal esophagus, while the type II esophageal microbiome was more relevant to the abnormal esophagus. The type I microbiome had a higher mean abundance of *Streptococcus*, while the type II microbiome had a higher level of microbial diversity and a higher average proportion of Gram-negative bacteria. They also concluded that the type II microbiome was mainly composed of Gram-negative anaerobes or microaerophiles, including *Veillonella, Prevotella, Neisseria, Haemophilus, Rothia, Granulicatella, Campylobacter, Fusobacterium, Porphyromonas,* and *Actinomyces.* The predominant organisms shifted from Gram-positive aerobic bacteria to Gram-negative anaerobic bacteria (Yang et al., 2009).

Similarly, increasing evidence has supported a shift toward some specific Gram-negative bacteria in the EAC cascade. It was reported that Gram-negative organisms colonizing the esophageal mucosa, especially *Campylobacters*, became increasingly in GERD and BE compared with healthy control groups (Blackett et al., 2013). Other studies found that there was a shift away from *Firmicutes* and toward Gram-negative *Fusobacteria, Sphingomonas, Proteobacteria* and an unclassified species of *Campylobacter* in BE compared to controls (Snider et al., 2019; Zhou et al., 2020). Of note, Lopetuso and colleagues found that the relative abundance of *Streptococcus* and *Granulicatella* decreased in the EAC mucosa compared with BE mucosa, with the relative abundance of *Prevotella* increased correspondingly. The authors considered EAC as an extreme dysbiotic perturbation of microbiota in BE mucosa which consisted largely of Gram-negative bacteria (Lopetuso et al., 2020). In summary, alteration of the human microbiota in EAC cascade was presented as decreased microbial diversity and enrichment of Gram-negative bacteria in esophagus as well as increased microbial diversity and enrichment of *Firmicutes, Tannerella forsythia, Actinomyces cardiffensis* in oral cavity (**Figure 2**).

HUMAN MICROBIOME AS POTENTIAL DIAGNOSTIC BIOMARKERS AND SCREENING TOOLS FOR ESOPHAGEAL ADENOCARCINOMA

Current screening tools have respective advantages and disadvantages. The gold-standard technique of EC and preinvasive lesions is endoscopy with adequate targeted biopsies. However, this method cannot be used extensively due to the time and expense. Esophageal tissue samples including sponges and inflatable balloons have good specificity but lack sensitivity (Lao-Sirieix and Fitzgerald, 2012). It has been confirmed some specific pathogens could promote the development of EC, while other pathogens could be a protective factor against the reduced risk of EC. As a result, some biomarkers have enormous potential as diagnostic biomarkers and screening tools for EAC (**Table 1**). Finding out a biomarker with excellent sensitivity and specificity is the key to extending the biomarker detection application field.

With the increase in antibiotic treatment in the mid-twentieth century, infections of *Helicobacter pylori* began to decline, then the incidence of esophageal adenocarcinoma and eosinophilic

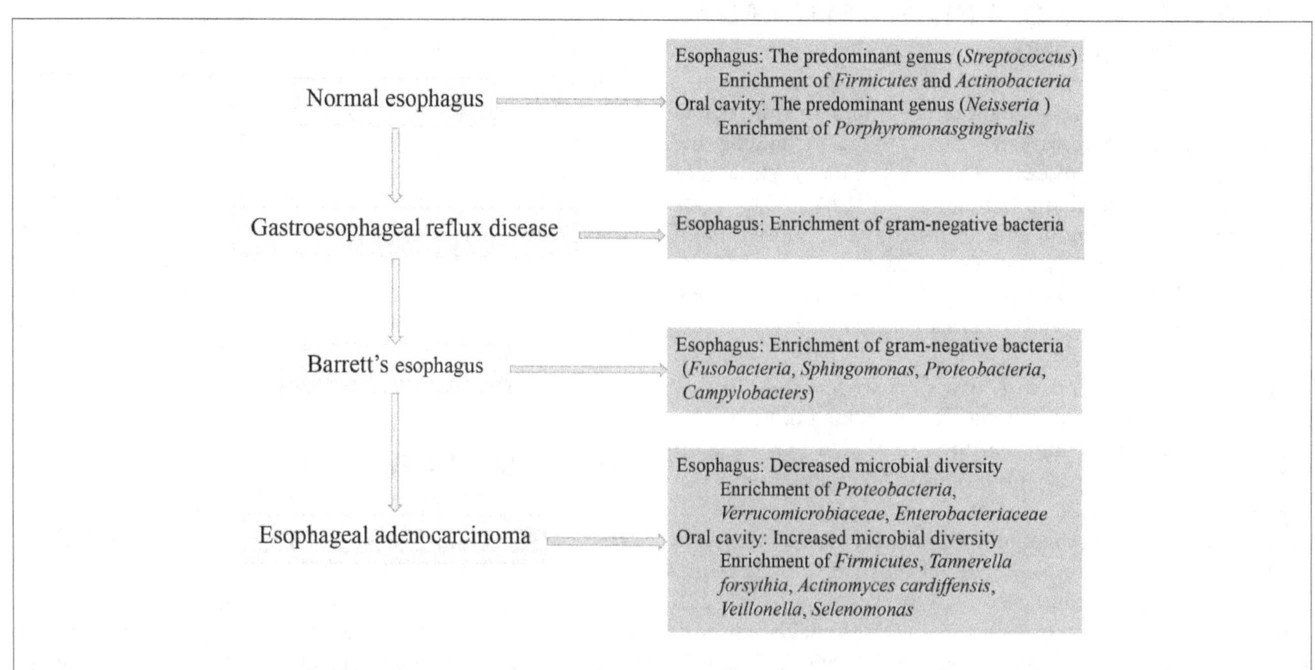

FIGURE 2 | The process of esophageal carcinogenesis and associated human microbiota. This figure describes specific human bacterial alternations in the normal esophagus, esophageal adenocarcinoma and its precursor lesion—gastroesophageal reflux disease and Barrett's esophagus.

TABLE 1 | Human microbiota studies for esophageal adenocarcinoma.

Study	Population(s)	Study sample size	Study period	Study platform	Sample type	Main findings	Tool type
Lopetuso et al., 2020	Rome	BE (*n* = 10); EAC (*n* = 6); controls (*n* = 16)	2020	16S rRNA	Esophageal mucosa	*Prevotella*, *Veillonella*, and *Leptotrichia* had higher abundance in EAC than that of CTRL, while *Streptococcus* had lower abundance.	Diagnosis
Zhou et al., 2020	Australia	RE (*n* = 20); BE (*n* = 17); EAC (*n* = 6); controls (*n* = 16)	2020	16S rRNA	Esophageal mucosa	Compared with CTRL, there was a reduction of *Actinobacteria* in EAC, with an increase of *Firmicutes* and *Proteobacteria*.	Diagnosis
Peters et al., 2017	America	EAC (*n* = 81); controls (*n* = 160)	2017	16S rRNA	Mouthwash samples	The abundances of species *Tannerella forsythia* were positive correlated with risk of EAC, while the abundances of the genus *Neisseria* and the species *Streptococcus pneumoniae* were inversely correlated with risk of EAC	Diagnosis
Snider et al., 2019	United States	LGD (*n* = 6); HGD (*n* = 5); BE (*n* = 14); EAC (*n* = 4); controls (*n* = 16)	2019	16S rRNA	Saliva samples	There was a shift toward *Enterobacteriaceae* and *Akkermansia muciniphila*, while away from *Firmicutes* in patients with HGD and EAC relative to controls	Diagnosis
Zhao et al., 2020	China	EC (*n* = 39); controls (*n* = 51)	2020	16S rDNA	Saliva samples	*Prevotella* was enriched in EC, while *Neisseria* was decreased.	Diagnosis
Peter et al., 2020	United Kingdom	IM (*n* = 10); LGD (*n* = 10); HGD (*n* = 10); EAC (*n* = 12); controls (*n* = 10)	2020	16S rDNA	Esophageal mucosa	The abundance of the phylum *Planctomycetes* and the archaean phylum *Crenarchaeota* in EAC was significantly lower than that in CTRL	Diagnosis
Deshpande et al., 2018	Australia	EoE (*n* = 1); GERD (*n* = 29); GM (*n* = 7); BE (*n* = 5); EAC (*n* = 1); CTRL (*n* = 59)	2018	16S rRNA; 18S rRNA; shotgun sequencing	Esophageal mucosa; esophageal brushings	An enrichment of Gram-negative bacteria associated with the oral cavity and microbial lactic acid production in the EAC cascade	Diagnosis
Elliott et al., 2017	United Kingdom	ND (*n* = 20); BE (*n* = 23); EAC (*n* = 19); CTRL (*n* = 20)	2017	16S rRNA	Esophageal mucosa; esophageal brushes; Cytosponge samples	*Lactobacillus fermentum* was enriched in EAC compared with controls	Diagnosis
Kawasaki et al., 2020	Japan	EC (*n* = 61); CTRL (*n* = 62)	2020	PCR	Subgingival dental plaque; saliva samples	The prevalence of *Tannerella forsythia*, *Streptococcus anginosus*, and *Aggregatibacter actinomycetemcomitans* was positively related to the presence of EC with high odds ratios, respectively	Diagnosis
Rajendra et al., 2013	Australia	BE (*n* = 77); BD (*n* = 35); EAC (*n* = 27); CTRL (*n* = 122)	2013	PCR; immunohistochemistry;	Esophageal mucosa; tumor specimens	High activity of *human papillomavirus* was strongly association with worse disease severity	Prognosis
Yamamura et al., 2016	Japan	EC (*n* = 325)	2016	PCR	Tumor specimens; tumor adjacent normal specimens	*Fusobacterium nucleatum* in EC was related to higher tumor stage and poor prognosis in the patients after the esophagus carcinoma resection	Prognosis

BEM, esophageal metaplastic samples; BE, Barrett's esophagus; IM, intestinal metaplasia; LGD, low-grade dysplasia; HGD, high-grade dysplasia; BD, Barrett's dysplasia; EC, esophageal cancer; EAC, esophageal adenocarcinoma; CTRL, healthy control samples; PCR, polymerase chain reaction.

esophagitis rises (May and Abrams, 2018). The large-scale pooled analysis found that *Helicobacter pylori* infection varied directly as the odds of BE and inversely proportional to the odds of GERD (Wang et al., 2018). However, Aghayeva and colleagues retrospectively analyzed cases in Azerbaijan, a high-prevalence region, and highlighted that there is no difference between the prevalence of *Helicobacter pylori* in BE and control group cases. The authors concluded that neither BE nor dysplasia is inversely associated with the prevalence of *Helicobacter pylori* (Aghayeva et al., 2019). Similarly, the hypothesis of the Swedish nationwide population-based cohort study was confirmed by calculating the standardized incidence ratios (SIRs), which were equal to the observed number of individuals in the *Helicobacter pylori* eradication cohort over the expected number of individuals in the Swedish background population. This study found that there is no evidence a gradually increased risk of BE or EAC is linked with *Helicobacter pylori* eradication treatment in spite of the increasing SIRs of BE and EAC after *Helicobacter pylori* eradication treatment (Doorakkers et al., 2020). Whether *Helicobacter pylori* infection influences EAC and its precursor is still a debatable point. However, it has been noted that *Helicobacter pylori* infection promotes Ki-67 expression in BE.

According to a meta-analysis with 1243 samples, Ki-67 showed a reasonable diagnostic odds ratio of 5.54, sensitivity of 82% and specificity of 48% in identifying high-risk patients of EAC in BE group (Altaf et al., 2017). In addition to *Helicobacter pylori*, other human microbiota-associated biomarkers may be reasonably efficient in EAC screening and diagnosis. As a result of significantly increased abundance of *Prevotella* at the genus level and family level that covered all samples, Zhao and colleagues indicated that *Prevotella* was may be used in the early prediction or prevention of EC (Zhao et al., 2020). Overall, *Prevotella* and Ki-67 may play an important role in the personalized precision diagnosis of EAC.

Several studies have also implicated periodontal pathogens as potential diagnostic biomarkers for EAC. As mentioned above, Peters and colleagues indicated that *Tannerella forsythia* was strongly related to EAC. They observed that the increased abundance of *Tannerella forsythia* was correlated to the higher risk of EAC, while the decreased abundance of Neisseria and *Streptococcus pneumoniae* was correlated to the lower risk of EAC (Peters et al., 2017). Similarly, the prevalence of *Tannerella forsythia* and *Aggregatibacter actinomycetemcomitans* with EC patients was significantly higher in the subgingival plaque compared with healthy controls (Kawasaki et al., 2020). It is now well accepted that both *Tannerella forsythia* and *Aggregatibacter actinomycetemcomitans* are Gram-negative periodontal pathogens that might contribute to the pathogenesis of periodontitis (Sharma, 2010; Gholizadeh et al., 2017). A previous study suggested a possible correlation between *Aggregatibacter actinomycetemcomitans* and the increasing risk of pancreatic cancer (Fan et al., 2018). An oral microbiome-based model containing a relative abundance of *Streptococcus*, *Lautropia*, and *Bacteroidales* discriminated between BE patients and controls with the ROC of 0.94, the sensitivity of 96.9%, and the specificity of 88.2% (Snider et al., 2018). Our findings suggest that periodontal pathogens, like *Tannerella forsythia* and *Aggregatibacter actinomycetemcomitans*, may be utilized as biomarkers for detecting EAC-associated changes in the human microbiota.

HUMAN MICROBIOTA FOR CLINICAL PROGNOSIS ANALYSIS OF ESOPHAGEAL ADENOCARCINOMA PATIENTS

The late presentation of symptoms and the aggressiveness of EAC results in poor prognosis (Coleman et al., 2018). Interestingly, *human papillomavirus* (HPV)-related biomarkers in pre-cancer lesions can become an important prognostic indicator of EAC. A previous study has demonstrated that head and neck squamous cell carcinoma (HNSCC) patients with HPV-positive have a higher rate of overall survival and a lower risk of recurrence compared with HPV-negative patients (Ragin and Taioli, 2007; O'Rorke et al., 2012). Given the well-established impact that HPV status has on the prognosis of HNSCC, it is highly plausible that HPV-related EAC would show a similar prognosis. A prospective study has identified that high-risk HPV with transcription activity is associated with BD and EAC. Biopsy samples were used for HPV DNA determination *via* PCR and viral transcriptional activity determination *via* E6/7 oncogene mRNA expression and $p16^{INK4a}$ immunohistochemistry. Compared with BE and controls, the proportion of HPV DNA-positive, $p16^{INK4a}$ positivity and oncogene expression in Barrett's dysplasia (BD) and EAC was significantly higher (Rajendra et al., 2013). The authors emphasized that HPV was strongly relevant to BD and EAC but irrelevant to BE and controls, which suggested the role of HPV in the pathogenesis of tumors. Based on preliminary studies, a retrospective case–control study assessed HPV-related biomarkers [retinoblastoma protein (pRb), cyclin D1 (CD1), Ki-67, and minichromosome maintenance protein (MCM2)] to estimate the prognostic value on the patients with BD and EAC. The authors found low expression of CD1 with a good prognosis in EAC (Rajendra et al., 2020). In contrast to HPV-negative patients, HPV-positive patients with low expression of CD1, high expression of MCM2, low expression of pRb, high expression of p16 and positive status of E6 and E7 mRNA had improved disease-free survival, suggesting HPV-positive EAC and HPV-negative EAC are two distinct diseases, exactly as in HNSCC (Rajendra et al., 2018).

Recently many studies about the relationship between *Fusobacterium nucleatum* and gastroenteric cancer have been reported. Yamamura and colleagues found the new application of *Fusobacterium nucleatum* DNA status in prognosis prediction in EC. The relative amounts of *Fusobacterium nucleatum* DNA were significantly higher in tumor tissue compared with adjacent normal tissue. The cancer-specific survival and OS were significantly shorter in *F. nucleatum*-positive individuals than that in *Fusobacterium nucleatum*-negative individuals. Similarly, the cancer-specific mortality was significantly higher in *Fusobacterium nucleatum*-positive individuals than that in *Fusobacterium nucleatum*-negative individuals. Thus, we consider this periodontal bacteria can be used for the clinical prognosis of the EC as an indicator (Yamamura et al., 2016).

A Japanese study has revealed that the presence of oropharyngeal allopatric flora was an independent predictive factor of post-esophagectomy pneumonia. The authors divided 675 patients into three groups by categorization of oropharyngeal flora, including indigenous flora (Ind group), antibiotic-sensitive microbes only (Allo-S group) and antibiotic-resistant microbes (Allo-R group). Compared with the Ind group, the incidence of postoperative pneumonia in the Allo-S and Allo-R groups increased markedly and the survival in the Allo-R group significantly decreased (Yuda et al., 2020). Hence, it is anticipated that we can prevent post-esophagectomy pneumonia from the classification of the oral microbiome someday.

POTENTIAL MECHANISMS OF MICROBE-MEDIATED ESOPHAGEAL CARCINOGENESIS

The molecular mechanisms by which the human microbiota could initiate and drive tumorigenesis have always been the focus.

Genomic integration, genotoxicity, inflammation, immunity and metabolism are major mechanisms (Lv et al., 2019; Scott et al., 2019). Given the well-established impact that the composition of human microbiota and its activity mediated inflammation and genotoxicity in tumorigenesis of many cancers, such as colon cancer, liver cancer and pancreatic cancer (Cani and Jordan, 2018), many investigators were making their attempts to elucidate the mechanism of human microbiota during carcinogenesis of EC, including metabolites, genotoxicity, inflammation and immune dysregulation. Here, we review the main microbiota-associated mechanisms which have been under extensive research in esophageal carcinogenesis (**Figure 3**). However, despite considerable evidence to suggest significant changes in human microbiota following EC, it remains to be determined whether these changes have a causal effect or are only correlative in nature.

The Human Microbiota, Inflammation and Esophageal Carcinogenesis

Specific Pathogens

Sustained infection or non-infectious factors may lead to various pro-inflammatory and oncogenic mediators in the process of chronic inflammation, eventually resulting in tumor promotion (Khandia and Munjal, 2020). Data from several studies suggested that *Campylobacters* may play an important role in the process of inflammation and esophageal carcinogenesis. With the dominant change of the appearance of *Campylobacters* during the disease states, Blackett and colleagues found IL-18 expression significantly increases in both GERD and BE colonized subjects compared with non-colonized subjects (Blackett et al., 2013). IL-18 is a multifunctional cytokine that induces pro-inflammatory cytokine expression and is associated with anti-tumor immunity. Many studies implicate that the serum IL-18 levels of EC patients were significantly higher than the control group, deficiency of IL-18 can aggravate the progression and development of EC and IL-18 signaling is strongly associated with BE and EAC (Diakowska et al., 2006; Babar et al., 2012; Li et al., 2018). The *Campylobacters* consist almost entirely of *Campylobacter concisus*, which virtually only appearing in the disease states. The cell culture model of Barrett's cell lines reported a marked increase and a time-dependent manner in the expression of pro-inflammatory mediators (IL-18 and TNF-α) and tumor suppressor gene (p53) in co-culture with *Campylobacter concisus* (Mozaffari Namin et al., 2015b). By means of a comprehensive analysis of *Campylobacter* species, a new viewpoint that *Campylobacter* species modulated the host inflammatory response, and then, it initiated the EAC cascade was presented theoretically

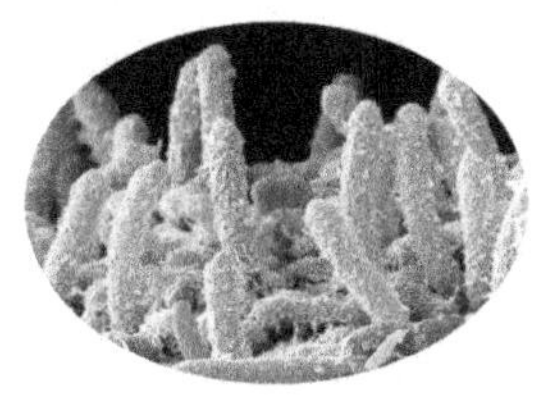

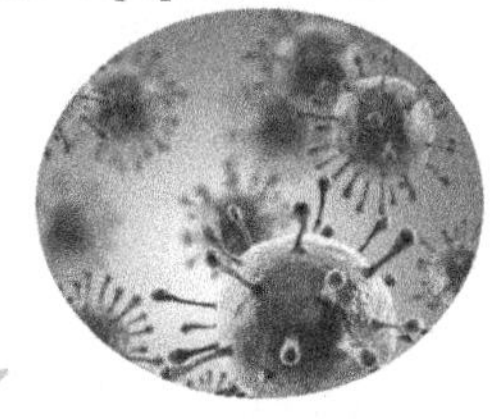

FIGURE 3 | The molecular mechanisms of microbe-mediated in EAC carcinogenesis. On the basis of the known contribution of human microbiota in esophageal carcinogenesis, the main mechanisms included inflammation, metabolism, and genotoxicity. Alteration of human microbiota in EAC showed a shift toward Gram-negative bacteria. Some specific pathogens, such as *Campylobacter concisus*, *Helicobacter pylori*, and *Escherichia coli*, involved in the process of inflammation and EAC cascade by regulating the expressions of toll-like receptors (TLRs) and pro-inflammatory mediators such as TNF-α, IL-18, COX-2, prostaglandins. And the components of Gram-negative bacteria activated the NLRP3 inflammasome and NF-κB pathway. Besides, detrimental metabolites, such as hydrogen sulfide, products of protein fermentation and bile acid metabolism, could play an important role in the initiation and progression of EAC. Some Gram-negative bacteria produced the cytolethal distending toxin (CDT), which could induce DNA damage and trigger EAC carcinogenesis. LPS, lipopolysaccharides; NF-κB, nuclear factor kappa B; TLRs, toll-like receptors; CDT, cytolethal distending toxin; TNF-α, tumor necrosis factor-α; IL, interleukin; COX, cyclooxygenase; PG, prostaglandin; p53, tumor protein 53; NLRP3, nucleotide-binding domain and leucine-rich repeat-containing protein 3.

(Kaakoush et al., 2015). Previous research has indicated that the colonization of *Helicobacter pylori* in the esophagus increased the incidence of BE and EAC (Liu et al., 2011). Subsequently, some researchers have implicated the possible role of *Helicobacter pylori* in the malignant progression of the esophagus by promoting the expression of gastrin, COX-2, prostaglandins and Ki-67 (Kountouras et al., 2019; Doorakkers et al., 2020). Similarly, investigators also explained the association between *Enterobacteriaceae* infection and esophageal carcinogenesis has been proposed. The expression of toll-like receptors (TLRs) 1–3, 6, 7, and 9 significantly increases in EAC rats (Zaidi et al., 2016), demonstrating an *Escherichia coli*-related esophageal carcinogenesis. As mentioned previously, *Campylobacters, Helicobacter pylori* and *Escherichia coli* seemed to be specifically involved in EAC cascade through pro-inflammatory cytokine expression. Nevertheless, it is not yet clear whether there is a causality between specific pathogens and EAC.

Microbial Metabolites

In addition to specific pathogens, human microbiota could trigger carcinogenesis as an integrated community. A quintessential example should be cited that microbiota dysbiosis and host–microbiota interactions seemed to promote colorectal tumorigenesis (Schwabe and Jobin, 2013). The metabolites play an important role in the initiation and progression of cancer. Protective metabolites are represented by short-chain fatty acids. And detrimental metabolites are represented by hydrogen sulfide, products of protein fermentation and bile acid metabolism (Louis et al., 2014). Evidence suggests that human microbiota contributes to esophageal tumorigenesis, not only *via* the inflammation of specific pathogens but also *via* the influence of its metabolome (Louis et al., 2014). Some bacteria produced certain compounds which might be a carcinogen. Bile acid metabolism is one of the most important microbial metabolism. Researchers found that chronic exposure to bile acids might result in esophageal carcinogenesis through over-expression of glucose-6-phosphate dehydrogenase and active nuclear factor-kB (NF-κB) (Munemoto et al., 2019). The toll-like receptor-4 ligand, named LPS, is produced by Gram-negative bacteria. LPS can activate the NOD-like receptor protein 3 inflammasome and NF-κB pathway. The esophageal microbiome, dominated by Gram-negative bacteria, might contribute to materializing the inflammation-mediated carcinogenesis in BE by LPS *via* relaxing the lower esophageal sphincter and delaying gastric emptying (Yang et al., 2012; Nadatani et al., 2016; Lv et al., 2019). This provides new evidence about the molecular mechanisms underlying the association between LPS and esophageal carcinogenesis.

The Human Microbiota, Genotoxicity and Esophageal Carcinogenesis

Genotoxicity refers to structural DNA damage (Scott et al., 2019). A multitude of Gram-negative bacteria mainly including *Escherichia coli*, *Actinobacillus actinomycetemcomitans*, Campylobacters and *Helicobacter pylori* could produced the cytolethal distending toxin (CDT), which could induce DNA damage and promote cancer (Nesiæ et al., 2004; He et al., 2019). Certain species within *Enterobacteriaceae* produced a DNA-alkylating genotoxin so that led to DNA damage, which might accelerate tumor progression (Wilson et al., 2019). *Helicobacter pylori* is prescribed for class I carcinogen. *Helicobacter pylori* toxin cytotoxin-associated gene A induced oxidative DNA damage and modulated the host inflammatory response in gastric carcinogenesis (Wroblewski et al., 2010). It continues to be controversial whether *Helicobacter pylori* influences the canceration course of esophageal. The study of esophageal epithelial cell transfection has demonstrated that *Helicobacter pylori* infection led to the up-regulated expression of microRNA-212-3p targeted COX2 and miR-361-3p targeted CDX2 through the translation inhibition of miRNAs, which contributed to the phenotypic transformation of esophageal epithelial cells (Teng et al., 2018).

THE HUMAN MICROBIOTA-BASED THERAPIES IN ESOPHAGEAL CANCER

The therapeutic principle of esophageal cancer is based on individualized comprehensive treatment. In fact, surgery combined with radiotherapy and chemotherapy has become the mainstay of clinical treatment for EC (Stahl et al., 2010). It is now well established that several healthy behaviors are helpful for cancer prevention, including a healthy diet, physical activity, weight control and alcohol consumption limit (Rock et al., 2020). In addition, some interventions related to the altered human microbial composition may become the new adjuvant treatment in EC, such as proton pump inhibitors, probiotics, mucosal protective agents, and chlorhexidine mouth rinse.

Oral Hygiene

A large body of published research has consistently demonstrated poor oral hygiene was associated with a higher risk of cancers, such as oral cancer (Deng et al., 2021), gastric cancer (Zhang et al., 2021), colorectal cancer (Wang et al., 2021). Based on the outcomes of two case–control studies, poor oral hygiene was an important risk factor for EC (Mmbaga et al., 2020; Poosari et al., 2021). And patients who received dental prophylaxis had a reduced risk of EC (Lee et al., 2014). The data highlighted the importance of adequate oral hygiene practices, which could be a simple means to prevent various cancers (Yano et al., 2021). The interdental brush is a form of toothbrush which could be inserted between the teeth in order to remove plaque (Worthington et al., 2019). Denis and colleagues demonstrated that toothbrushing and interdental brushing can decrease the number of oral bacteria in particular those who were associated with periodontal disease (Bourgeois et al., 2019a). The individuals may benefit from the daily use of toothbrushing and interdental brushing. Previous research has argued that interdental brush reduces interdental bleeding compared with manual toothbrush (Bourgeois et al., 2016). As for the frequencies of toothbrushing, it is suggested that toothbrushing twice daily for 2 min in order to prevent periodontal disease (Sälzer et al., 2020). Additionally, a randomized controlled trial analyzed the oral and esophageal microbiota and gene expression of the esophagus before and after treatment of chlorhexidine mouth rinse. The authors identified significant alterations in the oral and esophageal microbiota and demonstrated that the alterations of the esophageal microbiota could be closely related to changes in gene expression of the esophagus, suggest the clinical application of mouth rinse treatment in EC (Annavajhala et al., 2020).

Diet

Diet and nutrition are the major areas of interest within the prevention of chronic diseases and cancer. A healthy diet should include nutritious food, whole grains, fiber-rich legumes, a variety of vegetables and fruits (Rock et al., 2020). Several dietary patterns are representative, including Mediterranean, Dietary Approaches to Stop Hypertension, Okinawa and vegetarian diets. Many bioactive nutrients of these diets have played an effective role in the epigenetic modification and maintaining the balance of intestinal microbiota (Divella et al., 2020). Mediterranean diet (MD) is internationally regarded as a "long life" diet (Mentella et al., 2019; Martinon et al., 2021). The composition of Okinawa and Dietary Approaches to Stop Hypertension diets is similar to MD. Recent studies have shown that MD is associated with a decreased cancer mortality risk (Molina-Montes et al., 2020). Analyses indicated the decreased risk of gastro-intestinal cancer was associated with a vegetarian diet (Tantamango-Bartley et al., 2013). A low-fiber, high-fat, and high-refined-sugar diet might be responsible for the declining diversities (Lloyd-Price et al., 2016). Nevertheless, diet therapy is expected to be universally accepted low-risk and patient-friendly intervention to prevent chronic diseases and even cancer among the population, just as vaccines prevent flu. New therapeutic strategies of the EC could be proposed by targeted dietary intervention. Enteric pathogenic bacteria boosted their growth and pathogenicity by exploiting some short-chain fatty acids, microbiota-derived sources of carbon, and other nutrients (Bäumler and Sperandio, 2016). Host diet has a profound effect on the composition of the gut microbiota and its metabolites. Nobel and colleagues found a negative correlation between fiber intake and the relative abundance of Gram-negative bacteria, most notably *Betaproteobacteria* (Nobel et al., 2018). This study provided new evidence about the potential mechanisms underlying the association between dietary fiber and esophageal microbiome composition. Current consensus suggests that the risk of EAC could decrease after a reduction in total dietary fat, saturated fat, and cholesterol (Thrumurthy et al., 2019). Data from a study suggested that participants with reduced microbial gene richness presented more higher aberrant metabolism and low-grade inflammation, and weight-loss dietary intervention may succeed in improving these changes (Cotillard et al., 2013). Similarly, Münch and colleagues indicated that a high-fat diet led to the alterations of gut microbiota which accelerated inflammation and esophageal carcinogenesis in the mouse model which was irrelevant to obesity (Münch et al., 2019). In the future, a high fiber and low-fat diet may be helpful to prevent EC.

Physical Activity

Several studies have documented that exercise contributes to the human gut microbiota alternation (Shukla et al., 2015; Allen et al., 2018). Long-term regular exercise lead to higher diversity and significant shifts of major bacterial taxa in human gut microbiota, especially a higher relative abundance of the genus *Akkermansia* (Clarke et al., 2014). In addition, the role of physical activity in cancer prevention has received increased attention across a number of disciplines in recent years. There are consistent evidence that physical activity plays an important role in preventing cancer. An American roundtable report found that physical activity can reduce the risk of seven types of cancer including EAC (Patel et al., 2019). Aerobic exercise and muscle strength training before esophagectomy is useful for reducing the rates of postoperative respiratory complications in EC patients (Akiyama et al., 2021). Based on the preventive effect of exercise on EC, a study set it out to investigate the usefulness of evaluating the prognosis. The 6-min walking distance is a clinical examination gradually used to evaluate the prognosis of patients after surgery. It has the advantages of low cost and easy implementation. A retrospective cohort study has established that the 6-min walking distance is directly proportional to the overall survival in patients undergoing esophagectomy (Kondo et al., 2021).

Proton Pump Inhibitors and Mucosal Protective Agents

Proton pump inhibitors (PPIs) are used extensively for the full spectrum of gastric-acid-related diseases in clinic (Malfertheiner et al., 2017). It inhibits the activity of gastric H^+/K^+-adenosine triphosphatase, resulting in the inhibition of acid secretion from parietal cells (Rochman et al., 2021). Previous researches have established that long-term PPI use induces changes in the gut microbiota (Clooney et al., 2016; Malfertheiner et al., 2017). Compared with controls not using PPI, PPI users had decreased relative abundance of Gram-negative bacteria and increased relative abundance of *Streptococcus* (Snider et al., 2019). Changes in esophageal microbiota were observed before and after 8 weeks of PPI treatment. The predominant decreased taxa was *Comamonadaceae*, while the main increased taxa *were Clostridiaceae*, *Lachnospiraceae*, *Micrococcaceae*, *Actinomycetaceae*, *Gemellales*. As we discussed above, there was a shift toward Gram-negative bacteria in the EAC cascade. Although there is no direct evidence, PPI treatment may potentially benefit the patients with esophageal precancerous lesions (Amir et al., 2014). Similarly, mucosal protective agents are also applied extensively in the treatment of the gastric diseases (Haruma and Ito, 2003). In a murine Eosinophilic esophagitis (EoE) model, supplementation with *Lactococcus lactis* NCC 2287 attenuated esophageal eosinophilic inflammation (Holvoet et al., 2016). Recent research in a rat model suggests that rebamipide, a mucosal protective agent, can reduce BE development and alter the esophageal microbiome composition, in particular *Lactobacillus* and *Clostridium* (Kohata et al., 2015).

Probiotics

Probiotic is a major area of interest within the field of microbiotic therapy. Probiotics therapeutic tests showed a significant inhibitory effect on the expression of biomarkers that contribute

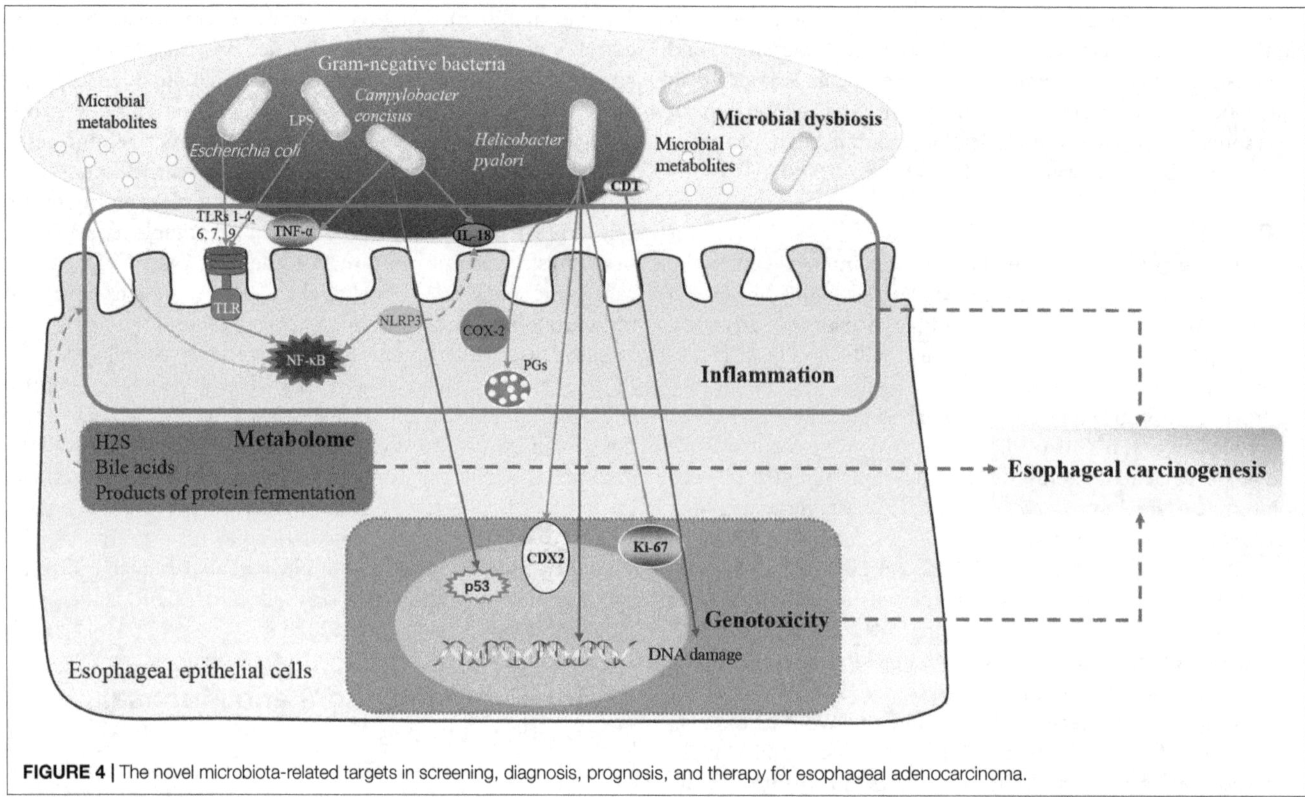

FIGURE 4 | The novel microbiota-related targets in screening, diagnosis, prognosis, and therapy for esophageal adenocarcinoma.

to BE transformation and indicated the possibility for the prevention of BE to EAC (Mozaffari Namin et al., 2015a). Besides, probiotics can be used to modulate the human microbiota in postoperative patients. A prospective trial evaluated the effect of probiotics on the prognosis of postoperative patients with EC (Lina et al., 2018). The result suggested that probiotics can reduce the rates of abdominal distension, constipation and gastric retention in postoperative patients with esophageal cancer.

CONCLUSION

The manuscript briefly summarizes our current knowledge regarding the relationship between human microbiota and the esophageal adenocarcinoma cascade. And it brings thinking from the fields of prevention, diagnosis, prognosis, and therapy for EAC (**Figure 4**). The current findings have identified decreased microbial diversity and altered human microbial communities in esophageal carcinogenesis, especially *Enterobacteriaceae*, *Campylobacters*, and acid-producing bacteria, periodontal pathogens (*Tannerella forsythia* and *Aggregatibacter actinomycetemcomitans*). *Helicobacter pylori*, *Prevotella*, *Tannerella forsythia*, and *Aggregatibacter actinomycetemcomitans* may be utilized as biomarkers for personalized precision diagnosis and screening of EAC. The expression of HPV-related biomarkers, the classification of the oral microbiome, and *Fusobacterium nucleatum* DNA status can become an important prognostic indicator of EAC. Notably, novel clinical interventions related to the human microbiota may also be used to treat EC, including adequate oral hygiene practices, a high fiber and low-fat diet, physical activity, PPI, mucosal protective agents and probiotics, which might benefit patients significantly. From this review, it emerged clearly that the human microbiota may impact the initiation and progression of EAC since it not only mediates inflammation and genotoxicity as specific pathogens, but also triggers detrimental metabolites as an integrated community. All mechanisms are not mutually exclusive and may be involved in tumorigenesis in a stage-specific and case-specific manner (Chen et al., 2017).

There were also certain limitations. Although preliminary studies have provided a comprehensive view of the role of the human microbiota in EAC development, information on causative effects on EAC cascade remained to be elucidated. This area needs more research to truly understand the complex mechanisms behind the impact of the human microbiota on tumorigenesis of EAC.

AUTHOR CONTRIBUTIONS

FP conceptualized the study, revised the manuscript, and supervised the study. WD drafted the manuscript and made the figures. LP and BY collected the literature and revised the manuscript. ZL improved the manuscript. All authors read and approved the final manuscript.

REFERENCES

1. Aghayeva, S., Mara, K. C., and Katzka, D. A. (2019). The impact of *Helicobacter* pylori on the presence of Barrett's esophagus in Azerbaijan, a high-prevalence area of infection. *Dis. Esophagus* 32:doz053. doi: 10.1093/dote/doz053
2. Akiyama, Y., Sasaki, A., Fujii, Y., Fujisawa, R., Sasaki, N., Nikai, H., et al. (2021). Efficacy of enhanced prehabilitation for patients with esophageal cancer undergoing esophagectomy. *Esophagus* 18, 56–64. doi: 10.1007/s10388-020- 00757-2
3. Allemani, C., Matsuda, T., Di Carlo, V., Harewood, R., Matz, M., Nikšiæ, M., et al. (2018). Global surveillance of trends in cancer survival 2000-14 (CONCORD- 3): analysis of individual records for 37 513 025 patients diagnosed with one of 18 cancers from 322 population-based registries in 71 countries. *Lancet* 391, 1023–1075. doi: 10.1016/s0140-6736(17)33326-3
4. Allen, J., Mailing, L., Niemiro, G., Moore, R., Cook, M., White, B., et al. (2018). Exercise alters gut microbiota composition and function in lean and obese humans. *Med. Sci. Sports Exerc.* 50, 747–757. doi: 10.1249/mss.0000000000001495
5. Altaf, K., Xiong, J. J., la Iglesia, D., Hickey, L., and Kaul, A. (2017). Meta-analysis of biomarkers predicting risk of malignant progression in Barrett's oesophagus. *Br. J. Surg.* 104, 493–502. doi: 10.1002/bjs.10484
6. Amir, I., Konikoff, F. M., Oppenheim, M., Gophna, U., and Half, E. E. (2014). Gastric microbiota is altered in oesophagitis and Barrett's oesophagus and further modified by proton pump inhibitors. *Environ. Microbiol.* 16, 2905–2914. doi: 10.1111/1462-2920.12285
7. Annavajhala, M. K., May, M., Compres, G., Freedberg, D. E., Graham, R., Stump, S., et al. (2020). Relationship of the esophageal microbiome and tissue gene expression and links to the oral microbiome: a randomized clinical trial. *Clin. Transl. Gastroenterol.* 11:e00235. doi: 10.14309/ctg.00000000000 00235
8. Arnold, M., Ferlay, J., van Berge Henegouwen, M. I., and Soerjomataram, I. (2020). Global burden of oesophageal and gastric cancer by histology and subsite in 2018. *Gut* 69, 1564–1571. doi: 10.1136/gutjnl-2020-321600
9. Babar, M., Ryan, A. W., Anderson, L. A., Segurado, R., Turner, G., Murray, L. J., et al. (2012). Genes of the interleukin-18 pathway are associated with susceptibility to Barrett's esophagus and esophageal adenocarcinoma. *Am. J. Gastroenterol.* 107, 1331–1341. doi: 10.1038/ajg.2012.134
10. Bashan, A., Gibson, T. E., Friedman, J., Carey, V. J., Weiss, S. T., Hohmann, E. L., et al. (2016). Universality of human microbial dynamics. *Nature* 534, 259–262. doi: 10.1038/nature18301
11. Bäumler, A. J., and Sperandio, V. (2016). Interactions between the microbiota and pathogenic bacteria in the gut. *Nature* 535, 85–93. doi: 10.1038/nature18849 Blackett, K. L., Siddhi, S. S., Cleary, S., Steed, H., Miller, M. H., Macfarlane, S., et al. (2013). Oesophageal bacterial biofilm changes in gastro-oesophageal reflux disease, Barrett's and oesophageal carcinoma: association or causality? *Aliment. Pharmacol. Ther.* 37, 1084–1092. doi: 10.1111/apt.12317
12. Bourgeois, D., Inquimbert, C., Ottolenghi, L., and Carrouel, F. (2019b). Periodontal pathogens as risk factors of cardiovascular diseases, diabetes, rheumatoid arthritis, cancer, and chronic obstructive pulmonary disease-is there cause for consideration? *Microorganisms* 7:424. doi: 10.3390/microorganisms7100424
13. Bourgeois, D., Bravo, M., Llodra, J., Inquimbert, C., Viennot, S., Dussart, C., et al. (2019a). Calibrated interdental brushing for the prevention of periodontal pathogens infection in young adults – a randomized controlled clinical trial. *Sci. Rep.* 9:15127. doi: 10.1038/s41598-019-51938-8
14. Bourgeois, D., Saliasi, I., Llodra, J., Bravo, M., Viennot, S., and Carrouel, F. (2016). Efficacy of interdental calibrated brushes on bleeding reduction in adults: a 3-month randomized controlled clinical trial. *Eur. J. Oral Sci.* 124, 566–571. doi: 10.1111/eos.12302
15. Cani, P., and Jordan, B. (2018). Gut microbiota-mediated inflammation in obesity: a link with gastrointestinal cancer. *Nat. Rev. Gastroenterol. Hepatol.* 15, 671– 682. doi: 10.1038/s41575-018-0025-6
16. Chen, J., Pitmon, E., and Wang, K. (2017). Microbiome, inflammation and colorectal cancer. *Semin. Immunol.* 32, 43–53. doi: 10.1016/j.smim.2017.09.006 Clarke, S., Murphy, E., O'Sullivan, O., Lucey, A., Humphreys, M., Hogan, A., et al. (2014). Exercise and associated dietary extremes impact on gut microbial diversity. *Gut* 63, 1913–1920. doi: 10.1136/gutjnl-2013-306541
17. Clooney, A., Bernstein, C., Leslie, W., Vagianos, K., Sargent, M., Laserna-Mendieta, E., et al. (2016). A comparison of the gut microbiome between long-termusers and non-users of proton pump inhibitors. *Aliment. Pharmacol. Ther.* 43, 974–984. doi: 10.1111/apt.13568
18. Coleman, H. G., Xie, S. H., and Lagergren, J. (2018). The epidemiology of esophageal adenocarcinoma. *Gastroenterology* 154, 390–405. doi: 10.1053/j.gastro.2017.07.046
19. Consortium, H. M. P. (2012). Structure, function and diversity of the healthy human microbiome. *Nature* 486, 207–214. doi: 10.1038/nature11234
20. Cotillard, A., Kennedy, S. P., Kong, L. C., Prifti, E., Pons, N., Le Chatelier, E., et al. (2013). Dietary intervention impact on gut microbial gene richness. *Nature* 500, 585–588. doi: 10.1038/nature12480
21. Deng, Q., Yan, L., Lin, J., Zhuang, Z., Hong, Y., Hu, C., et al. (2021). A composite oral hygiene score and the risk of oral cancer and its subtypes: a large- scale propensity score-based study. *Clin. Oral Invest.* doi: 10.1007/s00784-021- 04209-8
22. Deshpande, N. P., Riordan, S. M., Castaño-Rodríguez, N., Wilkins, M. R., and Kaakoush, N. O. (2018). Signatures within the esophageal microbiome are associated with host genetics, age, and disease. *Microbiome* 6:227. doi: 10.1186/ s40168-018-0611-4
23. Diakowska, D., Markocka-Maczka, K., Grabowski, K., and Lewandowski, A. (2006). Serum interleukin-12 and interleukin-18 levels in patients with oesophageal squamous cell carcinoma. *Exp. Oncol.* 28, 319–322.
24. Divella, R., Daniele, A., Savino, E., and Paradiso, A. (2020). Anticancer effects of nutraceuticals in the mediterranean diet: an epigenetic diet model. *Cancer Genomics Proteomics* 17, 335–350. doi: 10.21873/cgp.20193
25. Dominguez-Bello, M. G., Godoy-Vitorino, F., Knight, R., and Blaser, M. J. (2019). Role of the microbiome in human development. *Gut* 68, 1108–1114. doi: 10. 1136/gutjnl-2018-317503
26. Dong, L., Yin, J., Zhao, J., Ma, S. R., Wang, H. R., Wang, M., et al. (2018). Microbial similarity and preference for specific sites in healthy oral cavity and esophagus. *Front. Microbiol.* 9:1603. doi: 10.3389/fmicb.2018.01603
27. Doorakkers, E., Lagergren, J., Santoni, G., Engstrand, L., and Brusselaers, N. (2020). *Helicobacter* pylori eradication treatment and the risk of Barrett's esophagus and esophageal adenocarcinoma. *Helicobacter* 25:e12688. doi: 10.1111/hel.12688
28. Elliott, D. R. F., Walker, A. W., O'Donovan, M., Parkhill, J., and Fitzgerald, R. C. (2017). A non-endoscopic device to sample the oesophageal microbiota: a case- control study. *Lancet Gastroenterol. Hepatol.* 2, 32–42. doi: 10.1016/s2468- 1253(16)30086-3
29. Falony, G., Joossens, M., Vieira-Silva, S., Wang, J., Darzi, Y., Faust, K., et al. (2016). Population-level analysis of gut microbiome variation. *Science* 352, 560–564. doi: 10.1126/science.aad3503
30. Fan, X., Alekseyenko, A. V., Wu, J., Peters, B. A., Jacobs, E. J., Gapstur, S. M., et al. (2018). Human oral microbiome and prospective risk for pancreatic cancer: a population-based nested case-control study. *Gut* 67, 120–127. doi: 10.1136/ gutjnl-2016-312580
31. Fredricks, D. N., Fiedler, T. L., and Marrazzo, J. M. (2005). Molecular identification of bacteria associated with bacterial vaginosis. *N. Engl. J. Med.* 353, 1899–1911. doi: 10.1056/NEJMoa043802
32. Gholizadeh, P., Pormohammad, A., Eslami, H., Shokouhi, B., Fakhrzadeh, V., and Kafil, H. S. (2017). Oral pathogenesis of *Aggregatibacter actinomycetemcomitans*. *Microb. Pathog.* 113, 303–311. doi: 10.1016/j.micpath. 2017.11.001
33. Gilbert, J. A., Blaser, M. J., Caporaso, J. G., Jansson, J. K., Lynch, S. V., and Knight, R. (2018). Current understanding of the human microbiome. *Nat. Med.* 24, 392–400. doi: 10.1038/nm.4517
34. Gupta, V. K., Paul, S., and Dutta, C. (2017). Geography, ethnicity or subsistence- specific variations in human microbiome composition and diversity. *Front. Microbiol.* 8:1162. doi: 10.3389/fmicb.2017.01162
35. Haruma, K., and Ito, M. (2003). Review article: clinical significance of mucosal-protective agents: acid, inflammation, carcinogenesis and rebamipide. *Aliment. Pharmacol. Ther.* 18(Suppl. 1), 153–159. doi: 10.1046/j.1365-2036.18.s1.17.x
36. He, Z., Gharaibeh, R., Newsome, R., Pope, J., Dougherty, M., Tomkovich, S., et al. (2019). *Campylobacter jejuni* promotes colorectal tumorigenesis through the action of cytolethal distending toxin. *Gut* 68, 289–300. doi: 10.1136/gutjnl- 2018-317200
37. Holvoet, S., Doucet-Ladevèze, R., Perrot, M., Barretto, C., Nutten, S., and Blanchard, C. (2016). Beneficial effect of *Lactococcus lactis* NCC 2287 in a murine model of eosinophilic esophagitis. *Allergy* 71, 1753–1761. doi: 10.1111/ all.12951
38. Kaakoush, N. O., Castaño-Rodríguez, N., Man, S. M., and Mitchell, H. M. (2015). Is *Campylobacter* to esophageal adenocarcinoma as *Helicobacter* is to gastric adenocarcinoma? *Trends Microbiol.* 23, 455–462. doi: 10.1016/j.tim.2015.03. 009

39. Kageyama, S., Takeshita, T., Takeuchi, K., Asakawa, M., Matsumi, R., Furuta, M., et al. (2019). Characteristics of the salivary microbiota in patients with various digestive tract cancers. *Front. Microbiol.* 10:1780. doi: 10.3389/fmicb. 2019.01780
40. Kåhrström, C. T., Pariente, N., and Weiss, U. (2016). Intestinal microbiota in health and disease. *Nature* 535:47. doi: 10.1038/535047a
41. Kawasaki, M., Ikeda, Y., Ikeda, E., Takahashi, M., Tanaka, D., Nakajima, Y., et al. (2020). Oral infectious bacteria in dental plaque and saliva as risk factors in patients with esophageal cancer. *Cancer* 127, 512–519. doi: 10.1002/cncr.33316
42. Khandia, R., and Munjal, A. (2020). Interplay between inflammation and cancer. *Adv. Protein Chem. Struct. Biol.* 119, 199–245. doi: 10.1016/ bs.apcsb.2019.09. 004
43. Kohata, Y., Nakahara, K., Tanigawa, T., Yamagami, H., Shiba, M., Watanabe, T., et al. (2015). Rebamipide alters the esophageal microbiome and reduces the incidence of Barrett's esophagus in a rat model. *Dig. Dis. Sci.* 60, 2654–2661. doi: 10.1007/s10620-015-3662-4
44. Kondo, S., Inoue, T., Yoshida, T., Saito, T., Inoue, S., Nishino, T., et al. (2021). Impact of preoperative 6-minute walk distance on long-term prognosis after esophagectomy in patients with esophageal cancer. *Esophagus* doi: 10.1007/ s10388-021-00871-9
45. Kountouras, J., Doulberis, M., Papaefthymiou, A., Polyzos, S. A., Vardaka, E., Tzivras, D., et al. (2019). A perspective on risk factors for esophageal adenocarcinoma: emphasis on *Helicobacter* pylori infection. *Ann. N. Y. Acad. Sci.* 1452, 12–17. doi: 10.1111/nyas.14168
46. Lagergren, J., and Lagergren, P. (2013). Recent developments in esophageal adenocarcinoma. *CA: a cancer journal for clinicians* 63, 232–248. doi: 10.3322/ caac.21185.
47. Lamont, R., Koo, H., and Hajishengallis, G. (2018). The oral microbiota: dynamic communities and host interactions. *Nat. Rev. Microbiol.* 16, 745–759. doi: 10. 1038/s41579-018-0089-x
48. Lao-Sirieix, P., and Fitzgerald, R. C. (2012). Screening for oesophageal cancer. *Nat. Rev. Clin. Oncol.* 9, 278–287. doi: 10.1038/nrclinonc.2012.35
49. Lee, Y., Hu, H., Yang, N., Chou, P., and Chu, D. (2014). Dental prophylaxis decreases the risk of esophageal cancer in males; a nationwide population-based study in Taiwan. *PLoS One* 9:e109444. doi: 10.1371/journal. pone.0109444
50. Li, J., Qiu, G., Fang, B., Dai, X., and Cai, J. (2018). Deficiency of IL-18 aggravates esophageal carcinoma through inhibiting IFN-γ production by CD8(+)T cells and NK cells. *Inflammation* 41, 667–676. doi: 10.1007/s10753-017-0721-3
51. Lina, Z., Yufang, Z., Jiuchao, Z., Lijuan, C., and Xiaoyan, W. (2018). Effects of probiotics combined with enteral nutrition on gastrointestinal function of postoperative patients with esophageal cancer. *Chin. J. Microecol.* 30, 924–927.
52. Liu, F., Wang, W., Wang, J., Li, J., and Gao, P. (2011). Effect of *Helicobacter* pylori infection on Barrett's esophagus and esophageal adenocarcinoma formation in a rat model of chronic gastroesophageal reflux. *Helicobacter* 16, 66–77. doi: 10.1111/j.1523-5378.2010.00811.x
53. Liu, N., Ando, T., Ishiguro, K., Maeda, O., Watanabe, O., Funasaka, K., et al. (2013). Characterization of bacterial biota in the distal esophagus of Japanese patients with reflux esophagitis and Barrett's esophagus. *BMC Infect. Dis.* 13:130. doi: 10.1186/1471-2334-13-130
54. Lloyd-Price, J., Abu-Ali, G., and Huttenhower, C. (2016). The healthy human microbiome. *Genome Med.* 8:51. doi: 10.1186/s13073-016-0307-y
55. Lo, C. H., Kwon, S., Wang, L., Polychronidis, G., Knudsen, M. D., Zhong, R., et al. (2021). Periodontal disease, tooth loss, and risk of oesophageal and gastric adenocarcinoma: a prospective study. *Gut* 70, 620–621. doi: 10.1136/ gutjnl- 2020-321949
56. Lopetuso, L. R., Severgnini, M., Pecere, S., Ponziani, F. R., Boskoski, I., Larghi, A., et al. (2020). Esophageal microbiome signature in patients with Barrett's esophagus and esophageal adenocarcinoma. *PLoS One* 15:e0231789. doi: 10. 1371/journal.pone.0231789
57. Louis, P., Hold, G., and Flint, H. (2014). The gut microbiota, bacterial metabolites and colorectal cancer. *Nat. Rev. Microbiol.* 12, 661–672. doi: 10.1038/ nrmicro3344
58. Lv, J., Guo, L., Liu, J. J., Zhao, H. P., Zhang, J., and Wang, J. H. (2019). Alteration of the esophageal microbiota in Barrett's esophagus and esophageal adenocarcinoma. *World J. Gastroenterol.* 25, 2149–2161. doi: 10.3748/wjg.v25. i18.2149
59. Macfarlane, S., Furrie, E., Macfarlane, G. T., and Dillon, J. F. (2007). Microbial colonization of the upper gastrointestinal tract in patients with Barrett's esophagus. *Clin. Infect. Dis.* 45, 29–38. doi: 10.1086/518578
60. Malfertheiner, P., Kandulski, A., and Venerito, M. (2017). Proton-pump inhibitors: understanding the complications and risks. *Nat. Rev. Gastroenterol. Hepatol.* 14, 697–710. doi: 10.1038/nrgastro.2017.117
61. Mark Welch, J., Dewhirst, F., and Borisy, G. (2019). Biogeography of the oral microbiome: the site-specialist hypothesis. *Annu. Rev. Microbiol.* 73, 335–358. doi: 10.1146/annurev-micro-090817-062503
62. Martinon, P., Fraticelli, L., Giboreau, A., Dussart, C., Bourgeois, D., and Carrouel, F. (2021). Nutrition as a key modifiable factor for periodontitis and main chronic diseases. *J. Clin. Med.* 10:197. doi: 10.3390/jcm10020197
63. May, M., and Abrams, J. A. (2018). Emerging insights into the esophageal microbiome. *Curr. Treat. Options Gastroenterol.* 16, 72–85. doi: 10.1007/ s11938-018-0171-5
64. Mentella, M., Scaldaferri, F., Ricci, C., Gasbarrini, A., and Miggiano, G. (2019). Cancer and mediterranean diet: a review. *Nutrients* 11:2059. doi: 10.3390/ nu11092059
65. Mitra, A., MacIntyre, D. A., Lee, Y. S., Smith, A., Marchesi, J. R., Lehne, B., et al. (2015). Cervical intraepithelial Neoplasia disease progression is associated with increased vaginal microbiome diversity. *Sci. Rep.* 5:16865. doi: 10.1038/ srep16865
66. Mmbaga, B., Mwasamwaja, A., Mushi, G., Mremi, A., Nyakunga, G., Kiwelu, I., et al. (2020). Missing and decayed teeth, oral hygiene and dental staining in relation to esophageal cancer risk: ESCCAPE case-control study in Kilimanjaro, Tanzania. *Int. J. Cancer* 148, 2416–2428. doi: 10.1002/ijc.33433
67. Molina-Montes, E., Salamanca-Fernández, E., Garcia-Villanova, B., and Sánchez, M. (2020). The impact of plant-based dietary patterns on cancer-related outcomes: a rapid review and meta-analysis. *Nutrients* 12:2010. doi: 10.3390/ nu12072010
68. Mozaffari Namin, B., Soltan Dallal, M. M., and Ebrahimi Daryani, N. (2015b). The effect of *Campylobacter concisus* on expression of IL-18, TNF-α and p53 in Barrett's cell lines. *Jundishapur J. Microbiol.* 8:e26393. doi: 10.5812/jjm. 26393
69. Mozaffari Namin, B., Daryani, N. E., Mirshafiey, A., Yazdi, M. K. S., and Dallal, M. M. S. (2015a). Effect of probiotics on the expression of Barrett's oesophagus biomarkers. *J. Med. Microbiol.* 64(Pt. 4), 348–354. doi: 10.1099/ jmm.0.000039
70. Münch, N. S., Fang, H. Y., Ingermann, J., Maurer, H. C., Anand, A., Kellner, V., et al. (2019). High-Fat diet accelerates carcinogenesis in a mouse model of Barrett's esophagus *via* interleukin 8 and alterations to the gut microbiome. *Gastroenterology* 157, 492–506.e492. doi: 10.1053/j.gastro.2019.04.013
71. Munemoto, M., Mukaisho, K., Miyashita, T., Oyama, K., Haba, Y., Okamoto, K., et al. (2019). Roles of the hexosamine biosynthetic pathway and pentose phosphate pathway in bile acid-induced cancer development. *Cancer Sci.* 110, 2408–2420. doi: 10.1111/cas.14105
72. Nadatani, Y., Huo, X., Zhang, X., Yu, C., Cheng, E., Zhang, Q., et al. (2016). NOD-Like receptor protein 3 inflammasome priming and activation in Barrett's epithelial cells. *Cell. Mol. Gastroenterol. Hepatol.* 2, 439–453. doi: 10.1016/j. jcmgh.2016.03.006
73. Nesiæ, D., Hsu, Y., and Stebbins, C. (2004). Assembly and function of a bacterial genotoxin. *Nature* 429, 429–433. doi: 10.1038/nature02532
74. Nobel, Y. R., Snider, E. J., Compres, G., Freedberg, D. E., Khiabanian, H., Lightdale, C. J., et al. (2018). Increasing dietary fiber intake is associated with a distinct esophageal microbiome. *Clin. Transl. Gastroenterol.* 9:199. doi: 10.1038/s41424- 018-0067-7
75. Okereke, I. C., Miller, A. L., Hamilton, C. F., Booth, A. L., Reep, G. L., Andersen, C. L., et al. (2019). Microbiota of the oropharynx and endoscope compared to the esophagus. *Sci. Rep.* 9:10201. doi: 10.1038/s41598-019-46747-y
76. O'Rorke, M. A., Ellison, M. V., Murray, L. J., Moran, M., James, J., and Anderson, L. A. (2012). Human papillomavirus related head and neck cancer survival: a systematic review and meta-analysis. *Oral Oncol.* 48, 1191–1201. doi: 10.1016/j. oraloncology.2012.06.019
77. Patel, A., Friedenreich, C., Moore, S., Hayes, S., Silver, J., Campbell, K., et al. (2019). American college of sports medicine roundtable report on physical activity, sedentary behavior, and cancer prevention and control. *Med. Sci. Sports Exerc.* 51, 2391–2402. doi: 10.1249/mss.0000000000002117
78. Pei, Z., Bini, E. J., Yang, L., Zhou, M., Francois, F., and Blaser, M. J. (2004). Bacterial biota in the human distal esophagus. *Proc. Natl. Acad. Sci. U.S.A.* 101, 4250–4255. doi: 10.1073/pnas.0306398101
79. Peter, S., Pendergraft, A., VanDerPol, W., Wilcox, C. M., Kyanam Kabir Baig, K. R., Morrow, C., et al. (2020). Mucosa-Associated microbiota in Barrett's esophagus, dysplasia, and esophageal adenocarcinoma differ similarly compared with healthy controls. *Clin. Transl. Gastroenterol.* 11:e00199. doi: 10.14309/ctg. 0000000000000199

80. Peters, B. A., Wu, J., Pei, Z., Yang, L., Purdue, M. P., Freedman, N. D., et al. (2017). Oral microbiome composition reflects prospective risk for esophageal cancers. *Cancer Res.* 77, 6777–6787. doi: 10.1158/0008-5472.Can-17-1296
81. Plottel, C., and Blaser, M. (2011). Microbiome and malignancy. *Cell Host Microbe* 10, 324–335. doi: 10.1016/j.chom.2011.10.003
82. Poosari, A., Nutravong, T., Sa-Ngiamwibool, P., Namwat, W., Chatrchaiwiwatana, S., and Ungareewittaya, P. (2021). Association between infection with *Campylobacter* species, poor oral health and environmental risk factors on esophageal cancer: a hospital-based case-control study in Thailand. *Eur. J. Med. Res.* 26:82. doi: 10.1186/s40001-021-00561-3
83. Proctor, L. H. C. (2019). The integrative human microbiome project. *Nature* 569, 641–648. doi: 10.1038/s41586-019-1238-8
84. Qin, J., Li, Y., Cai, Z., Li, S., Zhu, J., Zhang, F., et al. (2012). A metagenome-wide association study of gut microbiota in type 2 diabetes. *Nature* 490, 55–60. doi: 10.1038/nature11450
85. Quante, M., Graham, T., and Jansen, M. (2018). Insights into the pathophysiology of esophageal adenocarcinoma. *Gastroenterology* 154, 406–420. doi: 10.1053/j. gastro.2017.09.046
86. Ragin, C. C., and Taioli, E. (2007). Survival of squamous cell carcinoma of the head and neck in relation to human papillomavirus infection: review and meta-analysis. *Int. J. Cancer* 121, 1813–1820. doi: 10.1002/ijc.22851
87. Rajendra, S., Sharma, P., Gautam, S. D., Saxena, M., Kapur, A., Sharma, P., et al. (2020). Association of biomarkers for human papillomavirus with survival among adults with Barrett high-grade dysplasia and esophageal adenocarcinoma. *JAMA Netw. Open* 3:e1921189. doi: 10.1001/jamanetwork open.2019.21189
88. Rajendra, S., Wang, B., Snow, E. T., Sharma, P., Pavey, D., Merrett, N., et al. (2013). Transcriptionally active human papillomavirus is strongly associated with Barrett's dysplasia and esophageal adenocarcinoma. *Am. J. Gastroenterol.* 108, 1082–1093. doi: 10.1038/ajg.2013.94
89. Rajendra, S., Xuan, W., Merrett, N., Sharma, P., Sharma, P., Pavey, D., et al. (2018). Survival rates for patients with Barrett high-grade dysplasia and esophageal adenocarcinoma with or without human papillomavirus infection. *JAMA Netw. Open* 1:e181054. doi: 10.1001/jamanetworkopen.2018.1054
90. Rochman, M., Xie, Y., Mack, L., Caldwell, J., Klingler, A., Osswald, G., et al. (2021). Broad transcriptional response of the human esophageal epithelium to proton pump inhibitors. *J. Allergy Clin. Immunol.* 147, 1924–1935. doi: 10.1016/j.jaci. 2020.09.039
91. Rock, C., Thomson, C., Gansler, T., Gapstur, S., McCullough, M., Patel, A., et al. (2020). American Cancer Society guideline for diet and physical activity for cancer prevention. *CA Cancer J. Clin.* 70, 245–271. doi: 10.3322/caac.21591
92. Sälzer, S., Graetz, C., Dörfer, C., Slot, D., and Van der Weijden, F. (2020). Contemporary practices for mechanical oral hygiene to prevent periodontal disease. *Periodontology 2000* 84, 35–44. doi: 10.1111/prd.12332
93. San-Millán, I., and Brooks, G. A. (2017). Reexamining cancer metabolism: lactate production for carcinogenesis could be the purpose and explanation of the Warburg Effect. *Carcinogenesis* 38, 119–133. doi: 10.1093/carcin/bgw127
94. Schwabe, R., and Jobin, C. (2013). The microbiome and cancer. *Nat. Rev. Cancer*13, 800–812. doi: 10.1038/nrc3610
95. Scott, A., Alexander, J., Merrifield, C., Cunningham, D., Jobin, C., Brown, R., et al. (2019). International Cancer Microbiome Consortium consensus statement on the role of the human microbiome in carcinogenesis. *Gut* 68, 1624–1632. doi: 10.1136/gutjnl-2019-318556
96. Segata, N., Haake, S., Mannon, P., Lemon, K., Waldron, L., Gevers, D., et al. (2012). Composition of the adult digestive tract bacterial microbiome based on seven mouth surfaces, tonsils, throat and stool samples. *Genome Biol.* 13:R42. doi: 10.1186/gb-2012-13-6-r42
97. Sharma, A. (2010). Virulence mechanisms of *Tannerella forsythia*. *Periodontol. 2000* 54, 106–116. doi: 10.1111/j.1600-0757.2009.00332.x
98. Shukla, S., Cook, D., Meyer, J., Vernon, S., Le, T., Clevidence, D., et al. (2015). Changes in gut and plasma microbiome following exercise challenge in myalgic encephalomyelitis/chronic fatigue syndrome (ME/CFS). *PLoS One* 10:e0145453. doi: 10.1371/journal.pone.0145453
99. Simard, E. P., Ward, E. M., Siegel, R., and Jemal, A. (2012). Cancers with increasing incidence trends in the United States: 1999 through 2008. *CA Cancer J. Clin.* 62, 118–128. doi: 10.3322/caac.20141
100. Snider, E. J., Compres, G., Freedberg, D. E., Khiabanian, H., Nobel, Y. R., Stump, S., et al. (2019). Alterations to the esophageal microbiome associated with progression from Barrett's esophagus to esophageal adenocarcinoma. *Cancer Epidemiol. Biomarkers Prev.* 28, 1687–1693. doi: 10.1158/1055-9965. Epi-19- 0008
101. Snider, E., Compres, G., Freedberg, D., Giddins, M., Khiabanian, H., Lightdale, C., et al. (2018). Barrett's esophagus is associated with a distinct oral microbiome. *Clin. Transl. Gastroenterol.* 9:135. doi: 10.1038/s41424-018-0005-8
102. Stahl, M., Budach, W., Meyer, H., and Cervantes, A. (2010). Esophageal cancer: clinical Practice Guidelines for diagnosis, treatment and follow-up. *Ann. Oncol.* 21(Suppl. 5), v46–v49. doi: 10.1093/annonc/mdq163
103. Sun, J., Tang, Q., Yu, S., Xie, M., Xie, Y., Chen, G., et al. (2020). Role of the oral microbiota in cancer evolution and progression. *Cancer Med.* 9, 6306–6321. doi: 10.1002/cam4.3206
104. Sung, H., Ferlay, J., Siegel, R.L., Laversanne, M., Soerjomataram, I., Jemal, A., et al. (2021). Global Cancer Statistics 2020: GLOBOCAN Estimates of Incidence and Mortality Worldwide for 36 Cancers in 185 Countries. *CA Cancer J. Clin.* 71, 209–249. doi: 10.3322/caac.21660.
105. Tantamango-Bartley, Y., Jaceldo-Siegl, K., Fan, J., and Fraser, G. (2013). Vegetarian diets and the incidence of cancer in a low-risk population. *Cancer Epidemiol. Biomarkers Prev.* 22, 286–294. doi: 10.1158/1055-9965. Epi-12-1060
106. Teng, G., Dai, Y., Chu, Y., Li, J., Zhang, H., Wu, T., et al. (2018). *Helicobacter* pylori induces caudal-type homeobox protein 2 and cyclooxygenase 2 expression by modulating microRNAs in esophageal epithelial cells. *Cancer Sci.* 109, 297–307. doi: 10.1111/cas.13462
107. Thrumurthy, S. G., Chaudry, M. A., Thrumurthy, S. S. D., and Mughal, M. (2019). Oesophageal cancer: risks, prevention, and diagnosis. *BMJ* 366:l4373. doi: 10. 1136/bmj.l4373
108. Tuominen, H., and Rautava, J. (2021). Oral microbiota and cancer development. *Pathobiology* 88, 116–126. doi: 10.1159/000510979
109. Turnbaugh, P. J., Ley, R. E., Hamady, M., Fraser-Liggett, C. M., Knight, R., and Gordon, J. I. (2007). The human microbiome project. *Nature* 449, 804–810. doi: 10.1038/nature06244
110. Wang, Y., Zhang, Y., Wang, Z., Tang, J., Cao, D., Qian, Y., et al. (2021). *Desulfovibrio desulfuricans*A clinical nomogram incorporating salivary level and oral hygiene index for predicting colorectal cancer. *Ann. Transl. Med.* 9:754. doi: 10.21037/atm-20-8168
111. Wang, Z., Shaheen, N. J., Whiteman, D. C., Anderson, L. A., Vaughan, T. L., Corley, D. A., et al. (2018). *Helicobacter* pylori infection is associated with reduced risk of Barrett's esophagus: an analysis of the Barrett's and esophageal adenocarcinoma consortium. *Am. J. Gastroenterol.* 113, 1148–1155. doi: 10. 1038/s41395-018-0070-3
112. Wilson, M. R., Jiang, Y., Villalta, P. W., Stornetta, A., Boudreau, P. D., Carrá, A., et al. (2019). The human gut bacterial genotoxin colibactin alkylates DNA. *Science* 363:eaar7785. doi: 10.1126/science.aar7785
113. Worthington, H., MacDonald, L., Poklepovic Pericic, T., Sambunjak, D., Johnson, T., Imai, P., et al. (2019). Home use of interdental cleaning devices, in addition to toothbrushing, for preventing and controlling periodontal diseases and dental caries. *Cochr. Database Syst. Rev.* 4:CD012018. doi: 10.1002/14651858. CD012018.pub2
114. Wroblewski, L., Peek, R., and Wilson, K. (2010). *Helicobacter* pylori and gastric cancer: factors that modulate disease risk. *Clin. Microbiol. Rev.* 23, 713–739. doi: 10.1128/cmr.00011-10
115. Yamamura, K., Baba, Y., Nakagawa, S., Mima, K., Miyake, K., Nakamura, K., et al. (2016). Human microbiome *Fusobacterium Nucleatum* in esophageal cancer tissue is associated with prognosis. *Clin. Cancer Res.* 22, 5574–5581. doi: 10.1158/1078-0432.Ccr-16-1786
116. Yang, L., Chaudhary, N., Baghdadi, J., and Pei, Z. (2014). Microbiome in reflux disorders and esophageal adenocarcinoma. *Cancer J.* 20, 207–210. doi: 10.1097/ ppo.0000000000000044 Yang, L., Francois, F., and Pei, Z. (2012). Molecular pathways: pathogenesis and clinical implications of microbiome alteration in esophagitis and Barrett esophagus. *Clin. Cancer Res.* 18, 2138–2144. doi: 10.1158/1078-0432.Ccr-11- 0934
117. Yang, L., Lu, X., Nossa, C. W., Francois, F., Peek, R. M., and Pei, Z. (2009). Inflammation and intestinal metaplasia of the distal esophagus are associated with alterations in the microbiome. *Gastroenterology* 137, 588–597. doi: 10. 1053/j.gastro.2009.04.046
118. Yano, Y., Abnet, C., Poustchi, H., Roshandel, G., Pourshams, A., Islami, F., et al. (2021). Oral health and risk of upper gastrointestinal cancers in a large prospective study from a high-risk region: Golestan cohort study. *Cancer Prev. Res. (Philadelphia, Pa.)* 14, 709–718. doi: 10.1158/1940-6207.Capr-20-0577

119. Yuda, M., Yamashita, K., Okamura, A., Hayami, M., Fukudome, I., Toihata, T., et al. (2020). Influence of preoperative Oropharyngeal microflora on the occurrence of postoperative pneumonia and survival in patients undergoing esophagectomy for esophageal cancer. *Ann. Surg.* 272, 1035–1043. doi: 10.1097/ sla.0000000000003287
120. Zaidi, A. H., Kelly, L. A., Kreft, R. E., Barlek, M., Omstead, A. N., Matsui, D., et al. (2016). Associations of microbiota and toll-like receptor signaling pathway in esophageal adenocarcinoma. *BMC Cancer* 16:52. doi: 10.1186/ s12885-016- 2093-8
121. Zhang, T., Yang, X., Yin, X., Yuan, Z., Chen, H., Jin, L., et al. (2021). Poor oral hygiene behavior is associated with an increased risk of gastric cancer: a population-based case-control study in China. *J. Periodontol.* doi: 10.1002/ jper. 21-0301
122. Zhao, Q., Yang, T., Yan, Y., Zhang, Y., Li, Z., Wang, Y., et al. (2020). Alterations of oral microbiota in Chinese patients with esophageal cancer. *Front. Cell. Infect. Microbiol.* 10:541144. doi: 10.3389/fcimb.2020.54 1144
123. Zhou, J., Shrestha, P., Qiu, Z., Harman, D. G., Teoh, W. C., Al-Sohaily, S., et al. (2020). Distinct microbiota dysbiosis in patients with non-erosive reflux disease and esophageal adenocarcinoma. *J. Clin. Med.* 9:2162. doi: 10.3390/ jcm907 2162

15

Alzheimer's Disease and Oral-Systemic Health: Bidirectional Care Integration Improving Outcomes

*Anne O. Rice**

Oral Systemic Seminars, Conroe, TX, United States

***Correspondence:**
Anne O. Rice
anneorice@gmail.com

Dentistry is an effective healthcare field that can impact Alzheimer's disease through prevention and education. Every day dental providers use an arsenal of assessment protocols directly coinciding with modifiable Alzheimer's risk factors. An innovative way to help in the prevention of Alzheimer's disease is to utilize oral health professionals who reach the public in ways other health care providers may not. Bidirectional care integration is needed to stifle many systemic diseases and Alzheimer's disease is no different. Ultimately with collaborative care the patient reaps the benefits. Alzheimer's is associated with many etiologies and pathophysiological processes. These include cardiovascular health, smoking, sleep, inflammatory pathogens, and diabetes. In the United States, dental providers assess each of these factors daily and can be instrumental in educating patients on the influence of these factors for dementia prevention. Globally, by 2025, the number of people with Alzheimer's disease is expected to rise by at least 14%. Such increases will strain local and national health care systems, but for the US if Medicare were expanded to include dental services, many older adults could be spared needless suffering. The goal of this perspective article is to highlight existing practices being used in the field of dentistry that can easily be adapted to educate patients in preventive care and treat risk factors. It is the duty of healthcare professionals to explore all opportunities to stem the advance of this disease and by integrating oral and systemic health into transdisciplinary science, health care and policy may do just that.

Keywords: Alzheimer's disease, medicare, sleep apnea, smoking, dentistry, pathogens, diabetes, cardiovascular disease

INTRODUCTION

Alzheimer's disease (AD) is a progressive mental deterioration that occurs in middle or old age due to the brain's degeneration [1]. Every 65 s, someone in the United States is diagnosed with Alzheimer's disease, the most common form of dementia, and it currently affects over 5.8 million people in the United States. The Alzheimer's Association projects by 2050 nearly 15 million people in the United States will receive an Alzheimer's diagnosis. The same report shows that a full half of primary care physicians feel unprepared to meet the demand of such a drastic increase [2]. In 2014, Rush University Medical Center analyzed death records nationally and found that most people who die from Alzheimer's have a recorded cause of death listed as respiratory or cardiac disease. When taking these numbers into account, AD would be elevated to the third leading cause of death in the United States [3].

Hundreds of billions of dollars in research and drug exploration have yielded a 99.6% drug failure rate [4]. While various drug developers are taking different approaches considering such near complete failure, many scientists and physicians are targeting prevention as the best strategy to reduce Alzheimer's cases [5–10]. In 2017, *The Lancet* Commission presented a report that stated more than one-third of global dementia cases may be preventable through addressing lifestyle factors that impact a person's risk [11]. The World Health Organization (WHO) agreed with this assessment and strongly recommended physical activity, quitting smoking, managing hypertension, and diabetes to reduce the risk of cognitive decline [12]. Disturbed sleeping patterns and periodontal disease have also been related to AD and accelerated cognitive decline rates [13–19].

The brain changes from Alzheimer's disease start at least a decade before symptoms show [20, 21], and as stated above, prevention is the best current defense against this disease. Prevention strategies should begin years before the typical onset presents, which is where dental providers can make the most significant contribution. Every day, dental professionals are performing vital tests, giving education on preventative measures, and prescribing medications in the line of treating and preventing dental health concerns that may also serve to reduce the risk of Alzheimer's. If dental professionals can use these routine tests to educate their patients and offer counseling on risk and preventative measures, more ways may be found to reduce the human suffering caused by AD. Even simply good oral health can have a positive effect on brain health [22]. This perspective focuses on the work that dental professionals regularly administer in the areas of cardiovascular health, smoking, sleep, inflammatory pathogens, and diabetes that can also serve in the prevention of Alzheimer's, with a special note on the benefit of Medicare spending in the dental field and Alzheimer's prevention.

HEALTH ISSUES AFFECTING ALZHEIMER'S DISEASE

Cardiovascular Health

Many factors related to cardiovascular health increase the risks of Alzheimer's [23, 24]. Midlife obesity, hypertension, and high cholesterol are all associated with an increased risk of dementia [25–27]. A study that followed Americans from 1987 to 2017 revealed that individuals with hypertension in midlife had a significant risk factor for cognitive decline [28]. In a 2014 study, Dr. Gottesman et al. found hypertension was associated with 39% greater odds of dementia [29]. Another study of over 500 people born the same week in 1946 measured blood pressure, cognitive assessments, and PET imaging at ages 36, 43, 53, 60–64, and 69 years. Results showed that elevated blood pressure in middle age resulted in drastic increases in dementia later in life, smaller brain volume, and increased blood vessel damage [30].

Discussion

Taking blood pressure is considered standard of care in dentistry. On every patient at every visit blood pressure is taken and recorded, which enables clinicians to see subtle increases that may indicate systemic issues. Dental providers see patients as often as four times more per year than their general practitioners. Panoramic radiographs are taken during regular assessments by most dental practices at initial visits, and every 3–5 years following. The radiographs allow practitioners to see cysts, tumors, wisdom teeth, the temporomandibular joint, and bone abnormalities, including bone loss from periodontal disease. The film can also detect any calcifications in the soft tissue area. Atherosclerotic lesions of the carotid artery occur at the bifurcation of the common carotid. When these lesions are calcified, they may present on panoramic radiographs as nodular calcifications or vertical radiopacities [31]. Often, these issues remain undetected, as they rarely produce symptoms. Ultimately, the interruption of blood flow to the brain causes a loss of neurological function and may lead to an ischemic or hemorrhagic stroke. Stroke is a strong, independent, and potentially modifiable risk factor for all-cause dementia [32]. People who have had a stroke have nearly double the risk of developing Alzheimer's disease [33]. Clinicians should be careful to evaluate panoramic radiographs in patients who have a history of cardiovascular disease, and other risk factors such as smoking, hypercholesteremia, being overweight or having diabetes. Calcifications are also associated with oral infections and increased mortality and clinicians should carefully assess panoramic radiographs to intercept calcified atherosclerotic lesions of the carotid artery [34]. By remaining vigilant while reviewing radiographs, dental professionals can help identify potential risk factors that may be early indicators of Alzheimer's.

Smoking

Smoking is linked to vascular problems, which is a contributor to Alzheimer's. This may be by way of strokes or smaller brain bleeds, but toxins in cigarette smoke increase oxidative stress and inflammation, which have been linked to Alzheimer's. A 2017 study found that a smoking habit increases the chance of dementia later in life [29]. Studies have found that smokers have reduced brain size, specifically in the cortex, which is responsible for many mental tasks including visual processing and complex abstract thinking [35]. Smoking is a leading cause of preventable death [36], so many smokers may actually die before they reach the age when dementia develops. Therefore, it is difficult for data to be conclusive as to how severely smoking is related to AD, but we know there is a strong correlation [37]. Fortunately, by quitting smoking, damage can at least be partially reversed [36].

Discussion

Smoking cessation programs within the dental practice are already being done, lending itself to individualized support. Dental practitioners have the availability to follow the 5 A's smoking cessation plan (ask, advise, assess, assist and arrange) developed by the US Public Health Service to enhance motivation for smokers to change their behavior [38]. Whether clinicians refer services, write a prescription, or perhaps even assess current smoking status by measuring exhaled carbon monoxide levels, they have the potential to change the lives of smoking patients. Through support, care, and education dental professionals can help to illustrate to patients the dangers of smoking concerning risk of AD.

Sleep

Sleep is critical to overall wellness [39, 40]. It helps to refresh the brain, clean out waste products [41], and replenishes nutrients. Impaired sleep effects the glymphatic system, the system that clears the brains waste products, and new research suggest that there may be a causal relationship between inadequate sleep and dementias [42]. Sleep cleans the hippocampus which facilitates consolidation of memories, which is a crucial step in being able to take in and process new information [43]. Getting proper amounts of sleep can help with most systemic ailments, from lowering blood pressure, reducing depression, obesity, regulating blood sugar, and strengthening the immune system. Proper sleep has been shown to increase amyloid clearance from the brain, and new research shows that people getting proper sleep make less amyloid [44–46]. Other studies have found that a lack of deep sleep is associated with higher tau levels, which forms toxic tangles inside brain cells and may be linked to Alzheimer's [47].

Sleep apnea, a condition that happens when the airway becomes blocked or collapses during the night, has been associated with numerous contributory factors for AD [48, 49]. According to the American Sleep Apnea Association, about 22 million Americans have sleep apnea [50]. A 2013 study found that older adults who experience fragmented sleep, such as that caused by sleep apnea, are more prone to develop Alzheimer's disease [13].

Discussion

Dentistry has become a force to help patients with sleep apnea Dental professional's contribution to patient care in this area should include assisting in diagnosing and to referring to other healthcare specialists, and to determining when dental therapies are of value, e.g., and even treating mild to moderate apnea with mandibular advancement devices [51, 52]. The collaboration between dentists and sleep physicians is growing stronger by the day. Being able to execute simple questionnaires like the STOP Bang and the Epworth Sleepiness Scale can help identify potential risk factors. Additionally, indicators of sleep disordered breathing, such as a scalloped tongue, large tonsils, a red beaten uvula, or grinding patterns [53], can be noted with a simple cursory look during an oral cancer exam. Two of the quickest and most simple assessments are the Malampatti score and tonsil grading that are incredible evaluators and teaching tools for the patient. Dental professionals are educators and pivotal in the discussion of risks, referrals, and treatment options of disordered sleep, which may help to lower patient's risk of developing Alzheimer's disease [54, 55].

Inflammatory Pathogens

Compelling active research regarding microbes, the immune system and the oral cavity and their interaction with inflammation keeps periodontal disease at the forefront of systemic discussions [56]. Many studies have shown that older people with periodontal disease may have an increased risk of Alzheimer's [57–59]. Inflammation causes neural damage from the cascade of events of the central nervous system starting with pro-inflammatory cytokines such as C-reactive proteins, tumor necrosis factor-a, interleukin-1 and interleukin-6 [60]. Periodontal pathogens such as Porphyromonas gingivalis, Treponema denticola, Prevotella intermedia, and even HSV1 (cold sores) may all be implicated in Alzheimer's [61–64].

Dr. Judith Miklossy has been studying spirochetes for 3 decades. She was one of the first to demonstrate spirochetes in brain matter. *In vivo* and *in vitro* spirochetes were able to reproduce the clinical, pathological and biological hallmarks of AD. These results fulfilled Hill's criteria and confirmed a causal relationship [65]. A 2021 report revealed *T. denticola* as a potential contributing factor, along with *P. gingivalis*, as risk factors for AD. The research group found that *T. denticola* had the ability to enter the brain and increased the expression of amyloid-β (the hallmark in AD), although the mechanism is unclear [66].

It has been reported that amyloid forms almost instantly around viruses and bacteria, and that infections, including mild ones that produce only minimal symptoms, fire up the immune system in the brain and leave a debris trail that is the hallmark for Alzheimer's [67, 68]. When a virus or bacterium sneaks past the blood-brain barrier, which becomes leaky with age, the brain's defense system is triggered. To combat the intruder, the brain makes amyloid to act as a sticky web to trap the intruder. The beta-amyloid is an antimicrobial peptide (basically, a protein) that the immune system creates to physically trap germs, so what is left is a webby plaque seen in the brains of those with Alzheimer's [69]. Some Alzheimer's researchers are convinced that microbes are causative in Alzheimer's [70, 71]. *P. gingivalis* is a high risk, red complex periodontal pathogen [72]. There is increasing evidence implicating the polymicrobial infection with *P. gingivalis* as playing a part in disease pathogenesis, not only from the low-grade inflammation but the actual translocation into the brain vasculature [64]. A link between Alzheimer's and *P. gingivalis* in the brain is consistent with this emerging model for microbes in the disease's etiology [58, 73–75].

Discussion

There is mounting evidence of periodontal disease impacting altering, systemic health negatively. There are independent associations between periodontal disease and a host of systemic diseases including but not limited to: diabetes, cardiovascular diseases, certain cancers, and cognitive diseases [76, 77]. The activities in health and disease within the gut, the brain and the oral cavity seem to have overlapping consequences. For example, individuals with chronic local inflammation due to periodontal disease have corresponding changes within the gut, to include a link to inflammatory bowel disease [78]. A growing body of clinical and experimental evidence suggests that gut microbiota may contribute to and influence brain disorders [79].

Treating patient's periodontal disease and preventing future events has long been a goal of dental professionals. The strong evidence that reducing oral inflammation, created by infections of the periodontia, contributes to a reduction in systemic inflammation, reinforces the concept that dental providers have a responsibility to help in treating a patient's total health, which in turn may reduce the possibility of many systemic diseases including Alzheimer's. We are the only licensed professionals with this capability, so it is essential to educate ourselves and our patients about Alzheimer's related risks and their periodontal health. Whether they are a causal agent, a contributory agent, or an exacerbator matters not, dentistry helps communities lower their risk. Our tools, from chairside pathogen testing to the use of ozone and lasers, not to be out done by education skills and behavior change strategies, can be put to use in ways to mitigate yet another disease.

Diabetes

Nearly 36% of all U.S. adults and 50% of those 60 years or older are estimated to have metabolic syndrome, a combination of health conditions such as obesity, high blood pressure, insulin resistance, type 2 diabetes, or a poor lipid profile [80]. The correlation between diabetes and risk for Alzheimer's has been the focus of numerous studies [81, 82]. Additionally, there is a new type of diabetes being studied, type 3, which is also strongly correlated with Alzheimer's [83]. People with type 2 diabetes may be twice as likely to develop Alzheimer's, and those with prediabetes or metabolic syndrome may have an increased risk for having predementia or mild cognitive impairment [84]. Those with high blood sugar, whether technically diabetic or not, have a faster cognitive decline rate than those with normal blood sugar [85].

Discussion

Oral health professionals have long been aware of the complications of hypoglycemia in patients with diabetes. Many oral health professionals scrutinize health histories, question patients, and check their blood glucose levels, yet there is a need to increase the monitoring of diabetes during dental visits. In 2018, the American Dental Association added CDT code D0411 for chairside HbA1c, and in 2019 code D0412 to check blood glucose levels. This was not put in place for the expectation to diagnose diabetes, but to help monitor patients during dental procedures. Chairside screening and referral may improve prediabetes and diabetes diagnosis. Point of care testing, specifically in dental practices, can play a vital role in the early detection of type 2 diabetes [86]. Many individuals may not seek diabetic testing due to fear. Dental practitioners often have strong, trusting relationships with patients that may help them feel more comfortable discussing health concerns, like diabetes and Alzheimer's. These are incredible opportunities for dental professionals to help in early detection.

Special Note on Medicare

Having access to dental care is difficult for many US populations especially the elderly and not having access is associated with cognitive decline [87]. It would be kinder and fiscally more responsible to extend Medicare benefits to dentistry if it lowers the cases of a disease projected to affect so many people in such a near future. In 2020, Alzheimer's and other dementias cost the nation ~$305 and $206 billion in Medicare and Medicaid payments [2]. If dental care were added to Medicare, it may help to reduce the flood of cases. Unless a treatment to slow, stop or prevent this disease is developed, in 2050, Alzheimer's cost is projected to exceed $1.1 trillion. This dramatic rise includes more than 4-fold increases in government spending under Medicare and Medicaid, and in out-of-pocket spending [2].

Medicare beneficiaries with Alzheimer's regularly have other chronic conditions, such as heart disease, diabetes, and kidney disease, and require more skilled nursing, home health, and hospital stays per year than other older people [2]. Not only are there regulations as to whether dental professionals can even do services in a care facility depending on state governing bodies, but there are minimal state and federal guidelines regarding dental care. The inclusion of dental services in Medicare may help to combat the ravages of Alzheimer's disease and curtail the rapid rise in diagnosis rates.

CONCLUSION

Successful healthcare is not just the proper management of disease, but it includes strong prevention strategies. Something must be done to spread knowledge on preventive measures to help slow down the rate of Alzheimer's disease. The goal of this perspective piece is to provide examples for the need to bring dentistry into the fold of interdisciplinary approaches in healthcare. The utilization of *all* healthcare providers is essential along with universal education, partnerships, and healthcare coverage. Many of our communities are left behind due to access and cost and many professionals are not willing to serve those regions. Dental professionals focus on disease prevention, health promotion and often form long-term relationships with their patients. The nature of these relationships can help dental professionals notice subtle changes that may be indicators of a future Alzheimer's diagnosis, and preventative care and education can then be advised. New roles are emerging to help address specific treatment needs and access to dental care, but much more must be done. Many dental hygienists are open to not only expanding services into the underserved communities but working within other healthcare areas such as hospitals and physicians' offices. Including dental care coverage to Medicare would be advantageous but making needed changes will not be easy. Innovative collaborative efforts must be made, and dental professionals are uniquely situated to help roll back the tide of this horrible disease.

For further information you may be interested in attend consensus conferences addressing oral systemic health, collaboration and integration principles. Some examples include, but not limited to, The Santa Fe Group *Oral Health into Overall Health* https://santafegroup.org/

events/ The American Academy of Oral Systemic Health *Collaboration Cures* https://www.aaosh.org/2021-scientific-session The Dental Integration Conference *A Time That's Come* https://www.dentalintegrationconference.com

AUTHOR CONTRIBUTIONS

AOR conceived and presented the idea and wrote the perspective article based upon their opinion and data supporting that opinion.

REFERENCES

1. *Encyclopedia of Neuroscience.* 1st ed. Available from: https://www.elsevier.com/books/encyclopedia-of-neuroscience/squire/978-0-08-044617-2 (accessed April 7, 2021).
2. *Facts and Figures. Alzheimer's Disease and Dementia.* Available from: https://www.alz.org/alzheimers-dementia/facts-figures (accessed February 28, 2021).
3. *Alzheimer's Disease a Much Larger Cause of Death Than Previously Recognized.* Available from: https://www.rush.edu/news/alzheimers-disease-much-larger-cause-death-previously-recognized (accessed February 28, 2021).
4. Cummings JL, Morstorf T, Zhong K. Alzheimer's disease drug-development pipeline: few candidates, frequent failures. *Alzheimers Res Ther.* (2014) 6:37. doi: 10.1186/alzrt269
5. Broom GM, Shaw IC, Rucklidge JJ. The ketogenic diet as a potential treatment and prevention strategy for Alzheimer's disease. *Nutrition.* (2019) 60:118–21. doi: 10.1016/j.nut.2018.10.003
6. Sun B-L, Li W-W, Zhu C, Jin W-S, Zeng F, Liu Y-H, et al. Clinical research on Alzheimer's disease: progress and perspectives. *Neurosci Bull.* (2018) 34:1111–8. doi: 10.1007/s12264-018-0249-z
7. Berkowitz CL, Mosconi L, Rahman A, Scheyer O, Hristov H, Isaacson RS. Clinical application of APOE in Alzheimer's prevention: a precision medicine approach. *J Prev Alzheimers Dis.* (2018) 5:245–52. doi: 10.14283/jpad.2018.35
8. *Diabetes and Alzheimer's Disease: Can Tea Phytochemicals Play a Role in Prevention?* IOS Press. Available from: https://content.iospress.com/articles/journal-of-alzheimers-disease/jad161200 (accessed April 6, 2021).
9. Mander BA, Winer JR, Jagust WJ, Walker MP. Sleep: a novel mechanistic pathway, biomarker, and treatment target in the pathology of Alzheimer's disease? *Trends Neurosci.* (2016) 39:552–66. doi: 10.1016/j.tins.2016.05.002
10. De la Rosa A, Olaso-Gonzalez G, Arc-Chagnaud C, Millan F, Salvador-Pascual A, García-Lucerga C, et al. Physical exercise in the prevention and treatment of Alzheimer's disease. *J Sport Health Sci.* (2020) 9:394–404. doi: 10.1016/j.jshs.2020.01.004
11. Livingston G, Huntley J, Sommerlad A, Ames D, Ballard C, Banerjee S, et al. Dementia prevention, intervention, and care: 2020 report of the Lancet Commission. *Lancet.* (2020) 396:413–46. doi: 10.1016/S0140-6736(20)30367-6
12. WHO. *Risk Reduction of Cognitive Decline Dementia.* WHO. World Health Organization. Available from: http://www.who.int/mental_health/neurology/dementia/guidelines_risk_reduction/en/ (accessed February 28, 2021).
13. Lim ASP, Kowgier M, Yu L, Buchman AS, Bennett DA. Sleep fragmentation and the risk of incident alzheimer's disease and cognitive decline in older persons. *Sleep.* (2013) 36:1027–32. doi: 10.5665/sleep.2802
14. Irwin MR, Vitiello MV. Implications of sleep disturbance and inflammation for Alzheimer's disease dementia. *Lancet Neurol.* (2019) 18:296–306. doi: 10.1016/S1474-4422(18)30450-2
15. Wennberg AMV, Wu MN, Rosenberg PB, Spira AP. Sleep disturbance, cognitive decline, and dementia: a review. *Semin Neurol.* (2017) 37:395–406. doi: 10.1055/s-0037-1604351
16. Ma Y, Liang L, Zheng F, Shi L, Zhong B, Xie W. Association between sleep duration and cognitive decline. *JAMA Netw Open.* (2020) 3:e2013573. doi: 10.1001/jamanetworkopen.2020.13573
17. Wang RP-H, Ho Y-S, Leung WK, Goto T, Chang RC-C. Systemic inflammation linking chronic periodontitis to cognitive decline. *Brain Behav Immun.* (2019) 81:63–73. doi: 10.1016/j.bbi.2019.07.002
18. Matsushita K, Yamada-Furukawa M, Kurosawa M, Shikama Y. Periodontal disease and periodontal disease-related bacteria involved in the pathogenesis of Alzheimer's disease. *JIR.* (2020) 13:275–83. doi: 10.2147/JIR.S255309
19. Gaur S, Agnihotri R. Alzheimer's disease and chronic periodontitis: is there an association? *Geriatr Gerontol Int.* (2015) 15:391–404. doi: 10.1111/ggi.12425
20. Beason-Held LL, Goh JO, An Y, Kraut MA, O'Brien RJ, Ferrucci L, et al. Changes in brain function occur years before the onset of cognitive impairment. *J Neurosci.* (2013) 33:18008–14. doi: 10.1523/JNEUROSCI.1402-13.2013
21. Younes L, Albert M, Moghekar A, Soldan A, Pettigrew C, Miller MI. Identifying changepoints in biomarkers during the preclinical phase of Alzheimer's disease. *Front Aging Neurosci.* (2019) 11:74. doi: 10.3389/fnagi.2019.00074
22. Kang J, Wu B, Bunce D, Ide M, Aggarwal VR, Pavitt S, et al. Bidirectional relations between cognitive function and oral health in ageing persons: a longitudinal cohort study. *Age Ageing.* (2020) 49:793–9. doi: 10.1093/ageing/afaa025
23. Lamar M, Boots EA, Arfanakis K, Barnes LL, Schneider JA. Common brain structural alterations associated with cardiovascular disease risk factors and Alzheimer's dementia: future directions and implications. *Neuropsychol Rev.* (2020) 30:546–57. doi: 10.1007/s11065-020-09460-6
24. Song R, Xu H, Dintica CS, Pan K-Y, Qi X, Buchman AS, et al. Associations between cardiovascular risk, structural brain changes, and cognitive decline. *J Am Coll Cardiol.* (2020) 75:2525–34. doi: 10.1016/j.jacc.2020.03.053
25. Anjum I, Fayyaz M, Wajid A, Sohail W, Ali A. Does obesity increase the risk of dementia: a literature review. *Cureus.* (2018) 10. doi: 10.7759/cureus.2660
26. Lennon MJ, Koncz R, Sachdev PS. Hypertension and Alzheimer's disease: is the picture any clearer? *Curr Opin Psychiatry.* (2021) 34:142–8. doi: 10.1097/YCO.0000000000000684
27. Sáiz-Vazquez O, Puente-Martínez A, Ubillos-Landa S, Pacheco-Bonrostro J, Santabárbara J. Cholesterol and Alzheimer's Disease risk: a meta-meta-Analysis. *Brain Sci.* (2020) 10:386. doi: 10.3390/brainsci10060386
28. Walker KA, Sharrett AR, Wu A, Schneider ALC, Albert M, Lutsey PL, et al. Association of midlife to late-life blood pressure patterns with incident dementia. *JAMA.* (2019) 322:535. doi: 10.1001/jama.2019.10575
29. Walker KA, Power MC, Gottesman RF. Defining the relationship between hypertension, cognitive decline, and dementia: a review. *Curr Hypertens Rep.* (2017) 19:24. doi: 10.1007/s11906-017-0724-3
30. Lane CA, Barnes J, Nicholas JM, Sudre CH, Cash DM, Parker TD, et al. Associations between blood pressure across adulthood and late-life brain structure and pathology in the neuroscience substudy of the 1946 British birth cohort (Insight 46): an epidemiological study. *Lancet Neurol.* (2019) 18:942–52. doi: 10.1016/S1474-4422(19)30228-5
31. Friedlander AH, Friedlander IK. Identification of stroke prone patients by panoramic radiography. *Aust Dent J.* (1998) 43:51–4. doi: 10.1111/j.1834-7819.1998.tb00153.x
32. Kuzma E, Lourida I, Moore SF, Levine DA, Ukoumunne OC, Llewellyn DJ. Stroke and dementia risk: a systematic review and meta-analysis. *Alzheimers Dement.* (2018) 14:1416–26. doi: 10.1016/j.jalz.2018.06.3061
33. Vijayan M, Reddy PH. Stroke and vascular dementia and Alzheimer's disease - molecular links. *J Alzheimers Dis.* (2016) 54:427–43. doi: 10.3233/JAD-160527
34. Paju S, Pietiäinen M, Liljestrand JM, Lahdentausta L, Salminen A, Kopra E, et al. Carotid artery calcification in panoramic radiographs associates with oral infections and mortality. *Int Endodon J.* (2021) 54:15–25. doi: 10.1111/iej.13451
35. Hanlon CA, Owens MM, Joseph JE, Zhu X, George MS, Brady KT, et al. Lower subcortical gray matter volume in both younger smokers and established smokers relative to non-smokers. *Addict Biol.* (2016) 21:185–95. doi: 10.1111/adb.12171
36. CDC Tobacco Free. *Fast Facts.* Atlanta, GA: Centers for Disease Control and Prevention (2020). Available from: https://www.cdc.gov/tobacco/data_statistics/fact_sheets/fast_facts/index.htm; https://www.cdc.gov/tobacco/data_statistics/fact_sheets/fast_facts/index.htm (accessed February 28, 2021).

37. Liu Y, Li H, Wang J, Xue Q, Yang X, Kang Y, et al. Association of cigarette smoking with cerebrospinal fluid biomarkers of neurodegeneration, neuroinflammation, and oxidation. *JAMA Netw Open.* (2020) 3:e2018777. doi: 10.1001/jamanetworkopen.2020.18777
38. *Five Major Steps to Intervention (The "5 A's").* Available from: http://www.ahrq.gov/prevention/guidelines/tobacco/5steps.html (accessed February 28, 2021).
39. Institute of Medicine (US) Committee on Sleep Medicine and Research. Sleep disorders and sleep deprivation: an unmet public health problem. In: Colten HR, Altevogt BM, editors. *The National Academies Collection: Reports funded by National Institutes of Health.* Washington, DC: National Academies Press (2006). Available from: http://www.ncbi.nlm.nih.gov/books/NBK19960/ (accessed April 6, 2021).
40. Wang Y-H, Wang J, Chen S-H, Li J-Q, Lu Q-D, Vitiello MV, et al. Association of longitudinal patterns of habitual sleep duration with risk of cardiovascular events and all-cause mortality. *JAMA Netw Open.* (2020) 3:e205246. doi: 10.1001/jamanetworkopen.2020.5246
41. Gordleeva S, Kanakov O, Ivanchenko M, Zaikin A, Franceschi C. Brain aging and garbage cleaning : modelling the role of sleep, glymphatic system, and microglia senescence in the propagation of inflammaging. *Semin Immunopathol.* (2020) 42:647–65. doi: 10.1007/s00281-020-00816-x
42. Nedergaard M, Goldman SA. Glymphatic failure as a final common pathway to dementia. *Science.* (2020) 370:50–6. doi: 10.1126/science.abb8739
43. Rasch B, Born J. About sleep's role in memory. *Physiol Rev.* (2013) 93:681–766. doi: 10.1152/physrev.00032.2012
44. Xie L, Kang H, Xu Q, Chen MJ, Liao Y, Thiyagarajan M, et al. Sleep drives metabolite clearance from the adult brain. *Science.* (2013) 342:373–7. doi: 10.1126/science.1241224
45. Spira AP, Gamaldo AA, An Y, Wu MN, Simonsick EM, Bilgel M, et al. Self-reported sleep and β-amyloid deposition in community-dwelling older adults. *JAMA Neurol.* (2013) 70:1537–43. doi: 10.1001/jamaneurol.2013.4258
46. Winer JR, Mander BA, Kumar S, Reed M, Baker SL, Jagust WJ, et al. Sleep disturbance forecasts β-amyloid accumulation across subsequent years. *Curr Biol.* (2020) 30:4291–4298.e3. doi: 10.1016/j.cub.2020.08.017
47. Lucey BP, McCullough A, Landsness EC, Toedebusch CD, McLeland JS, Zaza AM, et al. Reduced non-rapid eye movement sleep is associated with tau pathology in early Alzheimer's disease. *Sci Transl Med.* (2019) 11:eaau6550. doi: 10.1126/scitranslmed.aau6550
48. Liguori C, Maestri M, Spanetta M, Placidi F, Bonanni E, Mercuri NB, et al. Sleep-disordered breathing and the risk of Alzheimer's disease. *Sleep Med Rev.* (2021) 55:101375. doi: 10.1016/j.smrv.2020.101375
49. Tsai M-S, Li H-Y, Huang C-G, Wang RYL, Chuang L-P, Chen N-H, et al. Risk of Alzheimer's disease in obstructive sleep apnea patients with or without treatment: real-world evidence. *Laryngoscope.* (2020) 130:2292–8. doi: 10.1002/lary.28558
50. *Sleep Apnea Information for Clinicians.* sleepapnea.org. Available from: https://www.sleepapnea.org/learn/sleep-apnea-information-clinicians/ (accessed February 28, 2021).
51. Maggard MD, Cascella M. Upper airway resistance syndrome. In: *StatPearls.* Treasure Island, FL: StatPearls Publishing (2021). Available from: http://www.ncbi.nlm.nih.gov/books/NBK564402/ (accessed April 7, 2021).
52. Francis CE, Quinnell T. Mandibular advancement devices for OSA: an alternative to CPAP? *Pulm Ther.* (2020) 7:25–36. doi: 10.1007/s41030-020-00137-2
53. Schroeder K, Gurenlian JR. Recognizing poor sleep quality factors during oral health evaluations. *Clin Med Res.* (2019) 17:20–8. doi: 10.3121/cmr.2019.1465
54. Richards KC, Gooneratne N, Dicicco B, Hanlon A, Moelter S, Onen F, et al. CPAP adherence may slow 1-year cognitive decline in older adults with mild cognitive impairment and apnea. *J Am Geriatr Soc.* (2019) 67:558–64. doi: 10.1111/jgs.15758
55. Bubu OM, Andrade AG, Umasabor-Bubu OQ, Hogan MM, Turner AD, de Leon MJ, et al. Obstructive sleep apnea, cognition and Alzheimer's disease: a systematic review integrating three decades of multidisciplinary research. *Sleep Med Rev.* (2020) 50:101250. doi: 10.1016/j.smrv.2019.101250
56. Kleinstein SE, Nelson KE, Freire M. Inflammatory networks linking oral microbiome with systemic health and disease. *J Dent Res.* (2020) 99:1131–9. doi: 10.1177/0022034520926126
57. Leira Y, Domínguez C, Seoane J, Seoane-Romero J, Pías-Peleteiro JM, Takkouche B, et al. Is periodontal disease associated with Alzheimer's disease? A systematic review with meta-analysis. *Neuroepidemiology.* (2017) 48:21–31. doi: 10.1159/000458411
58. Dominy SS, Lynch C, Ermini F, Benedyk M, Marczyk A, Konradi A, et al. Porphyromonas gingivalis in Alzheimer's disease brains: evidence for disease causation and treatment with small-molecule inhibitors. *Sci Adv.* (2019) 5:eaau3333. doi: 10.1126/sciadv.aau3333
59. Oueslati Y, Oualha L, Touil D. Periodontal Disease and its Relevance in the Etiopathogenesis of Alzheimer's disease: A Systematic Review. In: *2018 Tunisian Annual Meeting.* Monastir: EC Dental Science (2019).
60. Tonsekar PP, Jiang SS, Yue G. Periodontal disease, tooth loss and dementia: is there a link? A systematic review. *Gerodontology.* (2017) 34:151–63. doi: 10.1111/ger.12261
61. Beydoun MA, Beydoun HA, Hossain S, El-Hajj ZW, Weiss J, Zonderman AB. Clinical and bacterial markers of periodontitis and their association with incident all-cause and Alzheimer's disease dementia in a Large National Survey. *J Alzheimers Dis.* (2020) 75:157–72. doi: 10.3233/JAD-200064
62. Piacentini R, De Chiara G, Li Puma DD, Ripoli C, Marcocci ME, Garaci E, et al. HSV-1 and Alzheimer's disease: more than a hypothesis. *Front Pharmacol.* (2014) 5:97. doi: 10.3389/fphar.2014.00097
63. Dioguardi M, Crincoli V, Laino L, Alovisi M, Sovereto D, Mastrangelo F, et al. The role of periodontitis and periodontal bacteria in the onset and progression of Alzheimer's disease: a systematic review. *J Clin Med.* (2020) 9:495. doi: 10.3390/jcm9020495
64. Wadhawan A, Reynolds MA, Makkar H, Scott AJ, Potocki E, Hoisington AJ, et al. Periodontal pathogens and neuropsychiatric health. *Curr Top Med Chem.* (2020) 20:1353–97. doi: 10.2174/1568026620666200110161105
65. Miklossy J. Alzheimer's disease - a neurospirochetosis. Analysis of the evidence following Koch's and Hill's criteria. *J Neuroinflamm.* (2011) 8:90. doi: 10.1186/1742-2094-8-90
66. Su X, Tang Z, Lu Z, Liu Y, He W, Jiang J, et al. Oral treponema denticola infection induces Aβ1-40 and Aβ1-42 accumulation in the hippocampus of C57BL/6 mice. *J Mol Neurosci.* (2021). doi: 10.21203/rs.3.rs-225008/v1. [Epub ahead of print].
67. Eimer WA, Vijaya Kumar DK, Navalpur Shanmugam NK, Rodriguez AS, Mitchell T, Washicosky KJ, et al. Alzheimer's disease-associated β-amyloid is rapidly seeded by herpesviridae to protect against brain infection. *Neuron.* (2018) 99:56–63.e3. doi: 10.1016/j.neuron.2018.06.030
68. Soscia SJ, Kirby JE, Washicosky KJ, Tucker SM, Ingelsson M, Hyman B, et al. The Alzheimer's disease-associated amyloid β-protein is an antimicrobial peptide. *PLoS ONE.* (2010) 5:e9505. doi: 10.1371/journal.pone.0009505
69. Carter CJ. Genetic, transcriptome, proteomic, and epidemiological evidence for blood-brain barrier disruption and polymicrobial brain invasion as determinant factors in Alzheimer's disease. *J Alzheimer Dis Rep.* (2017) 1:125–57. doi: 10.3233/ADR-170017
70. Fang P, Kazmi SA, Jameson KG, Hsiao EY. The microbiome as a modifier of neurodegenerative disease risk. *Cell Host Microbe.* (2020) 28:201–22. doi: 10.1016/j.chom.2020.06.008
71. Sochocka M, Zwolińska K, Leszek J. The infectious etiology of Alzheimer's disease. *Curr Neuropharmacol.* (2017) 15:996–1009. doi: 10.2174/1570159X15666170313122937
72. Holt SC, Ebersole JL. *Porphyromonas gingivalis, Treponema denticola,* and *Tannerella forsythia*: the "red complex", a prototype polybacterial pathogenic consortium in periodontitis. *Periodontol 2000.* (2005) 38:72–122. doi: 10.1111/j.1600-0757.2005.00113.x
73. Olsen I, Taubman MA, Singhrao SK. *Porphyromonas gingivalis* suppresses adaptive immunity in periodontitis, atherosclerosis, and Alzheimer's disease. *J Oral Microbiol.* (2016) 8:1. doi: 10.3402/jom.v8.33029
74. Costa MJF, de Araújo IDT, da Rocha Alves L, da Silva RL, Dos Santos Calderon P, Borges BCD, et al. Relationship of *Porphyromonas gingivalis* and Alzheimer's disease: a systematic review of pre-clinical studies. *Clin Oral Investig.* (2021) 25:797–806. doi: 10.1007/s00784-020-03764-w
75. Kanagasingam S, Chukkapalli SS, Welbury R, Singhrao SK. *Porphyromonas gingivalis* is a strong risk factor for Alzheimer's disease. *J Alzheimers Dis Rep.* (2020) 4:501–11. doi: 10.3233/ADR-200250
76. Genco RJ, Sanz M. Clinical and public health implications of periodontal and systemic diseases: an overview. *Periodontol 2000.* (2020) 83:7–13. doi: 10.1111/prd.12344

77. Hajishengallis G, Chavakis T. Local and systemic mechanisms linking periodontal disease and inflammatory comorbidities. *Nat Rev Immunol.* (2021) 1–15. doi: 10.1038/s41577-020-00488-6. [Epub ahead of print].
78. Kitamoto S, Nagao-Kitamoto H, Jiao Y, Gillilland MG, Hayashi A, Imai J, et al. The intermucosal connection between the mouth and gut in commensal pathobiont-driven colitis. *Cell.* (2020) 182:447–62.e14. doi: 10.1016/j.cell.2020.05.048
79. Marizzoni M, Cattaneo A, Mirabelli P, Festari C, Lopizzo N, Nicolosi V, et al. Short-chain fatty acids and lipopolysaccharide as mediators between gut dysbiosis and amyloid pathology in Alzheimer's disease. *J Alzheimers Dis.* (2020) 78:683–97. doi: 10.3233/JAD-200306
80. Aguilar M, Bhuket T, Torres S, Liu B, Wong RJ. Prevalence of the metabolic syndrome in the United States, 2003-2012. *JAMA.* (2015) 313:1973. doi: 10.1001/jama.2015.4260
81. Khan MSH, Hegde V. Obesity and diabetes mediated chronic inflammation: a potential biomarker in Alzheimer's Disease. *J Pers Med.* (2020) 10:42. doi: 10.3390/jpm10020042
82. Stanciu GD, Bild V, Ababei DC, Rusu RN, Cobzaru A, Paduraru L, et al. Link between diabetes and Alzheimer's disease due to the shared amyloid aggregation and deposition involving both neurodegenerative changes and neurovascular damages. *J Clin Med.* (2020) 9:1713. doi: 10.3390/jcm9061713
83. *Researchers Link Alzheimer's Gene to Type 3 Diabetes.* Available form: https://newsnetwork.mayoclinic.org/; https://newsnetwork.mayoclinic.org/discussion/researchers-link-alzheimers-gene-to-type-iii-diabetes/ (accessed February 28, 2021).
84. Panza F, Frisardi V, Seripa D, P Imbimbo B, Sancarlo D, D'Onofrio G, et al. Metabolic Syndrome, Mild Cognitive Impairment and Dementia. *Curr Alzheimer Res.* (2011) 8:492–509. doi: 10.2174/156720511796391818
85. Zheng F, Yan L, Yang Z, Zhong B, Xie W. HbA1c, diabetes and cognitive decline: the english longitudinal study of ageing. *Diabetologia.* (2018) 61:839–48. doi: 10.1007/s00125-017-4541-7
86. Montero E, Matesanz P, Nobili A, Luis Herrera-Pombo J, Sanz M, Guerrero A, et al. Screening of undiagnosed hyperglycaemia in the dental setting: the DiabetRisk study. A field trial. *J Clin Periodontol.* (2021) 48:378–88. doi: 10.1111/jcpe.13408
87. Han SH, Wu B, Burr JA. Edentulism and trajectories of cognitive functioning among older adults: the role of dental care service utilization. *J Aging Health.* (2020) 32:744–52. doi: 10.1177/0898264319851654

16

Can the Salivary Microbiome Predict Cardiovascular Diseases? Lessons Learned from the Qatari Population

*Selvasankar Murugesan[1], Mohammed Elanbari[2], Dhinoth Kumar Bangarusamy[1], Annalisa Terranegra[1] and Souhaila Al Khodor[1]**

[1] *Mother and Child Health Department, Sidra Medicine, Doha, Qatar,* [2] *Clinical Research Center Department, Sidra Medicine, Doha, Qatar*

Correspondence:
Souhaila Al Khodor
salkhodor@sidra.org

Background: Many studies have linked dysbiosis of the gut microbiome to the development of cardiovascular diseases (CVD). However, studies assessing the association between the salivary microbiome and CVD risk on a large cohort remain sparse. This study aims to identify whether a predictive salivary microbiome signature is associated with a high risk of developing CVD in the Qatari population.

Methods: Saliva samples from 2,974 Qatar Genome Project (QGP) participants were collected from Qatar Biobank (QBB). Based on the CVD score, subjects were classified into low-risk (LR < 10) ($n = 2491$), moderate-risk (MR = 10–20) ($n = 320$) and high-risk (HR > 30) ($n = 163$). To assess the salivary microbiome (SM) composition, 16S-rDNA libraries were sequenced and analyzed using QIIME-pipeline. Machine Learning (ML) strategies were used to identify SM-based predictors of CVD risk.

Results: *Firmicutes* and *Bacteroidetes* were the predominant phyla among all the subjects included. Linear Discriminant Analysis Effect Size (LEfSe) analysis revealed that *Clostridiaceae* and *Capnocytophaga* were the most significantly abundant genera in the LR group, while *Lactobacillus* and *Rothia* were significantly abundant in the HR group. ML based prediction models revealed that *Desulfobulbus, Prevotella*, and *Tissierellaceae* were the common predictors of increased risk to CVD.

Conclusion: This study identified significant differences in the SM composition in HR and LR CVD subjects. This is the first study to apply ML-based prediction modeling using the SM to predict CVD in an Arab population. More studies are required to better understand the mechanisms of how those microbes contribute to CVD.

Keywords: CVD, salivary microbiome, precision medicine, machine learning, QGP

INTRODUCTION

Non-communicable Diseases (NCDs) are the leading cause of death globally (Allen et al., 2017). According to the World Health Organization [WHO] (2013) report, the global burden of non-communicable diseases (NCDs) raised to 82% by 2020. The most common NCDs are cardiovascular diseases (CVD), cancer, respiratory disorders, and diabetes (Balakumar et al., 2016).

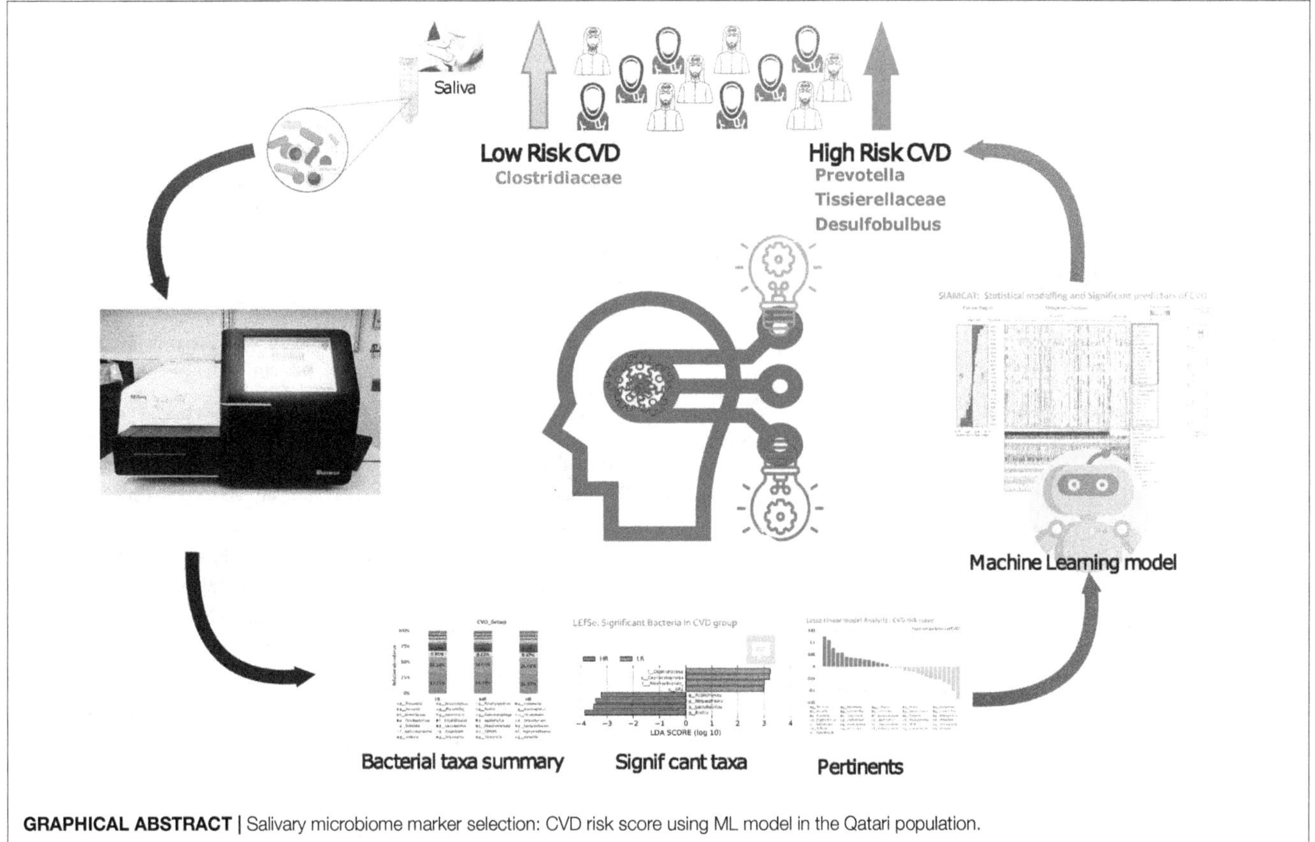

GRAPHICAL ABSTRACT | Salivary microbiome marker selection: CVD risk score using ML model in the Qatari population.

CVD comprises coronary heart disease, heart failure, stroke, rheumatic heart disease, and cardiomyopathies among others (Caldwell et al., 2019). CVD is the leading cause of death, claiming about 17.9 million deaths annually and increasing worldwide (Lear et al., 2017; Al-Shamsi et al., 2019).

In Qatar, NCDs are the leading cause of death for the past 10 years (Al-Kaabi and Atherton, 2015) with the CVD mortality rates reaching 8.3 per 100000 MOPH (2020). In addition, the 2006-World-Health-Survey revealed that the Qatari population suffers from various predisposing factors to CVD such as obesity (28.8%), high cholesterol (24.7%), diabetes (16.7%), and hypertension (14.4%) Haj Bakri and Al-Thani (2012).

In the past decade, advances in the multi-omics technologies have enhanced our chances to discover novel biomarkers (Olivier et al., 2019). Blood-based biomarkers are considered invasive, there is an urgent need to use non-invasive samples such as saliva to develop new disease biomarkers. In addition, the advance in Next-Generation Sequencing platforms (NGS) has enabled us to assess the human microbiome with an unprecedented resolution and depth. Using the human microbiome composition to identify disease biomarkers is the next chapter of precision medicine (Morganti et al., 2019; Zhong et al., 2021).

The human microbiome (HM) comprises trillions of bacteria, viruses, protozoa, and fungi that reside in and on our body surfaces (Amon and Sanderson, 2017). The HM is complex, dynamic, ubiquitous, and shows striking variability from one individual to another and between various body sites (Ursell et al., 2012; Aagaard et al., 2013). The HM has a wide array of roles ranging from digestion, protection from pathogens, immune-regulation, and metabolites production (Marchesi et al., 2016). The oral cavity harbors more than 700 diverse microorganisms and is considered the second most diverse site after the gut (Deo and Deshmukh, 2019). In healthy subjects, the core salivary microbiome (SM) includes genera *Streptococcus, Veillonella, Neisseria,* and *Actinomyces* (Zaura et al., 2009, 2014). In a large-scale population-based Japanese study, the authors showed that the SM is dominated by *Streptococcus, Neisseria, Rothia, Prevotella, Actinomyces, Granulicatella, Haemophilus,* and *Porphyromonas* (Yamashita and Takeshita, 2017). Our previous study aiming to characterize the salivary microbiome composition in the Qatari population (Murugesan et al., 2020) showed that *Bacteroidetes, Firmicutes, Actinobacteria,* and *Proteobacteria* were the common phyla, with *Bacteroidetes* being the most predominant (Murugesan et al., 2020). Dysbiosis in the SM is associated with oral diseases (Mashima et al., 2017; Davis et al., 2020) and systemic diseases like obesity, diabetes, and CVD (Wade, 2013; Kholy et al., 2015; Cortez et al., 2019).

Advances in Machine Learning (ML) technologies, an essential branch of artificial intelligence, have enabled researchers to build prediction biomarker models for various diseases such as arthritis, diabetes, and inflammatory bowel disease (Jamshidi et al., 2019; Aryal et al., 2020; Kohli et al., 2020). On the other hand, few studies have trained ML models using the gut microbiome profiles to identify predictors of atherosclerosis and CVD (Aryal et al., 2020; Liu et al., 2020) and none have used the SM so far.

This study aims to identify whether a predictive salivary microbiome signature is associated with a high risk of developing CVD in the Qatari population. We integrated the phenotypic, clinical, and microbiome data, and we identified SM-biomarkers associated with an increased risk to CVD using ML models.

MATERIALS AND METHODS

Ethics Statement

The study was approved by the Institutional Review Board (IRB) of Sidra Medicine under (protocol #1510001907) and by Qatar Biobank (QBB) (protocol #E/2018/QBB-RES-ACC-0063/0022. All study participants signed an informed consent before sample collection. All experiments were performed under the approved guidelines.

Clinical Data

We collected de-identified saliva samples, phenotypic and clinical data from a total of 2,974 participants enrolled in the Qatar genome project (QGP). QGP included any adult who is either a Qatari national or long-term resident (lived in Qatar for at least 15 years) and can contribute to QBB around 3 h of their time for answering all the questionnaires, complete measurements, imaging and fitness assessments, in addition to providing all the samples required including saliva. In the pilot phase, the cohort consisted of 1,432 males and 1,542 females (**Table 1**). Each subject's anthropometric and blood parameters were established by analyzing body mass index (BMI), total protein content, hemoglobin, albumin, ferritin, calcium, iron, vitamin-D, high or low-density lipoprotein cholesterol (HDL, LDL), triglycerides, and glucose levels.

Calculation of Cardiovascular Diseases Risk Score

Cox proportional-hazards regression has been used to evaluate the risk of developing CVD over 10-years. The CVD-risk score for 2974 patients was estimated using sex-specific multivariable factors consisting of age, total-Cholesterol, HDL, systolic blood pressure (BP), hypertension treatment, smoking, and diabetes status (HbA1C $\geq$ 6.5%, and participants who confirmed having diabetes). D'Agostino et al. (2013) adapted the regression coefficient for the functions from earlier analysis. This method uses the following equation:

$$\hat{p} = 1 - S_0(t)^{\exp(\sum_{i=1}^{p} \beta_i x_i - \sum_{i=1}^{p} \beta_i \bar{x}_i)}$$

Where $S_0(t)$, baseline survival at follow-up time t (here $t = 10$ years); β_i, estimated regression coefficient (log hazard ratio that is measured for all risk functions and sex-specific); x_i, log-transformed value of the ith risk factor; i, corresponding mean, p, number of risk factors.

Sample Collection

Qatar Biobank collected saliva samples according to standard procedure. They organized to collect 5 mL of spontaneous, whole, unstimulated saliva into a 50 mL sterile DNA-free Falcon tube from each participant by spitting. The samples were divided into 0.4 mL aliquots and stored at −80 C until further analysis. The aliquots were received from QBB for total salivary DNA extraction.

DNA Extraction and 16S rRNA Gene Sequencing

The total salivary DNA was extracted using automated QIAsymphony protocol (Qiagen, Hilden, Germany), following the Manufacturer's instructions. DNA purity was evaluated by the A260/A280 ratio using a NanoDrop 7000 Spectrophotometer (Thermo Fisher Scientific, Waltham, MA, United States), and the DNA integrity was checked on a 1% agarose by gel electrophoresis.

The V1–V3 regions of the 16S rRNA gene were amplified using Illumina NextEra XT library preparation Kit (FC-131-1002). Step 1 PCR is performed using 10 ng of template DNA for 50 μL PCR reaction using 2X Phusion Hot Start Ready mix (Thermo Fisher Scientific^{TM}). The following thermal cycling conditions were used: 5 min of initial denaturation at 94°C; 25 cycles of denaturation at 94 C for 30 s, annealing at 55°C for 30 s, extension at 72 C for 30 s; and a final extension at 72 C for 5 min. According to the Manufacturer's instructions, the amplified PCR products of approximately 550 bp in size was purified using AgenCourt AMPure XP magnetic beads (Beckman Coulter). Purified PCR products of STEP 1 was used as template for amplification of STEP 2 NextEra index PCR using thermocycling conditions of 5 min of initial denaturation at 94°C; 8 cycles of denaturation at 94 C for 30 s, annealing at 55°C for 30 s, extension at 72 C for 30 s; and a final extension at 72 C for 5 min. These PCR products were purified using AgenCourt AMPure XP magnetic beads and purified products were pooled in equimolar concentrations. High-throughput sequencing was performed using an Illumina MiSeq 2 × 300 platform following the manufacturer's instructions.

16S rRNA Sequencing Data Analysis

Demultiplexed sequence data were revised for quality control using FastQC (Andrews, 2010). PEAR tool was used to merge both forward and reverse sequence reads of respective samples (Zhang et al., 2014), and sequence reads of quality score <20 were discarded. All merged reads were trimmed to 160 bp > Reads < 500 bp using the Trimmomatic tool (Bolger et al., 2014). Trimmed FASTQ files were converted into FASTA files. Demultiplexed FASTA files were analyzed using Quantitative Insights Into Microbial Ecology (QIIME) v1.9.0 pipeline (Caporaso et al., 2010; Murugesan et al., 2020). Operational taxonomic units (OTUs) were generated by aligning against the Greengenes database (Version: 13_8) with a confidence threshold of 97% (DeSantis et al., 2006).

Statistical Taxonomic and Diversity Analyses

Linear Discriminant Analysis Effect Size (LEfSe) (Segata et al., 2011) was used to find differentially abundant taxa between the studied categories. Alpha diversity measures including Chao1, Observed, Shannon, and Simpson indices were calculated with R-phyloseq package (McMurdie and Holmes, 2013). The alpha

TABLE 1 | Clinical parameters of the study cohort.

	LR (*N* = 2491)	MR (*N* = 320)	HR (*N* = 163)	*P*-value
Male (*N* = 1432)	1184	161	87	<0.001[a***]
Female (*N* = 1542)	1307	159	76	<0.001[a***]
CVD score	2.78 ± 2.48	13.89 ± 2.75	31.76 ± 11.87	<0.001[b***]
BMI	28.37 ± 5.86	30.51 ± 4.76	31.18 ± 5.80	<0.001[b***]
Age	35.11 ± 10.22	50.89 ± 7.15	55.87 ± 8.14	<0.001[b***]
APT	33.82 ± 2.97	33.82 ± 2.97	33.13 ± 3.05	0.011[b*]
Albumin (gm/L)	44.30 ± 3.31	44.16 ± 3.16	43.14 ± 3.59	0.001[b**]
Alkaline phosphatase (U/L)	70.02 ± 20.66	75.71 ± 21.32	76.39 ± 21.70	<0.001[b***]
ALT (GPT) (U/L)	22.02 ± 16.54	28.67 ± 16.15	27.72 ± 15.11	<0.001[b***]
AST (GOT) (U/L)	19.89 ± 16.80	21.08 ± 7.83	20.39 ± 7.41	<0.001[b***]
Calcium (mmol/L)	2.29 ± 0.08	2.30 ± 0.095	2.32 ± 0.10	<0.001[b***]
Cholesterol total (mmol/L)	4.92 ± 0.93	5.37 ± 1.11	5.44 ± 1.28	<0.001[b***]
C-Peptide (ng/mL)	2.14 ± 1.30	2.88 ± 2.22	2.83 ± 1.38	<0.001[b***]
Creatinine (μmol/L)	65.24 ± 13.90	74.04 ± 13.91	77.71 ± 19.86	<0.001[b***]
Dihydroxy VitD Total (ng/mL)	17.65 ± 11.46	19.57 ± 11.35	19.13 ± 9.43	<0.001[b***]
Ferritin (mcg/L)	65.02 ± 105.93	109.76 ± 96.33	124.33 ± 101.1	<0.001[b***]
Fibrinogen (gm/L)	3.29 ± 0.68	3.40 ± 0.65	3.48 ± 0.67	0.001[b**]
Folate (nmol/L)	20.64 ± 7.51	22.42 ± 7.25	22.82 ± 7.44	<0.001[b***]
Free thyroxine (pmol/L)	12.96 ± 1.89	12.73 ± 1.85	12.82 ± 1.46	0.006[b**]
Glucose (mmol/L)	5.18 ± 1.50	6.71 ± 2.91	7.92 ± 3.79	<0.001[b***]
HbA1C	5.40 ± 0.83	6.28 ± 1.56	7.14 ± 1.95	<0.001[b***]
HDL-Cholesterol (mmol/L)	1.43 ± 0.38	1.19 ± 0.30	1.12 ± 0.29	<0.001[b***]
Hemoglobin (gm/dL)	13.44 ± 1.79	14.59 ± 1.44	14.45 ± 1.56	<0.001[b***]
Insulin (mcunit/mL)	12.31 ± 14.90	19.03 ± 27.04	16.25 ± 12.89	<0.001[b***]
INR	1.05 ± 0.09	1.01 ± 0.09	1.00 ± 0.10	<0.001[b***]
Iron (μmol/L)	14.92 ± 6.71	16.59 ± 5.75	16.18 ± 5.74	<0.001[b***]
LDL-Cholesterol (mmol/L)	2.96 ± 0.87	3.29 ± 1.20	3.37 ± 1.18	<0.001[b***]
Potassium (mmol/L)	4.36 ± 0.37	4.44 ± 0.38	4.51 ± 0.42	<0.001[b***]
Total protein (gm/L)	73.67 ± 3.90	73.26 ± 3.82	73.15 ± 3.81	0.083[b]
Triglyceride (mmol/L)	1.16 ± 0.69	1.81 ± 1.18	1.94 ± 1.15	<0.00[b***]
Urea (mmol/L)	4.21 ± 1.25	4.75 ± 1.21	5.07 ± 1.84	<0.001[b***]

APT, activated partial thromboplastin time; BMI, body mass index; INR, International Normalization Ration, PT, prothrombin time; TSH, thyroid stimulating Hormone; TIBC, total iron binding capacity.
[a]Chi-square test, [b]Kruskal–Wallis test.
**P-value < 0.05, **P-value < 0.01, ***P-value < 0.001.*

diversity statistical significance was calculated using Mann–Whitney test through Minitab-17 (2010). *P*-values less than 0.05 were considered statistically significant. Differences in the beta diversity were presented as principal coordinate analysis using QIIME. Analysis of similarities (ANOSIM) was used to calculate the distance matrix difference between the categories using Bray-Curtis metric (Caporaso et al., 2010).

Supervised Machine Learning Modeling

We applied four statistical ML methods for regularization and feature selection based on penalized least squares (**Figure 1B**). The methods are the Least Absolute Shrinkage and Selection Operator (Lasso), Smoothly Clipped Absolute Deviation Penalty (Zou and Li, 2008) (SCAD), Elastic Net (Zou and Hastie, 2005) (ENet), and Minimax concave penalty (Zhang, 2010) (MCP). The methods differ by the mathematical properties of the corresponding penalties: Lasso and ENet use convex penalties, while MCP and Scad use concave penalties. We applied two transformations to the abundance-counts as in: a binary transformation (Binary), and a variance-stability transformation (Arcsin), while the CVD-score outcome was log-transformed (Dong et al., 2020). Analyses were performed using the R-packages glmnet (Hastie and Qian, 2014) and ncvreg (Breheny, 2020). The graphics were generated using the R-packages ggplot2, RVenn, and ggpubr (Wickham, 2011; Akyol, 2019; Kassambara, 2020). We randomly split the data 50-times into a training set (80%) on which the predictive-models were build and a test-set (20%) on which we tested the performance of each model. Optimal tuning parameters were chosen *via* 10-fold cross-validation.

RESULTS

Demographic and Clinical Parameters of the Study Population

The study population was composed of 2,974 Qatari participants. The cohort was classified into three CVD groups as low-risk (LR) (CVD score < 10), moderate-risk (MR) (CVD score: 10–20), and high-risk (HR) (>20), as described in the section

"Materials and Methods." As a result, 2491 participants were LR, 320 were MR, and 163 were HR (**Table 1**). The average participant's age in the HR group (55.87 ± 8.14 years) was significantly higher than those in the MR (50.89 ± 7.15 years) and LR (35.11 ± 10.22 years) groups (**Table 1**). Moreover, the BMI was significantly higher in the HR group than in the MR and LR groups (**Table 1**). In addition, among the blood parameters tested, Alkaline phosphatase, Calcium, Total-Cholesterol, LDL, Creatinine, Ferritin, Fibrinogen, Folate, Glucose, HbA1C, Urea, and Triglycerides were significantly higher in the HR group (**Table 1**).

The Salivary Microbiome Composition Reveals Signatures for Cardiovascular Diseases

After stratifying the study cohort based on the CVD risk score, we assessed the SM composition in all subjects. Then, we compared the compositional changes between different study groups. A diagram that summarizes the study design is shown in **Figures 1A,B**. The microbial sequence data generated from all the participants revealed 22 bacterial phyla, 46 classes, 87 orders, 173 families, and 390 genera. *Bacteroidetes, Firmicutes, Actinobacteria*, and *Proteobacteria* were the most abundant phyla observed in the saliva samples collected from the Qatari subjects, covering approximately 90% of total microbial abundance (**Figure 2A**). In addition, our data showed that *Streptococcus, Prevotella, Porphyromonas, Granulicatella, and Veillonella* represent the salivary core microbiome members at the genus level (**Figure 2B**).

Differential Salivary Microbial Taxa Between the High-Risk and Low-Risk-Cardiovascular Diseases Groups

After assessing the study cohort's SM, LEfSe analysis compared the salivary microbiome compositions in the LR, MR, and HR (**Figure 3**). Our data indicated that *Capnocytophaga* and *Clostridiaceae* were significantly abundant in the LR group compared to the HR group ($p < 0.0001$). In contrast, *Lactobacillus* and *Rothia* were significantly enriched in the HR group ($p < 0.0001$) (**Figure 3A**) in comparison to the LR group. *Clostridiaceae* and *Porphyromonas* were significantly increased in the LR group than MR group. *Neisseria* and *Capnocytophaga* were greatly enriched in the MR group than HR group (**Figures 3B,C**).

Alpha and beta diversity measures were calculated to assess the changes in diversity among groups (**Supplementary Figure 1**). Alpha diversity parameters revealed no significant differences observed between all groups (**Supplementary Figure 1A**). We then performed beta diversity analysis to assess the divergence in the community composition between the groups using the Bray-Curtis distance metric (**Supplementary Figure 1B**). We showed that the salivary microbiome in HR and MR were

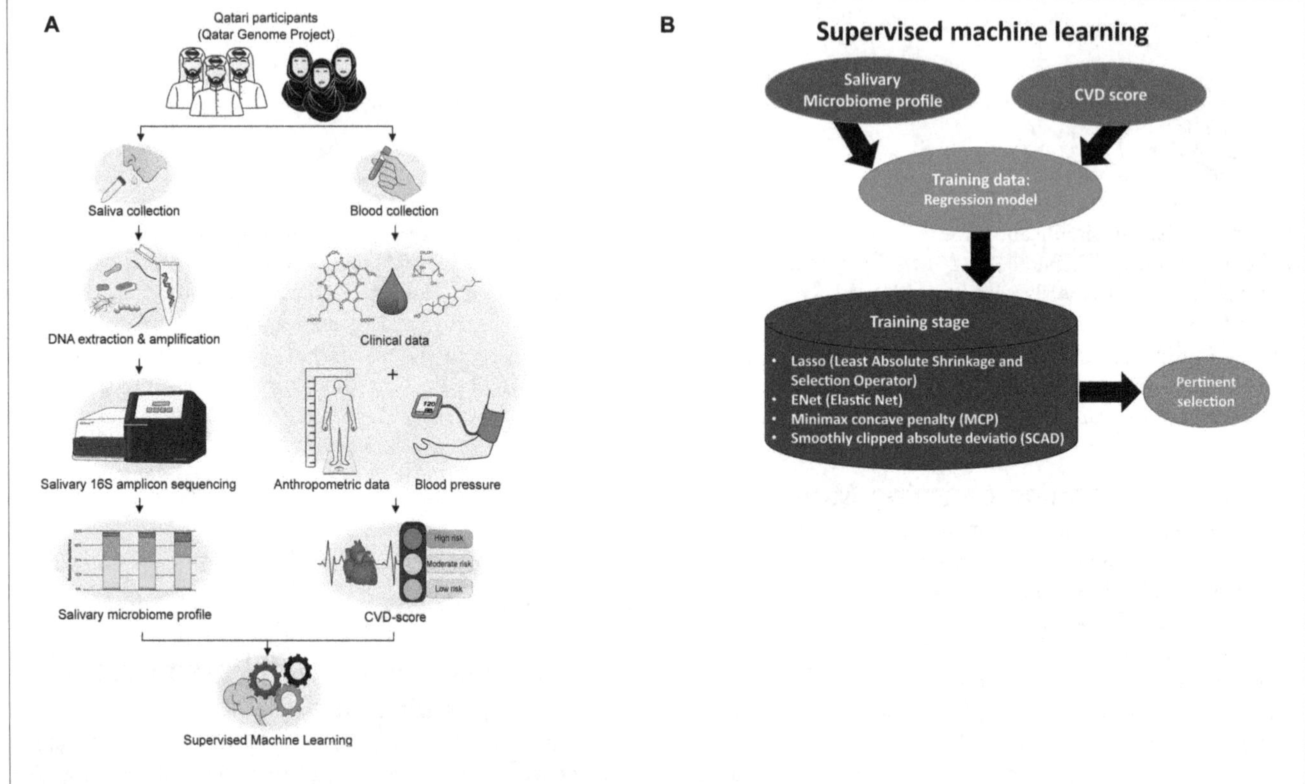

FIGURE 1 | Overall study design from participant recruitment to SM-based CVD marker selection. **(A)** The study workflow. **(B)** Strategies applied in Supervised machine learning (ML) to select pertinents.

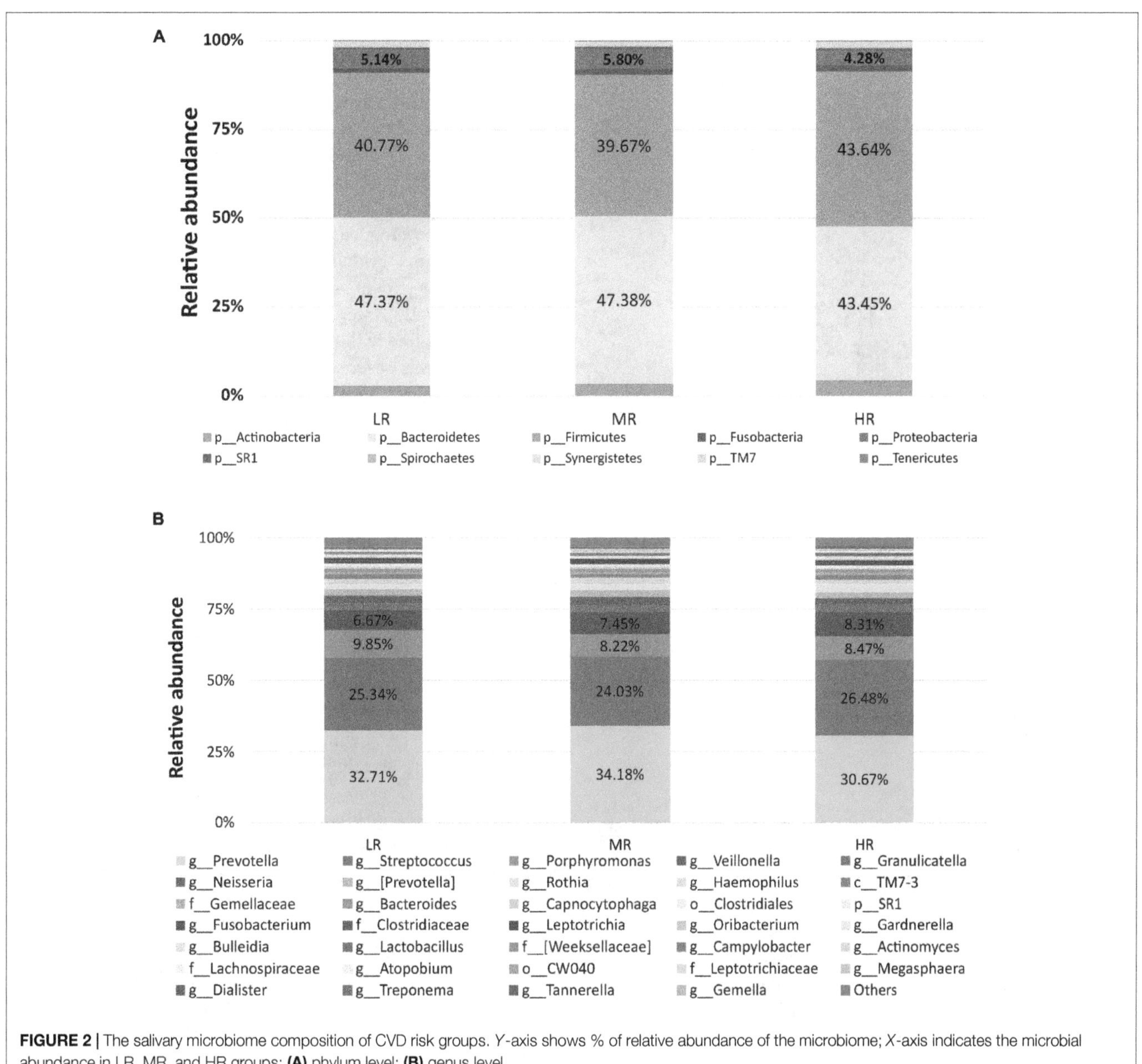

FIGURE 2 | The salivary microbiome composition of CVD risk groups. *Y*-axis shows % of relative abundance of the microbiome; *X*-axis indicates the microbial abundance in LR, MR, and HR groups; **(A)** phylum level; **(B)** genus level.

not significantly dissimilar from the LR group ($p = 0.085$) (**Supplementary Figure 1B**).

Identification of Pertinent Salivary Microbial Markers Associated With the Cardiovascular Diseases Score Using Machine Learning Models

The apparent differences between the study groups using alpha and beta diversity measures were not identified due to the significant sample size differences and imbalance. In this study, the participants were selected from the QGP Cohort, who provided saliva samples exclusively. QBB collected the biosamples from all volunteers as a sampling of Qatari population without focusing on CVD risk-based recruitment. We decided to use regression-based ML selection of pertinent SM biomarkers to avoid bias based on the sample size. The data were split 50-times randomly, using the four feature selection techniques, and the whole dataset was used without any exclusion (**Figure 1B**).

To search for pertinent variables, we focused on the abundances of SM selected at least 80% of the time among the 50-random splits of the data and the four feature selection techniques as described in the section "Materials and Methods." Our results are shown in **Figure 4**. Seven microbes were selected at least 80% of the time using the binary and Arcsin transformations by all the ML methods (Lasso, SCAD, ENet, and MCP) (**Figures 4A,B**). Three microbes were presented at all the tested models and both transformations (**Figures 4C,D**). In comparison, four microbes were specific to the binary transformation and four were particular to the Arcsin transformation (**Figure 4D**).

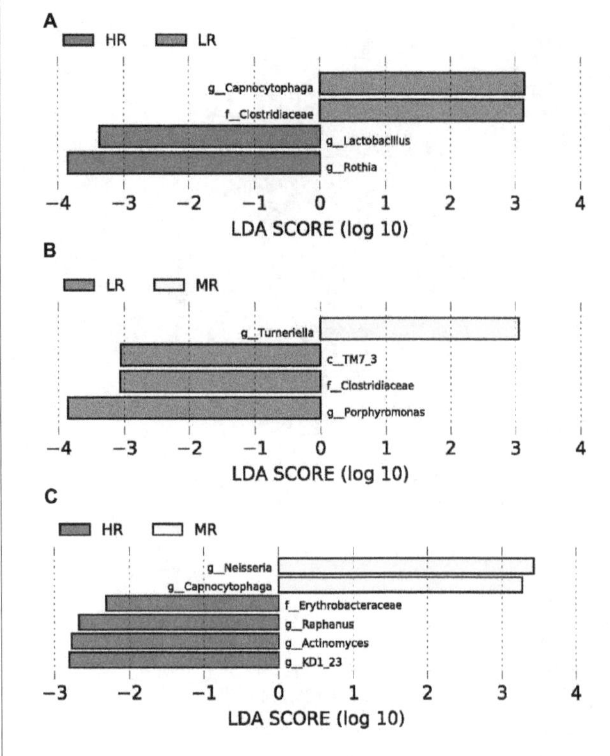

FIGURE 3 | Graphs of linear discriminant analysis (LDA) scores for differentially enriched bacterial genera among the groups. **(A)** LR (green) vs. HR (red) groups; **(B)** LR (green) vs. MR (Yellow) groups; **(C)** HR (red) vs MR (Yellow) groups.

The common microbes were *Prevotella, Tissierellaceae,* and *Desulfobulbus* (**Figure 4D**). To better understand how these microbes affect the CVD-score, we counted the sign of the regression coefficients number of times, Positive, Negative, or Zero (**Figure 4E**). From this analysis, the three microbes mentioned above contribute to an increase in the CVD score (**Figure 4E**). At the same time, our data showed that an increase in *Clostridiaceae* level contributed to a decrease in CVD-score (**Figure 4F**). Assessment using the Mean squared error (MSE) method disclosed that binary transformation has better prediction accuracy than Arcsin (**Figure 4G**).

DISCUSSION

The need for practical, non-invasive tools for predicting and preventing CVD risk has led to concerted research efforts in recent years to identify and characterize biomarkers associated with the disease as a step forward toward precision medicine. In addition, recent studies on the microbiome have enlightened its role in human health and disease (Solbiati and Frias-Lopez, 2018). Despite that, the diversity of the gut microbiome is affected by several factors like gender, ethnicity, age, and environmental factors; it was found to be associated with many diseases, including CVD and IBD using ML-models (Gulden, 2018; Chang and Kao, 2019). However, the potential use of the SM composition in assessing CVD is still lacking.

This study evaluated whether the SM composition can predict a high risk for developing CVD in a diverse Qatari population. Using a large cohort of 2,974 Qatari participants and based on the CVD risk score, we showed for the first time that the SM composition in LR and HR individuals is different (LefSe analysis). A significant SM alteration was observed between LR, MR, and HR groups (**Figures 3A–C**). Furthermore, *Capnocytophaga* and *Clostridiaceae* were significantly enriched in the LR group (**Figure 3A**). While no studies are addressing the role of *Capnocytophaga* in health and disease, a study among Japanese patients showed that non-ischemic heart failure is associated with lower levels of *Clostridiaceae* (Katsimichas et al., 2018). In line with our findings, a significant reduction of *Clostridiaceae* was observed in the HR-CVD group in the Qatari population (**Figures 3A,4D,F**).

Moreover, our data showed that *Lactobacillus* and *Rothia* were enriched in the HR group compared to the LR group (**Figure 3A**). Similarly, a study aiming to utilize the gut microbiome as a diagnostic marker of coronary artery disease (CAD) in the Japanese population has revealed that *Lactobacilli* were more abundant in patients with CAD than their matching controls (Emoto et al., 2017). On the other hand, *Rothia,* a nitrate-reducing bacterium, was enriched in hypertensive patients (Wang et al., 2021).

Next, we employed a novel approach of regression-based machine learning by combining the entire dataset of 16S rDNA sequencing data with ML models to identify the potential predictors of HR CVD without stratifying the cohort to mask the bias due to sample size differences among groups. We found that three microbes (*Prevotella, Tissierellaceae,* and *Desulfobulbus)* were represented by binary and Arcsin transformations and different training model techniques. Those were associated with high CVD-score (**Figure 4**). The Bogalusa Heart Study aimed to associate the lifetime CVD risk among the participants using the gut microbes revealed that the genus *Prevotella* was significantly enriched in the CVD HR participants (Kelly et al., 2016). Also, the role of gut microbiome in Chinese CVD patients with cardiac valve calcification revealed that *Prevotella* is a potential pathogen that is positively correlated with LDL (Liu et al., 2019). Moreover, hypertensive rats had a significant increase of *Tissierellaceae* in the gut microbiome (Sherman et al., 2018). Furthermore, *Tissierella soehngenia* was more abundant in rats with acute myocardial infarction than in the control groups (Wu et al., 2017). *Tissierellaceae* produces trimethyl amino N-oxide (TMAO), a known microbial metabolite associated with heart attack, stroke, and chronic kidney disease (Al-Obaide et al., 2017). Our study showed that *Desulfobulbus* - sulfidogenic bacterium (Devkota et al., 2012) has a positive regression coefficient with CVD scores in both trained models (**Figures 4C,D**). The elevated level of *Desulfobulbus* is known to trigger proinflammatory cytokines in patients with rheumatoid arthritis and periodontitis (Eriksson et al., 2019). Moreover, its abundance is positively correlated with age rendering it an excellent predictor to diagnose systemic diseases like diabetes and CVD (Tomas et al., 2012).

To our knowledge, this study is the first to demonstrate the promising potential of artificial intelligence *via* ML modeling for a convenient prediction screening of CVD based on the SM

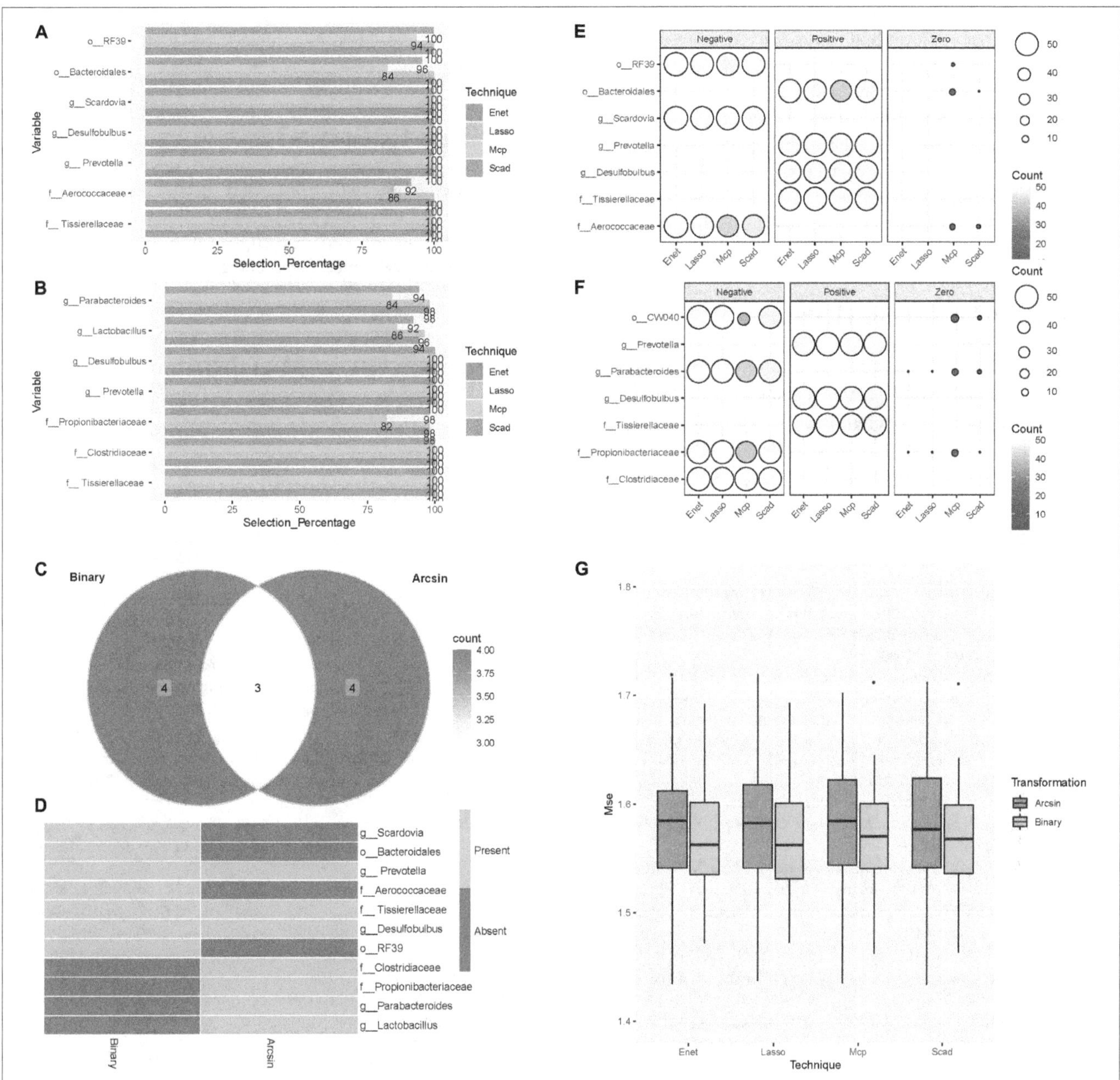

FIGURE 4 | Machine learning models. Barplots representing the selection percentages of the microbes selected at least 80% of the time by the four methods over the 50 random splits of the data. **(A)** Binary transformation. **(B)** Arcsin transformation. **(C)** Venn Diagram showing the number of microbes. **(D)** Heatmap [presence (green)/absence (red)] of selected microbes using Binary and Arcsin transformations. **(E)** Balloon plot representing sign counts of the regression coefficients: Binary transformation **(F)** Arcsin transformation. The size of circles represents the number of splits. The color represents the number of counts. **(G)** Box plots of the MSE for the four-methods and the two transformations applied to the microbiome abundance data. Each point of the boxplot represents the MSE on the test-set.

composition in the Arab population. While most ML strategies based on the health records (including age, sex, smoking habit, systolic BP, total cholesterol, HDL, cholesterol, BP treatment, and diabetes), fewer studies used gut microbiome profiles to predict IBD and CVD with an AUC of ≈0.70 and 0.90, respectively (Masetic and Subasi, 2016; Weng et al., 2017; Aryal et al., 2020; Tsoi et al., 2020; Manandhar et al., 2021). A pilot study of Japanese patients with atherosclerotic cardiovascular disease (ACVD) revealed that SM could be used as an optimal marker of ACVD with an AUC of 0.933 (Kato-Kogoe et al., 2021). It is a promising finding to enable the discovery of non-invasive biomarkers that can predict the risk of the disease before it occurs. This study is novel, and the outcomes will be a step toward developing new biomarkers for early non-invasive testing aiming to reduce the CVD burden. The main limitation of this study is the single time point recruitment of the participants without any follow-up on the participants, in addition to the imbalance in the sample size between the groups. This study mainly focuses on the

SM shift with a change in CVD-score. In this study, we did not consider the other confounding factors such as chronic diseases like diabetes, arthritis, and hypertension and their treatment, which can also influence the SM shift.

Further studies are warranted to confirm our findings and the potential use of these microbial signatures as diagnostic or prognostic markers. In addition, more investigation of these biomarkers for their mechanistic and pathophysiological evidence could be helpful in the personalized approach to treat CVD.

AUTHOR CONTRIBUTIONS

SAK designed the study, obtained funds for the project, reviewed the data, and finalized the manuscript. SM processed the samples, analyzed the data, and wrote the initial draft. AT and DB calculated the CVD scores and reviewed the data and the manuscript. ME analyzed the data using ML techniques. All authors reviewed and accepted the final version of the manuscript.

ACKNOWLEDGMENTS

Samples were collected from QGP participants. Data and samples used in this study were obtained from QBB (www.qatarbiobank.org.qa). Sample processing for DNA extraction was performed by members from the Omics Core at Sidra Medicine.

SUPPLEMENTARY MATERIAL

Supplementary Figure 1 | (A) Alpha diversity measures for the LR, MR, and HR groups. **(B)** Principal Coordinates Analysis (PCoA) based on Bray-Curtis distances of SM.

REFERENCES

1. Aagaard, K., Petrosino, J., Keitel, W., Watson, M., Katancik, J., Garcia, N., et al. (2013). The Human Microbiome Project strategy for comprehensive sampling of the human microbiome and why it matters. *FASEB J.* 27, 1012–1022. doi: 10.1096/fj.12-220806
2. Akyol, T. Y. (2019). *RVenn: An R Package for Set Operationson Multiple Sets.*
3. Allen, L., Williams, J., Townsend, N., Mikkelsen, B., Roberts, N., Foster, C., et al. (2017). Socioeconomic status and non-communicable disease behavioural risk factors in low-income and lower-middle-income countries: a systematic review. *Lancet Glob. Health* 5, e277–e289. doi: 10.1016/S2214-109X(17) 30058-X
4. Al-Kaabi, S. K., and Atherton, A. (2015). Impact of noncommunicable diseases in the State of Qatar. *Clinicoecon. Outcomes Res.* 7, 377–385. doi: 10.2147/CEOR. S74682
5. Al-Obaide, M. A. I., Singh, R., Datta, P., Rewers-Felkins, K. A., Salguero, M. V., Al-Obaidi, I., et al. (2017). Gut microbiota-dependent trimethylamine-N-oxide and serum biomarkers in patients with T2DM and advanced CKD. *J. Clin. Med.* 6:86. doi: 10.3390/jcm6090086
6. Al-Shamsi, S., Regmi, D., and Govender, R. D. (2019). Incidence of cardiovascular disease and its associated risk factors in at-risk men and women in the United Arab Emirates: a 9-year retrospective cohort study. *BMC Cardiovasc. Disord.* 19:148. doi: 10.1186/s12872-019-1131-2
7. Amon, P., and Sanderson, I. (2017). What is the microbiome? *Arch. Dis. Child. Educ. Pract. Ed.* 102, 257–260.
8. Andrews, S. (2010). *FastQC: A Quality Control Tool for High Throughput Sequence Data.*
9. Aryal, S., Alimadadi, A., Manandhar, I., Joe, B., and Cheng, X. (2020). Machine learning strategy for gut microbiome-based diagnostic screening of cardiovascular disease. *Hypertension* 76, 1555–1562. doi: 10.1161/ HYPERTENSIONAHA.120.15885
10. Balakumar, P., Maung, U. K., and Jagadeesh, G. (2016). Prevalence and prevention of cardiovascular disease and diabetes mellitus. *Pharmacol. Res.* 113, 600–609. doi: 10.1016/j.phrs.2016.09.040
11. Bolger, A. M., Lohse, M., and Usadel, B. (2014). Trimmomatic: a flexible trimmer for Illumina sequence data. *Bioinformatics* 30, 2114–2120. doi: 10. 1093/bioinformatics/btu170
12. Breheny, P. J. (2020). *Regularization Paths for SCAD and MCP Penalized Regression Models. CRAN 3.12.0.*
13. Caldwell, M., Martinez, L., Foster, J. G., Sherling, D., and Hennekens, C. H. (2019). Prospects for the primary prevention of myocardial infarction and stroke. *J. Cardiovasc. Pharmacol. Ther.* 24, 207–214. doi: 10.1177/1074248418817344
14. Caporaso, J. G., Kuczynski, J., Stombaugh, J., Bittinger, K., Bushman, F. D., Costello, E. K., et al. (2010). QIIME allows analysis of high-throughput community sequencing data. *Nat. Methods* 7, 335–336. doi: 10.1038/nmeth.f. 303
15. Chang, C. S., and Kao, C. Y. (2019). Current understanding of the gut microbiota shaping mechanisms. *J. Biomed. Sci.* 26:59. doi: 10.1186/s12929-019-0554-5
16. Cortez, R. V., Taddei, C. R., Sparvoli, L. G., Angelo, A. G. S., Padilha, M., Mattar, R., et al. (2019). Microbiome and its relation to gestational diabetes. *Endocrine* 64, 254–264. doi: 10.1007/s12020-018-1813-z
17. D'Agostino, R. B. Sr., Pencina, M. J., Massaro, J. M., and Coady, S. (2013). Cardiovascular disease risk assessment: insights from Framingham. *Glob. Heart* 8, 11–23. doi: 10.1016/j.gheart.2013.01.001
18. Davis, E., Bakulski, K. M., Goodrich, J. M., Peterson, K. E., Marazita, M. L., and Foxman, B. (2020). Low levels of salivary metals, oral microbiome composition and dental decay. *Sci. Rep.* 10:14640. doi: 10.1038/s41598-020-71495-9
19. Deo, P. N., and Deshmukh, R. (2019). Oral microbiome: unveiling the fundamentals. *J. Oral Maxillofac. Pathol.* 23, 122–128. doi: 10.4103/jomfp. JOMFP_304_18
20. DeSantis, T. Z., Hugenholtz, P., Larsen, N., Rojas, M., Brodie, E. L., Keller, K., et al. (2006). Greengenes, a chimera-checked 16S rRNA gene database and workbench compatible with ARB. *Appl. Environ. Microbiol.* 72, 5069–5072. doi: 10.1128/AEM.03006-05
21. Devkota, S., Wang, Y., Musch, M. W., Leone, V., Fehlner-Peach, H., Nadimpalli, A., et al. (2012). Dietary-fat-induced taurocholic acid promotes pathobiont expansion and colitis in Il10$^{-/-}$ mice. *Nature* 487, 104–108. doi: 10.1038/ nature11225
22. Dong, M., Li, L., Chen, M., Kusalik, A., and Xu, W. (2020). Predictive analysis methods for human microbiome data with application to Parkinson's disease. *PLoS One* 15:e0237779. doi: 10.1371/journal.pone.0237779
23. Emoto, T., Yamashita, T., Kobayashi, T., Sasaki, N., Hirota, Y., Hayashi, T., et al. (2017). Characterization of gut microbiota profiles in coronary artery disease patients using data mining analysis of terminal restriction fragment length polymorphism: gut microbiota could be a diagnostic marker of coronary artery disease. *Heart Vessels* 32, 39–46. doi: 10.1007/s00380-016- 0841-y
24. Eriksson, K., Fei, G., Lundmark, A., Benchimol, D., Lee, L., Hu, Y. O. O., et al. (2019). Periodontal health and oral microbiota in patients with rheumatoid arthritis. *J. Clin. Med.* 8:630. doi: 10.3390/jcm8050630
25. Gulden, E. (2018). Lifestyle factors affecting the gut microbiota's relationship with type 1 diabetes. *Curr. Diab. Rep.* 18:111. doi: 10.1007/s11892-018-1098-x
26. Haj Bakri, A., and Al-Thani, A. (2012). *Chronic Disease Risk Factor Surveillance. Qatar STEPwsie Report 2012.* Doha: The Supreme Council of Health. Hastie, T., and Qian, J. (2014). *Glmnet Vignette*, 1–30.
27. Jamshidi, A., Pelletier, J. P., and Martel-Pelletier, J. (2019). Machine-learning-based patient-specific prediction models for knee osteoarthritis. *Nat. Rev. Rheumatol.* 15, 49–60. doi: 10.1038/s41584-018-0130-5
28. Kassambara, A. (2020). *ggpubr: 'ggplot2' Based Publication Ready Plots. R Package Version 0.3.0.*

29. Kato-Kogoe, N., Sakaguchi, S., Kamiya, K., Omori, M., Gu, Y. H., Ito, Y., et al. (2021). Characterization of salivary microbiota in patients with atherosclerotic cardiovascular disease: a case-control study. *J. Atheroscler. Thromb.* doi: 10. 5551/jat.60608
30. Katsimichas, T., Ohtani, T., Motooka, D., Tsukamoto, Y., Kioka, H., Nakamoto, K., et al. (2018). Non-ischemic heart failure with reduced ejection fraction is associated with altered intestinal microbiota. *Circ. J.* 82, 1640–1650. doi: 10.1253/circj.CJ-17-1285
31. Kelly, T. N., Bazzano, L. A., Ajami, N. J., He, H., Zhao, J., Petrosino, J. F., et al. (2016). Gut microbiome associates with lifetime cardiovascular disease risk profile among Bogalusa heart study participants. *Circ. Res.* 119, 956–964. doi: 10.1161/CIRCRESAHA.116.309219
32. Kholy, K. E., Genco, R. J., and Van Dyke, T. E. (2015). Oral infections and cardiovascular disease. *Trends Endocrinol. Metab.* 26, 315–321.
33. Kohli, A., Holzwanger, E. A., and Levy, A. N. (2020). Emerging use of artificial intelligence in inflammatory bowel disease. *World J. Gastroenterol.* 26, 6923– 6928.
34. Lear, S. A., Hu, W., Rangarajan, S., Gasevic, D., Leong, D., Iqbal, R., et al. (2017). The effect of physical activity on mortality and cardiovascular disease in 130 000 people from 17 high-income, middle-income, and low-income countries: the PURE study. *Lancet* 390, 2643–2654. doi: 10.1016/S0140-6736(17)31634-3
35. Liu, S., Zhao, W., Liu, X., and Cheng, L. (2020). Metagenomic analysis of the gut microbiome in atherosclerosis patients identify cross-cohort microbial signatures and potential therapeutic target. *FASEB J.* 34, 14166–14181. doi: 10.1096/fj.202000622R
36. Liu, Z., Li, J., Liu, H., Tang, Y., Zhan, Q., Lai, W., et al. (2019). The intestinal microbiota associated with cardiac valve calcification differs from that of coronary artery disease. *Atherosclerosis* 284, 121–128. doi: 10.1016/j. atherosclerosis.2018.11.038
37. Manandhar, I., Alimadadi, A., Aryal, S., Munroe, P. B., Joe, B., and Cheng, X. (2021). Gut microbiome-based supervised machine learning for clinical diagnosis of inflammatory bowel diseases. *Am. J. Physiol. Gastrointest. Liver Physiol.* doi: 10.1152/ajpgi.00360.2020
38. Marchesi, J. R., Adams, D. H., Fava, F., Hermes, G. D., Hirschfield, G. M., Hold, G., et al. (2016). The gut microbiota and host health: a new clinical frontier. *Gut* 65, 330–339. doi: 10.1136/gutjnl-2015-309990
39. Masetic, Z., and Subasi, A. (2016). Congestive heart failure detection using random forest classifier. *Comput. Methods Programs Biomed.* 130, 54–64. doi: 10.1016/j. cmpb.2016.03.020
40. Mashima, I., Theodorea, C. F., Thaweboon, B., Thaweboon, S., Scannapieco, F. A., and Nakazawa, F. (2017). Exploring the salivary microbiome of children stratified by the oral hygiene index. *PLoS One* 12:e0185274. doi: 10.1371/ journal.pone.0185274
41. McMurdie, P. J., and Holmes, S. (2013). phyloseq: an R package for reproducible interactive analysis and graphics of microbiome census data. *PLoS One* 8:e61217. doi: 10.1371/journal.pone.0061217
42. Minitab-17 (2010). *Minitab 17 Statistical Software [Computer Software]*. State College, PA: Minitab, Inc.
43. MOPH (2020). *Ministry of Public Health: Cardiovascular Diseases.* Available online at: https://www.moph.gov.qa/english/strategies/ Supporting-Strategies-and- Frameworks/QatarPublicHealthStrategy/Pages/ Cardiovascular-diseases.aspx
44. Morganti, S., Tarantino, P., Ferraro, E., D'Amico, P., Viale, G., Trapani, D., et al. (2019). Complexity of genome sequencing and reporting: next generation sequencing (NGS) technologies and implementation of precision medicine in real life. *Crit. Rev. Oncol. Hematol.* 133, 171–182. doi: 10.1016/j. critrevonc.2018. 11.008
45. Murugesan, S., Al Ahmad, S. F., Singh, P., Saadaoui, M., Kumar, M., and Al Khodor, S. (2020). Profiling the salivary microbiome of the Qatari population. *J. Transl. Med.* 18:127. doi: 10.1186/s12967-020-02291-2
46. Olivier, M., Asmis, R., Hawkins, G. A., Howard, T. D., and Cox, L. A. (2019). The need for multi-omics biomarker signatures in precision medicine. *Int. J. Mol. Sci.* 20:4781. doi: 10.3390/ijms20194781
47. Segata, N., Izard, J., Waldron, L., Gevers, D., Miropolsky, L., Garrett, W. S., et al. (2011). Metagenomic biomarker discovery and explanation. *Genome Biol.* 12:R60. doi: 10.1186/gb-2011-12-6-r60
48. Sherman, S. B., Sarsour, N., Salehi, M., Schroering, A., Mell, B., Joe, B., et al. (2018). Prenatal androgen exposure causes hypertension and gut microbiota dysbiosis. *Gut Microbes* 9, 400–421. doi: 10.1080/19490976.2018.14 41664
49. Solbiati, J., and Frias-Lopez, J. (2018). Metatranscriptome of the oral microbiome in health and disease. *J. Dent. Res.* 97, 492–500. doi: 10.1177/00220345187 61644
50. Tomas, I., Diz, P., Tobias, A., Scully, C., and Donos, N. (2012). Periodontal health status and bacteraemia from daily oral activities: systematic review/ meta- analysis. *J. Clin. Periodontol.* 39, 213–228. doi: 10.1111/j.1600-051X.2011. 01784.x
51. Tsoi, K. K. F., Chan, N. B., Yiu, K. K. L., Poon, S. K. S., Lin, B., and Ho, K. (2020). Machine learning clustering for blood pressure variability applied to Systolic Blood Pressure Intervention Trial (SPRINT) and the Hong Kong community cohort. *Hypertension* 76, 569–576. doi: 10.1161/HYPERTENSIONAHA.119. 14213
52. Ursell, L. K., Clemente, J. C., Rideout, J. R., Gevers, D., Caporaso, J. G., and Knight, R. (2012). The interpersonal and intrapersonal diversity of human-associated microbiota in key body sites. *J. Allergy Clin. Immunol.* 129, 1204–1208. doi: 10.1016/j.jaci.2012.03.010
53. Wade, W. G. (2013). The oral microbiome in health and disease. *Pharmacol. Res.* 69, 137–143.
54. Wang, P., Dong, Y., Zuo, K., Han, C., Jiao, J., Yang, X., et al. (2021). Characteristics and variation of fecal bacterial communities and functions in isolated systolic and diastolic hypertensive patients. *BMC Microbiol.* 21:128. doi: 10.1186/ s12866-021-02195-1
55. Weng, S. F., Reps, J., Kai, J., Garibaldi, J. M., and Qureshi, N. (2017). Can machine-learning improve cardiovascular risk prediction using routine clinical data? *PLoS One* 12:e0174944. doi: 10.1371/journal.pone.017 4944
56. Wickham, H. (2011). ggplot2. *Wiley Interdiscip. Rev. Comput. Stat.* 3, 180–185. World Health Organization [WHO] (2013). *Global Action Plan for the Prevention and Control of Noncommunicable Diseases 2013-2020.* Geneva: WHO, 55.
57. Wu, Z. X., Li, S. F., Chen, H., Song, J. X., Gao, Y. F., Zhang, F., et al. (2017). Thechanges of gut microbiota after acute myocardial infarction in rats. *PLoS One*12:e0180717. doi: 10.1371/journal.pone.0180717
58. Yamashita, Y., and Takeshita, T. (2017). The oral microbiome and human health.*J. Oral Sci.* 59, 201–206.
59. Zaura, E., Keijser, B. J., Huse, S. M., and Crielaard, W. (2009). Defining the healthy "core microbiome" of oral microbial communities. *BMC Microbiol.* 9:259. doi: 10.1186/1471-2180-9-259
60. Zaura, E., Nicu, E. A., Krom, B. P., and Keijser, B. J. (2014). Acquiring and maintaining a normal oral microbiome: current perspective. *Front. Cell. Infect. Microbiol.* 4:85. doi: 10.3389/fcimb.2014.00085
61. Zhang, C.-H. (2010). Nearly unbiased variable selection under minimax concave penalty. *Ann. Stat.* 38, 894–942.
62. Zhang, J., Kobert, K., Flouri, T., and Stamatakis, A. (2014). PEAR: a fast and accurate Illumina paired-end reAd mergeR. *Bioinformatics* 30, 614–620. doi: 10.1093/bioinformatics/btt593
63. Zhong, Y., Xu, F., Wu, J., Schubert, J., and Li, M. M. (2021). Application of next generation sequencing in laboratory medicine. *Ann. Lab. Med.* 41, 25–43. doi: 10.3343/alm.2021.41.1.25
64. Zou, H., and Hastie, T. (2005). Regularization and variable selection *via* the elastic net. *J. R. Stat. Soc. Ser. B Stat. Methodol.* 67, 301–320. doi: 10.1093/ brain/awv075
65. Zou, H., and Li, R. (2008). One-step sparse estimates in nonconcave penalized likelihood models. *Ann. Stat.* 36, 1509–1533. doi: 10.1214/ 009053607000000802

17

Urban-Rural Disparities in Dental Services Utilization Among Adults in China's Megacities

Xiang Qi[1†], *Xiaomin Qu*[2*†] *and Bei Wu*[1*†]

[1] *Rory Meyers College of Nursing, New York University, New York, NY, United States,* [2] *School of Social Development, East China University of Political Science and Law, Shanghai, China*

Correspondence:
Xiaomin Qu
millie_qu@163.com
Bei Wu
bei.wu@nyu.edu

Objective: China's dental care system is bifurcated between urban and rural areas. However, very few studies have examined the dental services utilization inequities in China's megacities, particularly in these urban and rural areas. This study aims to examine the urban-rural disparities in dental services utilization among adults living in China's megacities based on the Andersen dental services utilization model.

Methods: This study used data from 4,049 residents aged 18–65 who participated in the "2019 New Era and Living Conditions in Megacities Survey." Multivariate logistic regressions were employed to examine the associations between place of residence and dental services utilization for individuals from ten megacities in China. Predisposing variables (age, gender, marital status, living arrangement, and education), enabling variables (socioeconomic status, occupational status, income, insurance coverage, health attitude, and health behavior), and need variables (self-rated health, oral health status, gum bleeding) were controlled for.

Results: The mean age of the 4,049 adults was 45.2 (standard deviation = 13.0), and 30.4% (n = 1,232) had no dental visits at all. Adults who resided in urban areas were more likely to use dental services [odds ratio (OR) = 1.57, 95% confidence interval (CI) = 1.30 to 1.91] than those residing in rural areas after controlling for key covariates. Factors associated with higher odds of visiting dentists include having a higher income (OR = 1.44, $P < 0.001$), higher education level (OR = 1.53, $P = 0.042$), being covered by insurance for urban residents/employees (OR = 1.49, $P = 0.031$), having a positive attitude toward healthy diets (OR = 1.43, $P < 0.001$), attending regular physical examination (OR = 1.66, $P < 0.001$), having more tooth loss (OR = 1.05, $P < 0.001$), and having frequent gum bleeding (OR = 2.29, $P < 0.001$).

Conclusion: The findings confirm that place of residence is associated with dental services utilization while adjusting for key covariates. Despite rapid economic development in China, many adults had never visited dentists at all. More efforts should be taken to encourage widespread dental care, such as providing more dental coverage and better access to dental care services.

Keywords: urban-rural, oral health, dental care use, dental visit, Chinese

INTRODUCTION

Oral health problems and disorders are common among adults in the Chinese population. According to the 4th National Oral Health Epidemiology Survey conducted between 2015 and 2016 in China, the prevalence of dental caries is more than 90.0% for adults between the ages of 35 and 74 years old [1]. Furthermore, the prevalence of periodontitis among middle-aged adults ranging from 35 to 44 years old is 52.8% [2]. Such oral health diseases and problems are associated with a lack of dental services utilization [3–5]. Moreover, the use of dental care services among the Chinese population is very low compared to those in developed countries [6–10]. Due to its direct association with the persistence of oral health issues, it is important to identify factors associated with dental services utilization in China. The knowledge generated in this area would provide a better understanding of service utilization patterns, assist in designing a cost-effective dental care system and promote policy change in the future.

Despite China's significant economic development in the past three decades, large disparities in income, infrastructure, and social services between urban and rural areas remain. For example, the ratio of urban to rural income was 1.86 in 1985, and it increased to 2.56 in 2019 [11]. According to the Chinese Health Statistics Yearbook of 2018, urban areas had 535 hospitals specializing in dental treatments in 2017; in contrast, rural areas only had 154 dental hospitals. People living in urban areas are more likely to have higher levels of income and education than their rural counterparts, as well as have retirement pensions [12, 13]. Additionally, rural residents encounter barriers in obtaining basic public services and welfare, such as the healthcare system and social security coverage [14]. Such urban-rural disparities impose a significant barrier that hinders individuals residing in rural areas from accessing dental care; studies have generally reported a lower use of dental care services in rural areas [8, 15–17]. Due to the unbalanced development across urban and rural areas, dental health resources, including the dental department and dental workforce, are insufficient and distributed unevenly between the two areas [18]. Although there are no national statistics on the dental care expenses in China, some estimates suggest that 85% of dental care cost is paid out-of-pocket [18, 19]. Rural residents are more likely to postpone dental appointments due to the inaccessibility of dental services and their inability to pay out-of-pocket dental care expenses [7].

The urban-rural divide also exists in megacities that exhibit a higher development level than other areas of China [20]. A megacity is defined as containing over five million residents [21], and under this definition there were 16 megacities in China in 2019 [22]. Unlike developed countries, all of China's megacities are metropolitan regions that include urban, peri-urban and rural land, and all have rural populations within the city boundaries. Because their development level is higher than other parts of China, the urban-rural divide in China's megacities has significantly narrowed with respect to income, education level, housing, and social welfare programs since 1990 [20, 23, 24]. However, the reduced urban-rural income divide does not significantly diminish the urban-rural disparities in healthcare service allocation and distribution [25]. Understanding the dental services utilization in China's megacities is of particular importance because of their mega-sized populations, rapid economic development, and millions of rural migrants without urban household registration status [20]. Nonetheless, very few studies have been conducted on dental services utilization among adults in China's megacities.

This study aimed to address the knowledge gap by examining how dental service utilization was associated with place of residence among adult populations in China's megacities. Based on existing literature on dental services use [6–10], we hypothesized that dental services utilization would be associated with urban area residence after controlling for key covariates.

METHODS

Samples and Data Collection

This study used the data from the "2019 New Era and Living Conditions in Megacities Survey (NELCMS)." This survey is a cross-sectional observational study using a multi-stage, stratified sampling design and focuses on policy issues related to social structure and social mobility among adults in China's megacities. It was conducted in ten megacities in China, including the most economically developed megacities characterized by a Gross Domestic Product (GDP) per capita higher than 134,000 RMB (equivalent to 19,619 U.S. dollars). Namely, the megacities surveyed were Beijing, Shanghai, Guangzhou, Shenzhen, Tianjin, Hangzhou, Chongqing, Chengdu, Wuhan, and Changsha. The questionnaire consists of two volumes, including 418 items. The main contents included the following aspects: demographic characteristics, work and social security, socioeconomic status, living and household conditions, activities of daily living assessment, and health status and behavior habits.

Using the probability-proportional-to-size sampling method, researchers selected participants through four stages: city, community, household, and individual. Forty communities were randomly selected from each city. Twenty-five households were randomly selected from the housing registration database obtained from each community. One individual was randomly selected from each household. The study was approved by the Ethics Committee of Shanghai University (ECSHU 2020–096).

Inclusion criteria for participation were: (a) self-identified as Chinese and able to communicate in Mandarin; (b) full-time residence in this city for more than 6 months in the past year; (c) age between 18 and 65; (d) capable of answering interview questions. In this survey, questionnaires included Volume A and Volume B. Volume A is the core interview that focuses on social mobility and social structure. Volume B covers individuals' health-related questions, such as health status, health insurance, and health care utilization. Participants were randomly selected to complete either Volume A or Volume B. To address the study aim, only participants who completed Volume B were selected.

In full accordance with ethical principles, well-trained interviewers collected the data during in-home interviews in Mandarin. The informed consent was obtained prior to the data collection. The interviews lasted about 45–60 min. To ensure that the questionnaire was reliable and valid, we conducted a pilot

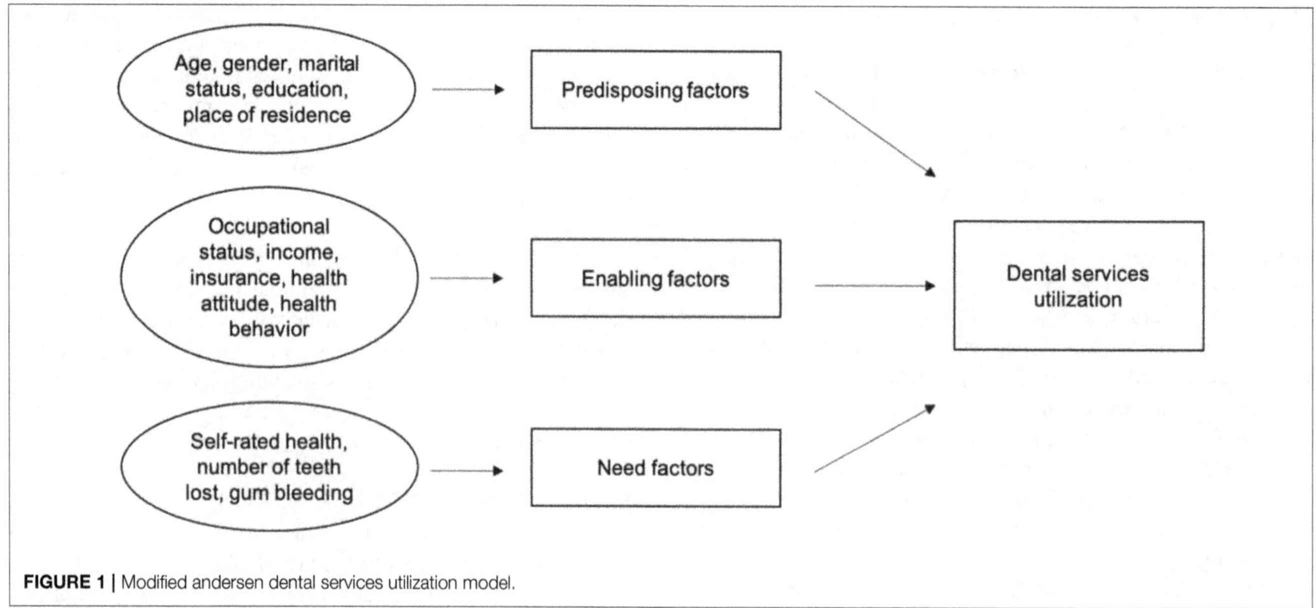

FIGURE 1 | Modified andersen dental services utilization model.

study on 50 adults. Based on their feedback and suggestions, the questionnaire was revised and finalized before the formal data collection. From July 2019 to August 2019, the research team collected data from a total of 5,000 participants who filled out Volume B of the questionnaire. After excluding 815 participants with missing values on the individual's and father's International Socio-Economic Index of Occupational Status (ISEI) and 136 participants with missing values on the study variables, the final analytical sample consisted of 4,049 respondents.

Measures

Dependent and Independent Variables

The dependent variable in our analysis is dental services utilization. The survey asked, "how often do you visit a dentist for dental care?" The responses are the frequency of dental visits (0 = never, 1 = rarely, 2 = less than once every two years, 3 = at least once every 2 years, 4 = at least once a year, 5 = twice a year). Dental care utilization in China is at a very low level; a national survey in 2015-2016 found that 78.6% of adults aged 35–44 and 79.3% of older adults aged 65–74 had not used dental care services in the past 12 months [17]. We therefore dichotomized the responses into 1 = "never" and 0 = "otherwise." The independent variable, place of residence, was dichotomized into 1 = urban or 0 = rural.

Covariates

This study applies the Andersen Healthcare Utilization Model (**Figure 1**) [26, 27] to guide the selection of variables. According to this model, people's use of dental services over a given period is a function of predisposing factors, enabling factors, and need factors.

Predisposing Factors

Demographic information includes age (18–25, 26–30, ..., 61–65 years old, nine categories ranging from 18 to 65), gender (0 = female, 1 = male), marital status (1 = married or living with partner, 0 = otherwise), and education (0 = illiterate/elementary school, 1 = middle/high/vocational school, 3 = 3 years college or more).

Enabling Factors

Early-life and current socioeconomic status include the father's and individual's occupational status determined by the International Socio-Economic Index of Occupational Status (ISEI) developed by Ganzeboom et. al. [28], and individual's annual income (0 = $<$ 78,000 RMB, 1 = $\geq$ 78,000 RMB). To facilitate interpretation of findings, ISEI were dichotomized into 2 groups [0 = $<$ 54 (low), 1 = $\geq$ 54 (high)]. Health insurance coverage consists of 0 = no health insurance, 1 = New Cooperative Medical Scheme for rural residents, 2 = Urban Residents Basic Medical Insurance, 3 = Urban Employees Basic Medical Insurance, and 4 = other insurance (mostly commercial insurance). In addition, we measured the respondents' health attitude by asking whether they are concerned about eating a healthy diet. The response was coded as 0 = no, and 1 = yes. Health behaviors were measured by the regularity of attending physical exams (having physical exam once a year, 0 = no, 1 = yes).

Need Factors

Self-rated health was measured by nine questions acquired from the Self-Rated Health Measurement Scale [29]. Each item was scored on a scale of 0–10, with higher values representing better self-rated health. The potential range of the scale is 0 to 90. The Cronbach's alpha for the measure was 0.833, which showed a high internal consistency. Oral health status was determined by self-reported tooth loss (the number of missing teeth), and self-reported gum bleeding (0 = never/hardly, 1 = occasionally/frequently/always).

Statistical Analysis

Post-stratification individual-level sampling weights were used to adjust for differences in the individual-by-household-by-community-by-city distribution between the sample and the general population in the ten megacities in the study [30]. We defined city as sampling unit (n = 10), and neighborhood as strata (n = 40). All analyses presented in **Tables 1, 2** and **Figure 2** were adjusted for sampling weight.

We first used descriptive statistics, including proportions and 95% confidence intervals (CIs), to consider the complex sampling and sampling weights. Bivariate analyses were conducted using Chi-Square tests to estimate urban-rural disparities in dental visits. Multivariate stepwise logistic regressions were conducted, according to the Andersen Healthcare Utilization Model [27] and previous literature [16, 31]. We only included the place of residence in the first step (Model 1). In the second step, we entered predisposing factors, including age, gender, marital status, and education. Next, we added enabling factors, which consisted of the father's and individual's occupational class, income, insurance, health attitude, and health behavior (Model 3). In the final Model 4, we added need factors, including self-rated health and oral health status of the participants.

We used margins post estimation to examine whether the urban-rural disparities in dental services utilization were associated with a change in age after controlling for other covariates [32, 33]. We used STATA (Version 15.0) for all statistical analyses. A P-value ≤ 0.05 was considered significant.

RESULTS

The sample characteristics are summarized in **Table 1**. In the weighted analytical sample, 28.23% of urban residents and 17.58 % of rural residents had at least one dental visit per year. In addition, 637 (23.82%) urban residents and 595 (43.27%) rural residents never had any dental visits.

Bivariate analyses did not find urban-rural differences in the distributions of gender, age, and marital status. However, in comparison to residents in urban areas, those in rural areas were less likely to have dental visits [76.18% (urban) vs. 56.73% (rural)]. Rural residents had lower income, lower levels of education, and lower levels of father's and individual's occupational status. Additionally, rural residents were less concerned about eating a healthy diet and less likely to have regular physical exams compared with their urban counterparts. No significant urban-rural difference was found in self-rated health and oral health status.

Table 2 presents the results from the stepwise logistic regression models on visiting a dentist for Chinese adults in megacities. Place of residence had a significant association with dental visits in Model 1 (including the variable on place of residence only) [Odds Ratio (OR) = 2.44, 95% CI = 2.10 to 2.85].

In Model 2, male adults were less likely to visit a dentist (OR = 0.81, 95% CI = 0.69 to 0.95). Education beyond three-year college was significantly associated with dental visits (OR = 2.17, 95% CI = 1.57 to 2.99).

Individuals with a higher level of socioeconomic status (i.e., education, income, and occupational status) were more likely to visit a dentist ($P < 0.05$) (Model 3). Additionally, in comparison with those who did not have insurance, residents with the New Cooperative Medical Scheme (health insurance for rural residents) had similar odds of visiting a dentist. Individuals who were more concerned about a healthy diet and had regular physical examinations were more likely to visit a dentist.

Among need variables, self-rated health was not related to dental visits. In the fully specified model (Model 4), the odds of visiting a dentist were 57.3% higher for urban residents than their rural counterparts (OR = 1.57, 95% CI = 1.30 to 1.91). Moreover, individuals with fewer remaining teeth (OR = 1.05, 95% CI = 1.02 to 1.09) and gum bleeding symptoms were more likely to visit a dentist (OR = 2.29, 95% CI = 1.95 to 2.68).

Adjusting for other covariates (demographics, socioeconomic status, health attitude and behavior, self-rated health, and oral health status), **Figure 2** shows the margins post estimation of predicted probability of visiting a dentist across age groups and by place of residence. Overall, rural residents were less likely to use dental care compared with their urban counterparts in all age groups.

DISCUSSION

This study has provided a better understanding of dental services utilization in megacities by demonstrating that place of residence was associated with dental services utilization while adjusting for key covariates. Data from ten megacities in China were employed, and the individuals' socioeconomic conditions, health insurance, health attitude and behaviors, and oral health status were found to be significant explanatory variables. In addition, the urban-rural disparities in dental services utilization remained regardless of age.

Never visiting a dentist is a common phenomenon among the adult population in China. Our study showed that 30.4% of the respondents had never experienced a dental visit. Furthermore, a study conducted in China using national data found the rates of not visiting a dentist in the past 12 months were relatively high—78.6% for adults aged 35 to 44, and 79.3% for older adults aged 65 to 74 [17]. According to the data from the National Health and Nutrition Examination Survey (NHANES) conducted in the U.S. from 2011 to 2014, 33.8% of adults aged over 30 reported not having a dental visit in the past 12 months [6]. Our study shows that even in these highly economically developed megacities in China, the rate of dental visits is much lower than those in developed or high-income countries [9, 10].

Urban-rural disparities are reflected by the predisposing factors. Affordability of dental service could be another significant reason for the limited dental visits, particularly among residents from rural areas. This is consistent with a study conducted in 14 European countries among older adults that found older adults with lower income were less likely to seek dental care [9]. Our study found that the type of health insurance possessed by an individual strongly associated with dental services utilization. Although the Chinese government has

TABLE 1 | Sample characteristics ($N = 4,049$, weighted).

	Total sample	Residents with dental visits ($N = 2,817$)		Residents with no dental visits ($N = 1,232$)	
	$N = 4,049$	Urban ($N = 2,037$)	Rural ($N = 780$)	Urban ($N = 637$)	Rural ($N = 595$)
	%/Mean (SD)	%/Mean (SD)	%/Mean (SD)	%/Mean (SD)	%/Mean (SD)
PREDISPOSING VARIABLES					
Gender					
Male	46.6	44.1	46.0	51.8	50.3
Age					
18–25	6.3	5.2	8.6	4.4	9.1
26–30	10.7	9.6	14.3	8.3	12.3
31–35	11.8	10.9	12.9	12.4	12.9
36–40	10.8	11.3	11.0	10.6	8.8
41–45	10.3	10.3	10.1	9.0	12.4
46–50	12.0	11.9	12.0	10.7	13.8
51–55	9.7	8.3	10.9	10.6	11.8
56–60	10.8	11.9	7.1	12.5	9.7
61–65	17.6	20.6	13.1	21.5	9.2
Marital status					
Married/living with partner	80.1	79.6	79.7	79.4	83.3
Education					
Illiterate/elementary school	8.7	3.7	14.3	6.4	20.6
Middle/high/vocational school	50.6	43.9	56.1	54.6	62.1
3 years college or more	40.7	52.4	29.6	39.0	17.3
ENABLING VARIABLES					
Father's occupational status (ISEI)					
High (≥54)	31.1	40.3	16.8	36.3	13.1
Individual's occupational status (ISEI)					
High (≥54)	33.3	44.2	24.2	28.4	13.4
Income					
High (≥78,000)	32.2	37.9	31.6	29.7	16.1
Insurance					
No health insurance	8.5	5.6	10.2	10.4	14.0
New Cooperative Medical Scheme	11.1	1.2	25.4	2.2	35.4
Urban Resident Basic Medical Insurance	22.0	23.9	18.9	24.6	16.8
Urban Employee Basic Medical Insurance	51.7	60.6	40.7	56.2	30.8
Other medical insurance	6.7	8.7	4.8	6.6	3.0
Regular physical exam					
Yes	60.7	72.5	54.5	55.0	34.4
Care about eating a healthy diet					
Yes	56.9	64.5	54.9	50.9	40.0
NEED VARIABLES					
Self-rated health					
SRHMS (range:0–90)	61.5 (12.7)	61.0 (12.4)	61.2 (12.4)	61.8 (13.2)	63.1 (13.2)
Tooth loss					
Number of missing teeth (range:0-28)	1.5 (3.3)	1.7 (3.4)	1.5 (2.8)	1.3 (3.4)	1.0 (3.0)
Gum bleeding					
Yes (occasionally/frequently/always)	50.9	56.1	59.1	37.4	36.6

SD, standard deviation; ISEI, international socio-economic index of occupational status; SRHMS, self-rated health measurement scale.

TABLE 2 | Multivariate logistic regression models of having dental services utilization at least once (*N* =4,049, weighted).

	Model 1		Model 2		Model 3		Model 4	
	OR	**95% CI**	**OR**	**95% CI**	**OR**	**95% CI**	**OR**	**95% CI**
Place of residence (Ref. Rural)								
Urban	2.442***	2.095–2.845	1.731***	1.460–2.052	1.566***	1.299–1.889	1.573***	1.296–1.908
PREDISPOSING VARIABLES								
Gender (Ref. Female)								
Male			0.810**	0.691–0.949	0.773**	0.657–0.909	0.777**	0.658–0.918
Age (Ref. 18–25)								
26–30			1.079	0.726–1.603	1.006	0.680–1.488	0.976	0.658–1.448
31–35			0.909	0.604–1.367	0.855	0.571–1.281	0.819	0.545–1.230
36–40			1.232	0.812–1.871	1.160	0.767–1.756	1.068	0.702–1.625
41–45			1.196	0.780–1.833	1.101	0.719–1.684	1.053	0.688–1.611
46–50			1.359	0.891–2.072	1.270	0.837–1.927	1.146	0.752–1.745
51–55			1.243	0.797–1.936	1.209	0.780–1.873	1.044	0.669–1.631
56–60			1.206	0.784–1.855	1.181	0.771–1.807	0.969	0.627–1.498
61–65			1.504	0.992–2.279	1.485	0.986–2.236	1.185	0.777–1.806
Marital status (Ref. Otherwise)								
Married/living with partner			0.861	0.686–1.081	0.848	0.676–1.064	0.859	0.682–1.081
Education (Ref. Illiterate/elementary school)								
Middle/high/vocational school			1.301	0.988–1.713	1.203	0.910–1.590	1.225	0.913–1.643
3 years college or more			2.165***	1.567–2.993	1.537*	1.082–2.182	1.529*	1.061–2.205
ENABLING VARIABLES								
Father's ISEI (Ref. Low)								
High					1.010	0.844–1.209	1.014	0.844–1.218
Individual's ISEI (Ref. Low)								
High					1.422***	1.167–1.732	1.490***	1.222–1.817
Income (Ref. Low)								
High					1.382**	1.131–1.689	1.438***	1.175–1.760
Insurance (Ref. No health insurance)								
New Cooperative Medical Scheme					1.070	0.765–1.498	1.098	0.775–1.554
Urban Resident Basic Medical Insurance					1.474*	1.094–1.986	1.570**	1.154–2.135
Urban Employee Basic Medical Insurance					1.335*	1.011–1.763	1.383*	1.040–1.838
Other medical insurance					1.608*	1.053–2.455	1.763*	1.147–2.708
Regular physical exam (Ref. Low)								
Yes					1.669***	1.410–1.977	1.661***	1.399–1.972
Care about eating a healthy diet (Ref. No)								
Yes					1.457***	1.238–1.716	1.429***	1.209–1.689
NEED VARIABLES								
Self-rated health (SRHMS)							0.901	0.766–1.059
Tooth loss (Number of missing teeth)							1.053**	1.017–1.092
Gum bleeding (Ref. No)								
Yes (occasionally/frequently/always)							2.286***	1.948–2.682

*OR, odds ratio; CI, confidence interval. Significance level: *p < 0.05, **p < 0.01, ***p < 0.001. ISEI, international socio-economic index of occupational status; SRHMS, self-rated health measurement scale.*

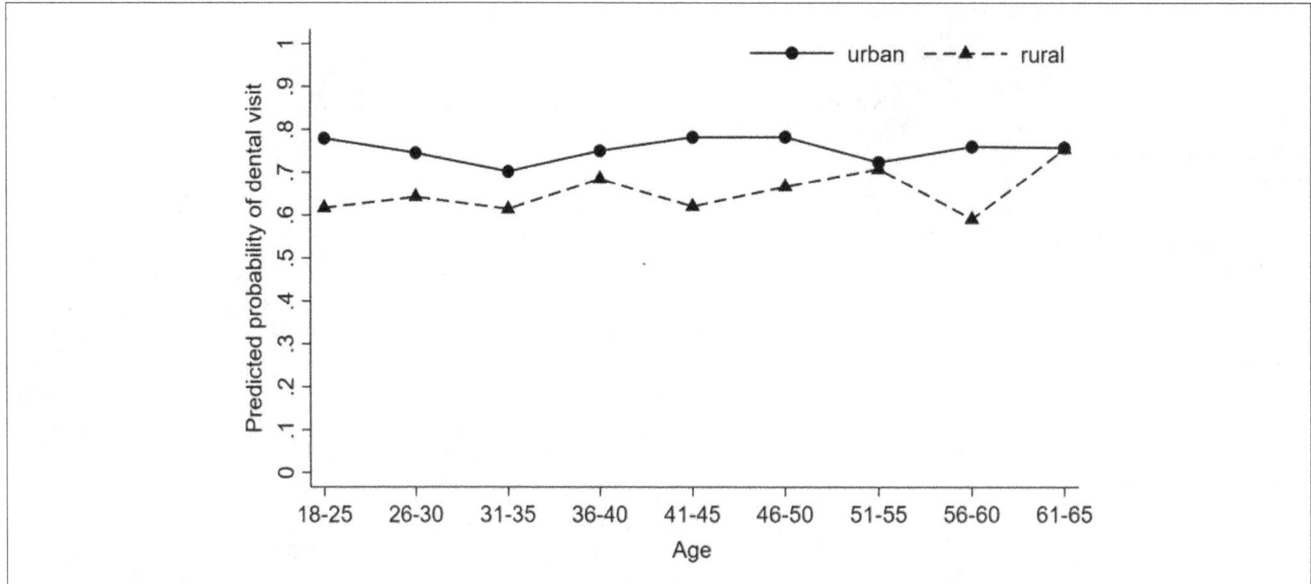

FIGURE 2 | Disparities in predicted probability of having dental visit by place of residence (urban vs. rural) with 95% confidence intervals (*N* = 4,049, weighted). All estimations include gender, marital status, education, attending the regular physical exam, care about eating a healthy diet, father's occupational status, individual's occupational status, income, insurance, self-rated health, tooth loss, and gum bleeding as covariates.

provided universal basic medical coverage since 2009 [34], no health insurance covers the expenses for preventative oral health services in China. There are still various out-of-pocket costs for dental visits, depending on the type of insurance. Compared with the Urban Resident Basic Medical Insurance (URBMI) and Urban Employee Basic Medical Insurance (UEBMI) for urban residents, the New Cooperative Medical Scheme (NCMS) for rural residents has less medical coverage. The NCMS also has complicated and ambiguous reimbursement procedures [14, 34, 35]. The NCSM covers only partial medical expenses and no dental treatment expenses [36]. This can be reflected in our study, as having NCSM did not increase the odds for dental visits. Thus, expanding dental services with a lower amount of out-of-pocket cost for adults could be a strategy to increase dental services utilization.

Within the enabling factors domain, the present study found that concerning about eating a healthy diet was significantly related to dental services utilization, consistent with previous studies [16, 31]. The Chinese population has a long tradition of attributing oral diseases to the food taken [37]. Oral health literacy has an important role in addressing oral health problems because it is associated with oral health behaviors (e.g., use of dental floss, regular toothbrushing) [38] and oral health-seeking behavior [39]. Similarly, having regular physical exams can reflect individuals' health literacy and health conscientiousness [40]. Adults living in urban areas have easier access to regular physical exams and are more likely to seek dental care. Studies have also indicated that oral health belief was associated with increased dental service use [4, 37]. Although a "National Love your Teeth Day" (September 20th) has been designated by the Chinese government to increase public awareness of oral health since 1989 [41], additional efforts are warranted to enhance public knowledge of oral diseases and problems and the importance of preventive dental visits.

Regarding the need factors for dental care, studies conducted in developed countries revealed that compromised oral health status was negatively associated with preventive dental services utilization [9]. Opposite from these previous findings, our study found that poorer oral health was positively associated with dental visits in China's megacities. Presumably, this contradictory finding could be attributed to the different approaches China and developed countries take in addressing oral health. Chinese dental visits are treatment-oriented and driven by severe dental symptoms, which means that people do not seek dental care unless they feel unbearable toothaches or experience severe periodontal symptoms [7]. On the other hand, in developed countries it is common to have regular dental visits that are prevention-oriented, such as tooth cleaning, dental check-ups, or examination [6]. Another factor could be that cultural attitudes toward oral health are different. Wu et al. [42] suggested that perceptions of oral health and oral health beliefs are embedded in social and cultural contexts. Most Chinese people tend to utilize traditional remedies such as drinking green tea and taking Vitamin C rather than seeking professional dental services for treatments [43].

The strengths of this study reside in its focus on the comparisons between urban and rural residents in China's megacities. This is one of the first studies devoted to revealing urban-rural disparities in dental services utilization among adult populations in China's megacities. This study is also unique in investigating whether the urban-rural disparities vary by age. In China, very few studies have been conducted on inequalities in dental services utilization. Moreover, the data were collected from ten megacities that can represent many regions of the urban areas in China.

There are a few limitations in this study that need to be acknowledged. First, this survey does not contain information on reasons for dental visits (preventive, treatment, or emergency visits), nor the time frame of each individual's dental visits. Second, respondents' health attitude was measured by asking whether they are concerned about eating a healthy diet. The absence of relevant information on oral health attitude is a limitation. Third, given the nature of the cross-sectional data, the possibilities of establishing a causal relationship between dental service utilization and the explanatory variables are precluded. Fourth, data in this study were derived from respondents' self-reports, which may lead to recall bias. Future studies should consider using objective measures of clinical oral examinations and including other factors that might influence an individual's dental services utilization, such as oral health literacy, personal health choices, and psychosocial factors. Furthermore, intervention strategies and related dental policies are warranted to ensure equitable access to and quality of dental services utilization in China.

CONCLUSIONS

This study has extended literature by showing that place of residence is associated with dental services utilization while controlling for key confounding factors using data from ten megacities in China. Despite rapid economic development in China, some adults had never visited a dentist, even in the most economically developed megacities. More efforts should be implemented to improve dental care use by providing more dental care coverage and better access to dental care services.

AUTHOR CONTRIBUTIONS

XgQ contributed to the acquisition, analysis and interpretation of data, and draft of the article. XnQ contributed to the acquisition, analysis and interpretation of data and draft of the article. BW contributed to the conceptualization and design of the study, interpretation of the results, and draft of the article. All authors contributed to the article and approved the submitted version.

ACKNOWLEDGMENTS

The 2019 New Era and Living Conditions in Megacities Survey (NELCMS) was designed and conducted by the Shanghai Social Science Survey Center, Shanghai University, and supported by the Shanghai Academy of Social Sciences. We thank them for making the data available for this study. Data were collected during in-home interviews by well-trained interviewers in full accordance with ethical principles. It was fully approved by the Ethics Committee of Shanghai University (ECSHU 2020-096). We would also like to thank Mackenzie Martinez (Duke University) for her editorial assistance.

REFERENCES

1. Si Y, Tai B, Hu D, Lin H, Wang B, Wang C, et al. Oral health status of Chinese residents and suggestions for prevention and treatment strategies. *Glob Health J.* (2019) 3:50–4. doi: 10.1016/j.glohj.2019.06.004
2. Jiao J, Jing W, Si Y, Feng X, Tai B, Hu D, et al. The prevalence and severity of periodontal disease in Mainland China: data from the fourth national oral health survey (2015–2016). *J Clin Periodontol.* (2021) 48:168–79. doi: 10.1111/jcpe.13396
3. Åstrøm AN, Ekback G, Ordell S, Nasir E. Long-term routine dental attendance: influence on tooth loss and oral health-related quality of life in S wedish older adults. *Community Dent Oral Epidemiol.* (2014) 42:460–9. doi: 10.1111/cdoe.12105
4. Broadbent JM, Zeng J, Foster Page LA, Baker SR, Ramrakha S, Thomson WM. Oral health–related beliefs, behaviors, and outcomes through the life course. *J Dent Res.* (2016) 95:808–13. doi: 10.1177/0022034516634663
5. Thomson WM, Williams SM, Broadbent JM, Poulton R, Locker D. Long-term dental visiting patterns and adult oral health. *J Dent Res.* (2010) 89:307–11. doi: 10.1177/0022034509356779
6. Adunola F, Garcia I, Iafolla T, Boroumand S, Silveira ML, Adesanya M, et al. Self-perceived oral health, normative need, and dental services utilization among dentate adults in the United States: national health and nutrition examination survey (NHANES) 2011-2014. *J Public Health Dent.* (2019) 79:79–90. doi: 10.1111/jphd.12300
7. Liu L, Zhang Y, Wu W, Cheng R. Characteristics of dental care-seeking behavior and related sociodemographic factors in a middle-aged and elderly population in northeast China. *BMC Oral Health.* (2015) 15:66. doi: 10.1186/s12903-015-0053-3
8. Qu X, Qi X, Wu B. Disparities in dental service utilization among adults in Chinese megacities: do health insurance and city of residence matter? *Int J Environ Res Public Health.* (2020) 17:6851. doi: 10.3390/ijerph17186851
9. Reda SM, Krois J, Reda SF, Thomson WM, Schwendicke F. The impact of demographic, health-related and social factors on dental services utilization: systematic review and meta-analysis. *J Dent.* (2018) 75:1–6. doi: 10.1016/j.jdent.2018.04.010
10. Wu Y, Zhang W, Wu B. Disparities in dental service use among adult populations in the U.S. *JDR Clin Trans Res.* (2020). doi: 10.1177/2380084421 1012660
11. PRC NBS. *People's Republic of China, National Bureau of Statistics (PRC NBS), China Statistical Yearbook 2020.* Beijing: China Statistics Press (2020).
12. Molero-Simarro R. Inequality in China revisited. The effect of functional distribution of income on urban top incomes, the urban-rural gap and the Gini index, 1978–2015. *China Econ Rev.* (2017) 42:101–17. doi: 10.1016/j.chieco.2016.11.006
13. Shi L. *Rising Inequality in China: Challenges to a Harmonious Society.* Cambridge: Cambridge University Press (2013). p. 499.
14. Li J, Shi L, Liang H, Ding G, Xu L. Urban-rural disparities in health care utilization among Chinese adults from 1993 to 2011. *BMC Health Serv Res.* (2018) 18:102. doi: 10.1186/s12913-018-2905-4
15. Li C, Yao NA, Yin A. Disparities in dental healthcare utilization in China. *Community Dent Oral Epidemiol.* (2018) 46:576–85. doi: 10.1111/cdoe.12394
16. Wu B. Dental service utilization among urban and rural older adults in China? A brief communication. *J Public Health Dent.* (2007) 67:185–8. doi: 10.1111/j.1752-7325.2007.00038.x
17. Xu M, Cheng M, Gao X, Wu H, Ding M, Zhang C, et al. Factors associated with oral health service utilization among adults and older adults in China, 2015-2016. *Community Dent Oral Epidemiol.* (2020) 48:32–41. doi: 10.1111/cdoe.12497
18. Hu D, Hong X, Li X. Oral health in China – trends and challenges. *Int J Oral Sci.* (2011) 3:7–12. doi: 10.4248/IJOS11006
19. Zhou X, Xu X, Li J, Hu D, Hu T, Yin W, et al. Oral health in China: from vision to action. *Int J Oral Sci.* (2018) 10:1. doi: 10.1038/s41368-017-0006-6
20. Chen C, LeGates R, Zhao M, Fang C. The changing rural-urban divide in China's megacities. *Cities.* (2018) 81:81–90. doi: 10.1016/j.cities.2018.03.017
21. People's Republic of China. *(PRC) State Council. National New Style Development Plan (NNSUP). 2014–2020.* Beijing: People's Publishing House (2015).

22. National Bureau of Statistics. *China Urban Construction Statistical Yearbook 2019.* Beijing: Ministry of Housing and Urban-Rural Development of People's Republic of China (2020).
23. Chen C, LeGates R, Fang C. From coordinated to integrated urban and rural development in China's megacity regions. *J Urban Aff.* (2019) 41:150–69. doi: 10.1080/07352166.2017.1413285
24. Huang L, Yan L, Wu J. Assessing urban sustainability of Chinese megacities: 35 years after the economic reform and open-door policy. *Landsc Urban Plan.* (2016) 145:57–70. doi: 10.1016/j.landurbplan.2015.09.005
25. Fu R, Wang Y, Bao H, Wang Z, Li Y, Su S, et al. Trend of urban-rural disparities in hospital admissions and medical expenditure in China from 2003 to 2011. *PLoS ONE.* (2014) 9:e108571. doi: 10.1371/journal.pone.0108571
26. Andersen RM, Davidson PL. Ethnicity, aging, and oral health outcomes: a conceptual framework. *Adv Dent Res.* (1997) 11:203–9. doi: 10.1177/08959374970110020201
27. Andersen RM. Revisiting the behavioral model and access to medical care: does it matter? *J Health Soc Behav.* (1995) 36:1. doi: 10.2307/2137284
28. Ganzeboom HBG, De Graaf PM, Treiman DJ. A standard international socio-economic index of occupational status. *Soc Sci Res.* (1992) 21:1–56. doi: 10.1016/0049-089X(92)90017-B
29. Xu J, Zhang J, Feng L, Qiu J. Self-rated health of population in southern China: association with socio-demographic characteristics measured with multiple-item self-rated health measurement scale. *BMC Public Health.* (2010) 10:393. doi: 10.1186/1471-2458-10-393
30. Caplan DJ, Slade GD, Gansky SA. Complex sampling: implications for data analysis. *J Public Health Dent.* (1999) 59:52–9. doi: 10.1111/j.1752-7325.1999.tb03235.x
31. Jang Y, Yoon H, Rhee M, Park NS, Chiriboga DA, Kim MT. Factors associated with dental service use of older Korean Americans. *Community Dent Oral Epidemiol.* (2019) 47:340–5. doi: 10.1111/cdoe.12464
32. Fereshtehnejad S-M, Garcia-Ptacek S, Religa D, Holmer J, Buhlin K, Eriksdotter M, et al. Dental care utilization in patients with different types of dementia: a longitudinal nationwide study of 58,037 individuals. *Alzheimers Dement.* (2018) 14:10–9. doi: 10.1016/j.jalz.2017.05.004
33. Rothman KJ, Greenland S, Lash TL. *Modern epidemiology. Third edition. Philadelphia Baltimore New York: Wolters Kluwer Health.* Philadelphia, PA: Lippincott Williams & Wilkins (2008). p. 758.
34. Meng Q, Fang H, Liu X, Yuan B, Xu J. Consolidating the social health insurance schemes in China: towards an equitable and efficient health system. *Lancet.* (2015) 386:1484–92. doi: 10.1016/S0140-6736(15)00342-6
35. Liu J, Zhang SS, Zheng SG, Xu T, Si Y. Oral health status and oral health care model in China. *Chin J Dent Res.* (2016) 19:207–15. doi: 10.3290/j.cjdr.a37145
36. You X, Kobayashi Y. The new cooperative medical scheme in China. *Health Policy.* (2009) 91:1–9. doi: 10.1016/j.healthpol.2008.11.012
37. Lin HC, Wong MCM, Wang ZJ, Lo ECM. Oral health knowledge, attitudes, and practices of chinese adults. *J Dent Res.* (2001) 80:1466–70. doi: 10.1177/00220345010800051601
38. Goodarzi A, Heidarnia A, Tavafian SS, Eslami M. Predicting oral health behaviors among Iranian students by using health belief model. *J Educ Health Promot.* (2019) 8:10. doi: 10.4103/jehp.jehp_10_18
39. Calvasina P, Lawrence HP, Hoffman-Goetz L, Norman CD. Brazilian immigrants' oral health literacy and participation in oral health care in Canada. *BMC Oral Health.* (2016) 16:18. doi: 10.1186/s12903-016-0176-1
40. Xu H, Straughan P, Pan W, Zhen Z, Wu B. Validating a scale of health beliefs in preventive health screenings among Chinese older adults. *J Transcult Nurs Off J Transcult Nurs Soc.* (2017) 28:464–72. doi: 10.1177/1043659616661392
41. Dai J, Hao Y, Li G, Hu D, Zhao Y. Love Teeth Day campaign in China and its impact on oral public health - the twentieth anniversary. *Br Dent J.* (2010) 209:523–6. doi: 10.1038/sj.bdj.2010.1039
42. Wu B, Plassman BL, Liang J, Remle RC, Bai L, Crout RJ. Differences in self-reported oral health among community-dwelling black, hispanic, and white elders. *J Aging Health.* (2011) 23:267–88. doi: 10.1177/0898264310382135
43. Dong M, Loignon C, Levine A, Bedos C. Perceptions of oral illness among Chinese immigrants in montreal: a qualitative study. *J Dent Educ.* (2007) 71:1340–7. doi: 10.1002/j.0022-0337.2007.71.10.tb04398.x

18

Saliva Quantification of SARS-CoV-2 in Real-Time PCR from Asymptomatic or Mild COVID-19 Adults

Florence Carrouel[1], Emilie Gadea[2,3], Aurélie Esparcieux[4], Jérome Dimet[5], Marie Elodie Langlois[6], Hervé Perrier[7], Claude Dussart[1] and Denis Bourgeois[1]*

[1] Health, Systemic, Process, UR4129 Research Unit, University Claude Bernard Lyon 1, University of Lyon, Lyon, France, [2] Equipe SNA-EPIS, EA4607, University Jean Monnet, Saint-Etienne, France, [3] Clinical Research Unit, Emile Roux Hospital Center, Le Puy-en-Velay, France, [4] Department of Internal Medicine and Infectious Diseases, Protestant Infirmary, Caluire-et-Cuire, France, [5] Clinical Research Center, Intercommunal Hospital Center of Mont de Marsan et du Pays des Sources, Mont de Marsan, France, [6] Department of Internal Medicine and Infectious Diseases, Saint Joseph Saint Luc Hospital, Lyon, France, [7] Clinical Research Unit, Protestant Infirmary, Lyon, France

***Correspondence:**
Florence Carrouel
florence.carrouel@univ-lyon1.fr

The fast spread of COVID-19 is related to the highly infectious nature of SARS-CoV-2. The disease is suggested to be transmitted through saliva droplets and nasal discharge. The saliva quantification of SARS-CoV-2 in real-time PCR from asymptomatic or mild COVID-19 adults has not been fully documented. This study analyzed the relationship between salivary viral load on demographics and clinical characteristics including symptoms, co-morbidities in 160 adults diagnosed as COVID-19 positive patients recruited between September and December 2020 in four French centers. Median initial viral load was 4.12 $\log_{10}$ copies/mL (IQR 2.95–5.16; range 0–10.19 $\log_{10}$ copies/mL). 68.6% of adults had no viral load detected. A median load reduction of 23% was observed between 0–2 days and 3–5 days, and of 11% between 3–5 days and 6–9 days for the delay from onset of symptoms to saliva sampling. No significant median difference between no-symptoms vs. symptoms patients was observed. Charge was consistently similar for the majority of the clinical symptoms excepted for headache with a median load value of 3.78 $\log_{10}$ copies/mL [1.95–4.58] ($P < 0.003$). SARS-CoV-2 RNA viral load was associated with headache and gastro-intestinal symptoms. The study found no statistically significant difference in viral loads between age groups, sex, or presence de co-morbidity. Our data suggest that oral cavity is an important site for SARS-CoV-2 infection and implicate saliva as a potential route of SARS-CoV-2 transmission.

Keywords: SARS-CoV-2, COVID-19, saliva, viral load, virus isolation, real-time reverse transcription PCR, infectivity, quantitative

INTRODUCTION

The fast spread of COVID-19 is related to the highly infectious nature of SARS-CoV-2. The disease is suggested to be transmitted through saliva droplets and nasal discharge (Li Y. et al., 2020). Indeed, SARS-CoV-2 is found in nasopharyngeal secretions, and its viral load is consistently high in the saliva, mainly in the early stage of the disease (Sapkota et al., 2020). In addition to saliva secreted by the major or minor salivary glands, saliva samples also contain secretions from the nasopharynx or from the lungs through the action of cilia lining the airway (Huang et al., 2021). Saliva can have potential applications in the context of COVID-19 by direct detection of the virus, quantification of the specific immunoglobulins produced against it, and for the evaluation of the non-specific, innate immune response of the patient (Ceron et al., 2020). Up to date, several cross-section and clinical trial studies published support the potential of detecting SARS-CoV-2 RNA in saliva as a biomarker for COVID-19, providing a self-collection, non-invasive, safe, and comfortable procedure (Caixeta et al., 2021; Carrouel et al., 2021).

Most published RT-qPCR assays for the diagnosis of SARS-CoV-2 are qualitative (Han et al., 2021). Considering the variability of viral load between and within patients, quantification of absolute viral load directly from pure raw saliva is important for COVID-19 diagnosis and monitoring (Vasudevan et al., 2021). Quantification of viral load has other objectives compared to screening. It gives an indication of the degree of contagiousness, provides guidance on the interest to predict contagiousness of patients and hence to guide epidemiological decisions, to evaluate different samples from different anatomical locations, to predict the patient prognosis and assess disease progression (Jacot et al., 2020). In this context, evidence reports on the salivary viral load or duration of viral detection or infectivity of COVID-19 to trace the disease and to implement strategies aimed at breaking the chain of disease transmission are particularly important (Huang et al., 2021). Overall, the studies were of low-to-moderate quality given that most of the included studies comprised case series and case reports at the early stages of the pandemic (Nasserie et al., 2021). Furthermore, given the number of studies analyzing the Chinese population, it is quite possible that the results cannot be generalized to other populations, especially to asymptomatic cases linked to 80% of disease transmission (Walsh et al., 2020). There is consensus that these results should be viewed with caution and should be confirmed by larger, more robust studies. It is clear that more research is needed on this topic to correlate viral load with symptoms and clinical outcomes (Mahallawi et al., 2021).

Hart et al. (2021) showed that about 65% of virus transmission occurs before symptoms develop. Thus, individuals circulate in the general community before their infections are detected (Hart et al., 2021). To better understand SARS-CoV-2 infectiousness before symptoms develop or with mild symptoms, we analyzed salivary viral load at the moment of disease. The purpose of this study is to outline the salivary SARS-CoV-2 viral load over the course of the infection in asymptomatic or mild COVID-19 adults.

MATERIALS AND METHODS

Study Design and Subjects

This analysis was a part of the randomized controlled trial BBCovid protocol published (Carrouel et al., 2020) and registered at ClinicalTrials.gov (NCT04352959). One hundred and sixty subjects diagnosed as COVID-19 positive patient were recruited between September and December 2020 in four French hospital centers. The study protocol was reviewed and approved by the National Ethics Committee "Committee for the Protection of Persons South Mediterranean III," France (2020.04.11 sept _20.04.06.46640). Written informed consent was obtained from all enrolled individuals. The study was conducted in accordance with the Declaration of Helsinki and the International Conference on Harmonization–Good Clinical Practice guidelines.

The inclusion criteria were: (i) age 18–85 years-old, (ii) RT-PCR positive COVID-19 nasopharyngeal swab, (iii) asymptomatic or mild clinical symptoms for less than 8 days.

The exclusion criteria were: (i) pregnancy, (ii) breastfeeding, (iii) risk of infectious endocarditis, (iii) use of mouthwash regularly (more than once a week), (iv) inability to comply with protocol, (v) lack of written agreement, (vi) unable to answer questions, and (vii) uncooperative patients.

Collecting of Demographic Data and Clinical Characteristics of Subjects

During the inclusion visit, demographic data (age, sex) and clinical characteristics (co-morbidities, symptoms, date of apparition of symptoms...) were collected from the subjects. Reporting of the nature of the symptoms was recorded at the time of the viral load measurement. An electronic medical record (e-CRF) permitted to record all these informations.

Quantification of SARS-CoV-2 Salivary Load

Saliva Sampling

At 9 a.m., each subject collected one salivary sample with an accredited health care professional using the Saliva Collection System kit (Greiner Bio-one, Kremsmünster, Austria). Only one sample was collected from each adult. Firstly, with the saliva extraction solution, the subject rinsed the oral cavity for 2 min. Secondly, the subject spit into a saliva-collection beaker, without coughing or scraping to clear the throat, to collect the non-stimulated and pure saliva (between 1 and 3.5 mL). Finally, the saliva sample transferred to a sterile tube and stored at 4°C until analysis.

Quantification of SARS-CoV-2 Viral Load by Real-Time RT-PCR

RNA was extracted from 200 μL of saliva sample using the NucliSens easyMAG instrument (bioMérieux, Marcy-l'Etoile, France), according to the manufacturer's guidelines. The RNA was eluted in 50 μL of water and used as a template for real-time (rt) RT-PCR.

Real-time RT-PCR assays were performed with the Invitrogen Superscript™ III Platinum One-Step qRT-PCR system (Invitrogen, Illkirch, France). The mix was composed of 5 μL of extracted RNA, 1 μL of Superscript III RT/Platinum Taq Mix, 12.5 μL of 2X reaction buffer, 0.4 μL of a 50 mM magnesium sulfate solution, 1 μL of RdRp-IP2 forward primer (0.4 μM), 1 μL of RdRp-IP2 reverse primer (0.4 μM), 1 μL of

RdRp-IP4 forward primer (0.4 μM), 1 μL of RdRp-IP4 reverse primer (0.4 μM). The primer and probe sequences correspond to the RdRp-IP2 and the RdRp-IP4 assays designed at The Institut Pasteur to target a section of the RdRp gene (nt 12621-12727 and 14010-14116 positions) based on the sequences of SARS-CoV-2 (NC_004718) made available on the Global Initiative on Sharing All Influenza Data data-base on 11 January 2020 (**Table 1**). These primers and probes were manufactured by Eurofins (Genomics, Germany).

The assays were performed on a Quant Studio 5 (Thermo Fisher Scientific, Dardilly, France) with the following program: 55°C for 10 min (reverse transcription), followed by 95°C for 2 min, and then 45 cycles of 95°C for 3 s and 58°C for 30 s. Each run included three negatives' samples bracketing unknown samples during RNA extraction, two positive controls, and one negative amplification control. When a sample was positive for RdRp-IP4, the quantification of the number of RNA copies was performed according to a scale ranging from 10^2 to 10^6 copies per μL. The SARS-CoV-2 viral load in saliva was calculated as the number of RNA copies per mL of saliva.

Statistical Analysis

SPSS Windows 20.0 (IBM, Chicago, IL, United States) was used for the descriptive statistics median values and interquartile range (IQR) and mean values with SD for the quantitative variables and percentages for categorical variables. One-way ANOVA was used to compare the differences of median between groups in a univariate analysis. Binary logistic regression analysis was used to model the relationship between viral load values as the dependent variable and the other parameters were entered individually as independent variables (adjusted for age and gender). The detailed statistical methods are indicated in the table footnotes. All data were considered statistically significant when $p < 0.05$.

RESULTS

Demographic Data and Clinical Characteristics of Subjects

The sex, the age and the clinical assessments of the study group are summarized in **Table 2**. The sample consisted of 160 subjects (55.97% of females and 44.03% of males) with a mean age of 43.62 ± 15.56 years. One co-morbidity was declared by 22.15% of subjects. The median time between symptoms onset and the positive nasopharyngeal RT-PCR was 4 days [IQR 3–5]. The median number of symptoms per subjects was 4 [IQR 2–5]. The most frequent symptoms described by 52.87% of subjects were the cough and the headache followed by myalgia in 48.41% of subjects. Fever was reported in 41.40% of subjects; anosmia in 40.13% of subjects; ageusia in 38.22% of subjects; dyspnea in 12.74% of subjects and; gastro intestinal symptoms in 8.92% of subjects. The absence of symptoms was only observed in 8.92% of subjects. For symptomatic subjects, the saliva sample was collected in median 6 days [IQR 5–7] after the onset of symptoms.

Quantification of SARS-CoV-2 Viral Load According to Demographics and Clinical Characteristics of Participants

Median initial viral load was 4.12 $\log_{10}$ copies/mL (IQR 2.95–5.16 $\log_{10}$ copies/mL, range 0–10.19 $\log_{10}$ copies/mL). The first quartile (Q1) corresponded to a viral load starting at 2.95 $\log_{10}$ copies/mL, whereas the second (Q2) corresponded to a viral load starting at 4.12 $\log_{10}$ copies/mL, and the third (Q3) corresponded to a viral load starting at 5.16 $\log_{10}$ copies/mL.

The SARS-CoV-2 salivary viral load according to demographics and clinical characteristics of participants are described in **Table 3** and **Figures 1, 2**. The median SARS-CoV-2 salivary viral load increased not significantly with age groups from 3.82 $\log_{10}$ copies/mL (18–34 years) to 4.31 $\log_{10}$ copies/mL (55–77 years). Salivary viral load was not associated with sex. The presence of co-morbidity or not, did not significantly modify the SARS-CoV-2 salivary viral load. Same observation was done for the time between RT-PCR and symptom onset, the delay from symptom onset to saliva sampling and for the number of symptoms per participants. Patients with symptoms demonstrated a median initial viral load of 4.12 $\log_{10}$ copies/mL (IQR 2.95–5.16; range 0–10.19 $\log_{10}$ copies/mL), while the no-symptoms patients had indices of 4.01 $\log_{10}$ copies/mL (IQR 0.56–5.75 $\log_{10}$ copies/mL, range 0–6.24 $\log_{10}$ copies/mL).

Determination of Factors Associated With SARS-CoV-2 Salivary Viral Load

The analysis of the mean difference of SARS-CoV-2 salivary load was reported in **Table 4**. For the delay from onset of symptoms

TABLE 1 | RT-PCR for the detection of SARS-CoV-2: primers and probes used.

Name	Sequences (5′–3′)	PCR product	References
RdRp gene/nCoV_IP2			
nCoV_IP2-12669Fw	ATGAGCTTAGTCCTGTTG	108 pb	CNR*
nCoV_IP2-12759Rv	CTCCCTTTGTTGTGTTGT		CNR*
nCoV_IP2-12669bProbe(+)	[5′]HEX-AGATGTCTTGTGCTGCCGGTA-[3′]BHQ-1		CNR*
RdRp gene/nCoV_IP4			
nCoV_IP4-14059Fw	GGTAACTGGTATGATTTCG	107 pb	CNR*
nCoV_IP4-14146Rv	CTGGTCAAGGTTAATATAGG		CNR*
nCoV_IP4-14084Probe(+)	[5′]Fam−TCATACAAACCACGCCAGG−[3′]BHQ-1		CNR*

**CNR: National Reference Center for Respiratory Viruses, Institut Pasteur, Paris, France.*

TABLE 2 | Baseline characteristics of enrolled patients with Coronavirus Disease 2019.

Variable	
Gender, n/N* (%)	
Male	70/159 (44.03%)
Female	89/159 (55.97%)
Age (years)	N = 158
Mean ± SD	43.62 ± 15.56
Median [IQR]	43 [30–55]
Age (class), n/N* (%)	
18–34 years	52/158 (32.91%)
35–54 years	65/158 (41.14%)
55–77 years	41/158 (25.95%)
Co-morbidity, n/N* (%)	33/149 (22.15%)
Time between positive RT-PCR and symptom onset (days)	N = 153
Mean ± SD	3.93 ± 1.46
Median [IQR]	4 [3–5]
Time between positive RT-PCR and symptom onset (class), n/N* (%)	
0–2 days	27/153 (17.65%)
3–5 days	108/153 (70.59%)
6–8 days	18/153 (11.76%)
Number of symptoms per subjects	N = 157
Mean ± SD	3.71 ± 2.27
Median [IQR]	4 [2–5]
Number of symptoms per subjects (class), n/N* (%)	
None	14/157 (8.92%)
1–4	40/157 (25.48%)
5–6	65/157 (41.40%)
7–9	38/157 (24.20%)
Symptoms, n/N* (%)	
None	14/157 (8.92%)
Fever	65/157 (41.40%)
Cough	83/157 (52.87%)
Dyspnea	20/157 (12.74%)
Headache	83/157 (52.87%)
Myalgia	76/157 (48.41%)
Gastro symptoms	14/157 (8.92%)
Anosmia	63/157 (40.13%)
Ageusia	60/157 (38.22%)
Delay from symptom onset to saliva sampling (days)	N = 141
Mean ± SD	5.55 ± 1.62
Median [IQR]	6 [5–7]
Delay from symptom onset to saliva sampling (class), n/N* (%)	
0–2 days	7/141 (4.96%)
3–5 days	57/141 (40.43%)
6–9 days	77/141 (54.61%)

n, Number of subjects, N, Total number of subjects.
**n/N, Number of subjects/Total number of subjects.*

to saliva sampling, the SARS-CoV-2 salivary load continuously decreased with the of the days. A median load reduction of 23% was observed between 0-2 days and 3-5 days, and of 11% between 3-5 days and 6-9 days. However, no significant difference between the groups was detected.

TABLE 3 | Association of viral Load with demographics and clinical parameters for all enrolled participants: N: number of subjects.

Variable	N	Viral load, median [95% CI]	*p*-value
Sex			0.290[a]
Male	70	4.48 [2.99–5.54]	
Female	89	4.02 [2.18–4.69]	
Age			0.290[b]
18–34 years	52	3.82 [2.89–4.57]	
35–54 years	65	4.14 [2.72–5.72]	
55–77 years	41	4.31 [2.94–5.62]	
Co-morbidity			0.856[a]
No	116	4.12 [2.95–5.15]	
Yes	33	4.12 [3.01–5.5]	
Time between positive RT-PCR and symptom onset			0.637[b]
0–2 days	27	4.33 [2.62–5.09]	
3–5 days	108	4.13 [2.94–5.48]	
6–8 days	18	4.08 [0.81–4.82]	
Delay from symptom onset to saliva sampling			0.206[c]
0–2 days	7	5.63 [3.91–5.88]	
3–5 days	57	4.34 [2.75–5.47]	
6–9 days	77	3.86 [2.96–4.72]	
Number of symptoms per subjects			0.573[b]
1–4	40	3.85 [2.16–4.75]	
5–6	65	4.29 [3.4–5.49]	
7–9	38	3.93 [2.98–5.16]	
None	14	4.01 [0.56–5.75]	
Symptoms			
Fever			0.504[a]
No	92	4.07 [2.6–5.01]	
Yes	65	4.24 [3.04–5.47]	
Cough			0.097[a]
No	74	3.83 [2.05–4.74]	
Yes	83	4.14 [3.03–5.48]	
Dyspnea			0.627[a]
No	137	4.12 [2.75–5.17]	
Yes	20	4.13 [2.77–5.04]	
Headache			0.004[a]
No	74	3.78 [1.95–4.58]	
Yes	83	4.51 [3.32–5.59]	
Myalgia			0.721[a]
No	81	4.14 [2.25–5.02]	
Yes	76	4.10 [2.98–5.29]	
Gastrointestinal symptoms			0.212[a]
No	143	4.12 [2.95–5.17]	
Yes	14	3.88 [0–4.57]	
Anosmia			0.126[a]
No	94	4.29 [2.95–5.5]	
Yes	63	3.78 [2.7–4.54]	
Ageusia			0.147[a]
No	97	4.26 [2.94–5.49]	
Yes	60	3.78 [2.71–4.59]	

[a] *Mann-Whitney test.*
[b] *Kruskal-Wallis test.*
[c] *ANOVA test.*

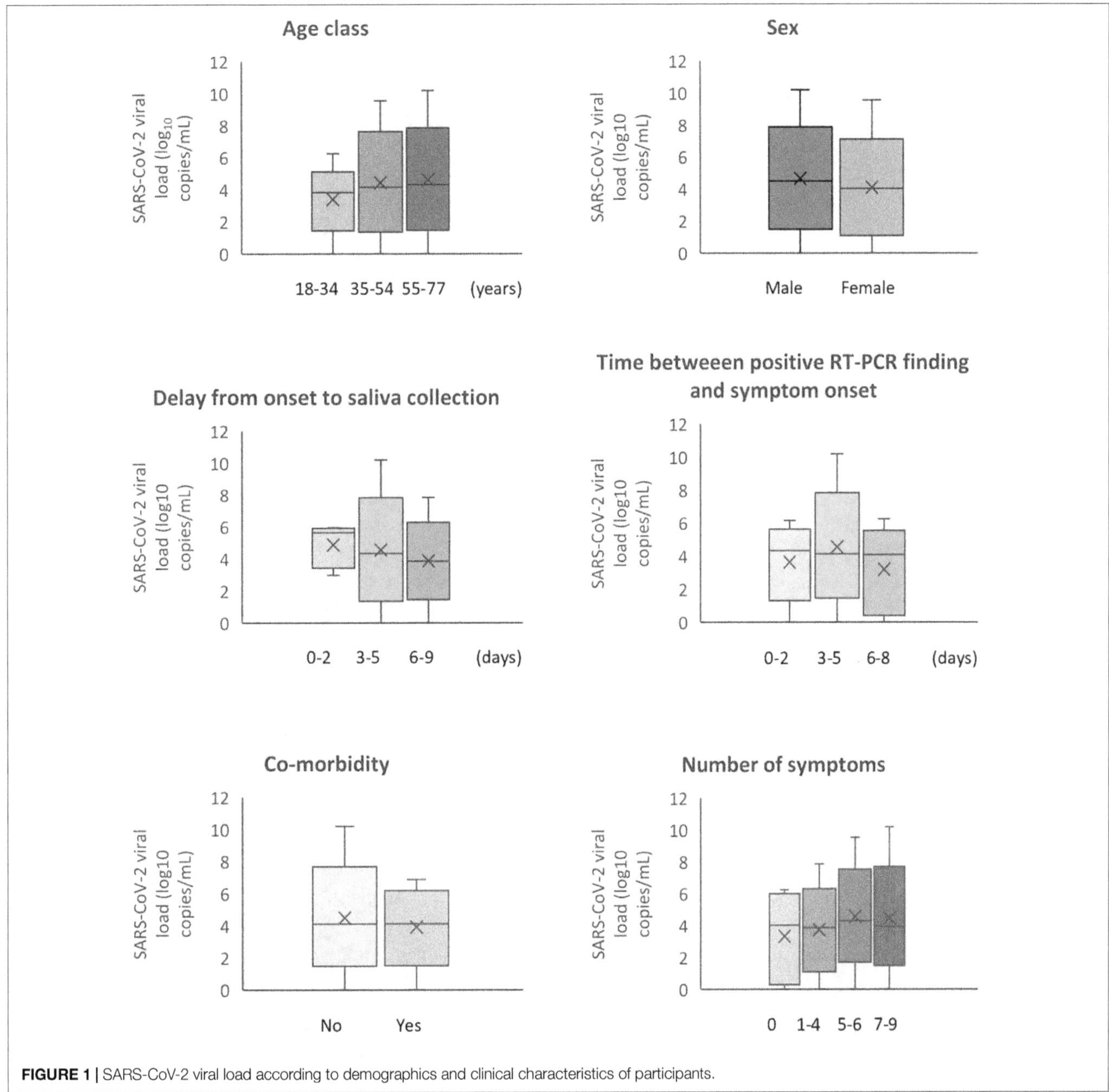

FIGURE 1 | SARS-CoV-2 viral load according to demographics and clinical characteristics of participants.

Concerning the time between positive RT-PCR and symptom onset, a non-significant decrease of −0.12 log_{10} copies/mL [IQR −0.34–0.10] was observed. First, an increase 0.26 log_{10} copies/mL [IQR −0.67–1.18] was observed at 3–5 days compared with 0–2 days. Then, a decrease of −0.39 log_{10} copies/mL [IQR −1.70–0.92] was observed at 6–8 days.

Between no-symptoms patients with an initially salivary SARS-CoV-2 load of 4.01 log_{10} copies/mL [IQR 0.56–5.75] and patients with symptoms (**Table 3**), there was no significant median difference in the viral load (**Table 4**). However, COVID-19 adults declaring 5–6 or 7–9 symptoms have a higher viral median difference charge of 0.56 log_{10} copies/mL [IQR −0.71–1.83] and 0.50 log_{10} copies/mL [IQR −0.85–1.85] respectively.

The salivary SARS-CoV-2 viral load was consistently similar for the majority of the clinical symptoms concerned even if SARS-CoV-2 salivary load increased in presence of fever 0.24 log_{10} copies/mL [IQR −0.46–0.93], cough 0.58 log_{10} copies/mL [IQR −0.10–1.26], dyspnea 0.50 log_{10} copies/mL [IQR −0.53–1.53] and myalgia 0.19 log_{10} copies/mL [IQR −0.50–0.88]. With a median difference increase of 1.04 log_{10} copies/mL [IQR 0.37–1.71], headache in confirmation of symptomatic cases influence significantly the salivary viral load ($P < 0.003$) (**Table 4**). The patients without headache had a mean salivary viral load of 3.78 log_{10} copies/mL [IQR 1.95–4.58] whereas patients with headache had a mean salivary viral load of 4.51 log_{10} copies/mL [IQR 3.32–5.59] (**Table 3**).

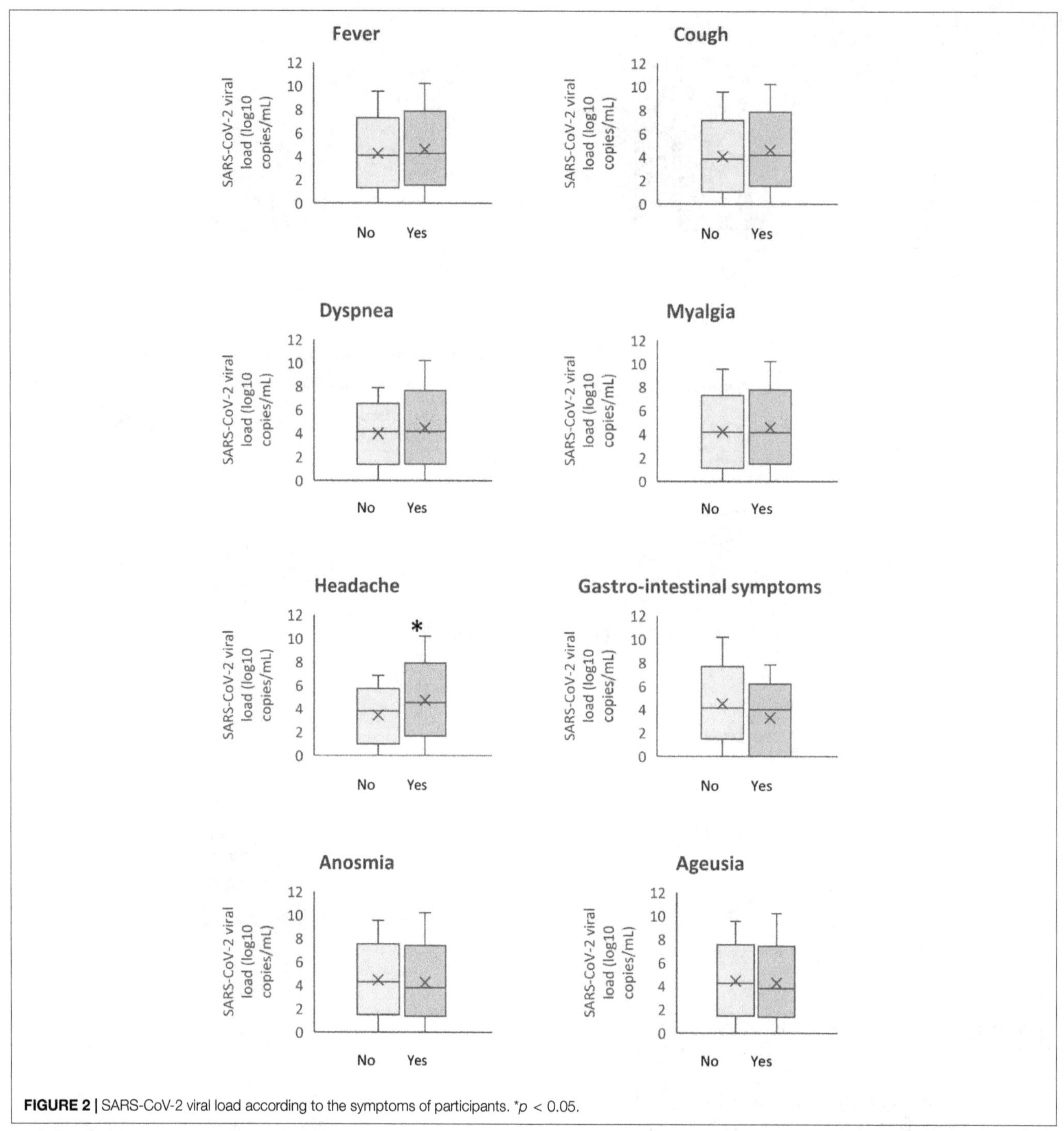

FIGURE 2 | SARS-CoV-2 viral load according to the symptoms of participants. $^*p < 0.05$.

In multivariate logistic regression analysis, the relation between salivary viral load and headache and GI symptoms remained significant after adjustment for age and sex ($P = 0.004$ and $P = 0.043$, respectively) (**Table 5**).

DISCUSSION

The present study was designed to explore the quantification of SARS-CoV-2 in pure saliva of adults with asymptomatic to mild COVID-19. This robust multicenter observational trial, including 160 individuals, is the first, to our knowledge, to target this specific population—mean age of patients was 43.62 ± 15.56 years- and to describe the sociodemographic and clinical characteristics of the salivary viral load. The load SARS-CoV-2 value of the whole sample ranged from 0.00 to 10.19 with a median of 4.12 $\log_{10}$ copies/mL (IQR 2.95–5.16 $\log_{10}$ copies/mL), 27/159 patients (16.98%) had no charge. Between no-symptoms patients with an initially salivary SARS and patients with symptoms, there was no significant

TABLE 4 | Association of viral load with sex, age, symptoms of severe acute respiratory syndrome coronavirus 2 (SARS-CoV-2) infection: univariable analysis.

Variable	References level	Class level	Mean difference [95% CI]	*p*-value
Age	CV		0.02 [−0.01–0.04]	0.179
Age (class)	18–34	35–54	0.40 [−0.40–1.20]	0.330
		55–77	0.42 [−0.48–1.32]	0.359
Gender	Male	Female	−0.60 [−1.28–0.08]	0.084
Co-morbidity	No	Yes	−0.01 [−0.83–0.81]	0.974
Time between positive RT-PCR and symptom onset	CV		−0.11 [−0.35–0.13]	0.354
Time between positive RT-PCR and symptom onset (class)	0–2 days	3–5 days	0.26 [−0.67–1.18]	0.583
		6–8 days	−0.39 [−1.70–0.92]	0.560
Delay from symptom onset to saliva sampling	CV		−0.12 [−0.34–0.10]	0.283
Delay from symptom onset to saliva sampling (class)	0–2 days	3–5 days	−0.87 [−2.55–0.81]	0.312
		6–9 days	−1.31 [−2.96–0.35]	0.124
Number of symptoms per subjects	CV		0.08 [−0.07–0.24]	0.275
Number of symptoms per subjects (class)	None	1–4	0.02 [−1.31–1.36]	0.973
		5–6	0.56 [−0.71–1.83]	0.387
		7–9	0.50 [−0.85–1.85]	0.468
Symptoms				
None	Yes	No	−0.39 [−1.60–0.81]	0.522
Fever	No	Yes	0.24 [−0.46–0.93]	0.504
Cough	No	Yes	0.58 [−0.10–1.26]	0.097
Dyspnea	No	Yes	0.50 [−0.53–1.53]	0.341
Headache	No	Yes	1.04 [0.37–1.71]	0.003
Myalgia	No	Yes	0.19 [−0.50–0.88]	0.589
Grasto-intestinal symptoms	No	Yes	−0.98 [−2.17–0.22]	0.112
Anosmia	No	Yes	−0.29 [−0.99–0.41]	0.423
Ageusia	No	Yes	−0.25 [−0.95–0.46]	0.497

CV: continuous variable.

TABLE 5 | Association of viral load with sex, age, symptoms of severe acute respiratory syndrome coronavirus 2 (SARS-CoV-2) infection: Multivariable Analysis.

Variable	References level	Class level	Mean difference [95% CI]	*p*-value
Age	CV		0.01 [−0.01–0.04]	0.188
Gender	Male	Female	−0.56 [−1.23–0.11]	0.102
Symptoms				
Cough	No	Yes	0.40 [−0.28–1.08]	0.250
Headache	No	Yes	1.02 [0.34–1.7]	0.004
Grasto-intestinal symptoms	No	Yes	−1.22 [−2.39−0.05]	0.043

CV, continuous variable.

median difference in the viral load. Collectively, these data show that the oral cavity is an important site for SARS-CoV-2 infection and implicate saliva as a potential route of SARS-CoV-2 transmission.

While self-collected saliva is a realistic alternative option for the diagnosis of COVID-19, there are no significant studies in the literature evaluating the salivary viral load of adults with asymptomatic, to mild COVID-19. If Huang et al. (2021) suggest two possible sources for SARS-CoV-2 in saliva: an acellular fraction from infected glands making virus *de novo* and a cellular fraction from infected and shed oral mucosa, little is known about the correlation between viral load and age, gender, symptoms, and comorbidity. The first study quantifying the salivary load of SARS-CoV-2 included 12 hospitalized patients with laboratory-confirmed COVID-19, with a median age of 62.5 years. SARS-CoV-2 was detected in 91.7% of throat saliva samples from COVID-19 patients, and the number was as high as 1–2 × 10^8 infectious copies per milliliter (To et al., 2020). Observational studies are subject to a number of different biases (Accorsi et al., 2021). Lecture of meta-analysis of diagnostic results from saliva (Moreira et al., 2021) reveals that no studies met our objective and methodological criteria.

So, studies included different subgroups categorized by gradation of disease severity, primarily in patients who developed severe disease admitted to intensive care during their hospital stay, and both inpatients with moderate disease symptoms (Alteri et al., 2020; Jeong et al., 2020; Kam et al., 2020; Kim et al., 2020; Lai et al., 2020; Pan et al., 2020; Pujadas et al., 2020; To et al., 2020; Yoon et al., 2020; Yu et al., 2020; Abasiyanik et al., 2021; Chua et al., 2021; Han et al., 2021;

Hasanoglu et al., 2021). Then, participants were included with a diverse range of COVID-19 disease severity, including in majority cases hospitalized, and individuals with resolved infection. So, different diagnosis methods were used in self-collected saliva as nucleic acid amplification testing, transcription mediated amplification, reverse transcription loop-mediated isothermal amplification, TRIzol-based RNA extraction, despite quantitative reverse transcription PCR is the diagnostic standard for SARS-CoV-2 (Nagura-Ikeda et al., 2020). Several papers used the naive Ct values from qualitative RT-PCR as a quantitation unit or use the ΔCt values with incorrect quantitation unit (Shen et al., 2020; Zou et al., 2020). Saliva collection protocols for included studies were assessed for differences with respect to asking patients to collect pure saliva or to cough or clear their throat before submission of enhanced sample likely mixed sputum and saliva specimen or deep throat saliva specimen or requesting the patients submit "drool" or "spit" (Carrouel et al., 2020; Khiabani and Amirzade-Iranaq, 2021).

With reference to viral load during infection in asymptomatic or mildly affected adults with COVID-19, we observed that viral load is generally high, although asymptomatic viral loads are not statistically different from symptomatic viral loads, tending, however, to be lower. These results highlight the potential infectivity of saliva although the possible threshold of transmissibility is not specified and there is no standard reference in this regard. In particular, these results suggest that expelled oral droplets containing infectious virus and infected cells may be a source of airborne transmission of SARS-CoV-2. SARS-CoV-2 transmission from people who are either asymptomatic or mild has implications for prevention. Social distancing measures will need to be sustained at some level because droplet transmission from close contact with people with asymptomatic and mild infection occurs (Bazant and Bush, 2021). Easing of restrictions will, however, only be possible with wide access to testing, contact tracing, and rapid isolation of infected individuals.

The mean age of patients in our study was 43.6 years. We found that gender and age are not factors affecting viral load. According to published data, younger patients would be more likely to be asymptomatic than older patients (Li Y. et al., 2020). Studies have shown that both older age and male gender are associated with severe disease (Qian et al., 2020). To et al. (2020) found similar results to Zheng et al. (2020) and both concluded that older age is associated with higher viral load. Mahallawi et al. (2021) studied the viral load of lower and upper respiratory tract specimens from 3,006 COVID-19 positive patients. They found no statistically significant difference between age groups, while the viral load was statistically significantly higher in women than in men.

Specific observational studies as well as modeling work have shown that the infection can be asymptomatic or paucisymptomatic (causing little or no clinical manifestations) in 30–60% of infected individuals, especially in young adults and adults (Plucinski et al., 2021). Asymptomatic individuals were the source for 69% (20–85%) of all infections (Emery et al., 2020). Saliva from asymptomatic individuals contains infectious virus. Surprisingly, the viral load was found to be significantly similar between asymptomatic and symptomatic patients infected with SARS-CoV-2 ($p = 0.573$). Since the beginning of the pandemic, there has been controversy about the infectivity of asymptomatic patients. With the aforementioned limitation on the robustness of existing studies which are based on considerably smaller data sets, most studies demonstrate more rapid viral clearance in asymptomatic individuals than in symptomatic ones (McEvoy et al., 2021). A large representative sample with longitudinal data has shown that both symptomatic and asymptomatic patients are often characterized by a similar amount of virus at the onset of infection (Lavezzo et al., 2020). It is reported that approximately 40–45% of patients infected with SARS-CoV-2 will remain asymptomatic (Oran and Topol, 2020). Additionally, individuals with mild, non-specific, asymptomatic symptoms are difficult to identify and quarantine (Han et al., 2021). The ambiguity surrounding both asymptomatic and presymptomatic conditions is highlighted. They are described as suggestive, and both inconclusive. Because of the high risk of silent spread by asymptomatic individuals, it is imperative that screening programs include those without symptoms (Oran and Topol, 2020; Almadhi et al., 2021).

Screening from symptoms could prioritize tests and increase diagnostic sensitivity (Lan et al., 2020). However, in our study, salivary load quantification is not discriminated on the number and nature of reported symptoms except for headache. General non-respiratory symptoms (eye pain, muscle pain, general malaise, fever, headache, and extreme fatigue), although not very specific, are the strongest independent predictors of positive tests (Tostmann et al., 2020). As a non-specific symptom, headache can occur not only in COVID-19 but also in other viral diseases. Therefore, headache alone may not raise suspicion of SARS-CoV-2 infection although headache was 1.7 times more common in patients with COVID-19 respiratory viral infection than in those with non-COVID-19 respiratory viral infection with $p = 0.04$ (Correia et al., 2020; Mutiawati et al., 2021). The presence of gastrointestinal symptoms associated with salivary viral load in COVID-19 patients raises questions about the impact of COVID-19 infection on the quality of life of at-risk subjects. It is quite plausible to observe the development of several gastro-intestinal symptoms induced by SARS-CoV-2 infection in patients, ranging from nausea, vomiting, and diarrhea to loss of appetite and abdominal pain (Yusuf et al., 2021).

Chemosensory dysfunctions, especially hyposmia, anosmia, hypogeusia, and ageusia, are one of the major symptoms of SARS-CoV2 infection (Srinivasan, 2021). Self-reported loss of smell and taste is a better prognosticator than other symptoms such as cough, fatigue, or fever for predicting symptomatic infection (Mastrangelo et al., 2021). Our results indicate that SARS-CoV-2 levels in saliva do not correlate with taste alterations.

First limitation of our study is that it focused on the second wave of the epidemic in the second half of 2020. Adaptation of salivary quantification guidelines in relation to newly detected SARS-CoV-2 variants is necessary. At the time of the study the variant circulating in France was predominantly the UK variant (B.1.1.7) and not the Delta variant (B.1.617.2) which is now detected in the majority of cases. Thus, it is likely that the results would be different if the study were conducted now since the delta variant has different characteristics (Mlcochova et al., 2021).

Secondly, we also clearly explained the ambiguity surrounding asymptomatic vs. presymptomatic status. We describe them as suggestive, not conclusive. While measuring viral load can be useful in clinical practice, a positive RT-qPCR result does not necessarily mean that the person is still infectious or still has significant disease. The RNA could be from a non-viable virus and/or the amount of live virus could be too low to allow transmission (Trunfio et al., 2021). Contacts of a carrier with a high viral salivary load may have a higher risk of acquiring infection, but to date there is no evidence that acquired infection will be more likely to be symptomatic or severe (Li R. et al., 2020; Hasanoglu et al., 2021; van Kampen et al., 2021).

Strengths of our study is that, although *post hoc* studies have revealed the importance of SARS-CoV-2 corona virus 2 transmission from both asymptomatic and mildly symptomatic cases, the virologic basis for their infectivity remains largely unquantified (Jones et al., 2021). Despite PCR method do not measure infectious virus, our study produces original and robust quantitative data applied to an ambulatory adult population susceptible to be the prime actor of transmission until effective vaccines have been distributed widely.

CONCLUSION

Our results raise the possibility that the oral cavity is an important site for SARS-CoV-2 infection and implicate saliva as a potential route of SARS-CoV-2 transmission. This result may have public health implications if enhanced saliva samples are used for asymptomatic screening. Considering oral SARS-CoV-2 infection and the ease of saliva for transmission, it remains critical to further understanding of the dominant modes of viral spread across the spectrum of asymptomatic, pre-symptomatic and symptomatic individuals.

South Mediterranean III, France. The patients/participants provided their written informed consent to participate in this study.

AUTHOR CONTRIBUTIONS

FC, DB, and CD proposed the original study idea and designed the trial and study protocol. DB and FC contributed to the data interpretation and wrote the first draft of the manuscript. FC, CD, and HP verified the data. EG, AE, ML, and JD were responsible for the site work including the recruitment, follow up and data collection. HP monitored the trial. DB did the main analysis. CD, EG, and JD contributed to the revision of the manuscript. All authors reviewed and accepted the manuscript before submission.

ACKNOWLEDGMENTS

We thank and acknowledge all the patients and trial team members. More particularly, Sophie Lengagne, Eva Geraud and Anthea Loiez from the Emile Roux Hospital Center (Le Puy-en-Velay, France); Louis Gauthier from the Protestant Infirmary (Lyon, France), Séverine Poupblanc, Anne-Hélène Boivin from the Intercommunal Hospital Center of "Mont de Marsan et du Pays des Sources" (Mont de Marsan, France); Armand Sophie, Caroline Gagneux, Adrien Didelot, Matthieu Pecquet, Marie Paul Perraud Josiane Thimonier (Cadres des services) from Saint Joseph Saint Luc Hospital (Lyon, France). We also thank all the technician from the CNR for their work. We thank Stéphane Morisset independent statistician and special adviser. We also extend our thanks to Eric Bomel, EZUS, University Lyon1 who provided central administrative support to the project, and Eric Gonzalez Garcia, from Greiner Bio-One GmbH (Kremsmuenster, Austria) who provided kindly technical support.

REFERENCES

1. Abasiyanik, M. F., Flood, B., Lin, J., Ozcan, S., Rouhani, S. J., Pyzer, A., et al. (2021). Sensitive detection and quantification of SARS-CoV-2 in saliva. *Sci. Rep.* 11:12425. doi: 10.1038/s41598-021-91835-7
2. Accorsi, E. K., Qiu, X., Rumpler, E., Kennedy-Shaffer, L., Kahn, R., Joshi, K., et al. (2021). How to detect and reduce potential sources of biases in studies of SARS- CoV-2 and COVID-19. *Eur. J. Epidemiol.* 36, 179–196. doi: 10.1007/s10654- 021-00727-7
3. Almadhi, M. A., Abdulrahman, A., Sharaf, S. A., AlSaad, D., Stevenson, N. J., Atkin, S. L., et al. (2021). The high prevalence of asymptomatic SARS-CoV-2 infection reveals the silent spread of COVID-19. *Int. J. Infect. Dis.* 105, 656–661. doi: 10.1016/j.ijid.2021.02.100
4. Alteri, C., Cento, V., Antonello, M., Colagrossi, L., Merli, M., Ughi, N., et al. (2020). Detection and quantification of SARS-CoV-2 by droplet digital PCR in real- time PCR negative nasopharyngeal swabs from suspected COVID-19 patients. *PLoS One* 15:e0236311. doi: 10.1371/journal.pone.0236311
5. Bazant, M. Z., and Bush, J. W. M. (2021). A guideline to limit indoor airborne transmission of COVID-19. *Proc. Natl. Acad. Sci. U.S.A.* 118:e2018995118. doi: 10.1073/pnas.2018995118
6. Caixeta, D. C., Oliveira, S. W., Cardoso-Sousa, L., Cunha, T. M., Goulart, L. R., Martins, M. M., et al. (2021). One-year update on salivary diagnostic of COVID-19. *Front. Public Health* 9:589564. doi: 10.3389/fpubh.2021. 589564
7. Carrouel, F., Valette, M., Perrier, H., Bouscambert-Duchamp, M., Dussart, C., Tramini, P., et al. (2021). Performance of self-collected saliva testing compared with nasopharyngeal swab testing for the detection of SARS-CoV-2. *Viruses* 13:895. doi: 10.3390/v13050895
8. Carrouel, F., Viennot, S., Valette, M., Cohen, J.-M., Dussart, C., and Bourgeois, D. (2020). Salivary and Nasal detection of the SARS-CoV-2 virus after antiviral mouthrinses (BBCovid): a structured summary of a study protocol for a randomised controlled trial. *Trials* 21:906. doi: 10.1186/s13063-020- 04846-6
9. Ceron, J. J., Lamy, E., Martinez-Subiela, S., Lopez-Jornet, P., Capela-Silva, F., Eckersall, P. D., et al. (2020). Use of saliva for diagnosis and monitoring the SARS-CoV-2: a general perspective. *J. Clin. Med.* 9:1491. doi: 10.3390/jcm9051491
10. Chua, G. T., Wong, J. S. C., To, K. K. W., Lam, I. C. S., Yau, F. Y. S., Chan, W. H., et al. (2021). Saliva viral load better correlates with clinical and immunological profiles in children with coronavirus disease 2019. *Emerg Microbes Infect.* 10, 235–241. doi: 10.1080/22221751.2021.1878937
11. Correia, A. O., Feitosa, P. W. G., Moreira, J. L., de, S., Nogueira, S. ÁR., Fonseca, R. B., et al. (2020). Neurological manifestations of COVID-19 and other coronaviruses: a systematic review. *Neurol. Psychiatry Brain Res.* 37, 27–32. doi: 10.1016/j.npbr.2020.05.008
12. Emery, J. C., Russell, T. W., Liu, Y., Hellewell, J., Pearson, C. A., Cmmid Covid-19 Working Group, et al. (2020). The contribution of asymptomatic SARS-CoV-2 infections to transmission on the diamond princess cruise ship. *Elife* 9:e58699. doi: 10.7554/eLife.58699
13. Han, M. S., Byun, J.-H., Cho, Y., and Rim, J. H. (2021). RT-PCR for SARS-CoV-2: quantitative versus qualitative. *Lancet Infect. Dis.* 21:165. doi: 10.1016/S1473- 3099(20)30424-2
14. Hart, W. S., Maini, P. K., and Thompson, R. N. (2021). High infectiousness immediately before COVID-19 symptom onset highlights the importance of continued contact tracing. *Elife* 10:e65534. doi: 10.7554/eLife.65534

15. Hasanoglu, I., Korukluoglu, G., Asilturk, D., Cosgun, Y., Kalem, A. K., Altas, A. B., et al. (2021). Higher viral loads in asymptomatic COVID-19 patients might be the invisible part of the iceberg. *Infection* 49, 117–126. doi: 10.1007/s15010-020- 01548-8
16. Huang, N., Pérez, P., Kato, T., Mikami, Y., Okuda, K., Gilmore, R. C., et al. (2021). SARS-CoV-2 infection of the oral cavity and saliva. *Nat. Med.* 27, 892–903. doi: 10.1038/s41591-021-01296-8
17. Jacot, D., Greub, G., Jaton, K., and Opota, O. (2020). Viral load of SARS-CoV-2 across patients and compared to other respiratory viruses. *Microbes Infect.* 22, 617–621. doi: 10.1016/j.micinf.2020.08.004
18. Jeong, H. W., Kim, S.-M., Kim, H.-S., Kim, Y.-I., Kim, J. H., Cho, J. Y., et al. (2020). Viable SARS-CoV-2 in various specimens from COVID-19 patients. *Clin. Microbiol. Infect.* 26, 1520–1524. doi: 10.1016/j.cmi.2020.07.020
19. Jones, T. C., Biele, G., Mühlemann, B., Veith, T., Schneider, J., Beheim-Schwarzbach, J., et al. (2021). Estimating infectiousness throughout SARS-CoV- 2 infection course. *Science* 373:eabi5273. doi: 10.1126/science.abi5273
20. Kam, K.-Q., Yung, C. F., Maiwald, M., Chong, C. Y., Soong, H. Y., Loo, L. H., et al. (2020). Clinical utility of buccal swabs for severe acute respiratory syndrome coronavirus 2 detection in coronavirus disease 2019-infected children. *J. Pediatr. Infect. Dis. Soc.* 9, 370–372. doi: 10.1093/jpids/piaa068
21. Khiabani, K., and Amirzade-Iranaq, M. H. (2021). Are saliva and deep throat sputum as reliable as common respiratory specimens for SARS-CoV-2 detection? A systematic review and meta-analysis. *Am. J. Infect. Control* 49, 1165–1176. doi: 10.1016/j.ajic.2021.03.008
22. Kim, S. E., Lee, J. Y., Lee, A., Kim, S., Park, K. H., Jung, S. I., et al. (2020). Viral load kinetics of SARS-CoV-2 infection in saliva in korean patients: a prospective multi-center comparative study. *J. Korean Med. Sci.* 35:e287. doi: 10.3346/jkms. 2020.35.e287
23. Lai, C. K. C., Chen, Z., Lui, G., Ling, L., Li, T., Wong, M. C. S., et al. (2020). Prospective study comparing deep throat saliva with other respiratory tract specimens in the diagnosis of novel coronavirus disease 2019. *J. Infect. Dis.* 222, 1612–1619. doi: 10.1093/infdis/jiaa487
24. Lan, F.-Y., Filler, R., Mathew, S., Buley, J., Iliaki, E., Bruno-Murtha, L. A., et al. (2020). COVID-19 symptoms predictive of healthcare workers' SARS-CoV-2 PCR results. *PLoS One* 15:e0235460. doi: 10.1371/journal.pone.0235460
25. Lavezzo, E., Franchin, E., Ciavarella, C., Cuomo-Dannenburg, G., Barzon, L., Del Vecchio, C., et al. (2020). Suppression of a SARS-CoV-2 outbreak in the Italian municipality of Vo'. *Nature* 584, 425–429. doi: 10.1038/s41586-020- 2488-1
26. Li, R., Pei, S., Chen, B., Song, Y., Zhang, T., Yang, W., et al. (2020). Substantial undocumented infection facilitates the rapid dissemination of novel coronavirus (SARS-CoV-2). *Science* 368, 489–493. doi: 10.1126/science. abb3221
27. Li, Y., Shi, J., Xia, J., Duan, J., Chen, L., Yu, X., et al. (2020). Asymptomatic and symptomatic patients with non-severe coronavirus disease (COVID-19) have similar clinical features and virological courses: a retrospective single center study. *Front. Microbiol.* 11:1570. doi: 10.3389/fmicb.2020.01570
28. Mahallawi, W. H., Alsamiri, A. D., Dabbour, A. F., Alsaeedi, H., and Al-Zalabani, A. H. (2021). Association of Viral Load in SARS-CoV-2 patients with age and gender. *Front. Med.* 8:608215. doi: 10.3389/fmed.2021.608215
29. Mastrangelo, A., Bonato, M., and Cinque, P. (2021). Smell and taste disorders in COVID-19: from pathogenesis to clinical features and outcomes. *Neurosci. Lett.* 748:135694. doi: 10.1016/j.neulet.2021.135694
30. McEvoy, D., McAloon, C., Collins, A., Hunt, K., Butler, F., Byrne, A., et al. (2021). Relative infectiousness of asymptomatic SARS-CoV-2 infected persons compared with symptomatic individuals: a rapid scoping review. *BMJ Open* 11:e042354. doi: 10.1136/bmjopen-2020-042354
31. Mlcochova, P., Kemp, S. A., Dhar, M. S., Papa, G., Meng, B., Ferreira, I. A. T. M., et al. (2021). SARS-CoV-2 B.1.617.2 delta variant replication and immune evasion. *Nature* 599, 114–119. doi: 10.1038/s41586-021-03944-y
32. Moreira, V. M., Mascarenhas, P., Machado, V., Botelho, J., Mendes, J. J., Taveira, N., et al. (2021). Diagnosis of SARS-Cov-2 infection by RT-PCR using specimens other than naso- and oropharyngeal swabs: a systematic review and meta- analysis. *Diagnostics* 11:363. doi: 10.3390/diagnostics11020363
33. Mutiawati, E., Syahrul, S., Fahriani, M., Fajar, J. K., Mamada, S. S., Maliga, H. A., et al. (2021). Global prevalence and pathogenesis of headache in COVID-19: a systematic review and meta-analysis. *F1000Res* 9:1316. doi: 10.12688/f1000research.27334.2
34. Nagura-Ikeda, M., Imai, K., Tabata, S., Miyoshi, K., Murahara, N., Mizuno, T., et al. (2020). Clinical evaluation of self-collected saliva by quantitative reverse transcription-PCR (RT-qPCR), Direct RT-qPCR, reverse transcription-loop-mediated isothermal amplification, and a rapid antigen test to diagnose COVID-19. *J. Clin. Microbiol.* 58:e01438-20. doi: 10.1128/JCM.01438-20
35. Nasserie, T., Hittle, M., and Goodman, S. N. (2021). Assessment of the frequency and variety of persistent symptoms among patients with COVID-19: a systematic review. *JAMA Netw. Open* 4:e2111417. doi: 10.1001/jamanetworkopen.2021.11417
36. Oran, D. P., and Topol, E. J. (2020). Prevalence of asymptomatic SARS-CoV-2 infection. *Ann. Intern. Med.* M20-3012. doi: 10.7326/M20-3012
37. Pan, Y., Zhang, D., Yang, P., Poon, L. L. M., and Wang, Q. (2020). Viral load of SARS-CoV-2 in clinical samples. *Lancet Infect. Dis.* 20, 411–412. doi: 10.1016/ S1473-3099(20)30113-4
38. Plucinski, M. M., Wallace, M., Uehara, A., Kurbatova, E. V., Tobolowsky, F. A., Schneider, Z. D., et al. (2021). Coronavirus disease 2019 (COVID-19) in Americans aboard the diamond princess cruise ship. *Clin. Infect. Dis.* 72, e448–e457. doi: 10.1093/cid/ciaa1180
39. Pujadas, E., Chaudhry, F., McBride, R., Richter, F., Zhao, S., Wajnberg, A., et al. (2020). SARS-CoV-2 viral load predicts COVID-19 mortality. *Lancet Respir. Med.* 8:e70. doi: 10.1016/S2213-2600(20)30354-4
40. Qian, J., Zhao, L., Ye, R.-Z., Li, X.-J., and Liu, Y.-L. (2020). Age-dependent gender differences in COVID-19 in Mainland China: comparative study. *Clin. Infect. Dis.* 71, 2488–2494. doi: 10.1093/cid/ciaa683
41. Sapkota, D., Søland, T. M., Galtung, H. K., Sand, L. P., Giannecchini, S., To, K. K. W., et al. (2020). COVID-19 salivary signature: diagnostic and research opportunities. *J. Clin. Pathol.* jclinpath-2020-206834. doi: 10.1136/jclinpath-2020-206834
42. Shen, C., Wang, Z., Zhao, F., Yang, Y., Li, J., Yuan, J., et al. (2020). Treatment of 5 critically Ill patients with COVID-19 with convalescent plasma. *JAMA* 323, 1582–1589. doi: 10.1001/jama.2020.4783
43. Srinivasan, M. (2021). Taste dysfunction and long COVID-19. *Front. Cell Infect. Microbiol* 11:716563. doi: 10.3389/fcimb.2021.716563
44. To, K. K.-W., Tsang, O. T.-Y., Leung, W.-S., Tam, A. R., Wu, T.-C., Lung, D. C., et al. (2020). Temporal profiles of viral load in posterior oropharyngeal saliva samples and serum antibody responses during infection by SARS-CoV-2: an observational cohort study. *Lancet Infect. Dis.* 20, 565–574. doi: 10.1016/S1473- 3099(20)30196-1
45. Tostmann, A., Bradley, J., Bousema, T., Yiek, W.-K., Holwerda, M., Bleeker-Rovers, C., et al. (2020). Strong associations and moderate predictive value of early symptoms for SARS-CoV-2 test positivity among healthcare workers, the Netherlands, March 2020. *Euro Surveill* 25:2000508. doi: 10.2807/1560-7917. ES.2020.25.16.2000508
46. Trunfio, M., Longo, B. M., Alladio, F., Venuti, F., Cerutti, F., Ghisetti, V., et al. (2021). On the SARS-CoV-2 "variolation hypothesis": no association between viral load of index cases and COVID-19 severity of secondary cases. *Front. Microbiol.* 12:646679. doi: 10.3389/fmicb.2021.646679
47. van Kampen, J. J. A., van de Vijver, D. A. M. C., Fraaij, P. L. A., Haagmans, B. L., Lamers, M. M., Okba, N., et al. (2021). Duration and key determinants of infectious virus shedding in hospitalized patients with coronavirus disease-2019 (COVID-19). *Nat. Commun.* 12:267. doi: 10.1038/s41467-020- 20568-4
48. Vasudevan, H. N., Xu, P., Servellita, V., Miller, S., Liu, L., Gopez, A., et al. (2021). Digital droplet PCR accurately quantifies SARS-CoV-2 viral load from crude lysate without nucleic acid purification. *Sci. Rep.* 11:780. doi: 10.1038/s41598- 020-80715-1
49. Walsh, K. A., Jordan, K., Clyne, B., Rohde, D., Drummond, L., Byrne, P., et al. (2020). SARS-CoV-2 detection, viral load and infectivity over the course of an infection. *J. Infect.* 81, 357–371. doi: 10.1016/j.jinf.2020. 06.067
50. Yoon, J. G., Yoon, J., Song, J. Y., Yoon, S. Y., Lim, C. S., Seong, H., et al. (2020). Clinical significance of a high SARS-CoV-2 viral load in the saliva. *J. Korean Med. Sci.* 35:e195. doi: 10.3346/jkms.2020.35.e195
51. Yu, F., Yan, L., Wang, N., Yang, S., Wang, L., Tang, Y., et al. (2020). Quantitative detection and viral load analysis of SARS-CoV-2 in infected patients. *Clin. Infect. Dis.* 71, 793–798. doi: 10.1093/cid/ciaa345
52. Yusuf, F., Fahriani, M., Mamada, S. S., Frediansyah, A., Abubakar, A., Maghfirah, D., et al. (2021). Global prevalence of prolonged gastrointestinal symptoms in COVID-19 survivors and potential pathogenesis: a systematic review and meta-analysis. *F1000Res* 10:301. doi: 10.12688/f1000research.52 216.1

19

Hyperphosphatemic Familial Tumoral Calcinosis Hidden in Plain Sight for 73 Years

Alisa E. Lee[1], *Iris R. Hartley*[1], *Kelly L. Roszko*[1], *Chaim Vanek*[2], *Rachel I. Gafni*[1] *and Michael T. Collins*[1*]

[1] National Institute of Dental and Craniofacial Research, National Institutes of Health, Bethesda, MD, United States, [2] Division of Endocrinology, Diabetes and Clinical Nutrition, Oregon Health and Science University, Portland, OR, United States

***Correspondence:**
Michael T. Collins
mcollins@mail.nih.gov

While dental pulp calcifications and root anomalies may be inconsequential incidental findings in dental radiographs, they can, especially in combination, represent a clue, hidden in plain sight, for the diagnosis of hyperphosphatemic familial tumoral calcinosis (HFTC). HFTC is an autosomal recessive disease of mineral metabolism characterized by sometimes massive, painful calcification around large joints, systemic inflammation, dental pulp calcification, and thistle-shaped roots. This paper describes a woman with HFTC who endured not only the symptoms of HFTC for decades, but also the frustration of not knowing the cause. The diagnosis was finally made at the age of 73 years, when the connection between a large right shoulder calcification and hyperphosphatemia was made. The dental findings were likely present on her initial radiographs taken in childhood. Increased awareness of the association between characteristic dental findings and HFTC may allow for earlier diagnosis and interventions to improve the care of patients with this rare condition.

Keywords: fibroblast growth factor 23, dental pulp calcification, root anomaly, phosphate metabolism, hyperphosphataemia

INTRODUCTION

In 2000, the U.S. Surgeon General's Report on Oral Health in America reported numerous ways in which oral and general health are interconnected (1). A thorough oral examination can reveal signs and symptoms of endocrinopathies, systemic infections, immunologic disorders, and nutritional deficiencies (2). Identifying these oral manifestations of systemic disorders may enable early diagnosis and treatment.

Hyperphosphatemic familial tumoral calcinosis (HFTC) is a rare autosomal recessive disease characterized by high blood phosphate, calcific masses, and dental anomalies (OMIM 211900) (3). The dental anomalies are the most penetrant phenotypic finding in the condition (4). The extra-dental clinical symptoms cover a broad spectrum, ranging from no significant involvement to lesions that are large, painful, and debilitating (5). HFTC is caused by deficiency of, or resistance to the phosphorus regulating hormone fibroblast growth factor 23 (FGF23) (6). Absence of FGF23 promotes renal tubule phosphate reabsorption that leads to hyperphosphatemia, which promotes ectopic calcifications in tissues exposed to trauma (7). Pathogenic variants in *FGF23*, *GALNT3*, or *KLOTHO*, have been found to cause HFTC (6); an acquired form due to FGF23 autoantibodies has also been described (8). Current treatment interventions focus on managing blood phosphate, reducing pain and inflammation, and addressing calcifications and their complications (6).

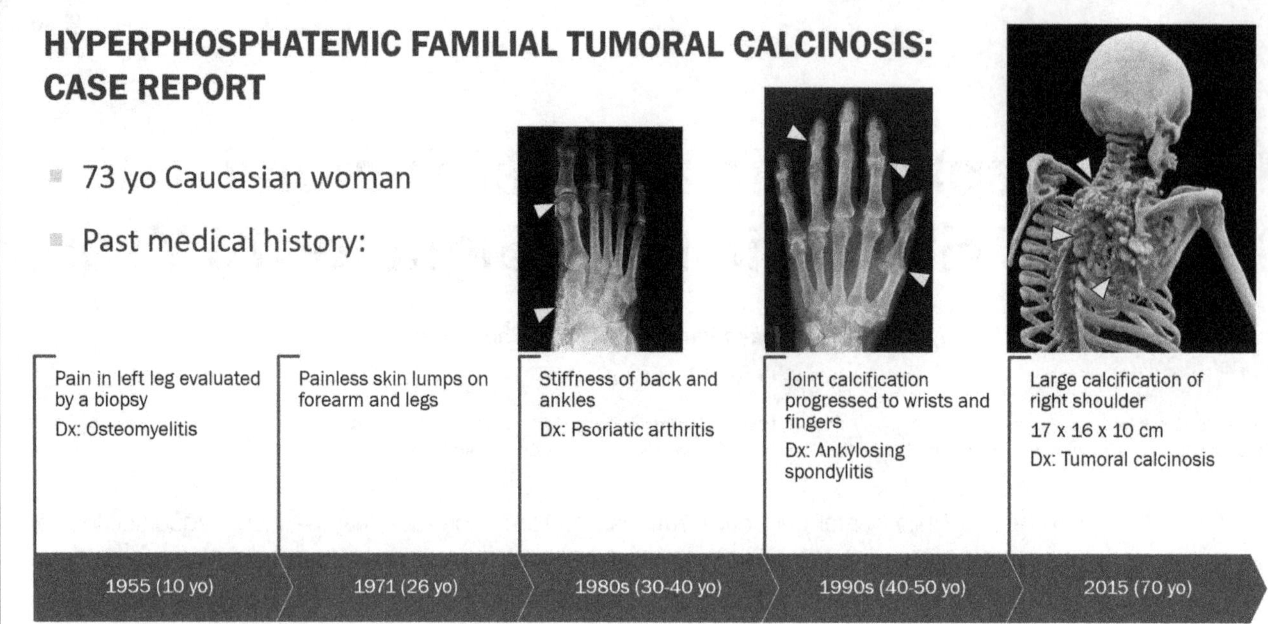

FIGURE 1 | Graphic representation of clinical course. At age 10 years, patient experienced unusual pain in her left leg that represented hyperostosis-hyperphosphatemia syndrome, which was evaluated with a biopsy and misdiagnosed as osteomyelitis. At age 26 years, she started noticing painless skin lumps on her forearm and legs. In her 30s, she started experiencing back pain and joint stiffness in her ankles and fingers. She was then evaluated by a rheumatologist and was diagnosed with an ill-defined rheumatologic disorder, possibly psoriatic arthritis. Over the next 30 years, the arthritis slowly progressed to involve almost all joints of her body. Eventually this was determined to be an aggressive form of osteoarthritis, currently felt not to be related to underlying HFTC. In 2015, a large bump appeared around her right shoulder, which was initially thought to be a sarcoma. Upon biopsy, bone calcifications were found with the possibility of tumoral calcinosis.

The unique dental phenotype of HFTC has been recently described in detail by our group (4). Internal pulp calcification and thistle-shaped, short roots with midroot bulging were most commonly observed in almost all of our cohort of 17 patients. The pulp can be partially to completely obliterated. Maxillary and mandibular premolars are most severely affected. In addition, primary dentition from pediatric patients with HFTC had findings similar to the permanent teeth.

Here we present a patient with hyperphosphatemic familial tumoral calcinosis who, despite numerous symptoms throughout her life, was not diagnosed with HFTC until the age of 73. Her diagnostic evaluation and treatment are presented and discussed.

CASE REPORT

A 73-year-old Caucasian woman was referred in December 2019 to the National Institute of Dental and Craniofacial Research at the National Institutes of Health by her endocrinologist at Oregon Health and Science University for evaluation of recently diagnosed HFTC. Review of the patient's medical history revealed several symptoms associated with HFTC that arose throughout her life since childhood (**Figure 1**). She had been in her usual state of health until age 10, when she experienced unusual pain in her left leg, which was evaluated with a biopsy and diagnosed as osteomyelitis. She received IV antibiotics for 10 days. As a teenager, she had no major health issues and participated in sports such as basketball and volleyball. During her regular dental checkups, she was told that she has abnormal pulp stones, but was not further evaluated (**Figure 2**).

At age 26, she started noticing painless skin lumps on her forearm and legs. In her 30s, she experienced back pain and joint stiffness in her ankles and fingers. She was then evaluated by a rheumatologist and was diagnosed with an ill-defined rheumatologic disorder. Over the next 30 years, the arthritis slowly progressed to involve almost all joints of her body. Her finger joints have fused, and she is unable to make a fist or pick up small items. She has been treated with prednisone, methotrexate, and infliximab. Multiple steroid injections in her back have provided temporary relief. On re-evaluation, the prevailing diagnosis of her rheumatologic findings is aggressive osteoarthritis, which is not believed to be related to the diagnosis of HFTC. In 2015, a large bump was noted around her right shoulder (**Figure 3**). Initial concern was that it might represent a sarcoma. On biopsy, paucicellular calcific material was seen, characteristic of tumoral calcinosis. In 2019, she was diagnosed with peripheral vascular disease requiring angioplasty.

Biochemical evaluation for causes of tumoral calcinosis revealed hyperphosphatemia and led to a referral to an endocrinologist in April 2019. HFTC was suspected and genetic testing identified two heterozygous variants in *GALNT3* (c.746_749del and c.926T>G), consistent with HFTC. The first change (c.746_749del) is in exon 4 of the *GALNT3* gene.

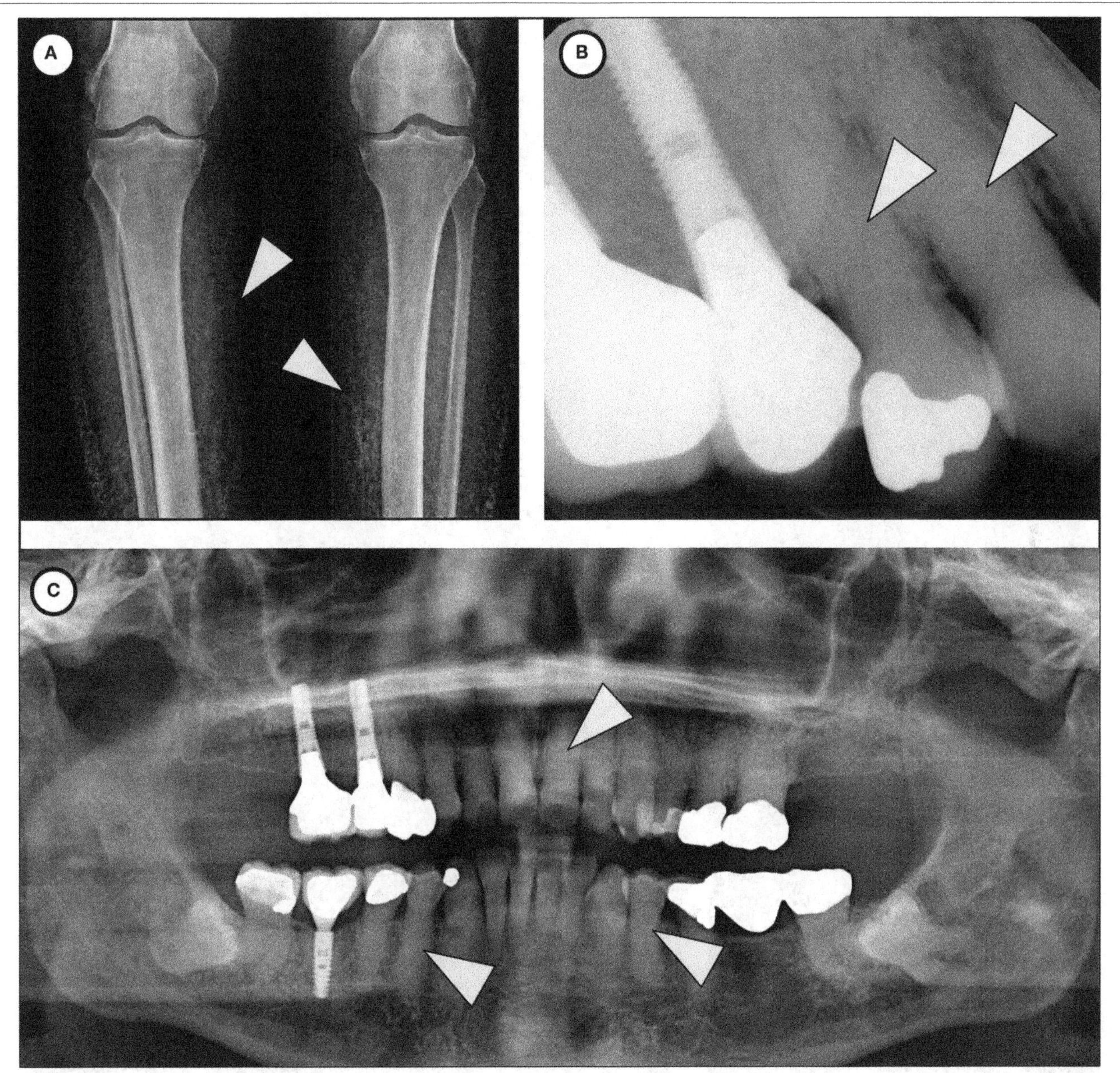

FIGURE 2 | Phenotypic features of HFTC. **(A)** Lower limb radiograph shows subcutaneous calcification of her legs, an unusual and rare finding seen in older patients with HFTC. **(B)** Periapical radiograph of teeth # 5 and 6 shows complete pulp obliteration and thistle-shaped roots. **(C)** Panoramic radiograph shows short bulbous root with complete pulp obliteration in all teeth.

This four-nucleotide deletion causes a frameshift and results in aberrant mRNA processing. This change has been previously reported as a variant associated with HFTC (9). The second change (c.926T>G) is in exon 5 of the *GALNT3* gene. This variant converts an isoleucine to arginine. To our knowledge, this change has not been previously reported as a disease-causing variant. Pathogenic variants in *GALNT3* often result in excessive cleavage of the active, intact FGF23 molecule, causing deficiency of functional FGF23 (10).

Following the diagnosis, the patient was referred to the NIH for further evaluation including blood and urine assessments and skeletal imaging. Laboratory studies showed elevated phosphorus 5.4 mg/dL (normal 2.5–4.5) and markers of systemic inflammation such as erythrocyte sedimentation rate 71 mm/h (0–42) and C-reactive protein 44 mg/L (0.00–4.99). Intact FGF23 was inappropriately low-normal 31 pg/mL (22–63) for the degree of hyperphosphatemia, while C-terminal FGF23 was markedly elevated 2,450 RU/mL (≤180), consistent with HFTC.

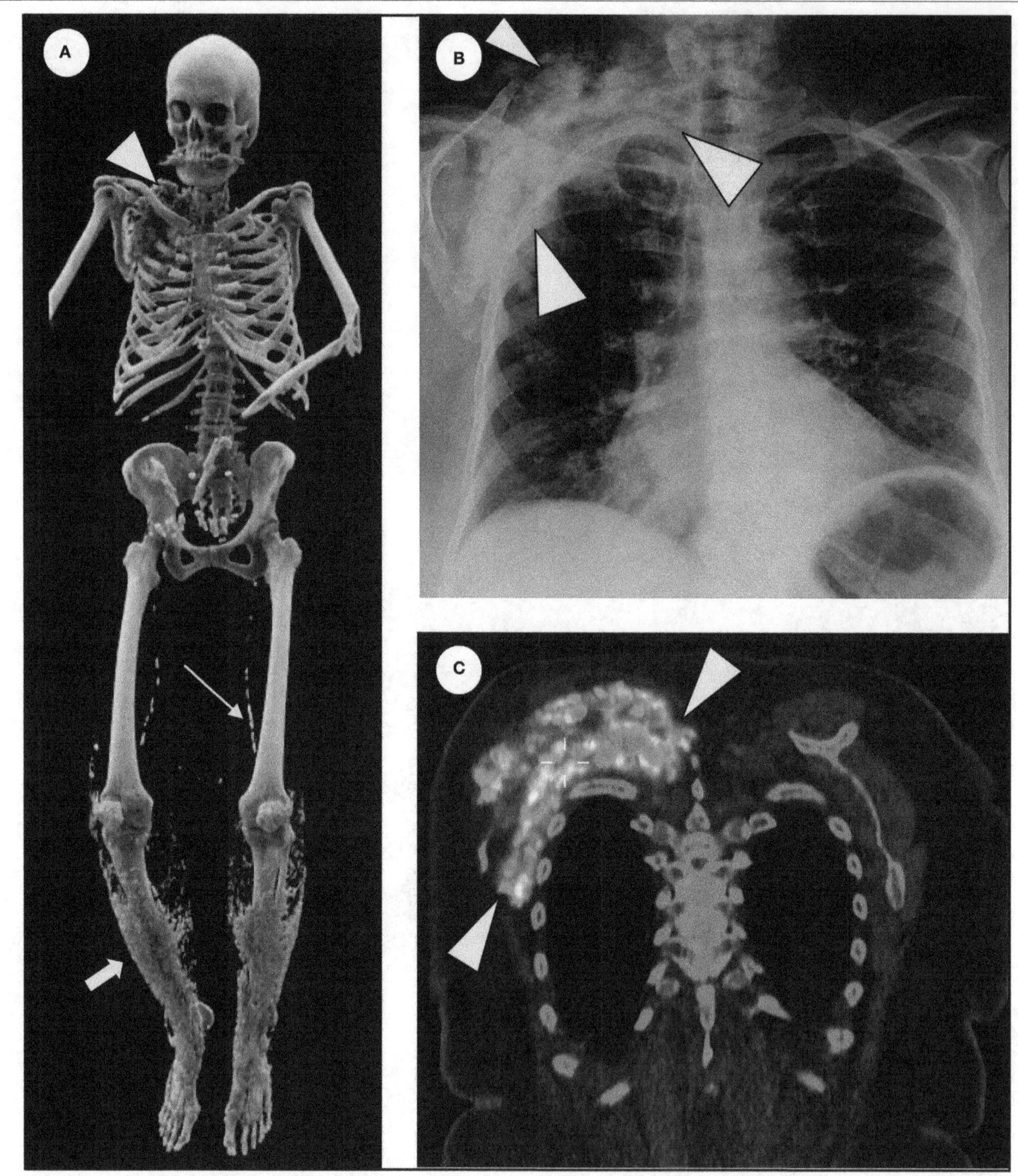

FIGURE 3 | Additional features of HFTC. **(A)** 3D reconstruction of a total body CT scan illustrates subcutaneous calcifications surrounding the right shoulder (arrowhead), superficial lacey calcification in the lower extremities bilaterally (short arrow), and calcifications of femoral arteries (long arrow). **(B)** Chest radiograph shows right shoulder calcification (arrowheads). **(C)** Coronal slice of the merged ^{18}F NaF PET/CT scan demonstrating intense tracer uptake in the actively forming calcific lesion seen in the chest radiograph (arrowheads).

Extraoral and intraoral examination revealed healthy mucosal tissues and well-restored permanent dentition. Panoramic radiograph showed moderate alveolar bone loss around mandibular anterior teeth, fully impacted # 17 and 32 with dilacerated roots, and changes in the roots consistent with HFTC (**Figure 2**). Complete pulp obliteration with short, thistle shaped

TABLE 1 | The diagnostic criteria of hyperphosphatemic familial tumoral calcinosis (HFTC).

Hyperphosphatemic familial tumoral calcinosis (HFTC)
Biochemical findings (common, required for diagnosis):
High serum phosphate
High C-terminal FGF23
Low/normal intact FGF23
Dental pathology (most common phenotypic feature):
Pulp calcification and thistle-shaped roots
Ectopic calcification (common):
Lateral hips, elbows, shoulders, hands, pressure/trauma points
Systemic inflammation (common, especially with new lesion formation):
Recurrent fevers, fatigue, anemia, polyarthritis, increased C-reactive protein and/or erythrocyte sedimentation rate
Vascular calcification:
Femoral/iliac arteries, aorta, carotids, cerebral vasculature
Hyperostosis (childhood only, often presenting symptom):
Tibiae (common), rarely ulnae, radii, and/or metacarpals
Stocking foot calcification (age-related/late finding):
Feet and legs
Ocular involvement (rare):
Calcification of eyelids/conjunctiva/cornea, retinal angioid streaks, vision loss

roots are observed in most of the teeth. Radiographs provided by her general dentist (taken 2008) also showed the altered tooth structure.

DISCUSSION

The earliest clinical features of HFTC can include characteristic dental findings, painful cortical hyperostosis of certain long bones (especially the tibiae), subcutaneous masses, and calcification around joints (especially the hips and/or shoulders) (**Table 1**) (6). Most diagnosed patients develop symptoms by 13 years of age (11). The patient in this case developed clinical symptoms at age 10, but it was not until the patient presented with a much larger calcification of her shoulder in combination with hyperphosphatemia that prompted genetic testing confirming the diagnosis of HFTC at age 73. The painful tibial lesions this patient experienced in childhood and misdiagnosed as osteomyelitis represented hyperostosis-hyperphosphatemia syndrome, one of the early manifestations and part of the spectrum of phenotypic findings of HFTC (OMIM 211900) (10). Despite the numerous symptoms throughout her life, the patient was not correctly diagnosed for many years partly due to the fact the mutation in *GALNT3* was not discovered until 2005 (12) and due to the rarity of the disorder.

Patients present with a moderate to severe dental phenotype with root bulging, pulp calcification and shortened thistle-shaped roots. It is believed that the severity of the dental phenotype in HFTC does not appear to progress over time, but there is insufficient longitudinal data to know definitively (4). Based on her current dental radiographs and review of past dental history, it is likely that the patient had similar dental findings in her primary dentition. Early identification and recognition of the dental phenotype of the disorder by an astute dentist may have contributed to a timelier diagnosis in this case.

In this case, we did not observe mineralization in the PDL space. The alveolar bone appears to be within normal limits as well. The patient has had multiple implants placed without complications. In addition, patients with HFTC have been able to get extractions without any complications and have had successful orthodontic treatment. In histological analysis of a previous study, widening of the cellular cementum layer was observed (4).

Upon review of the biochemical studies and confirmation of the diagnosis, the patient was encouraged to have routine evaluation of phosphorous and calcium metabolism. She was recommended to follow a low-phosphate diet, limiting meat, nuts, beans, and dairy, as well as avoiding excessive calcium and vitamin D supplements. The patient was encouraged to maintain physical activity as tolerated.

The patient was instructed to continue treatment with sevelamer, which reduces hyperphosphatemia by binding to dietary phosphate in the gut. The patient was started on anakinra, an interleukin-1 receptor antagonist, to address the marked degree of systemic inflammation. Infliximab was discontinued, but she remained on low dose prednisone and methotrexate. She had a significant degree of overall improvement in well-being on this regimen, probably related to the decrease in inflammation brought about by the anakinra.

In conclusion, this report describes the oldest known living patient with HFTC and highlights the importance of recognizing dental phenotypes that may be a sign of systemic disorders. In patients with HFTC, dental changes are often the first sign of disease. Dentists can contribute to early diagnosis and interdisciplinary care of systemic conditions that manifest in the oral cavity.

AUTHOR CONTRIBUTIONS

All authors contributed to manuscript preparation, revision, read, and approved the submitted version.

FUNDING

Work in the authors' laboratory was sponsored by the Intramural Research Program of the NIDCR, NIH (Grant# Z01 DE000649 25). This work was made possible through the National Institute of Health (NIH) Medical Research Scholars Program, a public-private partnership supported jointly by the NIH and contributions to the Foundation for the NIH from the Doris Duke Charitable Foundation, Genentech, the American Association for Dental Research, the Colgate-Palmolive Company, and other private donors (AEL). The funders were not involved in preparing this manuscript.

ACKNOWLEDGMENTS

We thank the patient and her family for their participation in the study. We thank Dr. Pamela Gardner for conducting the dental evaluation. We thank Dr. Martha Somerman for the invitation to contribute to this important research topic. We thank Dr. Emily Chu for providing guidance in manuscript preparation.

REFERENCES

1. Oral health in America: a report of the Surgeon General. *J Calif Dent Assoc.* (2000) 28:685–95.
2. Chi AC, Neville BW, Krayer JW, Gonsalves WC. Oral manifestations of systemic disease. *Am Fam Physician.* (2010) 82:1381–8.
3. Ramnitz MS, Gafni RI, Collins MT. Hyperphosphatemic familial tumoral calcinosis. In: Adam MP, Ardinger HH, Pagon RA, Wallace SE, Bean LJH, Mirzaa G, et al. editors. *GeneReviews((R)).* Seattle, WA: University of Washington (2018).
4. Lee AE, Chu EY, Gardner PJ, Duverger O, Saikali A, Wang SK, et al. A cross-sectional cohort study of the effects of FGF23 deficiency and hyperphosphatemia on dental structures in hyperphosphatemic familial tumoral calcinosis. *JBMR Plus.* (2021) 5:e10470. doi: 10.1002/jbm4.10470
5. Ichikawa S, Baujat G, Seyahi A, Garoufali AG, Imel EA, Padgett LR, et al. Clinical variability of familial tumoral calcinosis caused by novel GALNT3 mutations. *Am J Med Genet A.* (2010) 152A:896–903. doi: 10.1002/ajmg.a.33337
6. Boyce AM, Lee AE, Roszko KL, Gafni RI. Hyperphosphatemic tumoral calcinosis: pathogenesis, clinical presentation, and challenges in management. *Front Endocrinol (Lausanne).* (2020) 11:293. doi: 10.3389/fendo.2020.00293
7. Bhattacharyya N, Chong WH, Gafni RI, Collins MT. Fibroblast growth factor 23: state of the field and future directions. *Trends Endocrinol Metab.* (2012) 23:610–8. doi: 10.1016/j.tem.2012.07.002
8. Roberts MS, Burbelo PD, Egli-Spichtig D, Perwad F, Romero CJ, Ichikawa S, et al. Autoimmune hyperphosphatemic tumoral calcinosis in a patient with FGF23 autoantibodies. *J Clin Invest.* (2018) 128:5368–73. doi: 10.1172/JCI122004
9. Ramnitz MS, Gourh P, Goldbach-Mansky R, Wodajo F, Ichikawa S, Econs MJ, et al. Phenotypic and genotypic characterization and treatment of a cohort with familial tumoral calcinosis/hyperostosis-hyperphosphatemia syndrome. *J Bone Miner Res.* (2016) 31:1845–54. doi: 10.1002/jbmr.2870
10. Ichikawa S, Guigonis V, Imel EA, Courouble M, Heissat S, Henley JD, et al. Novel GALNT3 mutations causing hyperostosis-hyperphosphatemia syndrome result in low intact fibroblast growth factor 23 concentrations. *J Clin Endocrinol Metab.* (2007) 92:1943–7. doi: 10.1210/jc.2006-1825
11. Rafaelsen S, Johansson S, Raeder H, Bjerknes R. Long-term clinical outcome and phenotypic variability in hyperphosphatemic familial tumoral calcinosis and hyperphosphatemic hyperostosis syndrome caused by a novel GALNT3 mutation; case report and review of the literature. *BMC Genet.* (2014) 15:98. doi: 10.1186/s12863-014-0098-3
12. Frishberg Y, Topaz O, Bergman R, Behar D, Fisher D, Gordon D, et al. Identification of a recurrent mutation in GALNT3 demonstrates that hyperostosis-hyperphosphatemia syndrome and familial tumoral calcinosis are allelic disorders. *J Mol Med (Berl).* (2005) 83:33–8. doi: 10.1007/s00109-004-0610-8

20

Oral Microbiota is Associated with Immune Recovery in Human Immunodeficiency Virus-Infected Individuals

Yirui Xie[1], Jia Sun[2], Caiqin Hu[1], Bing Ruan[1] and Biao Zhu[1*]*

[1] State Key Laboratory for Diagnosis and Treatment of Infectious Diseases, Department of Infectious Diseases, National Clinical Research Center for Infectious Diseases, Collaborative Innovation Center for Diagnosis and Treatment of Infectious Diseases, School of Medicine, The First Affiliated Hospital, Zhejiang University, Hangzhou, China, [2] Ningbo Medical Center Lihuili Hospital, Ningbo, China

***Correspondence:**
Yirui Xie
1312019@zju.edu.cn
Biao Zhu
zhubiao1207@zju.edu.cn

The role of the oral microbiota in HIV-infected individuals deserves attention as either HIV infection or antiretroviral therapy (ART) may have effect on the diversity and the composition of the oral microbiome. However, few studies have addressed the oral microbiota and its interplay with different immune responses to ART in HIV-infected individuals. Salivary microbiota and immune activation were studied in 30 HIV-infected immunological responders (IR) and 34 immunological non-responders (INR) ($\geq$500 and $<$ 200 CD4 + T-cell counts/μl after 2 years of HIV-1 viral suppression, respectively) with no comorbidities. Metagenome sequencing revealed that the IR and the INR group presented similar salivary bacterial richness and diversity. The INR group presented a significantly higher abundance of genus *Selenomonas_4*, while the IR group manifested higher abundances of *Candidatus_Saccharimonas* and *norank_p_Saccharimonas. Candidatus_Saccharimonas* and *norank_p_Saccharimonas* were positively correlated with the current CD4 + T-cells. *Candidatus_Saccharimonas* was positively correlated with the markers of adaptive immunity CD4 + CD57 + T-cells, while negative correlation was found between *norank _p_Saccharimonas* and the CD8 + CD38 + T-cells as well as the CD4/CD8 + HLADR + CD38 + T-cells. The conclusions are that the overall salivary microbiota structure was similar in the immunological responders and immunological non-responders, while there were some taxonomic differences in the salivary bacterial composition. *Selenomona_4, Candidatus_Saccharimonas,* and *norank _p_Saccharimonas* might act as important factors of the immune recovery in the immunodeficiency patients, and *Candidatus_Saccharimonas* could be considered in the future as screening biomarkers for the immune responses in the HIV-infected individuals.

Keywords: HIV-1, oral microbiota, immunological responders, immunological non-responders, antiretroviral therapy

---

Abbreviations: HIV, human immunodeficiency virus; ART, antiretroviral therapy; HAART, highly active antiretroviral therapy; INR, immunological non-responders; IR, immunological responders; SLE, systemic lupus erythematosus; RDs, rheumatic diseases; ALL, acute lymphoblastic leukemia; RA, rheumatoid arthritis; BMI, body mass index; MSM, men who have sex with men; LPS, Lipopolysaccharide; PCoA, Principal coordinate analysis; LDA, Linear discriminant analysis; LEfSe, linear discriminant analysis effect size; OUT, operational taxonomic unit; 16S rRNA, 16S ribosomal RNA; ROC, receiver operating characteristic; NRTIs, nucleoside reverse transcriptase inhibitors; NNRTIs, non-nucleoside reverse transcriptase inhibitors; AZT, Zidovudine; TDF, Tenofovir Disoproxil Fumarate; 3TC, Lamivudine; EFV, Efavirenz; LPV/r, Lopinavir/ritonavir.

INTRODUCTION

The widespread use of potent antiretroviral therapy (ART) which has ability to achieve viral suppression and immune reconstitution has made human immunodeficiency virus (HIV) infection become a chronic manageable disease. ART can improve the immune function of HIV infected subjects, but significant individual difference exists in the extent of immunological recovery. Despite the persistent manifestation of virological suppression after receiving ART, HIV infected individuals with low increases of CD4 + T-cells are considered as immunological non-responders (INR), showing contrast to immunological responders (IR) (Cenderello and De Maria, 2016). An unanimously agreed definition of INR has not been reached by far. Therefore, the acceptable range of the prevalence of INR is from 10 to 40% in the cohorts (Yang et al., 2020). The most restrictive definition of INR refers to patients whose absolute CD4 + T-cells fail to reach 200 cells/μl with an undetectable plasma viral load after 2 years of receiving ART (Florence et al., 2003; Kaufmann et al., 2003; Tsukamoto et al., 2009).

Thanks to high-throughput sequencing, thorough and comprehensive studies of complex human microbiology have been conducted during the past years. In recent years, studies mainly focused on characterizing the impact of HIV infection on host–microbe interactions in the gut (Dillon et al., 2016) and some studies found that the gut microbiota are associated with immune recovery in HIV-infected patients (Ji et al., 2018; Lu et al., 2018; Xie et al., 2021). Oral microbiomes were also reported to have strong associations with human immune system functions, therefore, they were correlated with human immune system diseases such as rheumatic diseases (RDs), acute lymphoblastic leukemia (ALL), and HIV infection (Gao et al., 2018). Alterations in the oral microbiome distinguished individuals with rheumatoid arthritis (RA) from the healthy controls; correlations were shown between these alterations and clinical measures including immune response, and they could be used to stratify individuals based on their responses to the therapy, especially with microbial triggers being implicated in RA (Bellando-Randone et al., 2021). Furthermore, characterization of the oral microbiome in ALL patients demonstrated a structural imbalance of the oral microbiota, indicating the importance of immune status in shaping the structure of the oral microbiota. Although valuable insights on immune status have been presented by these studies, it is surprising that studies which focus on the role of the oral microbiome and their relationship with immune response in HIV are relatively rare. Few research addresses the overall oral microbiota structure in HIV infection; to our knowledge, the oral microbiota dysbiosis and the interaction with different immune responses to ART is still poorly defined. This study aims to evaluate the microbial composition in the salivary samples collected from HIV-infected immunological non-responders and immunological responders. We hypothesize that the compositional changes of the salivary microbiota could be associated with different immune responses of HIV-infected individuals receiving ART. The study adopted 16S ribosomal RNA (rRNA) targeted sequencing and flow cytometry to explore the oral microbiome and their relationship with immune activation in patients who are immunodiscordant and who are immunoconcordant. The compositional changes of salivary microbiota and their association with different immune responses in HIV-infected patients with ART is characterized for the first time in this study.

MATERIALS AND METHODS

Recruitment of Subjects

64 HIV-infected individuals who were diagnosed by the Disease Control and Prevention Center of Zhejiang Province (30 immunological responders and 34 immunological non-responders) were all recruited from the HIV clinic of the First Affiliated Hospital of Zhejiang University from November 2015 to October 2017. All subjects start ART during the chronic phase of HIV infection. In this study, IR and INR were defined as patients who with the average of the last two CD4 + T-cell counts/μl equal or is more than 500 or less than 200 and after 2 years of receiving complete viral suppression therapy, respectively. The selection excluded candidates with either one of the following conditions: below 18 years old; showing opportunistic infection symptoms; infected with hepatitis B or C; having history of using antibiotics, immunosuppressive regimen, probiotics, prebiotics, or symbiotics in the past 6 months; BMI higher than 30; showing oral active inflammation. None of the patients had obvious symptoms of oral mucosal diseases and periodontal disease (redness, swelling, and bleeding) when the clinical samples were collected. However, formal dental examinations were not performed to rule out the mild periodontal symptoms.

Ethics Statement

This study conforms to the ethical norms of the 1975 Helsinki Declaration. The research protocol was approved by the Institutional Review Committee of The First Affiliated Hospital of Zhejiang University on October 7, 2015. All participants provided written informed consents before participating in the study. All the data used for analysis were anonymized.

Salivary Samples Collection and DNA Extraction

Participants were required to refrain from eating, drinking, smoking before saliva collection. The amount of each salivary sample collected from participants before their clinic visit was 5 ml. The samples were stored in sterile containers of -80°C until DNA extraction by QiaAmp DNA Mini Kit (QIAGEN, Hilden, Germany) following instructions of the manufacturer. NanoDrop (Thermo Fisher Scientific) was used to determine the concentration and purity of DNA as well as 1.0% agarose gel electrophoresis for the integrity and size of DNA. After the procedures above, the DNA samples were frozen at -20°C for further analysis.

16S Ribosomal RNA Gene Sequencing

The bacterial 16S rRNA gene high-throughput sequencing was conducted by Shanghai Majorbio Bio-Pharm Technology Co.,

Ltd. (Shanghai, China). The bacterial 16S rRNA gene sequences spanning the variable regions V3–V4 were amplified using the primer 338F (5′- ACTCCTACGGGAGGCAGCAG-3′), and 806R (5′-GGACTACHVGGGTWTCTAAT-3′) as previous recorded (Xie et al., 2021). The amplicons were extracted from 2% agarose gels, purified by the AxyPrep DNA Gel Extraction Kit (Axygen Biosciences, Union City, CA, United States) and quantified using QuantiFluor™-ST (Promega, United States) based on the guidelines of the manufacturer's protocol. In equimolar amounts, purified amplicons were sent to paired-end sequencing (2 × 300) on an Illumina MiSeq platform (Illumina, San Diego, United States).

Bacterial Translocation, Viral Load, and Flow Cytometry

Sera samples of immunological responders and non-responders were collected to measure the bacterial translocation markers. Following the standard protocols, human Lipopolysaccharides (LPS) ELISA Kit (CUSABIO; Wuhan, China) and Human soluble CD14 (sCD14) ELISA Kit (MultiSciences, Hangzhou, China) were used to test plasma LPS and sCD14. Flow cytometry and Cobas Amplicor (Roche Molecular Systems Inc., Branchburg, New Jersey, United States) were used to quantify CD4 + /CD8 + T-cells and HIV-1 RNA, respectively. Fresh anticoagulated whole blood was used to quantify the expressing markers of immune activation (CD25 +, CD38 +, HLADR +, or CD38 + /HLA-DR +) of CD4 + and CD8 + T-cells and immune senescence (CD57 +) by BD FACS Canto II flow cytometer (BD Biosciences, California, United States). The antibodies needed during the experiment were purchased from Biolegend (San Diego, CA), including CD3-FITC, CD4- PerCP/Cy5.5, CD8-Brilliant Violet 510™, CD38-Brilliant Violet 421, CD25-PE, HLA-DR-APC/Fire™ 750, and CD57-allophycocyanin (APC).

Bioinformatics and Statistics

The 16S rRNA high-throughput sequencing raw fastq files were demultiplexed and quality-filtered by QIIME (version 1.9.1).[1] Operational taxonomic units (OTUs) were clustered with a 97% similarity cut-off using UPARSE.[2] The taxonomy of each 16S rRNA gene sequence was analyzed using the RDP Classifier (version 2.2)[3] and compared with the SILVA rRNA database[4] with the confidence threshold being 70%. After eliminating the interference sequence, alpha diversity estimator calculations were performed using Mothur v.1.30.2. Phylogenetic beta diversity measures, such as Bray-Curtis distance metrics analysis; the representative sequences of OTUs were used for each sample, respectively. Principal Coordinates analysis (PCoA) was performed to visualize the microbial communities following the distance matrices, as well as Linear discriminant analysis effect size (LEfSe) on Galaxy to calculate bacteria taxa with significantly different abundances between groups (Segata et al., 2011). In this study, alpha values for the factorial Kruskal Wallis at 0.05 and linear discriminant analysis (LDA) effect size threshold of 2.0 for discriminative features were applied for all bacteria that were discussed. The calculation of correlations between the variables were conducted with Spearman's rank-correlation analysis. Spearman correlation matrix with p-adjust lower than 0.05 and ρ-value above 0.2 were used to filter strong correlations. The discriminatory function of the biomarkers was evaluated through calculating the area under the receiver operating characteristic (ROC) curve (AUC) using pROC of R package. The comparisons between groups were conducted through the Chi-square test, Independent-Samples T-test, Wilcoxon rank sum test and Mann-Whitney U-test in the R package and SPSS 21.0 software (SPSS Inc., Chicago, IL, United States). Differences were considered significant when $P < 0.05$.

[1] http://qiime.org/install/index.html
[2] http://drive5.com/uparse/
[3] http://rdp.cme.msu.edu/
[4] http://www.arb-silva.de

RESULTS

General Clinical Features of the Patients

The cross-sectional study subjects included 30 immunological responders and 34 immunological non-responders with HIV infection. The characteristics such as gender, age, body mass index (BMI), and smoking status are relatively matched between the two groups (**Table 1**). The MSM transmission route rate is 53.3% vs. 44.1% (p = 0.461).

ART medications were composed by two Nucleoside/nucleotide reverse transcriptase inhibitors (NRTIs) and a non-nucleoside reverse transcriptase inhibitor (NNRTI), or a ritonavir-boosted protease inhibitor (PI). No differences are observed in the duration of ART and the type of ART drugs between the IR and the INR groups (p = 0.193 and p = 0.821). The HIV RNA viral load levels were considered as undetectable (<20 copies/ml) in all samples of the patients. In the IR group,

TABLE 1 | Clinical characteristics data summary.

Characteristics	IR (n = 30)	INR (n = 34)	P-value
Age, (years), mean ± SD	36.97 ± 9.91	38.59 ± 9.45	0.506
Gender male/female	27/3	33/1	0.224
BMI, mean ± SD	21.31 ± 2.60	20.67 ± 2.58	0.368
Mode of transmission, MSM, N (%)	16 (53.3%)	15 (44.1%)	0.461
Smoking, N (%)	0 (0%)	1 (2.94%)	0.096
HAART months (mean ± SD)	37.60 ± 13.21	33.61 ± 10.20	0.193
Ongoing ART regimen, N (%)			
NNRTI-based	27 (90.0%)	30 (88.2%)	0.821
PI-based	3 (10.0%)	4 (11.8%)	0.821
Nadir CD4 + T cell count, /mm^3, median (IQR)	298 (200, 371)	42.5 (13, 140.3)	**<0.001**

Continuous variables were compared using Independent-Samples t-test or the Mann-Whitney U-test. Categorical variables were compared using Chi-square test or Fisher's exact test. BMI, body mass index; MSM, men who sex with men; NNRTI, Non-nucleoside reverse transcriptase inhibitors; PI, Protease inhibitor; IR, immunological responders; INR, immunological non-responders. Bold values indicate P < 0.05.

TABLE 2 | Salivary microbiota 16S rRNA gene high-throughput sequencing data summary.

Characteristics	IR (*n* = 30)	INR (*n* = 34)	*P*-value
Sobs index#	268.93 ± 45.29	262.79 ± 40.93	0.716
Shannon index#	3.56 ± 0.27	3.50 ± 0.29	0.471
Simpson index#	0.06 ± 0.02	0.07 ± 0.02	0.245
ACE#	306.14 ± 49.96	295.87 ± 44.66	0.497
Chao 1 index#	310.13 ± 54.65	301.49 ± 48.64	0.568
Good's coverage (%)#	99.85 ± 0.04	99.84 ± 0.03	0.404

#Indicate the diversity and richness was calculated after the reads number of each sample were equalized. IR: immunological responders; INR: immunological non-responders.

the number of Nadir CD4 + T cell is greatly higher than that in the INR group (298 vs. 42.5, $p < 0.001$) (**Table 1**).

Salivary Microbiota Analysis in the Immunological Responders and Immunological Non-responders Groups

To characterize the salivary microbiota composition, 3,884,775 high-quality16S rRNA sequences were obtained from all 64 participants. An average length of 445 bp and an average of 60,700 sequences per sample were adopted for further analysis. Rarefaction was conducted on the OTU table to 27,986 reads per sample to avoid any methodological artifacts. Specifically, 504 OTUs in the IR group and 503 OTUs in the INR group were defined at a similarity level of 97%. The diversity (Sobs index, Simpson's index of diversity and Shannon index) and richness (Chao1, ACE estimator and Good's coverage) of the salivary microbiota in each group at the OTU level were analyzed, and the IR group present similar Alpha and Beta diversity compared to the INR group (**Table 2**). It can be seen from the principal coordinate (PCoA) analysis by Bray-Curtis matrices that there is no significant difference between the two groups (PERMANOVA, pseudo-F: 1.64608, $R^2 = 0.02586$, $p = 0.109$, **Figure 1**). Visualization of the relative abundances of dominant taxa at the genus level in the oral microbiome is presented in **Figure 2**. In order to identify the key phylotypes responsible for the difference in distinguishing the saliva microbiota between the two groups, linear discriminant analysis (LDA) effect size (LEfSe) was performed and the threshold was 2. The INR group present a significantly higher abundance of genus *Selenomonas_4*, while the IR group has higher abundances of genus *Candidatus_Saccharimonas, norank _p_Saccharimonas,*

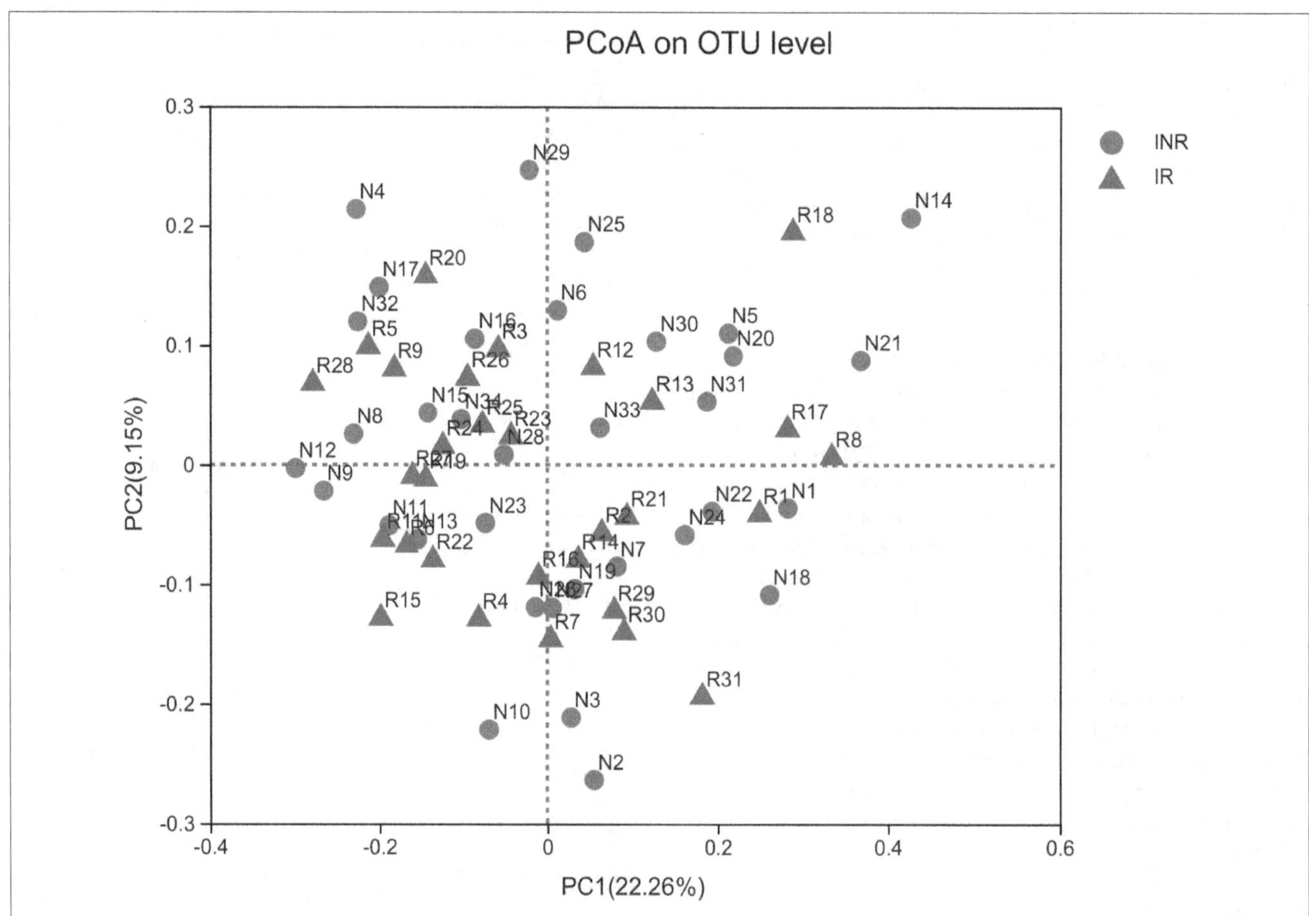

FIGURE 1 | Principal coordinates analysis (PCoA) of salivary microbiota in the IR and INR groups. No significant difference of bacterial communities between the immunological responders (IR) and immunological non-responders (INR) groups. IR, immunological responders; INR, immunological non-responders.

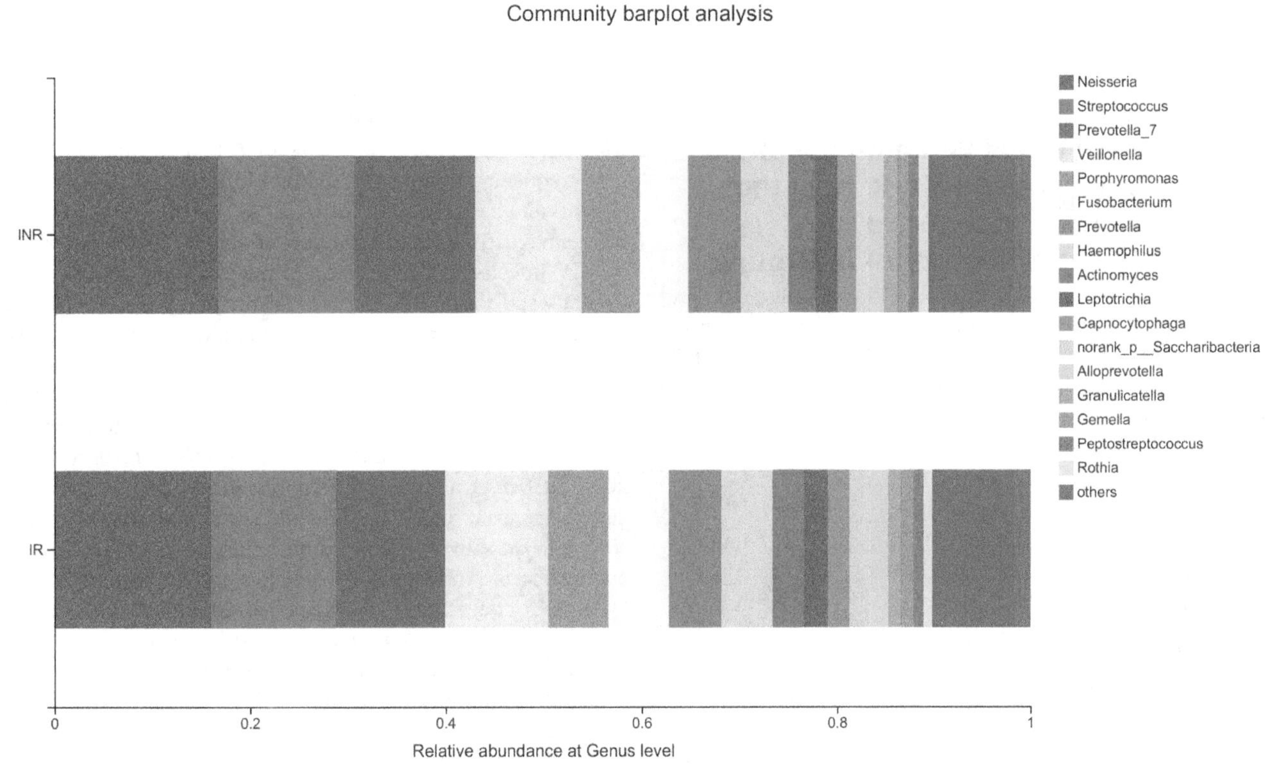

Community barplot analysis
INR
IR
0
0.2
0.4
0.6
0.8
1
Relative abundance at Genus level
Neisseria
Streptococcus
Prevotella_7
Veillonella
Porphyromonas
Fusobacterium
Prevotella
Haemophilus
Actinomyces
Leptotrichia
Capnocytophaga
norank_p__Saccharibacteria
Alloprevotella
Granulicatella
Gemella
Peptostreptococcus
Rothia
others

FIGURE 2 | The salivary microbiota composition at genus level in the IR and INR groups. IR, immunological responders; INR, immunological non-responders.

LEfSe Bar
INR
IR
g__Selenomonas_4
p__Saccharibacteria
g__norank_p__Saccharibacteria
f__norank_p__Saccharibacteria
o__norank_p__Saccharibacteria
c__norank_p__Saccharibacteria
o__Unknown_Order_c__Unknown_Class_p__Saccharibacteria
f__Unknown_Family_o__Unknown_Order_c__Unknown_Class_p__Saccharibacteria
c__Unknown_Class_p__Saccharibacteria
g__Candidatus_Saccharimonas
g__Desulfobulbus
f__Desulfobulbaceae
o__Desulfobacterales
4.0 3.5 3.0 2.5 2.0 1.5 1.0 0.5 0.0 0.5 1.0 1.5 2.0 2.5 3.0 3.5 4.0
LDA SCORE(log10)

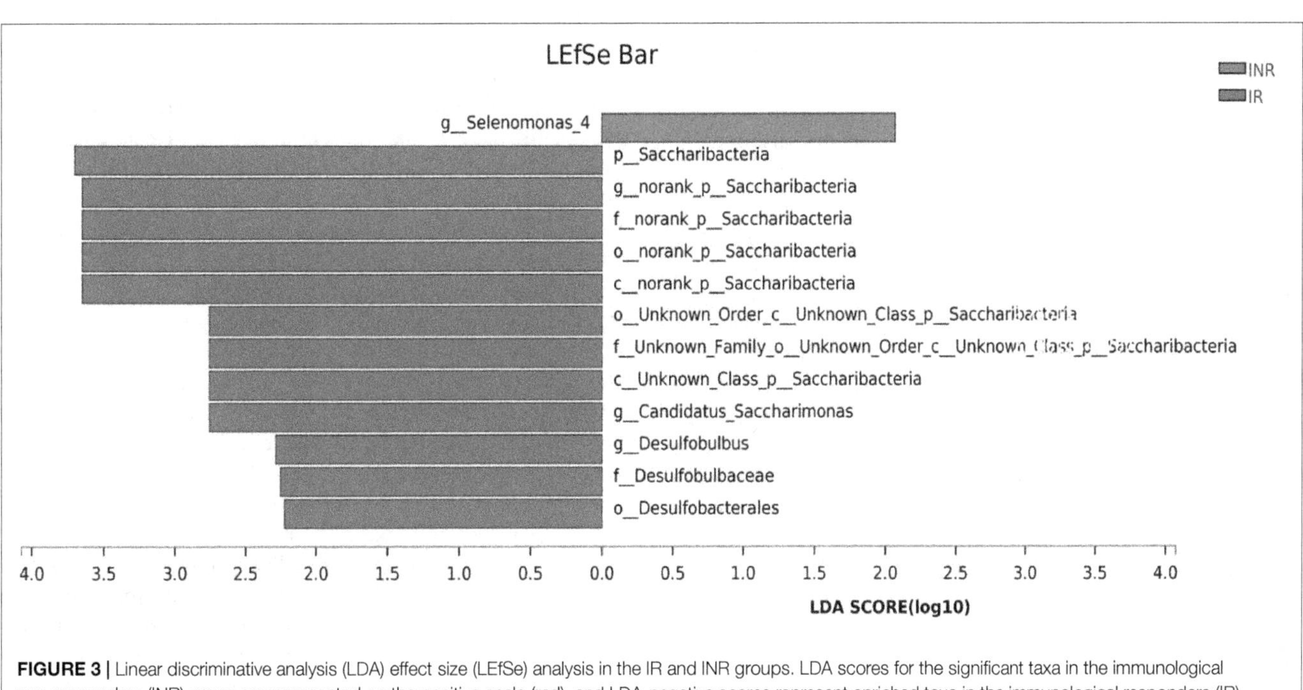

FIGURE 3 | Linear discriminative analysis (LDA) effect size (LEfSe) analysis in the IR and INR groups. LDA scores for the significant taxa in the immunological non-responders (INR) group are represented on the positive scale (red), and LDA-negative scores represent enriched taxa in the immunological responders (IR) group (blue). IR, immunological responders; INR, immunological non-responders.

and *Desulfobulbus* (**Figure 3**). The Wilcoxon Rank Sum test was also used to detect the taxa with significant differences in the relative abundances between the two groups (using confidence interval method). The abundance of *Saccharimonas* is more abundant in the IR group than the INR group at the phylum level (**Figure 4A**). Compared with the INR group, the abundances of genus *Candidatus_Saccharimonas* and *norank_p_Saccharimonas* are dramatically increased in the IR group, while the abundance of genus *Selenomonas_4* is dramatically decreased in the IR group (**Figure 4B**).

Comparison of Adaptive Immunity and Bacterial Translocation Markers in the Immunological Responders and Immunological Non-responders Groups

As expected, the amount of the current CD4 + T-cell counts and the CD4/CD8 ratio in the INR group is lower than those in the IR group ($p < 0.001$). The proportion of the CD8 + CD38 + T-cell and the CD8 + CD57 + T-cell is significantly higher in the INR group than those in the IR group ($p = 0.032$ and $p = 0.001$). The proportion level of the CD4 + immune activation (CD4 + T-cell by the expression of CD25 +, HLA-DR +, CD38 +, or HLA-DR + /CD38 +) shows similarity in the INR and IR groups. Lipopolysaccharide (LPS), which is commonly used as the major antigens driving chronic immune activation, is significantly higher in the INR group compared with that in the IR group ($p = 0.027$) (**Table 3**).

Associations Between Oral Microbiome and Adaptive Immunity

The Spearman's correlation test was used to investigate the correlation between the relative abundance of the different genera and adaptive immunity markers. The *p*-value was corrected by FDR, *p*-adjust lower than 0.05 with ρ-value above 0.2 were considered relevant and showed in **Figure 5**. As the abundance of genus *Selenomonas_4* is low in the two groups, the multiple correlation analyses were not performed. *Candidatus_Saccharimonas* and *norank _p_Saccharimonas* are positively correlated with the current CD4 + T cells (*p*-adjust = 0.033 and 0.025, respectively). *Candidatus_Saccharimonas* is positively correlated with the markers of the adaptive immunity CD4 + CD57 + T-cells (*p*-adjust = 0.049), while *norank _p_Saccharimonas* is negatively correlated with the CD8 + CD38 + T-cells and the CD4/CD8 + HLADR + CD38 + T-cells, respectively (*p*-adjust = 0.001 and 0.032, respectively) (**Figure 5**). To explore the potential function of the saliva microbiome for discriminating the IR and INR status, a random forest model was created based on the microbiome and the top 5 genus was shown in **Figure 6A**. The ROC analysis shows that *Candidatus_Saccharimonas* could be used to discriminate the IR from the INR group [ROC-plot AUC value of 0.7 (95% CI, 0.56–0.83), **Figure 6B**].

DISCUSSION

It is well-known that there is a dynamic interaction between the host and the microbiota, which is a major factor of people's health (Dethlefsen et al., 2007). Current available studies have confirmed that discernible alterations of the composition of the salivary microbiota are inherent to a range of systemic disorders. Studies on oral microbiomes of human immune system diseases such as RA, ALL, and HIV have also indicated that the oral microbiota is strongly related to the immune responses in immunodeficiency patients (Acharya et al., 2017; Corrêa et al., 2017; Annavajhala et al., 2020; Bellando-Randone et al., 2021). Furthermore, the hypothesis that oral microbiota is associated with different immune responses to ART is supported by the high frequency of opportunistic oral infections in HIV-infected patients and its association with CD4 + T cells levels (Berberi and Noujeim, 2015). As stated, the role of the oral microbiota played in HIV-infected patients deserves much attention because the diversity and composition of the oral microbiome can be changed by HIV infection or by ART (Heron and Elahi, 2017); however, the results are highly variable. Previous studies have observed the generally similar structure of salivary microbiota as well as the differences in the relative abundances of several bacterial taxa between HIV-infected subjects and uninfected controls (Li et al., 2014; Kistler et al., 2015; Mukherjee et al., 2018; Lewy et al., 2019). However, significant differences were also found by several studies in the saliva bacterial communities between HIV-infected and uninfected individuals (Hegde et al., 2014; Mukherjee et al., 2014; Beck et al., 2015; Goldberg et al., 2015; Kistler et al., 2015; Li et al., 2021). What's more, some studies reported significant distinctions in the prevalence and the distribution of the saliva bacterial communities among HIV-infected individuals before and after the antiretroviral therapy (Li et al., 2014; Kistler et al., 2015; Mukherjee et al., 2018). Few studies have addressed the interaction of oral microbiota with different immune responses to ART received by the HIV-infected individuals. In this paper, we demonstrate the oral microbiota structure and its relationship with immune response in HIV infection.

A previous study indicated that after receiving 24 weeks of ART, the salivary microbiome in the three HIV-infected participants with persistently low CD4 + T-cell count had significantly higher bacterial richness and Shannon diversity; when compared to those with CD4 counts that remained or recovered to greater than 200 cells/μl. Several taxa with different abundancies, such as *Porphyromonas* species, discriminated between the baseline and the posttreatment samples; this suggested that the salivary microbiome can be an important factor in the CD4 + T-cell count recovery after ART in the study (Presti et al., 2018). However, the major limitation of this study is the insufficient number of studied subjects and the short time period of patients receiving ART. Thus, more studies on larger cohorts are necessary for a better understanding of the potential roles of different immune responses to ART on oral microbiome. Making the most use of the non-invasive and unsuspicious functions of saliva sampling, we collected the salivary samples from the HIV-infected immunological non-responders and immunological responders and studied the salivary microbiome using high-throughput sequencing technology. To our knowledge, this is the first study that has fully utilized the next-generation sequencing technology to characterize and compare the community composition of the salivary microbiota in the higher number of HIV-infected immunological responders and non-responders. These findings are particularly important given that the adaptive immunity markers assessments were performed on all participants, offering

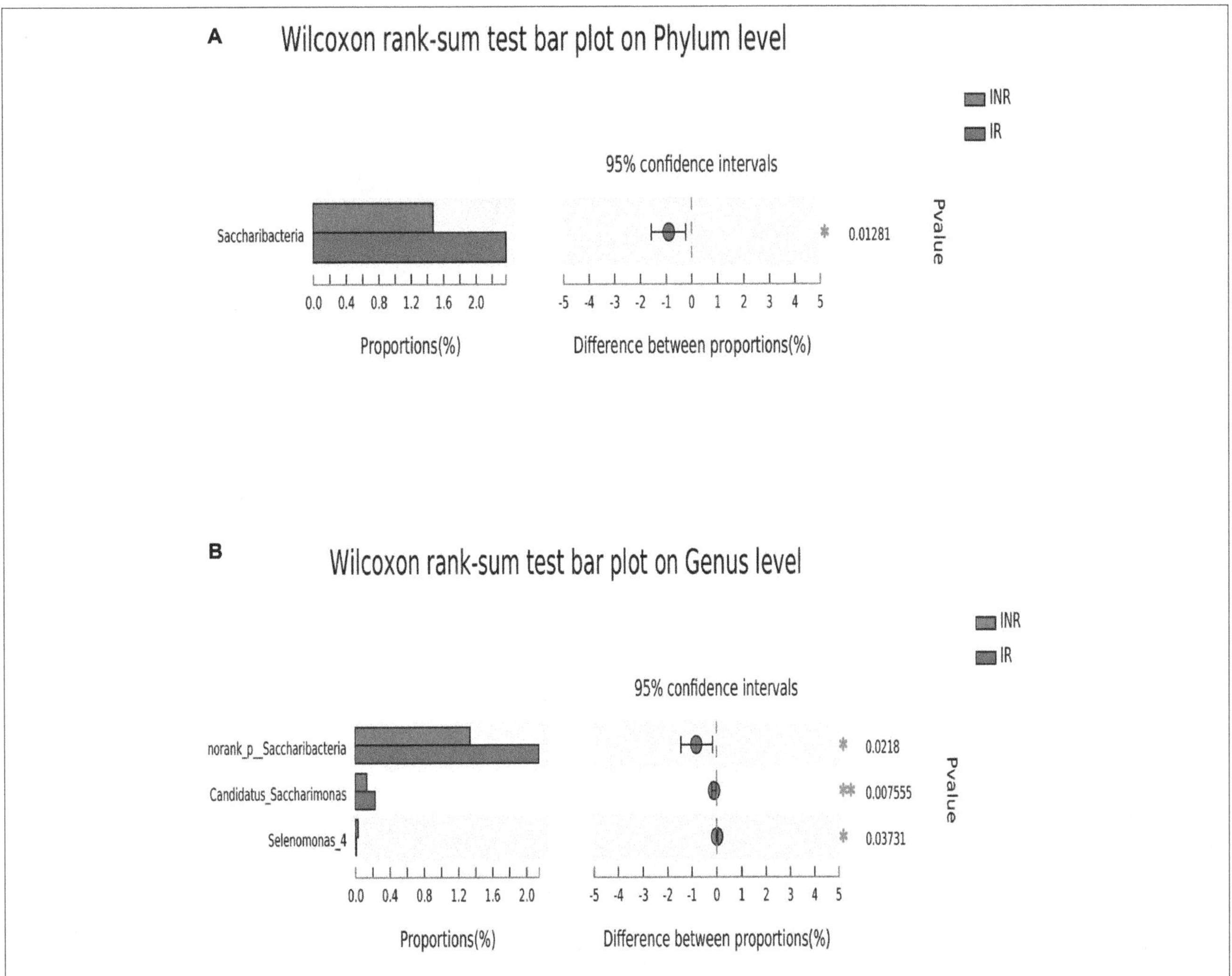

FIGURE 4 | The difference of saliva microbial taxa between the IR and INR groups at the phylum and genus levels. The Wilcoxon Rank Sum test was performed to detect taxa with significant differences in relative abundances at the phylum **(A)** and the genus levels **(B)** between the two groups (using confidence interval method). IR, immunological responders; INR, immunological non-responders. *$P < 0.05$ and **$P < 0.01$.

TABLE 3 | Comparison of adaptive immunity and bacterial translocation markers.

Characteristics	IR (n = 30)	INR (n = 34)	P-value
Current CD4 + T cell count,/mm^3, median (IQR)	597 (466.5, 666.5)	209 (163.3, 303)	**<0.001**
Current CD4 + /CD8 + T-cell ratio	0.9 (0.5, 1)	0.4 (0.2, 0.5)	**<0.001**
%CD4 + HLADR + CD38 +	7.2 (4.5, 10)	7.8 (4.7, 12.4)	0.418
%CD4 + CD25 +	1.1 (0.6, 1.5)	0.8 (0.3, 1.6)	0.388
%CD4 + CD57 +	2.3 (0.7, 4.1)	1.1 (0.2, 2.9)	0.083
%CD8 + CD38 +	31.6 (25.7, 39.2)	44.1 (28.0, 58.0)	**0.032**
%CD8 + HLADR + CD38 +	17.8 (13.1, 26.5)	23.7 (12.4, 35.7)	0.388
%CD8 + CD57 +	13.4 (10.5, 19.8)	21.7 (14.2, 34.5)	**0.001**
LPS (pg/ml, mean ± SD)	64.7 (50.6, 104.4)	90.1 (65.5, 152)	**0.027**
sCD14 (pg/ml, mean ± SD)	2052.1 (1797.7, 2413.5)	2319.8 (1878.1, 2654.4)	0.169

IR, immunological responders; INR, immunological non-responders. Bold values indicate $P < 0.05$.

an opportunity to evaluate the relationship between the salivary microbiota and the immunologic markers in the immunological responders and non-responders.

The IR group presented similar salivary bacterial richness and diversity when compared with the INR group in this study. A similar Alpha diversity of salivary bacterial community was

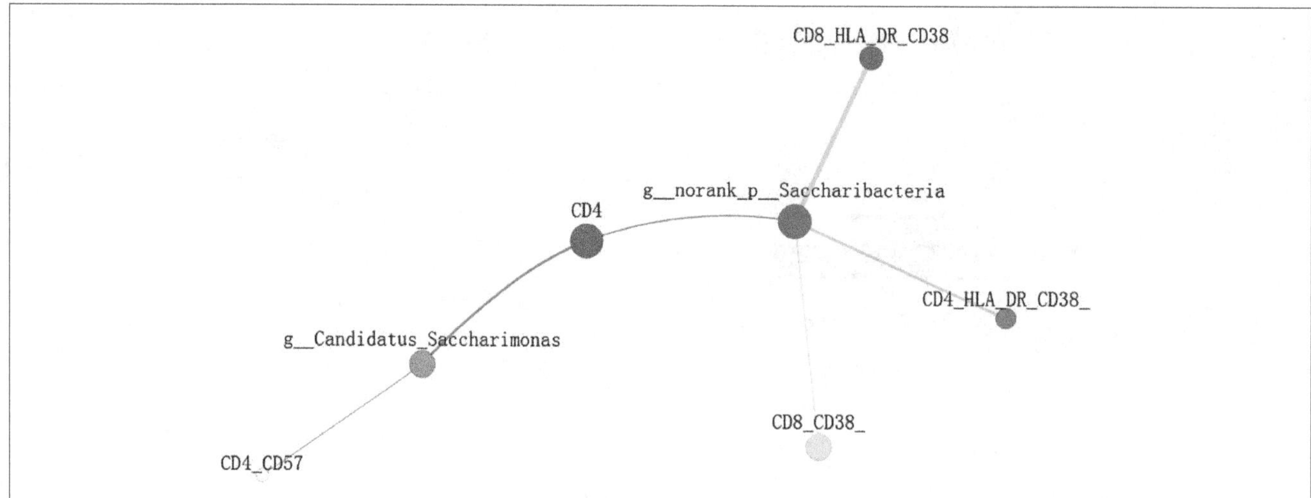

FIGURE 5 | Two-way correlation network analysis between the saliva microbiota and the adaptive immunity markers. Some adaptive immunity markers are correlated with the specific genera of saliva microbiota. Positive correlation is shown in the red line, negative correlation is shown in the green line. Spearman's correlation was used, and associations with p-adjust lower than 0.05 and ρ-value above 0.2 were considered relevant.

also described in the HIV-infected IR ($n = 18$) and INR ($n = 9$) individuals in a previous study (Jiménez-Hernández et al., 2019). While another study reported that the three HIV-infected participants with persistently low CD4 + T-cell counts had significantly higher salivary bacterial richness and Shannon diversity after their 24 weeks of ART, when compared with the participants whose CD4 + T-cell counts higher than 200 cells/μl (Presti et al., 2018). It claimed that the HIV infection and highly active antiretroviral therapy (HAART) had significant effects on salivary microbial colonization and composition, and *Selenomonas* noticeably increased after HAART (Li et al., 2014), which were reported to be depleted in the oral microbiome of the HIV-associated periodontitis (Noguera-Julian et al., 2017). For patients with systemic lupus erythematosus (SLE), increased numbers of *Selenomonas* were directly correlated with the elevated levels of inflammatory cytokines IL-6, IL-17, and IL-33 (Corrêa et al., 2017). In this study, when we visualized the relative abundances of dominant taxa at the genus level in the oral microbiome, we found that the INR group presented a significantly higher abundance of genus *Selenomonas_4.* Gut *Candidatus_Saccharimonas* was reported decreased in rats acute necrotizing pancreatitis (Chen et al., 2017), which indicated that *Candidatus_Saccharimonas* did play an important role in maintaining normal intestinal functions. A previously published study stated that the relative abundance of gut *Candidatus_Saccharimonas* was negatively correlated with the expression levels of cadherin-11, IL-17α, and TLR2 in the adjuvant-induced arthritis rat model (Huang et al., 2019). In this study, the IR group had higher abundances of genus *Candidatus_Saccharimonas* and *norank _p_Saccharimonas* when compared with the INR group. In addition, *Candidatus_Saccharimonas* had positive correlation with the CD4 + T-cells and CD4 + CD57 + T-cells, while *norank _p_Saccharimonas* was positively correlated with the CD4 + T-cells but negatively correlated with the CD8 + CD38 + T-cells and CD4/CD8 + HLADR + CD38 + T-cells. While host biomarkers were subjected to the individual biological variations, oral microbiome was relatively conserved among unrelated individuals. Recent advances of saliva analysis have played a key role in the definitions of biomarkers for the diagnosis, prognosis, and the treatment of human immune system diseases (Bellando-Randone et al., 2021). Expansion of specific microbial consortia in the saliva may act as imprints of the underlying immuno-inflammatory processes, especially in HIV. This study indicated that *Selenomona, Candidatus_Saccharimonas,* and *norank _p_Saccharimonas* might all played important roles in the immune recovery of the immunodeficiency patients, and *Candidatus_Saccharimonas* could be considered in the future as screening biomarkers for immune responses in HIV-infected individuals, leading to the future design of effective individualized treatment strategies such as probiotics for the immunological non-responders. However, a previous study on the effect of the prebiotic modulation of the salivary microbiota in HIV-infected patients with diverse immunopathogenesis stated that: *Streptococcus anginosus* was in correlation with the CD4 + T cells, *Veillonella parvula* with the CD4 + CD25 + T cells, and *Prevotella pallens, Prevotella copri, and Prevotella nigrencens* with the markers of adaptive immunity such as CD4 + CD25 + T cells, CD4 + CD57 + T cells, and CD4 + HLADR + CD38 + T cells, respectively (Jiménez-Hernández et al., 2019). The inconsistent results may be caused by the different number of subjects in the two studies and their different definitions of INR. More studies need to be carried out to determine the precise cause of this inconsistency.

This study provides a better understanding of the oral microbial profiles and their relationship with the immune responses in the immunocompromised patients. Although the correlations between the salivary microbiota and the biomarkers of adaptive immunity were observed, we could not establish a causal influence between the oral microbiome and the immune

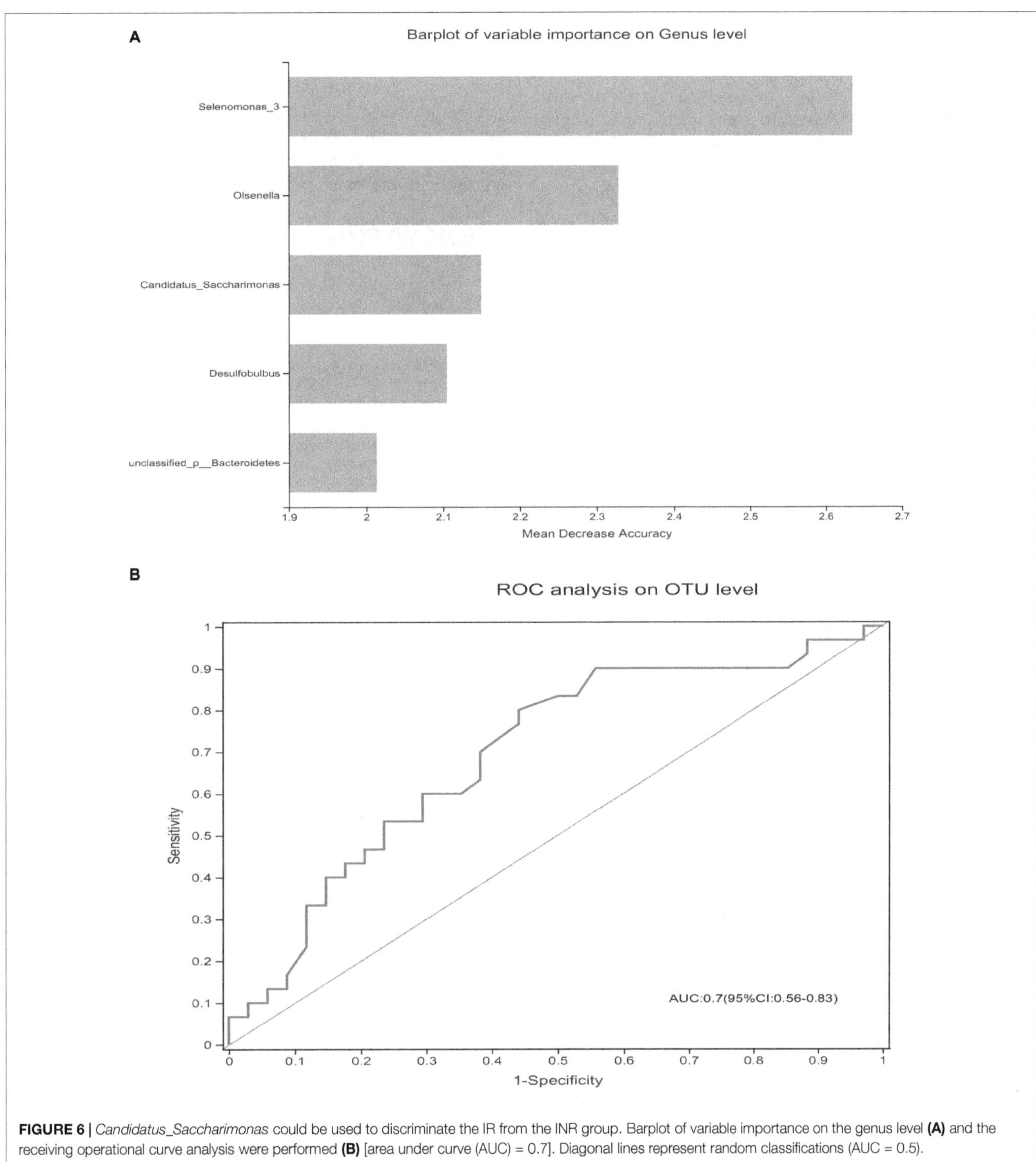

FIGURE 6 | *Candidatus_Saccharimonas* could be used to discriminate the IR from the INR group. Barplot of variable importance on the genus level **(A)** and the receiving operational curve analysis were performed **(B)** [area under curve (AUC) = 0.7]. Diagonal lines represent random classifications (AUC = 0.5).

system in the HIV-infected patients. Thus, further research on the exact mechanisms involved in the interaction between the immune system and oral microbiota is still required. We find the low number of participants, absence of control group, and cross-sectional analysis caused limitations to the explanation of our findings. Intra-person variability will need larger longitudinal studies with control group, which should involve plaque collection and the observation of the clinical and environmental changes that account for intra-person variability over time. Apart from taxonomic characterization, there should be more studies on identifying bacterial pathways and the resulting metabolites that promote disease and immunity.

In summary, this study focuses on the overall oral microbiota structure and its interactions with different immune responses

In summary, this study focuses on the overall oral microbiota structure and its interactions with different immune responses to ART. While there were some taxonomic differences in the salivary bacterial composition, the results suggested that the overall structure of the salivary microbiota in the immunological responders was similar with those that were in the immunological non-responders. *Selenomona_4, Candidatus_Saccharimonas,* and *norank_p_Saccharimonas* might act as important factors of the immune recovery in the immunodeficiency patients, and *Candidatus_Saccharimonas* could be considered in the future as screening biomarkers for immune responses in the HIV-infected individuals.

AUTHOR CONTRIBUTIONS

YX participated in the designing of the study and wrote the manuscript. JS performed the statistical analysis and revised the manuscript. JS and CH collected the biopsy samples and carried out the experiment. BR and BZ participated in the designing and reviewing of the manuscript. All authors read through and approved the final manuscript.

ACKNOWLEDGMENTS

This study gratefully acknowledges the patients who participated in the research.

REFERENCES

1. Acharya, A., Chan, Y., Kheur, S., Jin, L. J., Watt, R. M., and Mattheos, N. (2017). Salivary microbiome in non-oral disease: a summary of evidence and commentary. *Arch. Oral Biol.* 83, 169–173. doi: 10.1016/j.archoralbio.2017.07. 019
2. Annavajhala, M. K., Khan, S. D., Sullivan, S. B., Shah, J., Pass, L., Kister, K., et al. (2020). Oral and gut microbial diversity and immune regulation in patients with HIV on antiretroviral therapy. *mSphere* 5, e798–e719. doi: 10.1128/msphere. 00798-19
3. Beck, J. M., Schloss, P. D., Venkataraman, A., Twigg, H., Jablonski, K. A., Bushman, D., et al. (2015). Multicenter comparison of lung and oral microbiomes of HIV-infected and HIV-uninfected individuals. *Am. J. Respir. Crit. Care Med.* 192, 1335–1344. doi: 10.1164/rccm.201501-0128OC
4. Bellando-Randone, S., Russo, E., Venerito, V., Matucci-Cerinic, M., Iannone, F., Tangaro, S., et al. (2021). Exploring the oral microbiome in rheumatic diseases, state of art and future prospective in personalized medicine with an ai approach. *J. Pers. Med.* 11:625. doi: 10.3390/jpm11070625
5. Berberi, A., and Noujeim, Z. (2015). Epidemiology and Relationships between CD4+ Counts and Oral Lesions among 50 patients infected with human immunodeficiency virus. *J. Int. Oral Heal. JIOH* 7, 18–21.
6. Cenderello, G., and De Maria, A. (2016). Discordant responses to cART in HIV- 1 patients in the era of high potency antiretroviral drugs: clinical evaluation, classification, management prospects. *Expert Rev. Anti. Infect. Ther.* 14, 29–40. doi: 10.1586/14787210.2016.1106937
7. Chen, J., Huang, C., Wang, J., Zhou, H., Lu, Y., Lou, L., et al. (2017). Dysbiosis of intestinal microbiota and decrease in paneth cell antimicrobial peptide level during acute necrotizing pancreatitis in rats. *PLoS One* 12:e0176583. doi: 10. 1371/journal.pone.0176583
8. Corrêa, J. D., Calderaro, D. C., Ferreira, G. A., Mendonça, S. M. S., Fernandes, R., Xiao, E., et al. (2017). Subgingival microbiota dysbiosis in systemic lupus erythematosus: association with periodontal status. *Microbiome* 5:34. doi: 10.1186/s40168-017-0252-z
9. Dethlefsen, L., McFall-Ngai, M., and Relman, D. A. (2007). An ecological and evolutionary perspective on humang-microbe mutualism and disease. *Nature* 449, 811–818. doi: 10.1038/nature06245
10. Dillon, S. M., Frank, D. N., and Wilson, C. C. (2016). The gut microbiome and HIV-1 pathogenesis: a two-way street. *AIDS* 30, 2737–2751. doi: 10.1097/QAD. 0000000000001289
11. Florence, E., Lundgren, J., Dreezen, C., Fisher, M., Kirk, O., Blaxhult, A., et al. (2003). Factors associated with a reduced CD4 lymphocyte count response to HAART despite full viral suppression in the EuroSIDA study. *HIV Med.* 4, 255–262. doi: 10.1046/j.1468-1293.2003.00156.x
12. Gao, L., Xu, T., Huang, G., Jiang, S., Gu, Y., and Chen, F. (2018). Oral microbiomes: more and more importance in oral cavity and whole body. *Protein Cell* 9, 488–500. doi: 10.1007/s13238-018-0548-1
13. Goldberg, B. E., Mongodin, E. F., Jones, C. E., Chung, M., Fraser, C. M., Tate, A., et al. (2015). The oral bacterial communities of children with well-controlled HIV infection and without HIV infection. *PLoS One* 10:e0131615. doi: 10.1371/ journal.pone.0131615
14. Hegde, M. C., Kumar, A., Bhat, G., and Sreedharan, S. (2014). Oral microflora: a comparative study in HIV and normal patients. *Indian J. Otolaryngol. Head Neck Surg.* 66, 126–132. doi: 10.1007/s12070-011-0 370-z
15. Heron, S. E., and Elahi, S. (2017). HIV infection and compromised mucosal immunity: oral manifestations and systemic inflammation. *Front. Immunol.* 8:241. doi: 10.3389/fimmu.2017.00241
16. Huang, Y., Li, M., Zhou, L., Xu, D., Qian, F., Zhang, J., et al. (2019). Effects of qingluo tongbi decoction on gut flora of rats with adjuvant-induced arthritis and the underlying mechanism. *Evidence-Based Complement. Altern. Med.* 2019:6308021. doi: 10.1155/2019/6308021
17. Ji, Y., Zhang, F., Zhang, R., Shen, Y., Liu, L., Wang, J., et al. (2018). Changes in intestinal microbiota in HIV-1-infected subjects following cART initiation: influence of CD4+ T cell count article. *Emerg. Microbes Infect.* 7:113. doi: 10.1038/s41426-018-0117-y
18. Jiménez-Hernández, N., Serrano-Villar, S., Domingo, A., Pons, X., Artacho, A., Estrada, V., et al. (2019). Modulation of saliva microbiota through prebiotic intervention in HIV-Infected individuals. *Nutrients* 11:1346. doi: 10.3390/ nu11061346
19. Kaufmann, G. R., Perrin, L., Pantaleo, G., Opravil, M., Furrer, H., Telenti, A., et al. (2003). CD4 T-lymphocyte recovery in individuals with advanced HIV- 1 infection receiving potent antiretroviral therapy for 4 years: the Swiss HIV cohort study. *Arch. Intern. Med.* 163, 2187–2195. doi: 10.1001/archinte.163.18. 2187
20. Kistler, J. O., Arirachakaran, P., Poovorawan, Y., Dahlén, G., and Wade, W. G. (2015). The oral microbiome in human immunodeficiency virus (HIV)-positive individuals. *J. Med. Microbiol.* 64, 1094–1101. doi: 10.1099/jmm.0.00 0128
21. Lewy, T., Hong, B. Y., Weiser, B., Burger, H., Tremain, A., Weinstock, G., et al. (2019). Oral microbiome in HIV-infected women: shifts in the abundance of pathogenic and beneficial bacteria are associated with aging, HIV load, CD4 count, and antiretroviral therapy. *AIDS Res. Hum. Retroviruses* 35, 276–286. doi: 10.1089/aid.2017.0200
22. Li, S., Zhu, J., Su, B., Wei, H., Chen, F., Liu, H., et al. (2021). Alteration in oral microbiome among men who have sex with men with acute and chronic HIV infection on antiretroviral therapy. *Front. Cell. Infect. Microbiol.* 11:695515. doi: 10.3389/fcimb.2021.695515
23. Li, Y., Saxena, D., Chen, Z., Liu, G., Abrams, W. R., Phelan, J. A., et al. (2014). HIV infection and microbial diversity in saliva. *J. Clin. Microbiol.* 52, 1400–1411. doi: 10.1128/JCM.02954-13
24. Lu, W., Feng, Y., Jing, F., Han, Y., Lyu, N., Liu, F., et al. (2018). Association between gut microbiota and CD4 recovery in HIV-1 infected patients. *Front. Microbiol.* 9:1451. doi: 10.3389/fmicb.2018.01451
25. Mukherjee, P. K., Chandra, J., Retuerto, M., Sikaroodi, M., Brown, R. E., Jurevic, R., et al. (2014). Oral mycobiome analysis of HIV-infected patients: identification of pichia as an antagonist of opportunistic fungi. *PLoS Pathog.* 10:e1003996. doi: 10.1371/journal.ppat.1003996
26. Mukherjee, P. K., Chandra, J., Retuerto, M., Tatsuoka, C., Ghannoum, M. A., and McComsey, G. A. (2018). Dysbiosis in the oral bacterial and fungal microbiome of HIV-infected subjects is associated with clinical and immunologic variables of HIV infection. *PLoS One* 13:e0200285. doi: 10.1371/journal.pone.0200285

27. Noguera-Julian, M., Guillén, Y., Peterson, J., Reznik, D., Harris, E. V., Joseph, S. J., et al. (2017). Oral microbiome in HIV-associated periodontitis. *Medicine (United States)* 96:e5821. doi: 10.1097/MD.0000000000005821

28. Presti, R. M., Handley, S. A., Droit, L., Ghannoum, M., Jacobson, M., Shiboski, C. H., et al. (2018). Alterations in the oral microbiome in HIV- infected participants after antiretroviral therapy administration are influenced by immune status. *AIDS* 32, 1279–1287. doi: 10.1097/QAD.00000000000 01811

29. Segata, N., Izard, J., Waldron, L., Gevers, D., Miropolsky, L., Garrett, W. S., et al. (2011). Metagenomic biomarker discovery and explanation. *Genome Biol.* 12:R60. doi: 10.1186/gb-2011-12-6-r60

30. Tsukamoto, H., Clise-Dwyer, K., Huston, G. E., Duso, D. K., Buck, A. L., Johnson, L. L., et al. (2009). Age-associated increase in lifespan of naïve CD4 T cells contributes to T-cell homeostasis but facilitates development of functional defects. *Proc. Natl. Acad. Sci. U.S.A.* 106, 18333–18338. doi: 10.1073/pnas. 0910139106

31. Xie, Y., Sun, J., Wei, L., Jiang, H., Hu, C., Yang, J., et al. (2021). Altered gut microbiota correlate with different immune responses to HAART in HIV-infected individuals. *BMC Microbiol.* 21:11. doi: 10.1186/s12866-020-02 074-1

32. Yang, X., Su, B., Zhang, X., Liu, Y., Wu, H., and Zhang, T. (2020). Incomplete immune reconstitution in HIV/AIDS patients on antiretroviral therapy: challenges of immunological non-responders. *J. Leukoc. Biol.* 107, 597–612. doi: 10.1002/JLB.4MR1019-189R

21

Input from Practice: Reshaping Dental Education for Integrated Patient Care

R. Lamont (Monty) MacNeil and Helena Hilario*

University of Connecticut School of Dental Medicine, Farmington, CT, United States

Correspondence:
R. Lamont (Monty) MacNeil
macneil@uchc.edu

Among the primary challenges in advancing the practice of integrated primary dental and medical health care is the appropriate educational and clinical preparation of a dental workforce that can function and flourish within integrated care environments. Most dental schools teach to traditional concepts and standards of dental care delivery which may be inconsistent with those of integrated care and could deter the entry and retention of graduates in contemporary, non-traditional practice models. To better understand how the dental school curriculum should be modified to accommodate integrative care models, a number of patient care organizations actively engaged in dental-medical integration were site visited to gain insight into the readiness of newer graduates, with emphasis on the US DMD/DDS graduate, to function in integrated practice. Leaders, practicing clinicians and staff were interviewed and common observations and themes were documented. This manuscript will focus on those educational components that integrated care organizations identify as absent or inadequate in current dentist education which must be addressed to meet the unique expectations and requirements of integrated patient care. These changes appear pivotal in the preparation of a dental clinician workforce that is respectful and receptive to new practice concepts, adaptative to new practice models, and competent in new care delivery systems.

Keywords: integration, dentistry, medicine, health systems, interprofessional education, dental education

INTRODUCTION

Predoctoral (i.e., pre-DMD/DDS degree) dental education programs in the United States are in a perpetual mode of revision and adjustment as they attempt to respond to evolving change in society's needs and the practice of general dentistry [1–3]. Although these changes tend to emerge gradually, they are nevertheless real and compel dental schools to reconsider the knowledge, skills, abilities and values, collectively termed "competencies," required by new dental graduates [4]. There are many examples of change in dental practice: shifts in care emphasis from a repair/restoration focus to prevention and early interceptive treatment; growth in multi-provider group and corporate-affiliated practice; increased focus on the social determinants of health; employment of evidence-based decision making in treatment planning; and greater attention on the relationship of oral and overall systemic health. The emergence of new models of care delivery is linked to many of these drivers of change and is perhaps best exemplified in the growth of integrated dental-medical care practice [5].

Some of the changes pursued by dental schools have been self-inspired but many have been prompted by the advocacy of thought leaders and national dental organizations to instill necessary updates in prevailing dental accreditation standards [6–8]. In response to professional and community input, the Commission on Dental Education (CODA) has introduced a number of new standards over the past several decades which, in turn, have prompted dental schools to modify curriculum, clinical practices and community interaction [9]. Several newer standards were informed by the embryogenesis of integrated dental-medical care and the opinion held by many in the profession that its continued development in both traditional and non-traditional models of practice could significantly improve health care outcomes [10, 11]. The following are examples of modified or new accreditation standards that refer to those competencies considered essential in integrated care delivery:

- Standard 2-15: *Graduates must be competent in the application of biomedical science knowledge in the delivery of patient* care[1].
- Standard 2-19: *Graduates must be competent in applying the basic principles and philosophies of practice management, models of oral health care delivery and how to function successfully as the leader of the oral health care team.*
- Standard 2-20: *Graduates must be competent in communicating and collaborating with other members of the healthcare team to facilitate the provision of healthcare*[2].

These and other accreditation standards and intent statements have led to the adoption of new educational approaches in US dental schools. One major initiative has been the development of interprofessional education (IPE) activities wherein dental students at timepoints within the typical four-year DMD/DDS curriculum are brought together in learning experiences with students from the other health professions including but not limited to medicine, nursing and pharmacy [12–14]. The objective is that these students learn together, better understand the relationship with and scope of other health professions, develop interprofessional communication skills and, optimally, co-participate in the coordinated care of patients [15]. Beginning in 2009, several health professions education organizations including the American Dental Education Association (ADEA) began to formally organize around these initiatives leading to the creation of the Interprofessional Education Collaborative, or IPEC, which currently includes 21 national health profession associations. In 2011, the first IPEC competencies were adopted [16], expanding in 2016 to four core competencies described by IPEC as essential for students in the health professions to succeed in interprofessional collaborative practice [17].

Beyond these particular changes, recommendations continue to be voiced on how dental schools can best respond to changes in the needs of society and the emergence of new healthcare systems and models of practice [4]. Schools have been moderately successful in analyzing their success in the implementation of curricular revisions but much less so on the impact of these responses on the preparedness of new graduates to function and succeed within new models of dental care especially those characterized by high levels of interprofessional interaction such as that observed in integrated dental-medical practice [18, 19].

Consequently, this project was undertaken to gain input from leaders of dental care entities with high levels of integrated care activity about the readiness of new DMD/DDS graduates for this unique form of practice.

METHODS

Study Construct

During 2018-2019, the American Dental Education Association (ADEA), under the direction of its Chair of the Board of Directors, initiated the project with the goal to gain a better understanding about how US dental education institutions were currently preparing graduates for integrated care practice and possible areas where improvement in curriculum and/or clinical training was necessary [20]. As an initial step, the authors sought to identify dental practices and health care organizations that were actively engaged in a meaningful level of integrated care activity. The SAMHSA-HRSA Center for Integrated Health Solutions (CIHS) framework for levels of integrated health care [21] served as a reference to assess level of integrated care. Potential practices were identified by conducting literature searches of peer- reviewed publications and abstracts and by scanning conferences proceedings, meeting presentations, professional monographs and marketing materials. Entities appearing to have a moderate-to-high degree of integrated care activity and approaching CIHS's Levels 4-6 of collaboration/integration were targeted (i.e., Level 4- Close collaboration onsite with some systems integration; Level 5- Close collaboration approaching integrated practice; Level 6- Full collaboration in a transformed/merged integrated practice). In total, thirteen entities were identified and then contacted directly for further review. Two entities did not respond, one expressed a low level of interest in the project and three others were considered to have a relatively small amount of integrated activity. Based on initial response and interest in the project, seven entities remained and agreed to participate.

Each practice organization was site visited over a period of 1–2 days by one of the authors (RLMN) and included interactions with directors, care providers and support staff.

In the case of multi-site practices, a representative number of satellite locations were visited along with the primary site of care delivery. Structured questions (**Table 1**) were proposed to the chief administrative leaders. Interviews with clinical providers and auxiliary staff were less formal and more conversational in nature.

[1]Each CODA standard is accompanied by an Intent Statement(s). The Intent Statement within standard 2-15 is that the graduate can "*... integrate new medical knowledge and therapies relative to oral health care*".

[2]An Intent Statement within standard 2-20 is that students should "*... have educational experiences, particularly clinical experiences, that involve working with other healthcare professional students and practitioners. Students should have educational experiences in which they coordinate patient care with the healthcare system relative to dentistry*".

TABLE 1 | Interview guide for integrated care practice leaders.

1. Describe (in common language) the key characteristics of your oral health care delivery approach/model and how it differs from a traditional (large) group dental practice?
2. Was your organization integrated from its inception? If so, what factors drove that integration? If not, when did your organization or group become interested in integration or greater connectivity with the larger health system and why? What were your key drivers? Who were your key "connected" health partners?
3. How are you connected to your other healthcare colleagues, and how do functionally communicate with them?
4. In terms of your initial goals, at what phase are you in your integration efforts?
5. At your current and unique phase of integration or connectivity, what do you see as the major, unique advantages of your delivery approach?
6. How have your integration efforts benefited your patients?
7. How have your integration efforts benefited the dental providers and staff?
8. How have your integration efforts benefited your other health care colleagues?
9. Are the competencies/skills needed by dentists in this system different than that needed in a traditional group practice? If so, what must dental providers bring to your practice approach in order to be successful within it?
10. How can dental academic institutions better prepare their graduates to be successful in organizations such as yours?
11. What advice can you provide to dental schools or academic health centers considering a more integrated approach in their clinical endeavors?

The focus of the interviews and interactions was to determine how the participants viewed the preparedness of recent dental school graduates, specifically dentists, for professional activity within an active, integrated care environment, and where gaps in the educational process were evident. "Recent graduate" was defined as a dentist graduating from a US DMD/DDS degree program within the past 5 years. The site visit also served to assess the level of integrated dental-medical care by the selected entity.

The seven care groups visited included two large managed care/HMO type organizations, a multi-site hospital/federally qualified health center (FQHC) care entity, a hospital-based system with a general practice residency program serving as its chief dental care arm, a benefits organization with an expanding care delivery network, and two large, multi-provider dental group practice. Sites spanned the Northeast, Midwest and Western region of the country. One site proved to have rather minimal integrated care activity, one declined to have its interview reports published, and two sites showed some integrated activity but substantially less than that of the three sites eventually selected as the key informants for the ADEA Association Report.

The three entities selected for reporting were Permanente Dental Associates (PDA) in Portland Oregon, Marshfield Clinic Health System in Marshfield, Wisconsin and HealthPartners in Minneapolis, Minnesota. The organizational construct, care philosophies and other characteristics of these three organizations are fully described in previous publications [22–24]. Following the site visits with these entities, summary notes taken by (RLMN) were shared with those interviewed to confirm accuracy. Using an inductive approach, responses to interview questions were grouped into common themes for further consideration. Conclusions and recommendations relative to new dentist preparedness and other aspects pertinent to dental education were then drafted, shared and finalized. A full description of these interviews and recommendations has been previously reported in a five-part Special Report in the Journal of Dental Education [22–26].

RESULTS/DISCUSSION

General Observations

In the initial scan of engaged sites, only a limited number were found to have meaningful and sustained integrative care activities with medical units or other health professions providers. A number of practices or organizations reporting integrated care were found to be practicing it at very low functional levels. Some were still in the planning stages while others were at the very early stages of implementation. This finding suggests that the dental profession is still very much at the embryonic stage of integrated practice. The apparently low number of active, functional sites poses certain limitations and challenges to dental education.

As the project got underway, several large multi-provider dental practices falling into the general description of dental service organizations, or DSOs, began reporting on increased engagement in integrated dental- medical care. At least one DSO practice reported that it had moved to better support its integration efforts through conversion of its dental electronic health record (EHR) to a fully integrated, nationally recognized EHR used by a large number of US hospitals and medical care networks [27]. Unfortunately, the current project was not able to include these organizations and their engagement could potentially have expanded the site visit pool and the diversity of perspectives gained.

Perspectives and Recommendations From the Field

The following is a summary of the most common findings and suggestions gained through site visits at the three organizations described above and reported in greater detail in a special report of the Journal of Dental Education [22–26].

Interprofessional Education Must Be Improved Through Reinforcing Clinical Experiences

Organization leaders reported little difference in the preparedness of recent dental school graduates for integrated care practice compared to providers joining their organizations who graduated much earlier or who were engaged in prior traditional practice ("Recent graduate" was defined as a graduate of a dental school within the previous 5 years, between 2013 and 2018). This perspective was unanticipated as more recent graduates were expected to have had greater exposure to aspects of interprofessional education during their dental school training. Those interviewed were aware that dental schools had increased their emphasis on IPE in response to new accreditation standards and increased educational emphasis on IPE over the last decade. In general, they failed to see how that experience was translating into a different type of new provider or one more prepared for integrated care. Concern was expressed that IPE might be occurring in what one leader described as an "educational silo" [28], not strongly linked with active patient care and reinforcing clinical experiences, more formally termed interprofessional collaborative care (IPCC).

Based on the considerable investment that many schools have made in IPE, these comments should evoke reaction within the educational community. While the goals and objectives of IPE extend far beyond readying graduates for specific care environments, preparedness for delivery of integrated care represents a unique opportunity to measure IPE's impact in the form of a practical outcome. A strong recommendation from those interviewed in this project was that the IPE experience in dental schools not occur too distant or detached from the clinical practicum and that a good proportion of IPE should be embedded within clinical experiences where a measure of interprofessional collaborative care (IPCC) is practiced. This may be difficult for many schools with traditional intramural clinical operations, not part of an academic health center construct or not affiliated with other health professional schools or care units. Even for the approximate two-thirds of dental schools that are part of academic health centers, many have found it difficult to introduce and blend collaborative care activities with other health professions on campus. In some cases, it may be more feasible for dental schools to seek out extramural clinical sites where collaborative integrated care is active and could be modeled. One major limitation as previously noted is the relative paucity of dental settings where integrated care is active and institutionally supported.

Hospital- or Medically-Focused Residency Training Improves Preparedness

A correlate recommendation from those interviewed was that new providers with interest in integrated care practice should pursue advanced training of at least 1 year in a hospital-based general practice or pediatric dentistry residency program, representing the two chief elements of primary dental care. Graduates of general practice residency (GPR) programs that are closely aligned with hospital or medical operations and which provide coordinated care for inpatient populations were viewed as distinguishable from other new dental providers. The respondents felt that this was likely the result of the professional interactions between dentistry, medicine and the other health professions required within these types of programs. Not surprisingly, all three organizations had moved to placing substantial emphasis on a GPR experience as part of new provider recruitment. One organization felt that graduates of a particular US dental school were much better prepared for their brand of integrated practice; this particular school places senior students in extended community health center rotations and in several different locations nationally during the majority of the fourth year of their DMD/DDS education. This organization felt that these experiences exposed students to the dynamics of oral health inequities, health care disparities, economic/social/cultural determinants of health, and the treatment of acute dental disease, all which were an important part of their operational mantra. A general recommendation was that dental schools should sustain, if not expand, the amount of clinical time spent at community-based sites and, if possible, at FQHCs where medical and dental units support an integrative care philosophy and approach.

Maintain a Strong Curricular Experience in the Medical Sciences but Ensure an Applied, Practical Focus

The interviews identified a concern that dental schools were downscaling their basic and applied medical science curriculum in favor of competing curricular interests. The following examples were articulated: schools providing students with earlier clinical experience by transferring curricular time traditionally devoted to medical science instruction to the clinical practicum; a greater proportion of the available curriculum now devoted to exposure to and instruction in new chairside and laboratory technologies with focus on dental procedures; a fast-tracking of students through the core medical curriculum to meet the standards set by national boards but insufficient to provide the depth of knowledge needed for application in patient care; within the medical training of dental students insufficient emphasis placed on the discreet number of systemic conditions and diseases closely linked with oral health and provision of dental care. Some interviewed suggested that the dentist should be trained to the same level as primary care physicians relative to the limited number of medical conditions dominant within primary care and that consume the majority of integrated care communication and co-therapy planning such as diabetes, hypertension, and asthma. There was a perception that new dental providers have superficial knowledge across a wide range of medical conditions yet inappropriate depth and application ability in these common conditions. A prevailing opinion was that the foundational and applied medical curriculum within dental education must remain strong with emphasis on the possible unique role of dentists in the co-management of common medical conditions and the effective closure of gaps in disease prevention and health promotion strategies. The design of this type of curriculum requires effective communication between leaders of dental and other health professional schools and the coordinated participation of the entire dental faculty spanning generalist to specialist.

Invest in Integrated Electronic Health Records Allowing Communication Between Dental Medicine and the Other Health Professions

The issue of improving upon methods of professional communication was the strongest recommendation from our participants. It was strongly recommended that dental schools move toward participation in electronic health records (EHRs) shared with the medical community including hospitals and physician networks [29, 30]. The functional divide created by dental medicine and primary care medicine working from separate, unconnected EHRs was felt to be dramatically detrimental overall, placing dental practice in isolation from the surrounding and changing healthcare world. Optimism was expressed that several US dental schools recently moved away from dentistry-only EHRs to more broadly used health care platforms. While an expensive and challenging endeavor, this change was seen as essential if integrated care is to grow and new dental providers are prepared to be actively engaged. Of note, the three organizations surveyed here each employ a unifying EHR with integrated medical and dental components.

Provide Practical Experience in the Use of Health Analytic Tools

Contributors stressed the importance of the modern dental care provider being versed in the use of health analytic tools. These tools are often supported by contemporary, integrated EHRs, yet another reason for student exposure to such records. It was anticipated that providers will be more motivated to pursue innovative care strategies if they can witness the results of these efforts in improved quality care metrics. One example was the demonstrated ability by one organization to close gaps in certain medical preventive care protocols by the engagement of the dental team [22]. Those interviewed expressed that dental providers must feel comfortable and confident in accessing these analytic tools and in interpreting the data.

Educate Students About New Dental Practice and Compensation Models

Questions were raised about the efficiency of dental schools in providing practice management concepts that vary from the traditional, prevailing fee-for-service, independent contractor model of dental practice. As integrated medical-dental care is further pursued, and as the dental profession shifts from a repair/restore emphasis to a more prevention/early disease interception mode, it is probable that other business models of practice will emerge. For example, it is predicted that group practices will likely grow in size and number [31] and more third-party plans will incorporate value-based reimbursement approaches. Within these changes, our interviewees predicted that outcomes-focused, incentive-based formulas tightly linked to the ability of the dental provider to practice in diverse teams that include non-dental professionals will capture a larger part of the compensation landscape. Dental students must be exposed to these concepts so that as new graduates they can understand their relative strengths and weaknesses and make informed decisions on the type of practice that best matches their preferences and shifts in future dental care.

Stress the Power and Art of Effective Interprofessional Communication

A common thread across these interviews was the critical importance the individual provider to effectively communicate with all members of the care team in order to flourish in a more integrative model of care. There was a position that most schools could still improve upon training in both intraprofessional (i.e., within the dental team proper) and interprofessional communication. In a number of the practices visited, auxiliary personnel including dental hygienists, licensed practical nurses (LPNs) and medical assistants (MAs) performed a large portion of the integrated care effort including identification of medical/dental risk, gaps in care, and in the clinical provision of services such as blood pressure monitoring, blood draws and vaccine administration. The importance of effective communication between the supervising

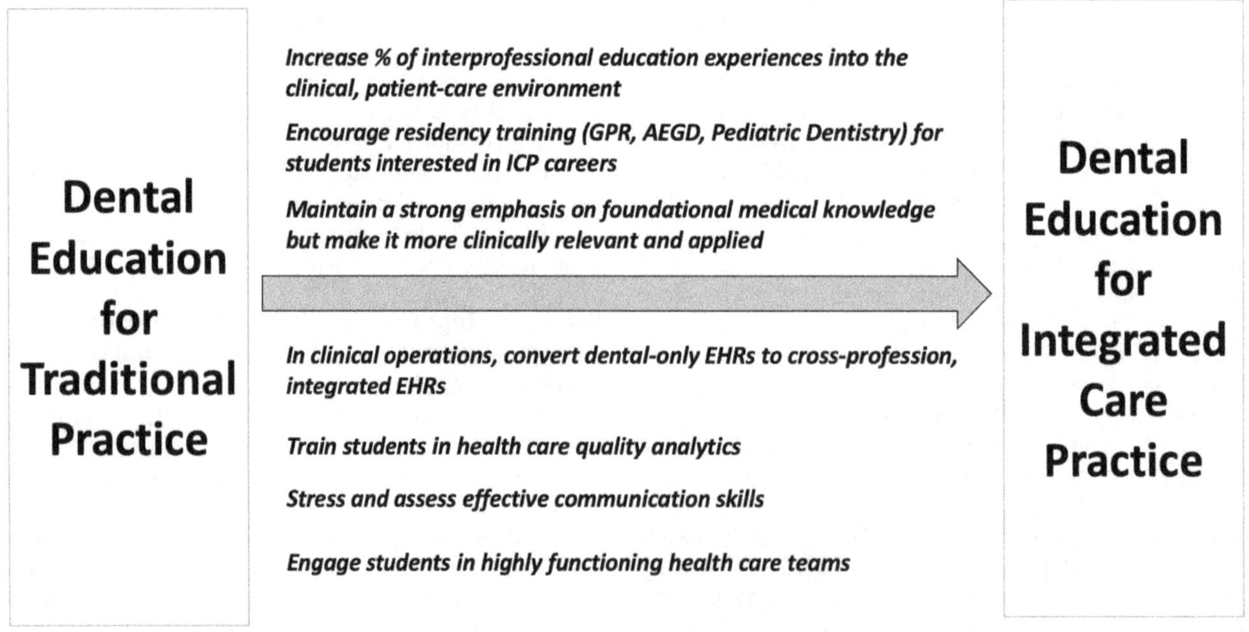

FIGURE 1 | Integrated care practice leader recommendations for improvement in the education and preparedness of dentists for future practice.

dentist and auxiliary staff is essential, as is the necessary interprofessional communication with correlate members of the primary care medical team. It was advised that increased efforts be made to prepare dental students to consistently and accurately use contemporary medical terminology to ensure the effective and safe transfer of information across the integrated team.

Engage Students in Highly Functioning, Intraprofessional and Interprofessional Teams, and Incentivize Effective Teamwork

An overwhelming recommendation from the interviews was that dental curricula further advance the concept of team-based care as essential to traditional and contemporary forms of practice. Students must be exposed to dynamic team environments where they practice as authentic members of a team in the care of patients. While simulated environments may be useful in this task, exposure to working examples of active teamwork was deemed critical. It was recognized, however, that identification of these examples may be difficult but must be pursued. Again, dental schools may need to move outside their intramural systems of care and explore external, community- based models to achieve this goal.

CONCLUSION

The recommendations emanating from this interview survey with leaders of integrated care practices (summarized in **Figure 1**) suggest that despite efforts to adequately prepare graduates for interprofessional collaborative care, improvements are necessary. Institutional responses to recent accreditation standards and national initiatives such as those emphasizing interprofessional education have undoubtedly had an impact but perhaps not to the extent envisioned. The dental education community should consider the presented recommendations and continue to advocate for advancement of current programs and continual refinement in the guidelines and principles upon which future program development is propelled. This report suggests that interprofessional education must move to the forefront and that greater efforts be undertaken to identify examples of integrated practice in the community where interprofessional, collaborative care is actively and effectively modeled.

These recommendations may present additional challenge for dental education as it attempts to respond to and address the many diverse drivers and indicators for change in the dental curriculum. Several of these recommendations will not align easily or fluidly with other shifts currently being witnessed or suggested (see Fontana). For example, devoting more curricular time to applied medical science and interprofessional collaborative care could be viewed as incongruent with expansion and earlier introduction of clinical care hours devoted to traditional care and greater immersion in new dental technologies. Experimentation with collaborative team models where appropriate compensation strategies have not yet been developed may be deemed inconsistent with the urgency to create more sustainable intramural clinical care systems and improved net clinical revenues. Investments in expensive universal EHRs will undoubtedly prove difficult as dental institutions attempt to curtail or reduce the rising cost of dental education. Despite these challenges, the promise and possibilities found within integrated dental-medical care demands that it be given high priority in dental education [3, 32]. New strategies will most likely require non-traditional approaches, innovation and significant adjustment in the current educational model, and in particular, the clinical practicum [33]. Therein lies the challenge for today's dental schools and leaders in dental education.

AUTHOR CONTRIBUTIONS

All authors listed have made a substantial, direct and intellectual contribution to the work, and approved it for publication.

ACKNOWLEDGMENTS

The authors would like to acknowledge the contributions and insights provided by the following: John J. Snyder, DMD (Permanente Dental Associates, Portland, OR); Amit Acharya BDS, MS, PhD, Megan M. Ryan DMD, Ingrid Glurich PhD, Greg R. Nycz (Marshfield Clinics, Marshfield, WI); David Gesko DDS, Todd Thierer, DDS (HealthPartners, Bloomington, MN).

REFERENCES

1. Formicola AJ, Bailit HL, Weintraub JA, Fried JL, Polverini PJ. Advancing dental education in the 21st century: phase 2 report on strategic analysis and recommendations. *J Dent Educ.* (2018) 82:eS1–32. doi: 10.21815/JDE.018.109
2. Haden NK, Catalanotto FA, Alexander CJ, Bailit H, Battrell A, Broussard J, et al. Improving the oral health status of all Americans: roles and responsibilities of academic dental institutions. *J Dent Educ.* (2003) 67:563–83. doi: 10.1002/j.0022-0337.2003.67.5.tb03658.x
3. Lamster IB, Tedesco LA, Fournier DM, Goodson JM, Gould AR, Haden NK, et al. New opportunities for dentistry in diagnosis and primary health care. *J Dent Educ.* (2008) 72:66–72. doi: 10.1002/j.0022-0337.2008.72.2_suppl.tb04483.x
4. Fontana M, González-Cabezas C, de Peralta T, Johnsen DC. Dental education required for the changing health care environment. *J Dent Educ.* (2017) 81:eS153–161. doi: 10.21815/JDE.017.022
5. Jones JA, Snyder JJ, Gesko DS, Helgeson MJ. Integrated medical-dental delivery systems: models in a changing environment and their implications for dental education. *J Dent Educ.* (2017) 81:eS21–9. doi: 10.21815/JDE.017.029
6. Haden NK, Andrieu SC, Chadwick DG, Chmar JE, Cole JR, George MC, et al. The dental education environment. *J Dent Educ.* (2006) 70:1265–70. doi: 10.1002/j.0022-0337.2006.70.12.tb04228.x
7. Hunt RJ, Bushong M. ADEA CCI vision focuses on preparing graduates for discoveries of the future. *J Dent Educ.* (2010) 74:819–23. doi: 10.1002/j.0022-0337.2010.74.8.tb04937.x
8. Kassebaum DK, Tedesco LA. The 21st-century dental curriculum: a framework for understanding current models. *J Dent Educ.* (2017) 81:eS13–21. doi: 10.21815/JDE.017.002

9. Commission on Dental Accreditation. *Accreditation Standards For Dental Education Programs.* (2019). Available online at: https://www.ada.org/~/media/CODA/Files/predoc_standards.pdf?la=en (accessed January 11, 2021).
10. Atchison KA, Rozier RG, Weintraub JA. Integration of oral health and primary care: communication, coordination, and referral. In: *NAM Perspectives.* Washington, DC: Discussion Paper, National Academy of Medicine (2018). doi: 10.31478/201810e
11. Donoff RB, McDonough JE, Riedy CA. Integrating oral and general health care. *N Engl J Med.* (2014) 371:2247–9. doi: 10.1056/NEJMp1410824
12. Andrews EA. The future of interprofessional education and practice for dentists and dental education. *J Dent Educ.* (2017) 81:eS186–92. doi: 10.21815/JDE.017.026
13. Formicola AJ, Andrieu SC, Buchanan JA, Childs GS, Gibbs M, Inglehart MR, et al. Interprofessional education in U.S. and Canadian dental schools: an ADEA team study group report. *J Dent Educ.* (2012) 76:1250–68. doi: 10.1002/j.0022-0337.2012.76.9.tb05381.x
14. Palatta A, Cook BJ, Anderson EL, Valachovic RW. 20 Years beyond the crossroads: the path to interprofessional education at U.S. dental schools. *J Dent Educ.* (2015) 79:982–6. doi: 10.1002/j.0022-0337.2015.79.8.tb05990.x
15. Institute of Medicine. *Interprofessional Education for Collaboration: Learning How to Improve Health from Interprofessional Models Across the Continuum of Education to Practice: Workshop Summary.* Washington, DC: The National Academies Press (2013).
16. Interprofessional Education Collaborative Expert Panel. *Core Competencies for Interprofessional Collaborative Practice: Report of an Expert Panel.* Washington, DC: Interprofessional Education Collaborative (2011).
17. Interprofessional Education Collaborative. *Core Competencies for Interprofessional Collaborative Practice: 2016 Update.* Washington, DC: Interprofessional Education Collaborative (2016).
18. Hammick M, Freeth D, Koppel I, Reeves S, Barr H. A best evidence systematic review of interprofessional education: BEME Guide no. 9. *Med Teach.* (2007) 29:735–51. doi: 10.1080/01421590701682576
19. Olson R, Bialocerkowski A. Interprofessional education in allied health: a systematic review. *Med Educ.* (2014) 48:236–46. doi: 10.1111/medu.12290
20. MacNeil RL. Address by chair of the ADEA board of directors. *J Dent Educ.* (2019) 83:720–2. doi: 10.1002/j.0022-0337.2019.83.7.tb06377.x
21. Heath B, Wise Romero P, Reynolds K. *A Standard Framework for Levels of Integrated Healthcare.* Washington, DC: SAMHSA-HRSA Center for Integrated Health Solutions (2013).
22. MacNeil RL, Hilario H, Snyder JJ. The case for integrated oral and primary medical health care delivery: permanente dental associates. *J Dent Educ.* (2020) 84:920–3. doi: 10.1002/jdd.12284
23. MacNeil RL, Hilario H, Thierer TE, Gesko DS. The case for integrated oral and primary medical health care delivery: health partners. *J Dent Educ.* (2020) 84:932–5. doi: 10.1002/jdd.12288
24. MacNeil RL, Hilario H, Ryan MM, Glurich I, Nycz GR, Acharya A. The case for integrated oral and primary medical health care delivery: Marshfield clinic health system. *J Dent Educ.* (2020) 84:924–31. doi: 10.1002/jdd.12289
25. MacNeil RL, Hilario H. The case for integrated oral and primary medical health care delivery: an introduction to an examination of three engaged healthcare entities. *J Dent Educ.* (2020) 84:917–9. doi: 10.1002/jdd.12286
26. MacNeil RL, Hilario H. The case for integrated oral and primary medical health care delivery: synopsis and recommendations. *J Dent Educ.* (2020) 84:936–8. doi: 10.1002/jdd.12287
27. Monica K. *Pacific Dental Services to Implement Epic EHR System.* EHR Intelligence (2018). Available online at: https://ehrintelligence.com/news/pacific-dental-services-to-implement-epic-ehr-system (accessed January 11, 2021).
28. Bainbridge L. Interprofessional education in allied health: is this yet another silo? *Med Educ.* (2014) 48: 229–31. doi: 10.1111/medu.12414
29. Acharya A, Yoder N, Nycz G. An integrated medical-dental electronic health record environment: a Marshfield experience. In: Powell V, Din FM, Acharya A, Torres-Urquidy MH, editors. *Integration of Medical and Dental Care and Patient Data. Health Informatics.* London: Springer (2012). p. 331–51.
30. Acharya A, Shimpi N, Mahnke A, Mathias R, Ye Z. Medical care providers' perspectives on dental information needs in electronic health records. *J Am Dent Assoc.* (2017) 148:328–37 doi: 10.1016/j.adaj.2017.01.026
31. Vujicic M, Israelson H, Antoon J, Kiesling R, Paumier T, Zust M. A profession in transition. *J Am Dent Assoc.* (2014) 45:118–21. doi: 10.14219/jada.2013.40
32. Donoff RB, Daley GQ. Oral health care in the 21st century: it is time for the integration of dental and medical education. *J Dent Educ.* (2020) 84:999–1002. doi: 10.1002/jdd.12191
33. Bailit HL. The oral health care delivery system in 2040: executive summary. *J Dent Educ.* (2017) 81:1124–9. doi: 10.21815/JDE.017.068

22

Periodontal and Peri-Implant Microbiome Dysbiosis is Associated with Alterations in the Microbial Community Structure and Local Stability

Yuchen Zhang[1,2†], Yinhu Li[3†], Yuguang Yang[4], Yiqing Wang[5], Xiao Cao[1,2], Yu Jin[1,2], Yue Xu[1,6], Shuai Cheng Li[7] and Qin Zhou[1,2*]*

[1] Key Laboratory of Shaanxi Province for Craniofacial Precision Medicine Research, College of Stomatology, Xi'an Jiaotong University, Xi'an, China, [2] Department of Implant Dentistry, College of Stomatology, Xi'an Jiaotong University, Xi'an, China, [3] Shenzhen-Hong Kong Institute of Brain Science-Shenzhen Fundamental Research Institutions, The Brain Cognition and Brain Disease Institute, Shenzhen Institutes of Advanced Technology, Chinese Academy of Sciences, Shenzhen, China, [4] Department of Advanced Manufacturing and Robotics, College of Engineering, Peking University, Beijing, China, [5] Department of Prosthodontics, School and Hospital of Stomatology, Peking University, Beijing, China, [6] Department of General Dentistry and Emergency Room, College of Stomatology, Xi'an Jiaotong University, Xi'an, China, [7] Department of Computer Science, City University of Hong Kong, Kowloon, Hong Kong SAR, China

***Correspondence:**
Qin Zhou
zhouqin0529@126.com
Shuai Cheng Li
sc.li@cityu.edu.hk

† These authors have contributed equally to this work

Periodontitis and peri-implantitis are common biofilm-mediated infectious diseases affecting teeth and dental implants and have been considered to be initiated with microbial dysbiosis. To further understand the essence of oral microbiome dysbiosis in terms of bacterial interactions, community structure, and microbial stability, we analyzed 64 plaque samples from 34 participants with teeth or implants under different health conditions using metagenomic sequencing. After taxonomical annotation, we computed the inter-species correlations, analyzed the bacterial community structure, and calculated the microbial stability in supra- and subgingival plaques from hosts with different health conditions. The results showed that when inflammation arose, the subgingival communities became less connective and competitive with fewer hub species. In contrast, the supragingival communities tended to be more connective and competitive with an increased number of hub species. Besides, periodontitis and peri-implantitis were associated with significantly increased microbial stability in subgingival microbiome. These findings indicated that the periodontal and peri-implant dysbiosis is associated with aberrant alterations in the bacterial correlations, community structures, and local stability. The highly connected hub species, as well as the major contributing species of negative correlations, should also be given more concern in future studies.

Keywords: periodontitis, peri-implantitis, microbiome, community structure, metagenomic sequencing, dysbiosis, local stability

INTRODUCTION

Periodontitis is a prevalent disease in the human oral cavity and the major cause of dentition defects (Albandar, 2005). It is a complex infectious disease resulting from infection-induced inflammation and hyperimmune response toward various microbial pathogens (Kajiya et al., 2010; Bueno et al., 2015). Previous studies have proved that periodontitis is initiated with microbial dysbiosis in the periodontium (Kinane et al., 2017). The prevalence of periodontitis is estimated from 4 to 76.0% in developed countries and from over 50% to almost 90% in developing ones (Jiao et al., 2021). Approximately over 700 million adults are suffering from periodontitis worldwide (Kassebaum et al., 2014), which has become a severe burden in the oral health of humankind (Marcenes et al., 2013).

Peri-implantitis has been described as a pathological condition around dental implants where inflammation continuously affects connective tissue and finally leads to the loss of the supporting bone matrix (Schwarz et al., 2018). Similar to periodontitis, peri-implantitis is also caused by the hyper-inflammation in peri-implant tissue and the aberrant change in the microbial community (Alcoforado et al., 1991; Leonhardt et al., 1999; Wang et al., 2016). A meta-analysis in 2017 indicated that the weighted mean prevalence of peri-implantitis was around 19.83% at patient level (Lee et al., 2017). As implant-supported prostheses are being more and more widely used to replace missing teeth (Buser et al., 2017), there will be an increasing number of patients suffering from peri-implantitis in the coming future.

Periodontitis and peri-implantitis share many clinical and etiological features, including biofilm-mediated infection, hyperinflammatory reaction, and progressive absorption of alveolar bone (Berglundh et al., 2011; Carcuac and Berglundh, 2014; Liu et al., 2020). Most importantly, the accumulation of dental plaque and the following microbial dysbiosis are considered to be the initiation of both diseases (Ng et al., 2021). Given the shared nature as infectious diseases between periodontitis and peri-implantitis, it is necessary to delve into the microbial communities around teeth and implants to understand the two diseases further.

The stability of commensal microbial communities in human bodies has been proved essential to human health (Relman, 2012). However, previous studies investigating oral microbiota using high-throughput sequencing approaches have mainly focused on the taxonomical profile or microbial functionalities (Dabdoub et al., 2016; Ai et al., 2017; Babaev et al., 2017; Belstrom et al., 2017; Ghensi et al., 2020; Komatsu et al., 2020; Ng et al., 2021). Yet, the community structure and the microbial stability have not been fully illustrated, especially when the complexity of numerous bacterial correlations cannot be fully identified by isolating pairwise interactions. To fill this insufficiency, we analyzed 64 microbial samples from plaque around teeth and implants in different health conditions using metagenomic shotgun sequencing. We annotated taxonomical information at the species level, visualized the bacterial co-occurrence network, analyzed the community structure, and calculated the microbial stability of our samples to further our understanding of periodontitis and peri-implantitis.

MATERIALS AND METHODS

Participant Recruitment

This study enrolled 34 participants, including 19 subjects for the healthy group and 15 subjects with periodontitis or peri-implantitis for the diseased group (See **Supplementary Tables 1, 2**). All participants were Chinese natives who sought care at the College of Stomatology, Xi'an Jiaotong University, and provided written consents. Natural teeth were considered periodontal health when there was no bleeding on probing (BOP), no clinical attachment loss (CAL), or radiographic bone loss (RBL) and the maximum probing depth (PD) was less than 3 mm. Periodontitis was diagnosed with an increased PD of more than 4 mm, examinable RBL, and interdental CAL, which corresponded with the latest diagnostic criteria for Stage II-IV periodontitis (Papapanou et al., 2018). As for implants, subjects were considered peri-implant health when peri-implant tissue showed no redness, suppuration, BOP, and no more than 1-mm marginal RBL beyond bone remodeling. Peri-implantitis was diagnosed when there was clinical inflammation, increased PD of more than 6 mm, and radiographic evidence of more than 3 mm RBL compared to baselines (Lindhe et al., 2008). Detailed inclusion and exclusion criteria are listed in **Table 1**.

Clinical Examination and Sample Collection

Before sampling, full-mouth examinations were conducted on all subjects by the same calibrated clinician to record clinical and demographic features, including sex, age, PD, BOP, and RBL. Especially for subjects with implants, we also recorded their implant type, location, and functional time (**Supplementary Tables 1, 2**).

The selection of sampling sites followed the criteria in our **Supplementary Information**. When sampling commenced, patients first gargled with distilled water for 1 min. Then, we used cotton rolls to isolate the selected sites and sampled the supragingival plaque using sterile curettes by a single horizontal stroke on each site. Bacteria were washed off from the curettes by rinsing in 1.5-ml microcentrifuge tubes containing phosphate-buffered saline (PBS). The remaining supragingival plaque was then removed. Afterward, we used sterile endodontic paper points for subgingival sampling (Jervoe-Storm et al., 2007), by inserting paper points as deep as possible into the periodontal or peri-implant sulcus and staying for 20 seconds. After taking out, paper points were transferred into 1.5-ml microcentrifuge tubes containing PBS. All samples were stored at −80°C and were then sent to BGI Institute (BGI Group, Shenzhen, China) for genomic DNA extraction, metagenomic libraries preparation, and sequencing.

DNA Extraction and Metagenomic Sequencing

Genomic DNA of the samples was isolated using QIAmp DNA Micro Kit (Qiagen, Valencia, CA) with "Protocol: Isolation of Genomic DNA from Tissues" according to the handbook. The sequencing libraries were then prepared following BGI's

TABLE 1 | Detailed inclusion and exclusion criteria for subject recruitment.

Type	Health condition	Inclusion criteria	Exclusion criteria
Teeth	Periodontal health	• Individual normal occlusion with no less than 28 teeth left in dentition; • No RBL or examinable CAL; • Maximum PD $\leq$ 3 mm; • No BOP or redness examined.	• Diabetes mellitus or other severe systemic diseases; • HIV infection or other severe immune diseases; • A history of tobacco smoking; • A history of immunosuppressant therapy; • A history of bisphosphonates, steroids, or other therapy influencing bone metabolism; • Antibiotic therapy, oral antiseptic therapy, or oral prophylactic treatment undergoing or in recent 3 months; • Having other dentures in any form besides the selected dental implant; • Pregnancy or lactation; • Over 60 years old or below 20 years old.
	Periodontitis	• Individual normal occlusion with no less than 20 teeth left in dentition; • Examinable interdental CAL $\geq$ 3 mm; • PD $\geq$ 4mm; • Examinable RBL; • Existing BOP and/or suppuration.	
Implants	Peri-implant health	• A single implant with a single cement-retained crown seated to replace the missing tooth; • Implant in function for over 2 years; • Radiographic MBL $\leq$ 1 mm; • No redness, suppuration, or BOP examined around the implant.	
	Peri-implantitis	• A single bone-level implant with a single cement-retained crown seated to replace the missing tooth; • Implant in function for over 2 years; Radiographic MBL $\geq$ 3 mm compared to baseline; • PD $\geq$ 6 mm around the implant.	

instruction (BGI Group, Shenzhen, China). The libraries were sequenced on the BGI SEQ-500 sequencing platform (BGI Group, Shenzhen, China). Raw reads generated from the sequencing platform were then filtered and cleaned before further analysis.

Metagenomic Analysis

To obtain high-quality data, we firstly filtered the raw reads when they contained more than 10 low-quality bases (< Q20) or 15 bases of adapter sequences with a self-constructed script. Using BWA software (version 0.7.17), we aligned the read data to the human genome (hg19) and filtered the reads when the alignment length exceeds 40% of the read length (Li and Durbin, 2009). After the removal of host mapped reads, the clean metagenomic data were applied for the following metagenomic analysis.

Using MetaPhlAn3 (Truong et al., 2015), we aligned the filtered reads to the microbial database of specific marker genes (mpa_v30_CHOCOPhlAn_201901) and obtained the taxonomical annotation results. Based on the microbial profiling, we calculated the relative abundances of bacteria at phylum, class, order, family, genus, and species levels, respectively (see **Supplementary Data Sheet 1**). After the taxonomical annotation, we performed permutational multivariate analysis of variance (PERMANOVA) to evaluate the impact of environmental factors on the microbiome (permutation number equals 9,999), calculated alpha diversity using the Chao1 and Shannon indexes, and detected the Spearman correlation coefficients among the species with relative abundance over 0.01%. We kept the relations with coefficients <-0.6 or > 0.6 (adjusted p-value < 0.05) to construct the bacterial interacting matrix (**Supplementary Data Sheets 2, 3**) and to plot the bacterial co-occurrence networks by applying Gephi (version 0.4.2) and Cytoscape (version 3.8.2) for further analysis (Shannon et al., 2003; Bastian et al., 2009; Otasek et al., 2019). Species with more than 25 correlations were defined as hub species, which indicated their pivotal places in the bacterial co-occurrence networks. We screened and compared these species between different microbiomes.

Local Stability Analysis

Local stability measures the tendency of a community to return to its equilibrium after perturbation. The community is stable if it can return to its equilibrium after perturbation. Following the work by May and Allesina (May, 1972, 1973; Allesina and Tang, 2012), we used the community matrix generated from our co-occurrence network (**Supplementary Data Sheets 2, 3**) to analyze the local stability of oral microbiome (**Figure 1A**). The community matrix incorporates several structural properties, including the number of interacting species, the connectance, the types and strength of interactions, and the degree distribution. Connectance was defined as the fraction of non-zero off-diagonal elements of the community matrix (May, 1972, 1973), or briefly as the ratio of actual bacterial correlations to all topologically possible correlations. The types of interactions were extracted from our co-occurrence networks illustrated above. The degree of a species referred to the count of its correlations with other species. The local stability theory indicates that a stable system requires that all eigenvalues of the community matrix should have negative real parts (**Figure 1B**), which means the real part of the rightmost eigenvalue in the complex plane can be used to measure the extent of stability. A more negative real part corresponds to a more stable community, which grants it more robustness when resisting perturbations that tend to alter the abundance of its members (**Figure 1C**). Based on experimental data, we performed a series of simulations to show the differences in stability among different groups (see also **Supplementary Information**).

Statistics

For the Chao1 and Shannon indexes calculated for different groups, we performed the Wilcoxon rank-sum test to check whether significant differences exist between groups. All the

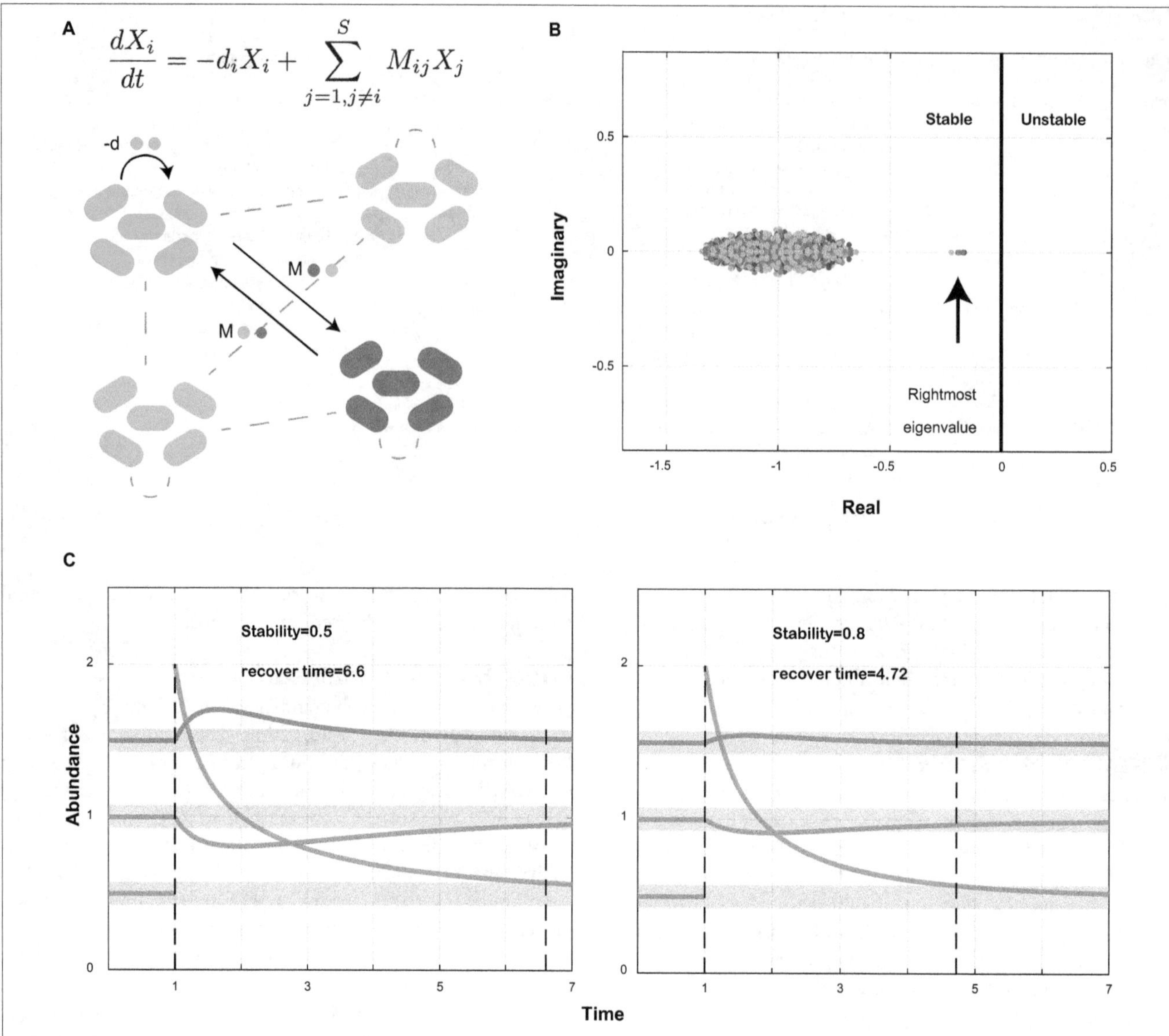

FIGURE 1 | Local stability theory. (A) A schematic diagram shows a small community with bacterial species interacting within themselves ($-d$) and with other species (M_{ij}). Ordinary differential equations measure the abundance change of species i after perturbation around the equilibrium point. X_i, abundance of species i; $-d_i$, self-regulating effect of species i; M_{ij}, effect of species j on species i. **(B)** All eigenvalues of community matrix M are shown in the complex plane. The community is stable if all eigenvalues have negative real parts. Therefore, the sign of the rightmost eigenvalue decides whether a community is stable or not, and the value of its real part decides how stable the community is: the more negative its real part, the more stable the community (see also **Supplementary Information**). **(C)** A community will return to its former equilibrium after perturbations if it is stable. A community with higher stability will recover faster than a less stable community.

Spearman correlation coefficients among the species were adjusted with Benjamini and Hochberg method (adjusted $p < 0.05$). As for the counts of negative and positive correlations, we applied the chi-square test for the detection of significant differences between the health and disease groups.

RESULTS

Taxonomical Annotation

After low-quality filtration and host-read removal, a total of 1,926,649,953 sequences were obtained from 64 samples, with an average of 30,103,906 sequences per sample (range from 1,004,522 to 77,090,552). Overall, 310 bacterial species have been identified (see **Supplementary Data Sheet 1**). The clinical and demographic characteristics of recruited subjects were summarized (**Supplementary Table 3**). There were no significant differences in mean age and sex distribution among all subjects, and functional time between healthy and diseased implants ($p > 0.05$).

PERMANOVA was performed to evaluate the differences in microbial communities contributed by several factors (**Supplementary Figure 1**). The results indicated a significant difference between the compositions of supra- and subgingival communities ($R^2 = 0.02631$, $p = 0.047$). Based on this finding, we therefore analyze and discuss supragingival and subgingival communities separately in the following procedures.

Using the interacting matrix extracted from our taxonomical annotations (see Materials and Methods), we plotted co-occurrence networks in healthy and diseased sites (**Figure 2**). In our networks, positive and negative coefficients represented potentially cooperative and competitive interactions between bacterial species, respectively. Overall, subgingival microbiome from periodontitis and peri-implantitis patients exhibited less connected and competitive bacterial networks. On the contrary, supragingival microbiome from the diseased subjects showed more connected and competitive bacterial networks when compared with their healthy controls.

Structural Properties of Bacterial Co-occurrence Networks

Besides the proportions of negative and positive interactions, we visualized more structural properties including the numbers of interacting species, the connectance, and the degree distributions of the networks using bar charts (**Figures 3A–D**), to further

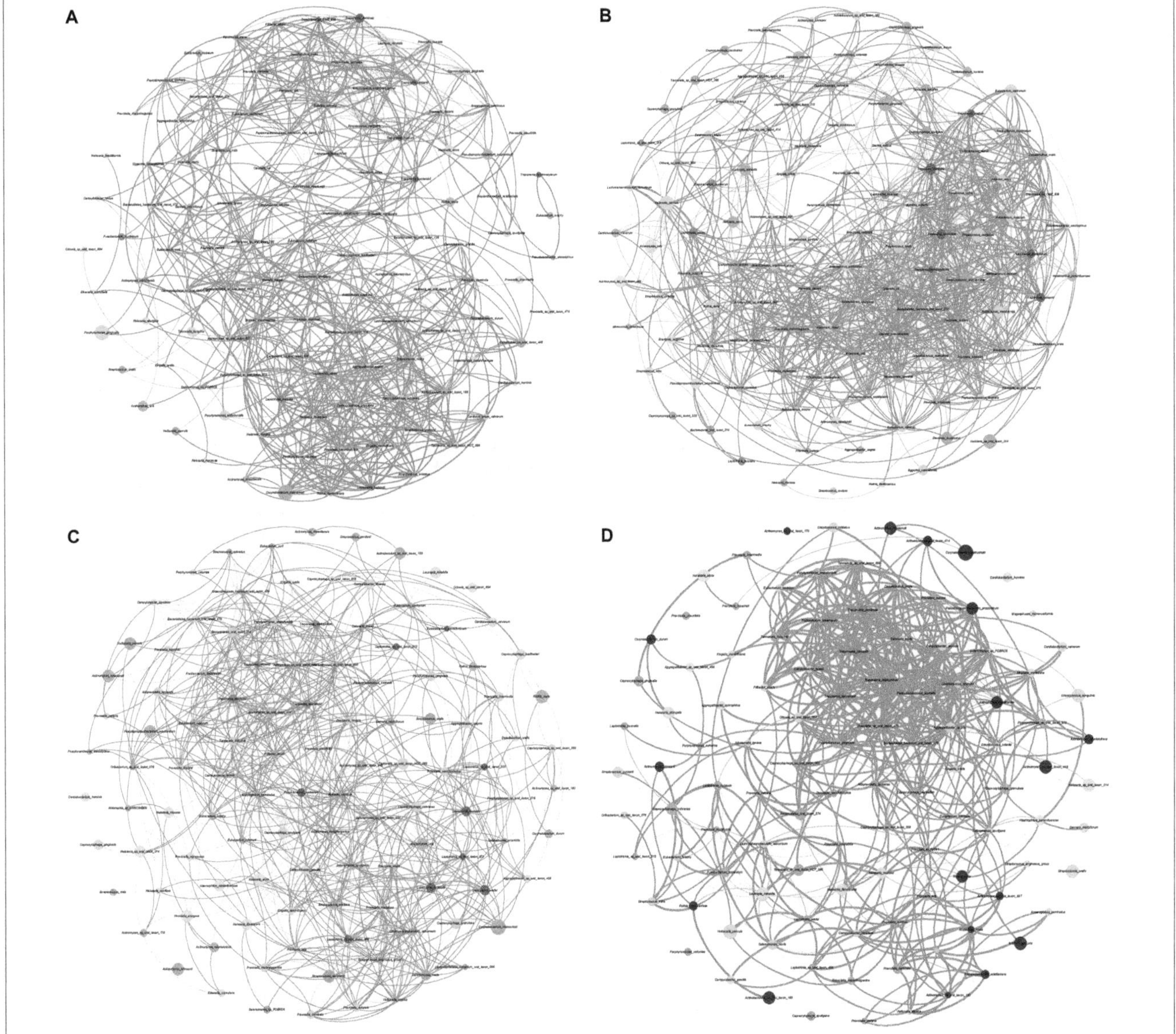

FIGURE 2 | Bacterial co-occurrence networks. **(A)** Network of diseased subgingival microbiome. **(B)** Network of healthy subgingival microbiome. **(C)** Network of diseased supragingival microbiome. **(D)** Network of healthy supragingival microbiome. Species from different phyla were marked in different colors. The larger nodes represented the higher mean relative abundance of the species. We selected those interactions with Spearman correlation coefficient <-0.6 or >0.6 (adjusted $p < 0.05$). Positive and negative correlations are shown in red and green lines, respectively. Thicker lines meant higher absolute values in Spearman coefficient. Generally, the healthy subgingival network was more complex than the diseased subgingival network, while the healthy supragingival network was less complex than the diseased supragingival network.

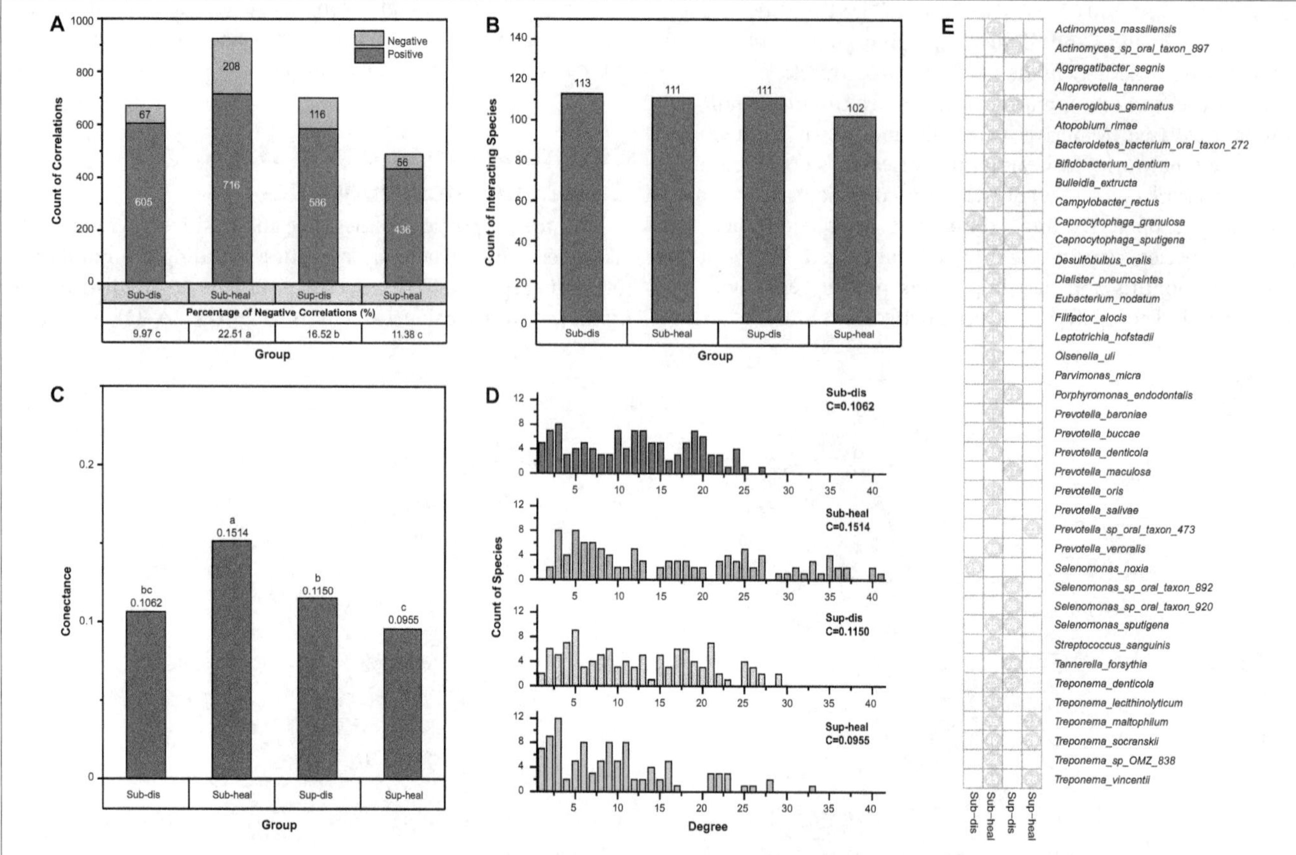

FIGURE 3 | Properties of the community structures in different microbiomes. **(A)** Positive and negative correlations were shown in red and blue, respectively. Positive correlations were predominant in all communities. The percentage of negative correlations in diseased subgingival communities was significantly lower than that in healthy subgingival communities. However, such difference was reversed between diseased and healthy supragingival communities ($p < 0.05$, Pearson chi-square). **(B)** All communities in our study had similar counts of interacting species ($p > 0.05$, Pearson chi-square). **(C)** When associated with periodontitis and peri-implantitis, the subgingival community exhibited a decrease in connectance while the supragingival community exhibited an increase in connectance. Significance of differences was marked in letters. **(D)** Degree distributions of the diseased subgingival, healthy subgingival, diseased supragingival, and healthy supragingival networks are shown in red, blue, yellow, and green bars, respectively. *C* stood for connectance. A conspicuous difference was observed in the degree distribution of healthy subgingival communities as there were significantly more high-degree (degree > 25) species ($p < 0.05$ Pearson chi-square). **(E)** Hub species in the diseased subgingival, healthy subgingival, diseased supragingival, and healthy supragingival microbiome are shown in the heatmap. A blue dot means the species had more than 25 interspecies correlations in the corresponding microbiome. Numbers within the dots showed the counts of correlations of the species.

dissect the community structure within these networks. In both supra- and subgingival samples, there are similar amounts of interacting species between healthy and diseased microbiome. However, in subgingival microbiome, healthy communities had higher connectance and more high-degree species than diseased communities ($p < 0.05$, Pearson chi-square and Fisher exact test). Besides, the healthy subgingival network had a larger proportion of negative correlations (22.51%, 208 of 924) than the diseased subgingival network (9.97%, 67 of 672) ($p < 0.05$, Pearson chi-square). As for supragingival microbiome, differences were reversed where healthy communities had lower connectance and exhibited a cluster in lower degrees when compared with diseased communities. Also, the healthy supragingival network showed a lower proportion of negative correlations (11.38%, 56 of 492) than the diseased supragingival network (16.52%, 116 of 702) ($p < 0.05$, Pearson chi-square).

Based on the degree distribution, we selected those hub species with more than 25 correlations (degree > 25) in each group. These hub species were the pivotal members in the co-occurrence networks which were highly connected with other species (**Figure 3E** and **Supplementary Table 5**). There were more hub species in the healthy subgingival microbiome than the diseased subgingival microbiome (31 in healthy microbiome and 2 in diseased microbiome). Such difference was again reversed in the supragingival group where diseased microbiome had more hub species (5 in healthy microbiome and 11 in diseased microbiome). The results above revealed distinct bacterial co-occurrence networks and community structures in different microbiomes and built the foundation for further stability analysis.

Alterations in Bacterial Interactions

Bacterial interactions are known to have an impact on oral health (Diaz and Valm, 2020), especially the competitive interactions which have been proved essential in preserving the fitness of microbial communities (Stacy et al., 2014). To evaluate how inflammation around teeth and implants would alter such bacterial interactions, we extracted all negative correlations unique to different health conditions for further comparison (**Figure 4**). As expected, there was a great change in the bacterial competition with the shift from health to disease. Each group had its own distinctive set of unique correlations.

In subgingival microbiome (**Figure 4A**), *Streptococcus sanguinis* ($l = 31$, number of negative linkages equal 31 with $R < -0.6$ and adjusted $p < 0.05$), *Streptococcus oralis* ($l = 17$), *Haemophilus parainfluenzae* ($l = 10$), *Rothia aeria* ($l = 12$), *Corynebacterium matruchotii* ($l = 18$), *Leptotrichia hofstadii* ($l = 11$), *Actinomyces massiliensis* ($l = 22$), and *Capnocytophaga sputigena* ($l = 14$) participated in a large number of negative correlations in healthy communities. When inflammation arose, the negative correlations were significantly weakened and those interactions associated with the above species were altered, among which *Corynebacterium matruchotii*, *Leptotrichia hofstadii*, *Actinomyces massiliensis*, and *Capnocytophaga sputigena* lost all their negative correlations, while *Streptococcus sanguinis* ($l = 10$), *Streptococcus oralis* ($l = 3$), *Haemophilus parainfluenzae* ($l = 5$), and *Rothia aeria* ($l = 2$) established fewer new negative correlations with other species. Instead, in the diseased communities, *Lautropia mirabilis* ($l = 15$), *Actinomyces naeslundii* ($l = 8$), and *Capnocytophaga gingivalis* ($l = 7$) emerged to become the concentrated nodes of negative correlations.

Changes in supragingival microbiome were quite different (**Figure 4B**), where healthy communities had significantly fewer negative correlations than diseased communities. *Kingella oralis* ($l = 3$), *Lautropia mirabilis* ($l = 9$), *Prevotella multiformis* ($l = 5$), and *Actinomyces massiliensis* ($l = 15$) were the major contributors of negative correlations in healthy communities, while in diseased communities, there were complex sets of negative correlations coming from *Streptococcus sanguinis* ($l = 14$), *Neisseria sicca* ($l = 10$), and *Capnocytophaga sputigena* ($l = 23$).

In contrast with alterations of negative correlations, there were also some correlations shared by all communities despite health conditions or sampling sites (**Figure 4C**). This shared network was mainly constructed by species from phyla *Bacteroidetes*, *Firmicutes*, and *Spirochaetes*. Different from the unique negative correlations which defined the health status of the microbiome, these shared correlations seemed to be constant and might have formed a fundamental framework for periodontal and peri-implant microbiome.

Stability Analysis

To compare the stability among different microbial communities, the above structural properties were required for numerical simulations. The number of interacting species, the connectance, and the types of interactions could be drawn directly from our taxonomical annotation and the co-occurrence networks. However, acquiring the strength of interactions would usually require a time-sequence analysis from longitudinal samples according to previous studies (Schloissnig et al., 2013; Stein et al., 2013; Oh et al., 2016). This seemed inapplicable to studying diseased subjects due to ethical reasons, as clinicians were supposed to treat the periodontitis or peri-implantitis rather than observing the diseased status without interference. In this scenario, we introduced a strategy to analyze the stability

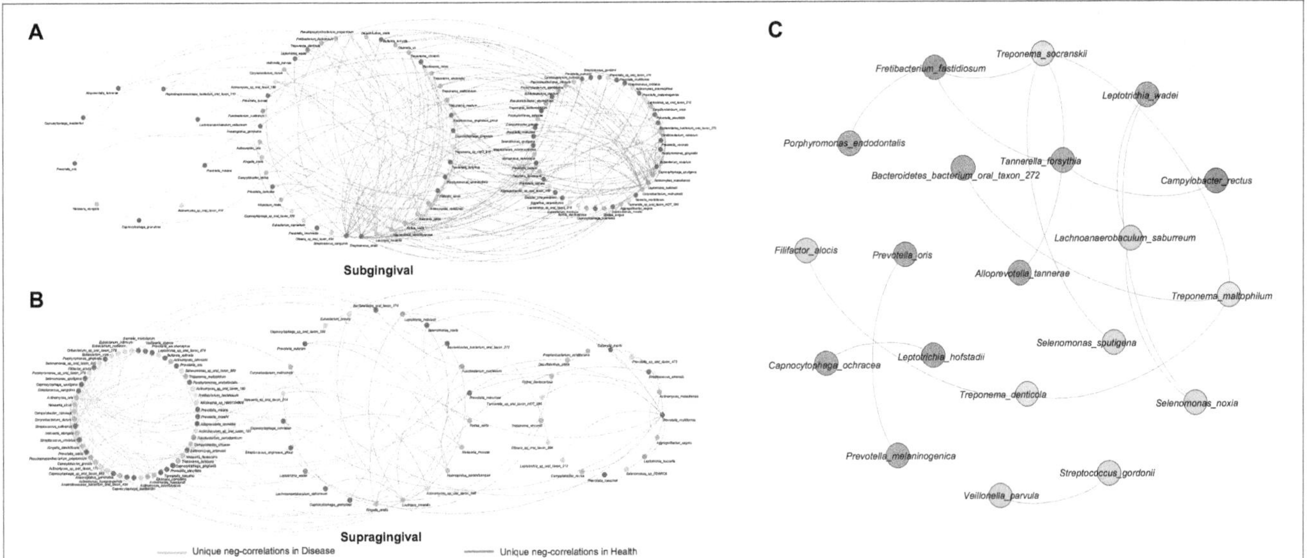

FIGURE 4 | Alterations in negative correlations from health to disease and the shared correlations. **(A)** Unique negative correlations of healthy and diseased subgingival communities. *Streptococcus sanguinis*, *Streptococcus oralis*, *Haemophilus parainfluenzae*, *Rothia aeria*, *Corynebacterium matruchotii*, *Leptotrichia hofstadii*, *Actinomyces massiliensis*, and *Capnocytophaga sputigena* were the concentrated nodes of negative correlations in health, while *Lautropia mirabilis*, *Actinomyces naeslundii*, and *Capnocytophaga gingivalis* were the concentrated nodes in disease. **(B)** Unique negative correlations of healthy and diseased supragingival communities. *Kingella oralis*, *Lautropia mirabilis*, *Prevotella multiformis*, and *Actinomyces massiliensis* were the concentrated nodes of negative correlations in health, while *Streptococcus sanguinis*, *Neisseria sicca*, and *Capnocytophaga sputigena* were the concentrated nodes of negative correlations in disease. **(C)** The shared correlations of all communities. All shared correlations were positive and were mainly constructed by phyla *Bacteroidetes*, *Firmicutes*, and *Spirochaetes*.

of microbial communities using cross-sectional samples based on Spearman coefficient (see Materials and Methods, see also **Supplementary Information**).

We assigned the strength of interactions following the assumptions by Allesina (Allesina and Tang, 2012) (see **Supplementary Information**) and mainly focused on comparing the stability among different communities rather than numerically calculating the absolute stability value of a specific community. Stability analysis showed that healthy subgingival communities had the worst stability among four groups while diseased subgingival communities possessed the highest stability (**Figure 5**). As for the supragingival group, the healthy and diseased supragingival communities showed similar stability in our analysis. We performed a series of simulations using different parameter sets and concluded the same result, which proved its robustness (**Figure 5**, see also **Supplementary Figure 3**).

To figure out why healthy subgingival microbiome was far less stable than the others, we generated unstructured ER (Erdős–Rényi) networks with the same amount of interacting species, connectance, and the positive–negative ratio of interactions as our original networks. Yet the sole different property was that these unstructured communities were distinguished from the original communities by having concentrated degree distributions (**Figure 6A**). Using the same method above, we compared the stability differences caused by distinct degree distributions between the original communities and the unstructured communities (**Figures 6B–E**). All original communities showed decreased stability when compared with their ER network counterparts in most parameter sets, while the healthy subgingival microbiome showed the largest extent of stability decrease. This indicated that the degree distributions of the original communities were somehow destabilizing,

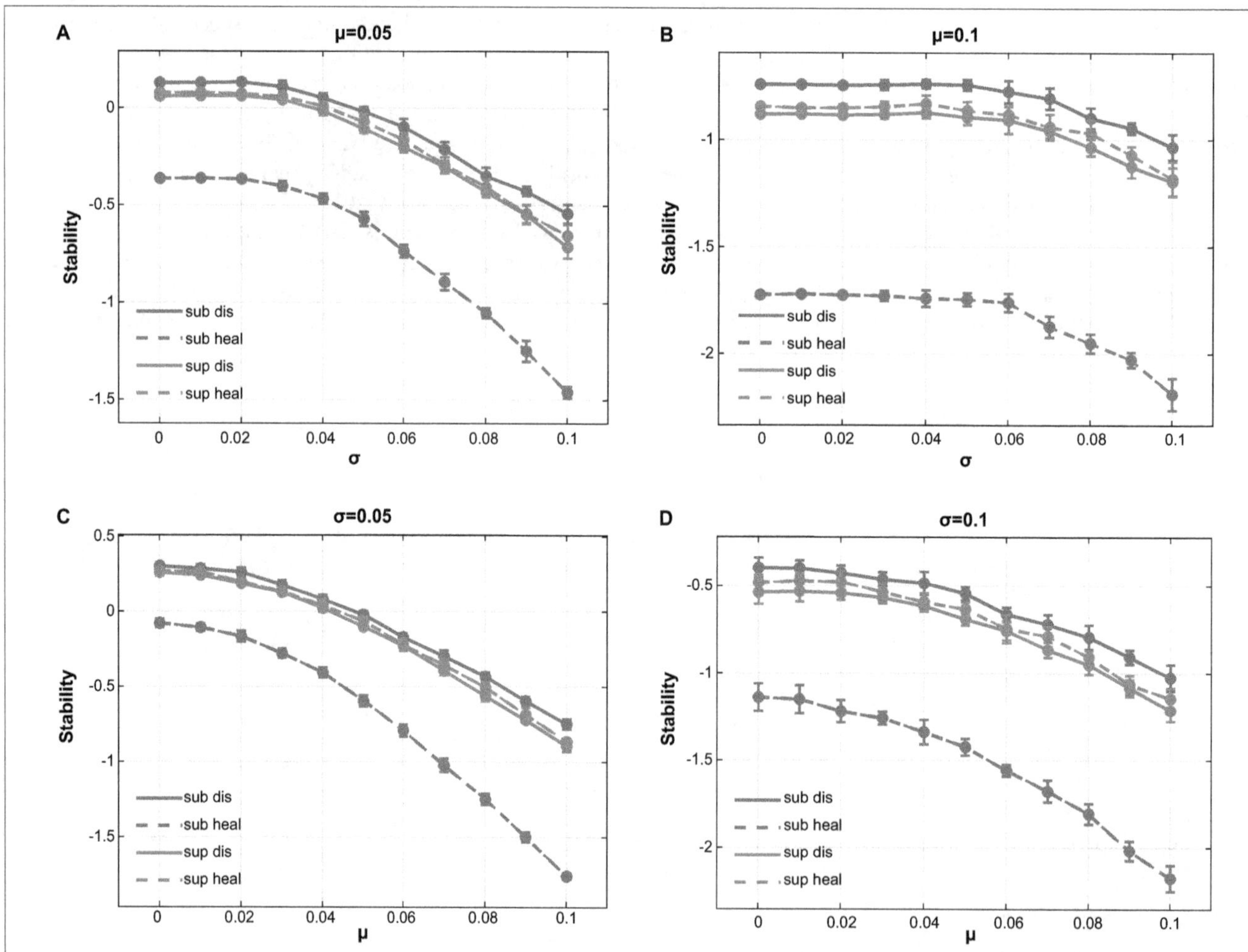

FIGURE 5 | Calculation of local stability. Red lines stood for supragingival communities while blue lines stood for subgingival communities. Healthy and diseased communities are shown in dotted and solid lines, respectively. Connectance, interacting species richness, and bacterial correlations were drawn directly from our interacting matrix. The strength of bacterial interactions was assigned to follow a normal distribution with mean μ and variance σ^2. By changing the value of μ and σ, we performed a series of calculations to compare the stability of our communities (see also **Supplementary Figure 3**). **(A)** μ = 0.05 with variable σ. **(B)** μ = 0.1 with variable σ. **(C)** σ = 0.05 with variable μ. **(D)** σ = 0.1 with variable μ. All calculations showed the same tendency that the healthy subgingival communities had the worst local stability while the diseased subgingival communities had the highest. However, the stability difference in supragingival communities was not as distinct as that in subgingival communities.

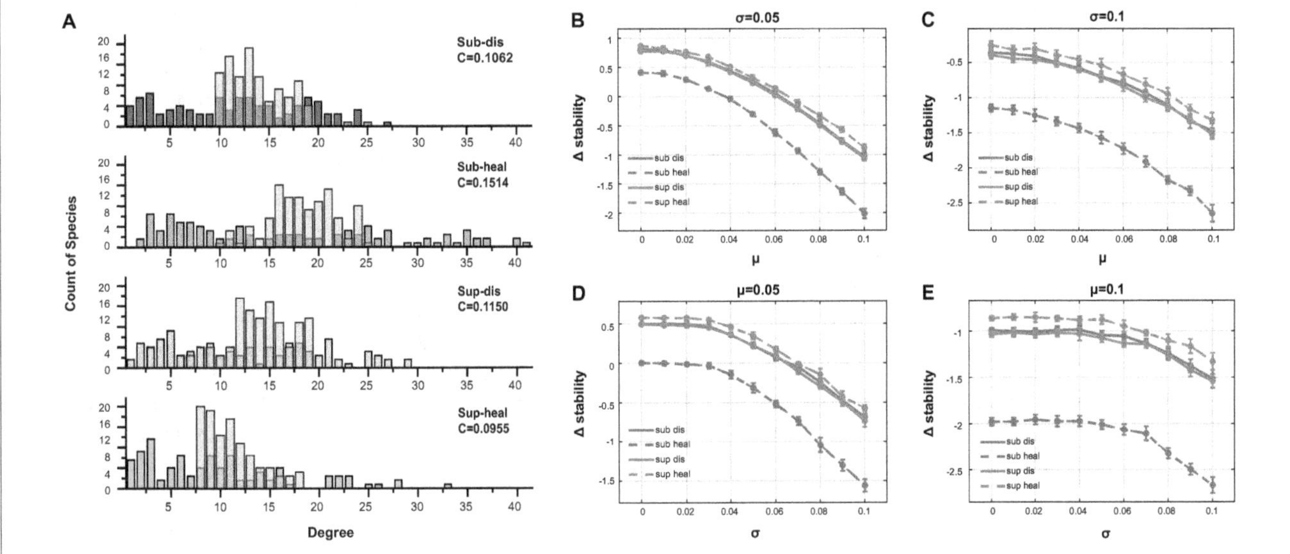

FIGURE 6 | Evaluation of the association between degree distribution and local stability. **(A)** The transparent pink bars showed the degree distribution of the ER networks while the opaque-colored bars showed the degree distribution of the original networks. The major difference was that the ER networks had concentrated degree distributions. **(B)–(E)** The vertical axis showed the stability change after ER randomization (Δ*stability*). Δ*stability* = $sta_{origin} - sta_{ER}$, in which sta_{origin} was the stability of the original communities, while sta_{ER} was the stability of the ER networks. It was clear that all original communities were less stable than their ER counterparts in all parameter sets (different μ and σ as in **Figure 5**), which indicated that their network structure tended to be destabilizing. The extent of stability decrease in the healthy subgingival group was much more than the other three groups, which meant that the network structure of the healthy subgingival community hampered stability the most.

among which the degree distribution of the healthy subgingival microbiome tended to hamper stability the most.

DISCUSSION

Distinct Structures Between Healthy and Diseased Communities

The oral microbiome is structurally and functionally organized, which means the properties of a microbial community are more than the sum of the components within it (Kuramitsu et al., 2007; Marsh and Zaura, 2017). To fully understand a microbial community, we are supposed to explore the whole structure and the aggregation of all interactions more than focusing on single or pairwise species. In this scenario, we investigated the bacterial co-occurrence networks and the community structures to explore the effect of periodontitis and peri-implantitis on the oral microbiome in a new perspective.

Our study revealed that when inflammation arose around teeth and implants, the subgingival bacterial networks tended to become less connected and less competitive. However, networks in supragingival communities seemed to shift in an opposite direction, with higher connectance and a larger proportion of competitive interactions in the diseased communities than their healthy counterparts.

Bacterial competition has been reported to be beneficial to both competitors involved and might even improve the fitness of the whole microbial community (Stacy et al., 2014), as they form a defensive mechanism in oral microbiome where the colonization of exogenous species was prevented (Marsh and Zaura, 2017). However, our results indicated that inflammation would alter the competition among species in periodontal and peri-implant microbiome. Such alterations could be observed in both supra- and subgingival microbiome and were not just in terms of number or proportion. In fact, the whole community seemed to reestablish a brand-new network with its own distinctive negative correlations and own centers for these correlations. These major changes in the community structure might lead to changes in the keystone compositions of the biofilm and come with the pathologic shift from health to disease (Marsh and Zaura, 2017).

The degree distribution of ecological networks is usually right-skewed with many low-degree vertices and only a small number of high-degree vertices (Girvan and Newman, 2002). Such was the case in our networks where the majority of the species were in low degrees. However, it was still clear that the degree distribution of the healthy subgingival microbiome distinguished itself among groups by having significantly more hub species, which also contributed to hampering the local stability of healthy subgingival community according to our further analysis.

The connectance was another important property of the community structure. Our result showed that when associated with periodontitis and peri-implantitis, the connectance of subgingival microbiome tended to decrease while the connectance of supragingival microbiome tended to increase. Previous studies proved that an ecosystem with higher connectance was more persistent when subjects to colonization–extinction dynamics (Gravel et al., 2011) and was less prone to losing hub species than systems with lower connectance (Kulkarni and De Laender, 2017). However, other studies on the dynamics of complex ecosystems showed that when connectance rose beyond a certain threshold, the local stability of the community would decrease rapidly (Gardner and Ashby, 1970). The healthy subgingival microbiome in our study had a larger number of hub species, which were sensitive to selective loss accordingly. Nonetheless, the high connectance helped prevent these species from losing. As for whether the connectance of our communities had crossed the threshold where local stability began to drop, we suggested that more studies were needed to draw the conclusion. However, we were able to plot the overall outcome of these factors and to compare the stability differences between the healthy subgingival microbiome and the other three groups (see below).

All findings above showed that healthy and diseased oral microbiome had distinct community structures. We addressed that these aberrant changes in bacterial competition, connectance, and degree distribution were crucially associated with the onset and progression of periodontitis and peri-implantitis. Among all communities in our study, we found that the differences between healthy and diseased subgingival microbiomes were most striking and complicated. Future studies should pay more attention to the relationship between community structures and oral infectious diseases, especially the changes in the community structure of subgingival microbiome.

Association Between Ecological Stability and Health Conditions

Patterns of the bacterial networks in supra- and subgingival microbiome were associated with health and disease. Moreover, the multiple interactions gave the community resilience to environmental perturbations (Marsh and Zaura, 2017). As mentioned above, the stability of a community mainly depends on its community matrix, which incorporates structural properties such as interaction types, connectance, and degree distribution. According to previous studies, competitive interactions tend to increase stability by decreasing diversity within the influence range of the competitors (Coyte et al., 2015), while connectance that reaches beyond a critical level might rapidly destabilize a microbial community (Gardner and Ashby, 1970; May, 1972). Interestingly, in our study, those communities with larger proportions of competitive interactions turned out to have higher connectance too. These communities, or more specifically, healthy subgingival communities and diseased supragingival communities, received antagonistic effects from both stronger competition within species and higher connectance. To plot the outcome of various effects on the stability in our study, we performed a series of simulations following the work of Allesina to compare the stability differences among our communities.

The result showed that healthy subgingival microbiome had the worst local stability among four groups while diseased subgingival microbiome had the highest. This meant that the equilibrium of healthy subgingival microbiome was more delicate and more prone to perturbations. When perturbations reached beyond resilience, equilibrium may break down with changes in microbial composition and shift in the community structure. That could be where dysbiosis happened and be the essence of the initiation of periodontal and peri-implant diseases. On the other hand, the high local stability in diseased subgingival microbiome explained why, if without interventions, the periodontal and peri-implant microbiome could not spontaneously change back to health once infected by periodontitis or peri-implantitis as the diseased equilibrium was very robust.

By comparing the stability between randomly generated ER communities and our original communities, we revealed that the degree distribution of healthy subgingival microbiome tended to be most destabilizing. As healthy subgingival microbiome was characterized by having more hub species, we hereby hypothesized that hub species were in some way a weak point during the breakdown of the current equilibrium, for changes in these highly connected species could trigger a massive alteration in the whole network. This explained why the stability of healthy subgingival microbiome was far lower than other microbiomes. In this scenario, we suggested that more caution should be raised toward these hub species together with their roles during the shift from health to disease.

Relationship Between Hub Species and Health Conditions

Hub species were those with a large number of interspecies correlations. Whether abundant or not, hub species played roles as "traffic centers" in the bacterial network. In one respect, these species were spatially or functionally related with many others and therefore contributed to the integration of the community. In another respect, they might also be responsible for destabilizing the community as mentioned above. Our study showed that the healthy subgingival microbiome had the highest count of hub species, of which species from genus *Prevotella* and *Treponema* made up a major part. In the diseased subgingival microbiome, there were only two hub species, *Capnocytophaga granulosa* and *Selenomonas noxia*. As for the supragingival microbiome, differences between healthy and diseased networks were not as distinct as subgingival microbiome and seemed to change in an opposite direction where the diseased network had more hub species than the healthy one. The supragingival hub species came from various genus including *Actinomyces*, *Aggregatibacter*, *Anaeroglobus*, *Bulleidia*, *Capnocytophaga*, *Porphyromonas*, *Prevotella*, *Selenomonas*, *Tannerella*, and *Treponema*.

The microbial community is extremely complex and sophisticated which subjects to numerous influences ranging from microbial compositions to environmental and genetic factors. It is difficult to explicitly address the role of a specific species in the community. Although most of the hub species of communities in our study had been proven associated with periodontal and peri-implant destruction (Morita et al., 1991; Ellen and Galimanas, 2000; Takeuchi et al., 2001; Ohishi et al., 2005), we suggested that their pivotal roles in the bacterial network should be treated dialectically, the roles that on the one hand contributed to their pathogenicity, but on the other hand, were also essential in integrating the community network. Future studies should pay more attention to the important roles of these hub species and associate the pivotal places in the network with their pathogenicity.

Limitations of the Study

One major limitation in this study is that the sample size, although equivalent to other congener studies (Dabdoub et al., 2016; Belstrom et al., 2017; Komatsu et al., 2020), is relatively small to describe the oral microbiome of the whole human population. As the oral microbiome is very individualized (Belibasakis et al., 2019), we suggest that future studies with a larger sample size are needed to further generalize our findings.

The strategy provided in this study is sound and rigorous in theoretical aspect. However, these methods were mainly based on taxonomical annotations. They revealed the phenomena observed from the samples within this study yet could not validate the mechanisms behind the phenomena in biochemistry or molecular view. We appeal that further studies using either *in vitro* models or *in vivo* trials are needed to figure out the detailed mechanisms and provide more clinical implications.

Predicting the stability of microbial community usually requires a time-sequence analysis from longitudinal samples, as longitudinal studies offer control for confounding factors including age, gender, diet and so on. Although cross-sectional samples can also provide prediction on community stability following our strategy, it can be less powerful than longitudinal ones (Knight et al., 2018).

CONCLUSION

In conclusion, we revealed distinct community structures in healthy and diseased microbial communities around teeth and implants. By extracting the bacterial correlation networks, we found that the subgingival microbiome tended to become less connective and competitive when inflammation arises. In contrast, the supragingival microbiome tended to become more connective and competitive. We also observed a great change in competitive interspecies correlations between healthy and diseased microbiome. These alterations contributed crucially to the shift from health to disease and were highly associated with periodontal and peri-implant microbiome dysbiosis in the aspect of community structures. Besides, by applying dynamic models on these microbial communities, we concluded that the healthy subgingival community was far less stable than the inflamed subgingival community. We also managed to prove that it was those highly connected species in the network that contributed to destabilizing the biofilm. Our results suggested these hub species should also be given more concern in future studies. Preserving these species and maintaining their normal functionalities might be of much meaning in preventing periodontal and peri-implant diseases. Combining the above findings, we revealed that microbiome dysbiosis in the periodontium was not limited to the changes in bacterial compositions. With durative perturbations from microbial pathogens, the former equilibrium broke down and the microbiomes formed new bacterial networks with distinct interspecies correlations and community structures. During this progress, the subgingival biofilm established a more stable and stubborn community with even higher resilience.

AUTHOR CONTRIBUTIONS

YZ designed the details of the study, conducted the statistical analysis, interpreted the analysis results, and wrote this manuscript. YL performed the bioinformatics analyses, interpreted the analysis results, and revised the manuscript. YY conducted mathematical simulations and interpreted the results. YW helped perform statistical analysis and revised the manuscript. XC and YX helped with the collection of samples and the revision of the manuscript. YJ revised the manuscript and performed statistical analysis. QZ and SCL supervised the whole project and polished the manuscript. All authors reviewed and approved the manuscript.

ACKNOWLEDGMENTS

We would like to thank Huizhen Ma and Shuqi Ma for their help in sample collection and storage. Special thanks go to Shengbin Li, Hongbo Zhang, and Liao Chang of Bio-evidence Sciences Academy, Xi'an Jiaotong University, for their valuable advice on the design and performance of this study. We would also like to thank all nurses in Department of Implantology, College of Stomatology, Xi'an Jiaotong University, for their assistance on sampling and clinical examinations.

REFERENCES

1. Ai, D., Huang, R., Wen, J., Li, C., Zhu, J., and Xia, L. C. (2017). Integrated metagenomic data analysis demonstrates that a loss of diversity in oral microbiota is associated with periodontitis. *BMC Genomics* 18(Suppl. 1):1041. doi: 10.1186/s12864-016-3254-5
2. Albandar, J. M. (2005). Epidemiology and risk factors of periodontal diseases. *Dent. Clin. North Am.* 49, 517–532, v-vi. doi: 10.1016/j.cden.2005.03.003
3. Alcoforado, G. A., Rams, T. E., Feik, D., and Slots, J. (1991). Microbial aspects of failing osseointegrated dental implants in humans. *J. Parodontol.* 10, 11–18.
4. Allesina, S., and Tang, S. (2012). Stability criteria for complex ecosystems. *Nature* 483, 205–208. doi: 10.1038/nature10832
5. Babaev, E. A., Balmasova, I. P., Mkrtumyan, A. M., Kostryukova, S. N., Vakhitova, E. S., Il'ina, E. N., et al. (2017). Metagenomic analysis of gingival sulcus microbiota and pathogenesis of periodontitis associated with Type 2 diabetes mellitus. *Bull. Exp. Biol. Med.* 163, 718–721. doi: 10.1007/s10517-017-3888-6
6. Bastian, M., Heymann, S., and Jacomy, M. (eds) (2009). "Gephi: an open source software for exploring and manipulating networks," in *Proceedings of the 3rd International AAAI Conference on Weblogs and Social Media* (Menlo Park, CA).
7. Belibasakis, G. N., Bostanci, N., Marsh, P. D., and Zaura, E. (2019). Applications of the oral microbiome in personalized dentistry. *Arch. Oral. Biol.* 104, 7–12. doi: 10.1016/j.archoralbio.2019.05.023
8. Belstrom, D., Constancias, F., Liu, Y., Yang, L., Drautz-Moses, D. I., Schuster, S. C., et al. (2017). Metagenomic and metatranscriptomic analysis of saliva reveals disease-associated microbiota in patients with periodontitis and dental caries. *NPJ Biofilms Microbiomes* 3:23. doi: 10.1038/s41522-017-0031-4
9. Berglundh, T., Zitzmann, N. U., and Donati, M. (2011). Are peri-implantitis lesions different from periodontitis lesions? *J. Clin. Periodontol.* 38(Suppl. 11), 188–202. doi: 10.1111/j.1600-051X.2010.01672.x
10. Bueno, A. C., Ferreira, R. C., Cota, L. O., Silva, G. C., Magalhaes, C. S., and Moreira, A. N. (2015). Comparison of different criteria for periodontitis

case definition in head and neck cancer individuals. *Support Care Cancer* 23, 2599–2604. doi: 10.1007/s00520-015-2618-8
11. Buser, D., Sennerby, L., and De Bruyn, H. (2017). Modern implant dentistry based on osseointegration: 50 years of progress, current trends and open questions. *Periodontol 2000* 73, 7–21. doi: 10.1111/prd.12185
12. Carcuac, O., and Berglundh, T. (2014). Composition of human peri-implantitis and periodontitis lesions. *J. Dent. Res.* 93, 1083–1088. doi: 10.1177/0022034 514551754
13. Coyte, K. Z., Schluter, J., and Foster, K. R. (2015). The ecology of the microbiome: networks, competition, and stability. *Science* 350, 663–666. doi: 10.1126/science. aad2602
14. Dabdoub, S. M., Ganesan, S. M., and Kumar, P. S. (2016). Comparative metagenomics reveals taxonomically idiosyncratic yet functionally congruent communities in periodontitis. *Sci. Rep.* 6:38993. doi: 10.1038/srep38993
15. Diaz, P. I., and Valm, A. M. (2020). Microbial interactions in oral communities mediate emergent biofilm properties. *J. Dent. Res.* 99, 18–25. doi: 10.1177/ 0022034519880157
16. Ellen, R. P., and Galimanas, V. B. (2000). Spirochetes at the forefront of periodontal infections. *Periodontology* 38, 13–32. doi: 10.1111/j.1600-0757.2005.00108.x Gardner, M. R., and Ashby, W. R. (1970). Connectance of large dynamic
17. (cybernetic) systems: critical values for stability. *Nature* 228:784. doi: 10.1038/ 228784a0
18. Ghensi, P., Manghi, P., Zolfo, M., Armanini, F., Pasolli, E., Bolzan, M., et al. (2020). Strong oral plaque microbiome signatures for dental implant diseases identified by strain-resolution metagenomics. *NPJ Biofilms Microbiomes* 6:47. doi: 10.1038/s41522-020-00155-7
19. Girvan, M., and Newman, M. E. (2002). Community structure in social and biological networks. *Proc. Natl. Acad. Sci. U S A.* 99, 7821–7826. doi: 10.1073/ pnas.122653799
20. Gravel, D., Canard, E., Guichard, F., and Mouquet, N. (2011). Persistence increases with diversity and connectance in trophic metacommunities. *PLoS One* 6:e19374. doi: 10.1371/journal.pone.0019374
21. Jervoe-Storm, P. M., Alahdab, H., Koltzscher, M., Fimmers, R., and Jepsen, S. (2007). Comparison of curet and paper point sampling of subgingival bacteria as analyzed by real-time polymerase chain reaction. *J. Periodontol.* 78, 909–917. doi: 10.1902/jop.2007.060218
22. Jiao, J., Jing, W., Si, Y., Feng, X., Tai, B., Hu, D., et al. (2021). The prevalence and severity of periodontal disease in Mainland China: data from the Fourth National Oral Health Survey (2015-2016). *J. Clin. Periodontol.* 48, 168–179. doi: 10.1111/jcpe.13396
23. Kajiya, M., Giro, G., Taubman, M. A., Han, X., Mayer, M. P., and Kawai, T. (2010). Role of periodontal pathogenic bacteria in RANKL-mediated bone destruction in periodontal disease. *J. Oral Microbiol.* 2:10.3402/jom. v2i0.5532. doi: 10.3402/jom.v2i0.5532
24. Kassebaum, N. J., Bernabe, E., Dahiya, M., Bhandari, B., Murray, C. J., and Marcenes, W. (2014). Global burden of severe periodontitis in 1990-2010: a systematic review and meta-regression. *J. Dent Res.* 93, 1045–1053. doi: 10.1177/ 0022034514552491
25. Kinane, D. F., Stathopoulou, P. G., and Papapanou, P. N. (2017). Periodontal diseases. *Nat. Rev. Dis. Primers* 3:17038.
26. Knight, R., Vrbanac, A., Taylor, B. C., Aksenov, A., Callewaert, C., Debelius, J., et al. (2018). Best practices for analysing microbiomes. *Nat. Rev. Microbiol.* 16, 410–422. doi: 10.1038/s41579-018-0029-9
27. Komatsu, K., Shiba, T., Takeuchi, Y., Watanabe, T., Koyanagi, T., Nemoto, T., et al. (2020). Discriminating microbial community structure between peri-implantitis and periodontitis with integrated metagenomic, metatranscriptomic, and network analysis. *Front. Cell Infect. Microbiol.* 10:596490. doi: 10.3389/fcimb.2020.596490
28. Kulkarni, D., and De Laender, F. (2017). The combined effects of biotic and abiotic stress on species richness and connectance. *PLoS One* 12:e0172828. doi: 10.1371/journal.pone.0172828
29. Kuramitsu, H. K., He, X., Lux, R., Anderson, M. H., and Shi, W. (2007). Interspecies interactions within oral microbial communities. *Microbiol. Mol. Biol. Rev.* 71, 653–670. doi: 10.1128/MMBR.00024-07
30. Lee, C. T., Huang, Y. W., Zhu, L., and Weltman, R. (2017). Prevalences of peri-implantitis and peri-implant mucositis: systematic review and meta-analysis. *J. Dent.* 62, 1–12. doi: 10.1016/j.jdent.2017.04.011
31. Leonhardt, A., Renvert, S., and Dahlen, G. (1999). Microbial findings at failing implants. *Clin. Oral Implants Res.* 10, 339–345. doi: 10.1034/j.1600-0501.1999. 100501.x
32. Li, H., and Durbin, R. (2009). Fast and accurate short read alignment with burrows- wheeler transform. *Bioinformatics* 25, 1754–1760. doi: 10.1093/ bioinformatics/ btp324
33. Lindhe, J., Meyle, J., Group, and DoEWoP. (2008). Peri-implant diseases: consensus report of the Sixth European Workshop on periodontology. *J. Clin. Periodontol.* 35 (8 Suppl), 282–285. doi: 10.1111/j.1600-051X.2008.01283.x
34. Liu, Y., Liu, Q., Li, Z., Acharya, A., Chen, D., Chen, Z., et al. (2020). Long non- coding RNA and mRNA expression profiles in peri-implantitis vs periodontitis. *J. Periodontal Res.* 55, 342–353. doi: 10.1111/jre.12718
35. Marcenes, W., Kassebaum, N. J., Bernabe, E., Flaxman, A., Naghavi, M., Lopez, A., et al. (2013). Global burden of oral conditions in 1990-2010: a systematic analysis. *J. Dent. Res.* 92, 592–597. doi: 10.1177/0022034513490168
36. Marsh, P. D., and Zaura, E. (2017). Dental biofilm: ecological interactions in health and disease. *J. Clin. Periodontol.* 44(Suppl. 18), S12–S22. doi: 10.1111/ jcpe. 12679
37. May, R. M. (1972). Will a large complex system be stable? *Nature* 238, 413–414. doi: 10.1038/238413a0
38. May, R. M. (1973). Stability and complexity in model ecosystems. *Monogr. Popul. Biol.* 6, 1–235.
39. Morita, M., Yamamoto, T., and Watanabe, T. (1991). Identification by biotinylated DNA probes of *Capnocytophaga species* isolated from supragingival calculus. *J. Dent. Res.* 70, 1048–1051. doi: 10.1177/00220345910700070601
40. Ng, E., Tay, J. R. H., Balan, P., Ong, M. M. A., Bostanci, N., Belibasakis, G. N., et al. (2021). Metagenomic sequencing provides new insights into the subgingival bacteriome and aetiopathology of periodontitis. *J. Periodontal. Res.* 56, 205–218. doi: 10.1111/jre.12811
41. Oh, J., Byrd, A. L., Park, M., Program, N. C. S., Kong, H. H., and Segre, J. A. (2016). Temporal stability of the human skin microbiome. *Cell* 165, 854–866. doi: 10.1016/j.cell.2016.04.008
42. Ohishi, K., Yamamoto, T., Tomofuji, T., Tamaki, N., and Watanabe, T. (2005). Isolation and characterization of aminopeptidase from *Capnocytophaga granulosa* ATCC 51502. *Oral. Microbiol. Immunol.* 20, 67–72. doi: 10.1111/j. 1399-302X.2005.00183.x
43. Otasek, D., Morris, J. H., Boucas, J., Pico, A. R., and Demchak, B. (2019). Cytoscape automation: empowering workflow-based network analysis. *Genome Biol.* 20:185. doi: 10.1186/s13059-019-1758-4
44. Papapanou, P. N., Sanz, M., Buduneli, N., Dietrich, T., Feres, M., Fine, D. H., et al. (2018). Periodontitis: consensus report of workgroup 2 of the 2017 World Workshop on the Classification of Periodontal and Peri-Implant Diseases and Conditions. *J. Periodontol.* 89(Suppl. 1), S173–S182.
45. Relman, D. A. (2012). The human microbiome: ecosystem resilience and health. *Nutr. Rev.* 70(Suppl. 1), S2–S9. doi: 10.1111/j.1753-4887.2012.00489.x
46. Schloissnig, S., Arumugam, M., Sunagawa, S., Mitreva, M., Tap, J., Zhu, A., et al. (2013). Genomic variation landscape of the human gut microbiome. *Nature* 493, 45–50. doi: 10.1038/nature11711
47. Schwarz, F., Derks, J., Monje, A., and Wang, H. L. (2018). Peri-implantitis. *J. Clin. Periodontol.* 45(Suppl. 20), S246–S266.
48. Shannon, P., Markiel, A., Ozier, O., Baliga, N. S., Wang, J. T., Ramage, D., et al. (2003). Cytoscape: a software environment for integrated models of biomolecular interaction networks. *Genome Res.* 13, 2498–2504. doi: 10.1101/ gr.1239303
49. Stacy, A., Everett, J., Jorth, P., Trivedi, U., Rumbaugh, K. P., and Whiteley, M. (2014). Bacterial fight-and-flight responses enhance virulence in a polymicrobial infection. *Proc. Natl. Acad. Sci. U S A.* 111, 7819–7824. doi: 10.1073/pnas.1400586111
50. Stein, R. R., Bucci, V., Toussaint, N. C., Buffie, C. G., Ratsch, G., Pamer, E. G., et al. (2013). Ecological modeling from time-series inference: insight into dynamics and stability of intestinal microbiota. *PLoS Comput. Biol.* 9:e1003388. doi: 10. 1371/journal.pcbi.1003388
51. Takeuchi, Y., Umeda, M., Sakamoto, M., Benno, Y., Huang, Y., and Ishikawa, I. (2001). *Treponema socranskii*, *Treponema denticola*, and *Porphyromonas gingivalis* are associated with severity of periodontal tissue destruction. *J. Periodontol.* 72, 1354–1363. doi: 10.1902/jop.2001.72.10.1354

23

Rare Presentation of Dentin Abnormalities in Loeys-Dietz Syndrome Type I

Priyam Jani[1], *Olivier Duverger*[1], *Rashmi Mishra*[1,2], *Pamela A. Frischmeyer-Guerrerio*[3] *and Janice S. Lee*[1*]

[1] *Craniofacial Anomalies and Regeneration Section, National Institute of Craniofacial and Dental Research, National Institutes of Health, Bethesda, MD, United States,* [2] *Department of Oral Medicine, University of Washington School of Dentistry, Seattle, WA, United States,* [3] *Food Allergy Research Unit, National Institute of Allergy and Infectious Diseases, National Institutes of Health, Bethesda, MD, United States*

***Correspondence:**
Janice S. Lee
janice.lee@nih.gov

Loeys-Dietz syndrome type 1 (LDS1) is caused by a mutation in the transforming growth factor-beta receptor 1 (*TGFBR1*) gene. We previously characterized the oral and dental anomalies in a cohort of individuals diagnosed with LDS and showed that LDS1 had a high frequency of oral manifestations, and most affected individuals had enamel defects. However, dentin anomalies were not apparent in most patients in the cohort. In this cohort, we had identified dentin anomalies in a patient with LDS1, harboring mutation *TGFBR1* c.1459C>T (p.Arg487Trp), and in this report, we present clinical and radiographic findings to confirm the dentin anomaly. The proband had gray-brown discoloration of most teeth typical for dentinogenesis imperfecta (DI). A radiographic exam revealed obliterated or very narrow pulp canals, with maxillary anterior teeth being affected more than the posterior teeth. The son of the proband, who also has the same mutation variant, had a history of DI affecting the primary teeth; however, his permanent teeth were normal in appearance at the time of exam. *TGFBR1* is expressed by odontoblasts throughout tooth development and deletion of *TGFBR1* in mouse models is known to affect dentin development. In this report, we present a rare case of abnormal dentin in two individuals with LDS1. These dental anomalies may be the first obvious manifestation of a life-threatening systemic disease and demonstrate the variable and multi-organ phenotypic effects in rare diseases.

Keywords: Loeys-Dietz syndrome, TGFBR1 mutation, TGF-beta signaling, dentin defect, dentinogenesis imperfecta, case report

INTRODUCTION

Transforming growth factor-beta (TGF-β) signaling plays a crucial role during mammalian development (1). It has been implicated to be critical to cell proliferation and maturation, including the craniofacial (2–5) and dental mineralized tissues (6, 7). More recently, mutations in the TGF-β family of genes were discovered in a cohort with Marfan-like features, and the disease was classified as Loeys-Dietz syndrome (LDS) (8). LDS is caused by mutations in genes encoding various components of the TGF-β signaling pathway (9) and is currently classified into six subtypes based on the gene involved. LDS1 (MIM# 609192) is associated with transforming growth factor-β receptor type I (*TGFBR1*), TGF-β receptor type II (*TGFBR2*) mutations are classified as LDS2

(MIM# 610168), mothers against decapentaplegic homolog 3 (*SMAD3*) mutations cause LDS3 (MIM# 613795) (10), LDS4 (MIM#61481) and LDS5 (MIM#615582) are caused by mutations in TGF-β2 (*TGFB2*) and the TGF-β3 (*TGFB3*) ligands, respectively (11–14). *SMAD2* mutations were recently found to cause LDS (LDS6, no MIM# assigned) (15).

We previously reported the oral manifestations in a cohort of 40 individuals with LDS from five subtypes (LDS1-5) and reported a high frequency of abnormal palate morphology, enamel defects, bifid uvula, or submucous cleft palate, malocclusion, dental crowding, and delayed eruption of permanent teeth (16). We concluded that individuals with LDS2 followed by LDS1 had the most severely affected oro-dental region, which is also true for the systemic manifestations reported in LDS literature. Additionally, we have also shown that these dental anomalies significantly worsen the oral health-related quality of life for individuals with LDS (17).

Dentinogenesis imperfecta (DI) is a rare hereditary condition affecting the teeth, which manifests as grayish or yellow-brown discoloration of teeth (18). The condition is characterized by abnormal dentin formation leading to weak teeth which are susceptible to fracture and breakage. DI is a common manifestation in individuals with osteogenesis imperfecta Type III or IV with mutations in Collagen type 1 (*COL1A1* or *COL1A2*) genes (19, 20). Mutations in dentin sialophosphoprotein (*DSPP*) may also lead to non-syndromic forms of DI (21). While several genes have been implicated in the manifestation of dentin abnormalities in human case reports (19, 22, 23), to date, there has been no report describing dentin abnormalities associated with the TGF-β pathway in humans. However, *TGFBR1* has been shown to play a role in dentin development in mouse models (24–26). In this report, we present a rare manifestation of dentin abnormality in two individuals with a diagnosis of LDS1. Additionally, we also present a comparison between the severity of oral manifestation and systemic manifestations in LDS1, reported in previous literature and individuals in this report.

METHODS

Study Participant

A 53-year-old male (II-1) with a diagnosis of LDS1 who was enrolled in the Natural History and Genetics of Food Allergy and Related Conditions study (NCT02504853) was seen in the NIDCR Dental Clinic along with his wife and 14-year-old affected son (III-1). All three participants agreed to enroll and consented to the Natural History of Craniofacial Anomalies and Developmental Growth Variants study (NCT02639312).

Genetic Test

Targeted mutation analysis for the LDS genes panel was performed for the proband and his family by the primary care physician through GeneDX (GeneDx Inc., Gaithersburg, Maryland). Subsequently, whole exome sequencing (WES) was performed through National Institute of Allery and Infectious Diseases (NIAID) Centralized Sequencing Initiative during their visit to the National Institutes of Health.

Genomic DNA was extracted from the submitted blood specimen of both individuals and subjected to massively parallel sequencing on an Illumina sequencing system. The exonic regions, flanking splice junctions, and both 5′ and 3′ untranslated regions (UTR) were sequenced with 100 bp or greater paired-end reads. Subsequently, the reads were aligned to the human genome build GRCh37/UCSC hg19, and analysis was performed using a custom-enhanced analysis tool (SEQR). The interpretation of the variants was performed according to the ACMG guidelines (27) and the nomenclature of the identified variants is consistent with the Human Genome Variation Society (HGVS) guidelines. Confirmation of potentially relevant findings was performed using capillary sequencing or other appropriate methods. Minimum coverage is 95% > x20 for targeted genomic regions.

Oral and Dental Evaluation

The oral and dental evaluation included a detailed clinical exam, performed by the NIH Craniofacial Anomalies Team (PJ, RM, and JSL). The intra-oral exam consisted of the inspection of the oral structures and soft tissue, including the palate, uvula, and gingiva for basic periodontal assessment without periodontal probing. The dental and hard tissue evaluation included the occlusion, eruption pattern, tooth morphology, jaw relationship, and TMJ function. A standardized oro-dental evaluation form was used in all cases.

Radiographic Evaluation

Cone beam computed tomography (CBCT) (Planmeca Promax 3D Max, 400 μm resolution; Planmeca USA Inc., IL) was performed to further assess dental phenotype including findings such as tooth impaction, dental decay, enamel or dentin defects, and alveolar bone loss. CBCT images were used to generate panoramic x-rays and individual tooth slices using Planmeca Romexis software.

Photography

Extraoral and intraoral photographs (Canon EOS 5D Mark II camera, Canon USA Inc., VA) were obtained for each participant. For each patient, seven intraoral photos were taken: the frontal view of dentition in occlusion, the frontal view of dentition at rest (2–3 mm leeway space), the maxillary arch, the mandibular arch, the left lateral view (maxillary and mandibular teeth in occlusion), the right lateral view, and the oropharyngeal region. Facial photos included frontal and profile views.

CASE REPORT

History of Present Illness

The proband (II-1), a 53-year-old male, was seen at the dental clinic for evaluation of his oral health and LDS-related manifestations. He presented with his wife (unaffected, 40 years old) and son (III-1, affected, 14 years old). The timeline for proband and son are shown in **Figure 1B**. At age 40, the proband suffered abrupt chest and tooth pain with subsequent diagnosis

Abbreviations: LDS, Loeys-Dietz syndrome; LDS1, Loeys-Dietz syndrome type 1; TGF-β, Transforming growth factor beta; TGFBR1, TGF-β receptor type I; DI, Dentinogenesis imperfecta; CBCT, Cone beam computed tomography.

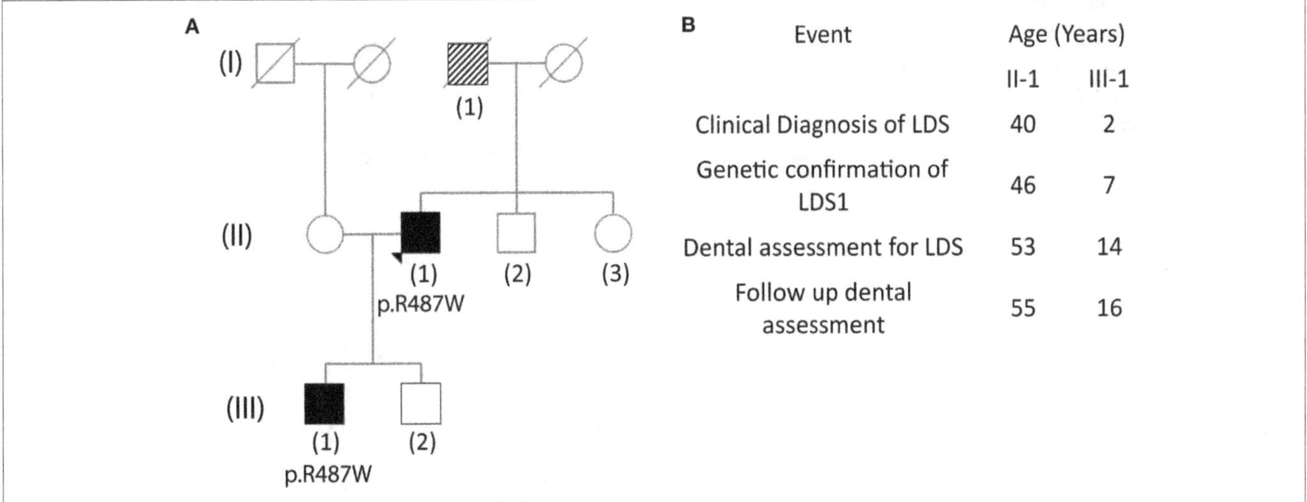

FIGURE 1 | Pedigree tree showing affected family members and timeline of events. **(A)** The (II-1) father of the proband is suspected of having Loeys-Dietz syndrome (LDS) as he died from an aneurysm at age 49. The mother of the proband has early-onset dementia. The brother of the proband is healthy, and the sister has skin carcinoma. Proband has two sons, one of whom (III-1) carries the LDS mutation. **(B)** Timeline of events for the proband (II-1) and the son of the proband (III-1) since diagnosis of LDS.

TABLE 1 | Comparison of oral manifestation with previously reported literature.

Systemic manifestation	TGFBR1 %	II-1	III-1	Oral manifestation	TGFBR1 %	II-1	III-1
Arterial tortuosity	75–100	+	+	Abnormal palate	100.0	+	+
Aortic root aneurysm	75–100	+	+	Retrognathic mandible	92.3	+	+
Pectus deformity	50–75	–	–	Gingivitis	61.5	–	+
Scoliosis	50–75	–	+	Class II malocclusion	61.5	+	–
Arachnodactyly	50–75	+	–	Enamel defects	46.1	+	–
Hernia	50–75	+	+	Submucosal cleft or bifid uvula	46.1	–	–
Osteoarthritis	25–50	–	–	TMJ abnormality	38.4	+	–
Striae	25–50	–	–	Deep bite	38.4	–	–
Dural ectasia	25–50	–	–	Dental crowding	7.6	–	+
Cervical spine malformation/instability	0–25	–	–	Delayed eruption	0	–	–
				Dentinogenesis imperfecta	0	+	+

–, Absent; +, Present. Systemic data for LDS1 adapted from (28); Oral data adapted from (16). Manifestation in bold are not previously reported in LDS.

of a type A aortic dissection. He underwent emergent aortic valve-sparing aortic root replacement. At age 46, his diagnosis of LDS1 was confirmed with a mutation in the *TGBR1* by candidate mutation analysis, specifically c.1459C>T, which resulted in the amino acid substitution p.R487W. At age 53, WES analysis was performed which confirmed the *TGFBR1* mutation but did not show the presence of any mutations in *DSPP*, the candidate gene for DI.

Family History

The father of the proband (I-1) died at 49 years of age from complications related to ruptured abdominal aorta; he had a history of myocardial infarction and pulmonary embolism. Although, the father did not have a known diagnosis of LDS, it is suspected retrospectively (**Figure 1A**). The proband (II-1) has two sons, one of whom shares the *TGFBR1* mutation (III-1). The wife of the proband and brother are healthy, whereas, his sister has a history of skin cancer.

Surgical History

The proband (II-1) had a history of Nissen fundoplication at age 36. He had undergone aneurysm repair at age 40 and mitral valve repair at age 51. He also had a history of inguinal hernia repair around age 45. The son of the proband (III-1) had a history of tympanostomy tube placement at age 1, inguinal hernia repair at age 9, and valve-sparing aortic root replacement at age 16. No adverse postsurgical outcomes were reported.

Systemic Findings

The proband (II-1) had multiple systemic findings including aneurysm in aorta, aneurysm in visceral/ileac arteries, atrial fibrillation, arterial tortuosity, mitral regurgitation, joint hyperflexibility, disc degeneration, translucent and stretchy skin, inguinal hernia, hiatal hernia, eosinophilic esophagitis, GERD, pes planus, asthma, and allergic rhinitis. Several of these findings were consistent with LDS (**Table 1**). More recently, at age 55, the proband was also diagnosed with Waldenstrom macroglobulinemia; however, its implications to oral health were uncertain as the proband was not aware of this diagnosis at the time of exam.

The son of the proband (III-1) presented with fewer systemic manifestations which included joint hyperflexibility, scoliosis, bone fracture, food allergies, atopic dermatitis, asthma, pes planus, translucent skin, arterial tortuosity, aortic root dilation, and inguinal hernia. These findings were also consistent with LDS.

Craniofacial/Extraoral Findings

The proband (II-1) had an oblong face with symmetrical soft and skeletal tissue. His vision was normal with the help of corrective lenses. He had significant bilateral ptosis and mild nystagmus. His midface and infraorbital projection were flat, and he was noted to have a retrognathic mandible. He had occasional temporomandibular joint (TMJ) pain and bilateral joint sounds (crepitus). He reported TMJ dislocation in the past.

The son of the proband (III-1) had an oblong face with a long lower third. He had bilateral nystagmus and mild ptosis. Both his ears were slightly lowest. He had a retrognathic mandible with normal TMJ function. He also had generalized acne on the cheeks, chin, and lips.

Overall, these patients were noted to be on the mild craniofacial spectrum compared to previous reports of craniofacial findings in LDS[1].

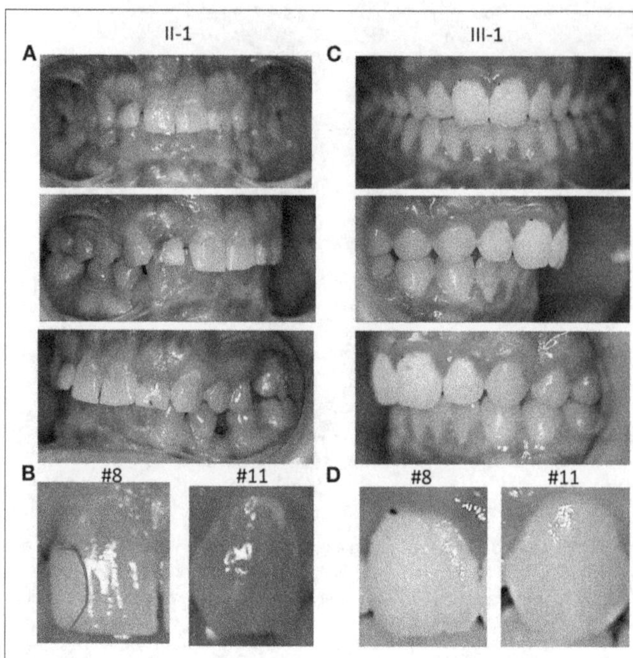

FIGURE 2 | Clinical oral manifestations. **(A)** Frontal, right lateral, and left lateral view of teeth showing tooth discoloration in proband II-1. **(B)** Magnified photos of tooth #8 and 11 with a red dotted line showing demarcation of the restoration on #8. **(C)** Frontal, right lateral, and left lateral view of teeth in the son of the proband III-1 **(D)** Magnified views of tooth #8 and 11 in III-1, showing normal appearance of teeth.

Intraoral Findings

The proband (II-1) had complete adult dentition with 28 teeth (wisdom teeth were extracted). He had a history of multiple cavities and had been told that his teeth are more susceptible to decay; root canal with tooth #7. His palate was high vaulted as seen in most other individuals affected by LDS. He had a Class II molar relationship with an increased overjet (7 mm) associated with mandibular retrognathia, a common feature in LDS. His teeth had grayish-brown discoloration which was unusual and prompted further investigation (**Figure 2A**). There were no signs of fracture or chipping of teeth, clinically, or radiographically. The discoloration affected the anterior teeth more than the posterior teeth which correlated with more restorations specifically in the anterior teeth (**Figure 2B**). He had mild enamel defects, grade 1 as per the enamel index (16). He did not report any bleeding of the gums and had no signs of gingivitis at the time of the exam. Mild plaque accumulation at the cervical margins of posterior teeth was noted.

The 14-year-old son of the proband (III-1) had an adult dentition with 28 teeth (**Figure 2C**); wisdom teeth were yet to erupt. He had a history of gray discoloration and early loss of his primary teeth. However, his permanent teeth did not have clinically discernable discoloration. He had a very mild anterior open bite with a parafunctional habit of resting his tongue in this space. He had mild crowding of teeth in the lower anterior region. He had a Class II molar relationship. He had mild generalized gingivitis and there was moderate plaque accumulation on most teeth; however, he did not report bleeding gums during routine activities like brushing his teeth. Thin occlusal enamel was noted on tooth #3, 14, 19, and 30 (first molars) with wear facets from opposing cusps which was unusual for his age. The anterior teeth did not have any apparent enamel defects, grade 0 as per the enamel index (**Figure 2D**). While both proband and his son had several features consistent with findings in LDS, they did not present with severe enamel defects or bifid uvula, common findings in LDS. Both individuals were seen after 2 years for a follow-up, but no changes in their oral health were noted.

Radiographic CBCT Exam

The missing teeth of proband (extractions) were confirmed in the panoramic image generated from CBCT images (**Figure 3A**). Bilateral tori on the medial surfaces of the mandible and small exostoses on the lateral surfaces were noted in the CBCT images (**Figure 3C**). Posterior teeth as well as mandibular anterior teeth showed thin pulp chambers (**Figure 3B**). All maxillary anterior teeth had narrow or obliterated pulp chambers indicating a phenotype mimicking DI Type II (**Figure 3D**). Small osteophytes involving the mandibular condyles and articular fossae were also visible explaining the TMJ abnormality experienced by the

[1]Almpani et al., 2021, Loeys-Dietz and Shprintzen-Goldberg Syndromes: analysis of TGF-β-opathies with craniofacial manifestations using innovative characterization methods, manuscript under revision.

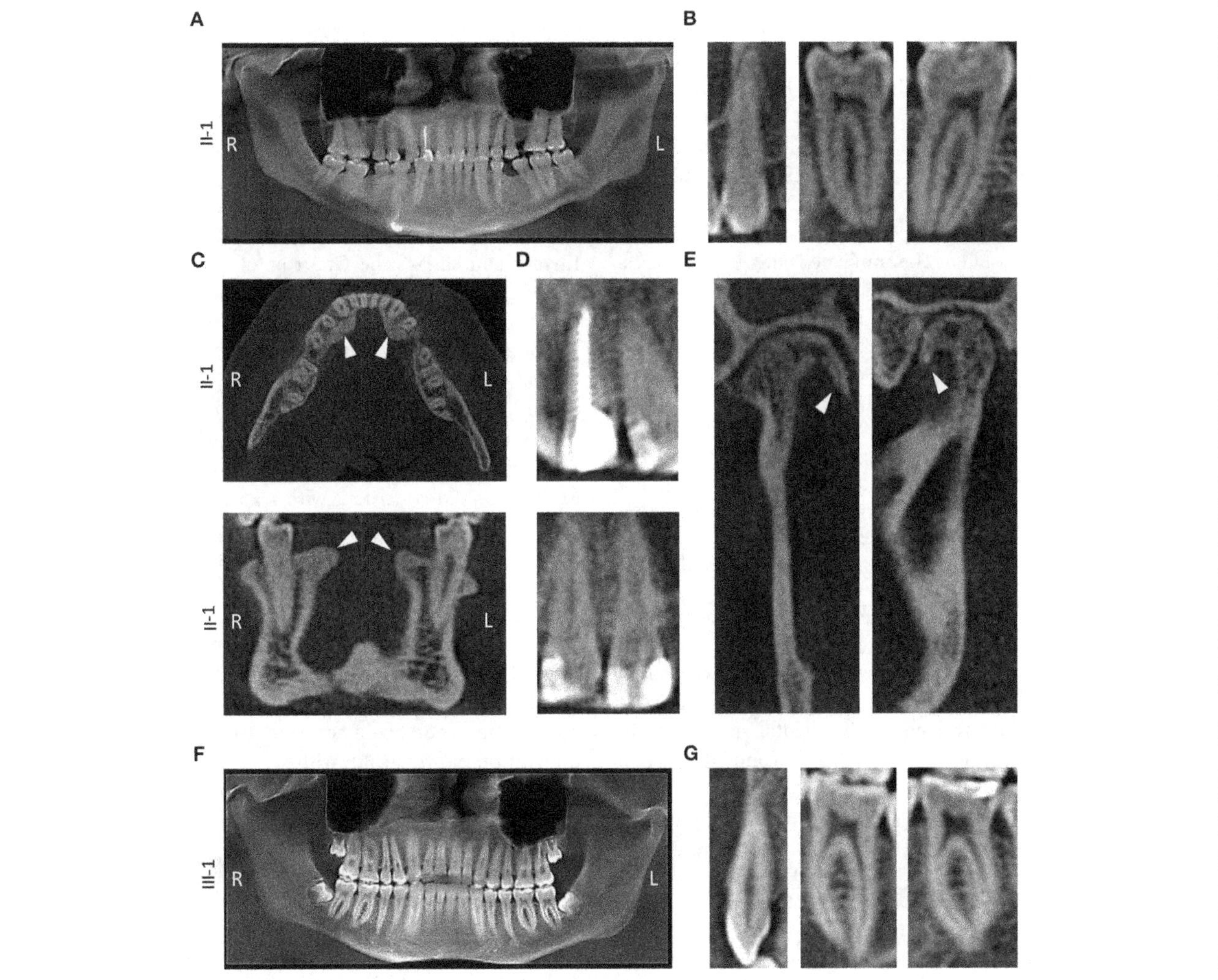

FIGURE 3 | Radiographic findings. **(A)** Panoramic x-ray from proband II-1 showing thickened dentin and obstructed pulp chambers. **(B)** 2D slices from II-1 cone beam computed tomography (CBCT) exam showing tooth # 11, 21, and 30 with constricted pulp canals. **(C)** Transverse (top) and a coronal (bottom) slice of the mandible showing lingual tori (white arrowheads). **(D)** Restorations in the teeth of proband with a root canal on tooth #7 (top) and class V restorations with teeth # 8 and 9 (bottom). **(E)** Coronal (left) and a sagittal (right) slice of the right mandibular condyle showing osteophytes (white arrowhead). **(F)** Panoramic x-ray from III-1. **(G)** 2D slices showing tooth # 11, 21, and 30.

proband (**Figure 3E**). Mild horizontal bone loss was noted in the CBCT images in both the upper and lower arch.

The son of the proband (III-I) had developing wisdom teeth visible in the radiographic exam (**Figure 3F**). His teeth did have long and slender roots with somewhat constricted pulp, although, not severe enough to be considered abnormal at the time of exam (**Figure 3G**). His alveolar bone was within normal limits and no bone loss was seen in the CBCT scans during the exam.

Correlation With Systemic Health

We analyzed the relationship between the systemic and oral manifestations in these two patients by linking the systemic findings (28) and oral findings (16) reported previously in LDS1 with the findings in these two patients (**Table 1**). While the proband (II-1) had multiple systemic conditions, several systemic findings were absent when compared to the LDS1 systemic findings reported in the literature (28). Similarly, the proband (II-1) had fewer oral manifestations compared to LDS1 affected individuals from the previous report (16), though, the DI in this individual is the first report of this dental finding in LDS. In the same fashion, the son of the proband (III-1) was on the milder spectrum of systemic and oral abnormalities, which may indicate that milder oral manifestations correlate with milder and fewer systemic conditions in individuals with LDS.

DISCUSSION

In this case report, we show the manifestation of dentin anomalies associated with LDS1. While enamel defects have been associated with LDS, and we also showed the correlation of enamel defect severity with mutations in LDS (16), it was not identified that dentin could also be adversely affected in individuals with LDS. To our knowledge, these are the only patients with LDS1 who exhibited a phenotype recapitulating DI type II with the pathognomonic tooth discoloration in this cohort. If a larger cohort of individuals with LDS were to be thoroughly examined for oral manifestations, more reports of dentin abnormalities are possible. Thus, individuals with LDS should be screened more thoroughly, both clinically and radiographically to rule out dentin abnormalities.

One limitation of this report is that the role of *TGBR1* in causing DI phenotype could not be confirmed with just two cases. As LDS is a rare disease with arterial aneurysms as a common finding, the oral findings and symptoms are often overlooked. We have studied the oral manifestations in LDS in detail in a cohort of 40 patients, including 15 patients with LDS1, and so far, these were the only two individuals with the manifestation of dentin abnormality. The dental manifestation reported in this case study may be unique to these two individuals or as more affected individuals are studied, more details about the dental abnormalities may be revealed. Nonetheless, screening more individuals with mutations in the TGF-β signaling pathway for oral manifestations is warranted. In addition to detailed dental history and a thorough clinical exam to confirm changes in dentin, a radiographic assessment should be performed to follow the progression of the disease. Moreover, advanced genetic analysis of the two patients affected with DI in this cohort will be necessary to investigate the presence of additional mutations that may be involved in this dental manifestation which is not common in LDS but is beyond the scope of this report.

The involvement of TGF-β signaling in dentin development is supported by numerous studies in mice (7, 29, 30). Odontoblasts are the cells that form dentin and line the inner wall of the pulp cavity. TGF-β ligands and receptors are known to be expressed by odontoblasts (26, 31, 32), and stimulate the secretion of predentin and dentin. The expression of TGF-β receptor 1 in human teeth has also been reported (32). These studies suggest that TGF-β signaling does play a vital role in dentin development. While we can confirm the dentin abnormality in these patients clinically and radiographically, further, ultrastructural and histological analysis of the teeth is necessary to investigate the effects of LDS-causing mutations on dentin formation. However, extraction of teeth is not an option unless clinically indicated. The son of proband did not clinically show the discoloration of his permanent teeth despite having a history of grayish discoloration of primary teeth. However, we suspect that the DI could be progressive and as the patient ages, his teeth may eventually discolor after pulp constriction.

The two individuals in this case report do not have the many systemic manifestations as other reported cohorts with LDS1 and their craniofacial findings are also on the milder spectrum for LDS (see footnote **1**). Similarly, the patients presented fewer and milder oral manifestations compared to the LDS1 cohort in the previous study (16). This suggests that the severity of oral manifestations may be related to the severity of systemic manifestations and a more thorough analysis of the correlations between oral health and systemic health is warranted. This report further emphasizes the vital role of diagnosing oral and dental abnormalities by dentists and physicians alike, as they may reflect the overall systemic health of an individual. Dental care providers could be the first to diagnose rare conditions based on the oral manifestations, following the accurate recording of history, thorough clinical exam, educating the patients about their oral conditions, and alerting the primary physicians of their findings. It is important to note that the unusual discoloration of the proband consistent with DI was likely visible well-before his aortic dissection was diagnosed and treated at age 40. As DI is relatively rare, this unusual presentation should alert clinicians and care providers that other systemic manifestations may need evaluation.

As science and medicine continue to move toward a multidisciplinary approach, dentists and oral health providers could play a critical role to advance the diagnosis, health management, and quality of life of the patient by considering the integration of oral health with systemic health and collaborating across disciplines and professions.

AUTHOR CONTRIBUTIONS

PJ, RM, and JL performed the clinical evaluation of patients. PJ and OD performed the analysis and interpretation of data. JL and PF-G obtained IRB approval, secured research funding, and identified and recruited LDS patients. PJ, OD, and JL wrote the manuscript. All the authors reviewed the manuscript critically for important intellectual content and approved the version to be published.

ACKNOWLEDGMENTS

We thank the personnel of the NIH Dental Clinic who were involved in the collection of the data and the patients who participated in the study.

REFERENCES

1. Massagué J, Blain SW, Lo RS. TGFβ signaling in growth control, cancer, and heritable disorders. *Cell.* (2000) 103:295–309. doi: 10.1016/S0092-8674(00)00121-5
2. Snider TN, Louie KaW, Zuzo G, de Oliveira Ruellas AC, Solem RC, Cevidanes LHS, et al. Quantification of three-dimensional morphology of craniofacial mineralized tissue defects in Tgfbr2/Osx-Cre mice. *Oral Sci Int.* (2021) 1–10. doi: 10.1002/osi2.1099
3. Ho T-V, Iwata J, Ho HA, Grimes WC, Park S, Sanchez-Lara PA, et al. Integration of comprehensive 3D microCT and signaling analysis reveals differential regulatory mechanisms of craniofacial bone development. *Dev Biol.* (2015) 400:180–90.: doi: 10.1016/j.ydbio.2015.02.010
4. Wu M, Chen G, Li Y-P. TGF-β and BMP signaling in osteoblast, skeletal development, and bone formation, homeostasis and disease. *Bone Research.* (2016) 4:16009. doi: 10.1038/boneres.2016.9
5. Ito Y, Yeo JY, Chytil A, Han J, Bringas P, Nakajima A, et al. Conditional inactivation of Tgfbr2 in cranial neural crest causes cleft palate and calvaria defects. *Development.* (2003) 130:5269–80. doi: 10.1242/dev.00708
6. Zhao H, Oka K, Bringas P, Kaartinen V, Chai Y. TGF-β type I receptor Alk5 regulates tooth initiation and mandible patterning

in a type II receptor-independent manner. *Dev Biol.* (2008) 320:19–29. doi: 10.1016/j.ydbio.2008.03.045

7. Wang Y, Cox MK, Coricor G, MacDougall M, Serra R. Inactivation of Tgfbr2 in osterix-cre expressing dental mesenchyme disrupts molar root formation. *Dev Biol.* (2013) 382:27–37. doi: 10.1016/j.ydbio.2013.08.003
8. Loeys BL, Chen J, Neptune ER, Judge DP, Podowski M, Holm T, et al. A syndrome of altered cardiovascular, craniofacial, neurocognitive and skeletal development caused by mutations in TGFBR1 or TGFBR2. *Nat Genet.* (2005) 37:275–81. doi: 10.1038/ng1511
9. Loeys BL, Schwarze U, Holm T, Callewaert BL, Thomas GH, Pannu H, et al. Aneurysm syndromes caused by mutations in the TGF-β receptor. *N Engl J Med.* (2006) 355:788–98. doi: 10.1056/NEJMoa055695
10. van de Laar IMBH, Oldenburg RA, Pals G, Roos-Hesselink JW, de Graaf BM, Verhagen JMA, et al. Mutations in SMAD3 cause a syndromic form of aortic aneurysms and dissections with early-onset osteoarthritis. *Nat Genet.* (2011) 43:121. doi: 10.1038/ng.744
11. Bertoli-Avella AM, Gillis E, Morisaki H, Verhagen JMA, de Graaf BM, van de Beek G, et al. Mutations in a TGF-β ligand, TGFB3, cause syndromic aortic aneurysms and dissections. *J Am Coll Cardiol.* (2015) 65:1324–36. doi: 10.1016/j.jacc.2015.01.040
12. Boileau C, Guo D-C, Hanna N, Regalado ES, Detaint D, Gong L, et al. TGFB2 mutations cause familial thoracic aortic aneurysms and dissections associated with mild systemic features of Marfan syndrome. *Nat Genet.* (2012) 44:916–21. doi: 10.1038/ng.2348
13. Lindsay ME, Schepers D, Bolar NA, Doyle JJ, Gallo E, Fert-Bober J, et al. Loss-of-function mutations in TGFB2 cause a syndromic presentation of thoracic aortic aneurysm. *Nat Genet.* (2012) 44:922. doi: 10.1038/ng.2349
14. Rienhoff HY Jr, Yeo C-Y, Morissette R, Khrebtukova I, Melnick J, Luo S, et al. A mutation in TGFB3 associated with a syndrome of low muscle mass, growth retardation, distal arthrogryposis and clinical features overlapping with marfan and loeys–dietz syndrome. *Am J Med Genet A.* (2013) 161:2040–6. doi: 10.1002/ajmg.a.36056
15. Micha D, Guo D-c, Hilhorst-Hofstee Y, van Kooten F, Atmaja D, Overwater E, et al. SMAD2 mutations are associated with arterial aneurysms and dissections. *Hum Mutat.* (2015) 36:1145–9. doi: 10.1002/humu.22854
16. Jani P, Nguyen QC, Almpani K, Keyvanfar C, Mishra R, Liberton D, et al. Severity of oro-dental anomalies in Loeys-Dietz syndrome segregates by gene mutation. *J Med Genet.* (2020) 57:699–707. doi: 10.1136/jmedgenet-2019-106678
17. Nguyen QC, Duverger O, Mishra R, Mitnik GL, Jani P, Frischmeyer-Guerrerio PA, et al. Oral health-related quality of life in Loeys-Dietz syndrome, a rare connective tissue disorder: an observational cohort study. *Orphanet J Rare Dis.* (2019) 14:291. doi: 10.1186/s13023-019-1250-y
18. Ivancie GP. Dentinogenesis imperfecta. *Oral Surg Oral Med Oral Pathol.* (1954) 7:984–92. doi: 10.1016/0030-4220(54)90298-4
19. Pallos D, Hart PS, Cortelli JR, Vian S, Wright JT, Korkko J, et al. Novel COL1A1 mutation (G599C) associated with mild osteogenesis imperfecta and dentinogenesis imperfecta. *Arch Oral Biol.* (2001) 46:459–70. doi: 10.1016/S0003-9969(00)00130-8
20. Malmgren B, Lindskog S. Assessment of dysplastic dentin in osteogenesis imperfecta and dentinogenesis imperfecta. *Acta Odontol Scand.* (2003) 61:72–80. doi: 10.1080/00016350310001398
21. Zhang X, Zhao J, Li C, Gao S, Qiu C, Liu P, et al. DSPP mutation in dentinogenesis imperfecta Shields type II. *Nat Genet.* (2001) 27:151–2. doi: 10.1038/84765
22. Aubin I, Adams CP, Opsahl S, Septier D, Bishop CE, Auge N, et al. A deletion in the gene encoding sphingomyelin phosphodiesterase 3 (Smpd3) results in osteogenesis and dentinogenesis imperfecta in the mouse. *Nat Genet.* (2005) 37:803–5. doi: 10.1038/ng1603
23. Beattie ML, Kim J-W, Gong S-G, Murdoch-Kinch CA, Simmer JP, Hu JC-C. Phenotypic variation in dentinogenesis imperfecta/dentin dysplasia linked to 4q21. *J Dent Res.* (2006) 85:329–33. doi: 10.1177/154405910608500409
24. D'Souza RN, Cavender A, Dickinson D, Roberts A, Letterio J. TGF-β1 is essential for the homeostasis of the dentin-pulp complex. *Eur J Oral Sci.* (1998) 106(Suppl. 1):185–91. doi: 10.1111/j.1600-0722.1998.tb02174.x
25. Smith AJ, Matthews JB, Hall RC. Transforming Growth Factor-β1 (TGF-β1) in dentine matrix. *Eur J Oral Sci.* (1998) 106(Suppl. 1):179–84. doi: 10.1111/j.1600-0722.1998.tb02173.x
26. Sloan AJ, Matthews JB, Smith AJ. TGF-β receptor expression in human odontoblasts and pulpal cells. *Histochem J.* (1999) 31:565–9. doi: 10.1023/A:1003852409574
27. Richards S, Aziz N, Bale S, Bick D, Das S, Gastier-Foster J, et al. Standards and guidelines for the interpretation of sequence variants: a joint consensus recommendation of the American College of Medical Genetics and Genomics and the Association for Molecular Pathology. *Genet Med.* (2015) 17:405–23. doi: 10.1038/gim.2015.30
28. Camerota L, Ritelli M, Wischmeijer A, Majore S, Cinquina V, Fortugno P, et al. Genotypic categorization of Loeys-Dietz syndrome based on 24 novel families and literature data. *Genes.* (2019) 10:764. doi: 10.3390/genes10100764
29. Oka S, Oka K, Xu X, Sasaki T, Bringas P, Chai Y. Cell autonomous requirement for TGF-β signaling during odontoblast differentiation and dentin matrix formation. *Mech Dev.* (2007) 124:409–15. doi: 10.1016/j.mod.2007.02.003
30. Ahn YH, Kim TH, Choi H, Bae CH, Yang YM, Baek JA, et al. Disruption of Tgfbr2 in odontoblasts leads to aberrant pulp calcification. *J Dent Res.* (2015) 94:828–35. doi: 10.1177/0022034515577427
31. Cassidy N, Fahey M, Prime SS, Smith AJ. Comparative analysis of transforming growth factor-β isoforms 1–3 in human and rabbit dentine matrices. *Arch Oral Biol.* (1997) 42:219–23. doi: 10.1016/S0003-9969(96)00115-X
32. Sloan AJ, Perry H, Matthews JB, Smith AJ. transforming growth factor-β isoform expression in mature human healthy and carious molar teeth. *Histochem J.* (2000) 32:247–52. doi: 10.1023/A:1004007202404

24

Dentists as Primary Care Providers: Expert Opinion on Predoctoral Competencies

Sara C. Gordon[1*†], *Linda M. Kaste*[2†], *Wendy E. Mouradian*[3,4], *Phyllis L. Beemsterboer*[5], *Joel H. Berg*[3] *and Carol Anne Murdoch-Kinch*[6]

[1] Department of Oral Medicine, School of Dentistry, University of Washington, Seattle, WA, United States, [2] Department of Oral Biology, College of Dentistry, University of Illinois Chicago, Chicago, IL, United States, [3] Department of Pediatric Dentistry, School of Dentistry, University of Washington, Seattle, WA, United States, [4] The Santa Fe Group, New York, NY, United States, [5] Center for Ethics in Healthcare, School of Dentistry, Oregon Health & Science University, Portland, OR, United States, [6] School of Dentistry, Indiana University, Indianapolis, IN, United States

***Correspondence:**
Sara C. Gordon
gordons@uw.edu

† These authors have contributed equally to this work and share first authorship

Dentistry and medicine traditionally practice as separate professions despite sharing goals for optimal patient health. Many US residents experience both poor oral and general health, with difficulty accessing care. More efficient collaboration between these professions could enhance health. The COVID-19 pandemic disclosed further disparities while underscoring concerns that physician supply is inadequate for population needs. Hence, enhancing healthcare provider education to better meet the public's health needs is critical. The proposed titles "Oral Physician" or "Oral Health Primary Care Provider" (OP-PCP) acknowledge dentist's capacity to diagnose and manage diseases of the orofacial complex and provide some basic primary healthcare. The US Surgeon General's National Prevention Council and others recommend such models. Medical and dental education already overlap considerably, thus it is plausible that dental graduates could be trained as OP-PCPs to provide primary healthcare such as basic screening and preventive services within existing dental education standards. In 2018, 23 dental and medical educators participated in an expert-opinion elicitation process to review educational competencies for this model. They demonstrated consensus on educational expansion and agreed that the proposed OP-PCP model could work within existing US Commission on Dental Accreditation (CODA) standards for predoctoral education. However, there were broader opinions on scope of practice details. Existing CODA standards could allow interested dental programs to educate OP-PCPs as a highly-skilled workforce assisting with care of medically-complex patients and to helping to reduce health disparities. Next steps include broader stakeholder discussion of OC-PCP competencies and applied studies including patient outcome assessments.

Keywords: oral physician, primary care dentist, dental student, oral health primary care provider (OP-PCP), oral-systemic, interprofessional education/care (IPE/IPC), dental education, dentistry

INTRODUCTION

Definition of the Problem

Many Americans experience poor health and lack adequate access to care. This is especially true for underserved populations such as low-income and minority groups. Dentistry and medicine practice as separate professions despite their shared missions to optimize their patients' health. Yet more efficient interprofessional collaboration could broaden access to oral and general healthcare, potentially reducing disparities and costs (1–4). Dental team disease screening could save between $42.4 million and $102.6 million in U.S. healthcare costs annually (5). The U.S. Surgeon General's National Prevention Council and others support the use of dentists in primary care roles (6–8). Meanwhile, concerns about lack of an adequate physician supply in the US have only increased during the COVID-19 pandemic.

This paper was submitted in response to a Frontiers in Dental Medicine challenge to "contribute to the development of evidence-based, cost-effective disease prevention and healthcare strategies applicable across diverse populations" on integrating oral and systemic health (9). It evaluates new dental education competency statements for training dentists to provide primary care tasks. To make this curriculum more cost-effective, it proposes to deliver this education during predoctoral education, within existing Commission on Dental Education (CODA) Standards (10). Hence, this educational action step augments recently published aspects of dental and medical integration related to the challenge (3, 4, 11–15).

Oral Health Primary Care Provider

"Oral Physician" or "Oral Health Primary Care Provider" (OP-PCP) are potential titles acknowledging general dentist's prospective expanded roles in basic primary healthcare (16–18). The American Dental Association (ADA) refers to dentists as "doctors who specialize in oral health" (19). The OP-PCP would be an enhanced dental practitioner functioning as part of an interprofessional healthcare team, connected virtually or in-person (20).

When dentists perform a thorough examination of dental patients, they typically assess the patient's blood pressure, and review medical, pharmaceutical, and psychosocial histories. They examine the oral cavity and head and neck, looking for oral diseases ranging from gingivitis to oral cancer. Dentists may detect signs and symptoms of other diseases beyond the oral cavity such as diabetes (21–24), cardiovascular disease (25–27), substance abuse (28, 29), eating disorders (30, 31) and child abuse or intimate partner violence (32–34), among others (35).

At the same time, an increasingly complex patient population requires dentists to become more sophisticated providers with greater knowledge of systemic conditions, and to be familiar with emerging approaches such as precision healthcare, salivary diagnostics, and new medical therapeutics (12). It is within the current legal scope of practice for dentists to diagnose and manage oral manifestations of systemic diseases, and to detect and help prevent systemic manifestations of oral diseases (14, 26, 36).

Appropriately trained dentists could build on these procedures to include some basic primary care in an integrated oral health practice, as described by Myers-Wright and Lamster (1). Expansion of primary screening within dental practice has been shown to be acceptable to the public. For example, random blood glucose testing in the dental office was well accepted by American patients and clinicians (21). Saudi Arabian patients accepted screening for hypertension and diabetes from dentists (37). In response to the pandemic, viral screening and immunizations became part of dentistry's scope of practice in many states (38).

The establishment of OP-PCPs within dentistry could shift dentistry's primary focus from restoring patient's oral health to maintaining their overall health. They could spend more time examining, diagnosing, and counseling patients and less time performing interceptive procedures. As leaders of dental teams, they can selectively delegate care to dental hygienists, expanded function dental assistants, or dental therapists as permitted by law (5, 20) and this could free their time to accommodate this expanded scope. Referral of more complex procedures to specialists makes room for more prevention in their practices an option (20).

Recent Changes and Timelines

The COVID-19 pandemic caused major disruptions in higher education, creating financial and logistical challenges for dental and other health professional schools. As schools struggled to provide adequate patient experiences while maintaining infrastructure and meeting other requirements, challenges led to innovation.

At the University of Washington (UW), the advent of the pandemic coincided with the construction of a new interprofessional health sciences education building, sparking new interprofessional bonds. The Health Sciences deans designed the building together to foster shared education and began planning a merged core curriculum in which dentistry is an equal partner with the other health professions. With the pandemic, scope of dental practice was already changing at the policy level. In Washington, dentists were permitted to prescribe or administer coronavirus screening (39). UW School of Dentistry successfully proposed that the state allow dentists, dental students, and dental hygienists to administer COVID-19 vaccines (40). Subsequently all UW health professions schools attended hands-on vaccination trainings together (with some dentist-trainers).

Immunization and disease testing by dentists are not new concepts. In 2005, Illinois Public Act 49-409 gave dentists status as "emergency dental responders" (Illinois Public Act 99-0025 changed this term to "dental responders") who could provide emergency medical care, triage, and immunizations during a disaster if appropriately certified (41). Illinois dentists were authorized to provide influenza vaccines in 2016 (41) and Oregon has permitted dentists to vaccinate patients since 2019 (42). The US Public Readiness and Emergency Preparedness (PREP) Act extended COVID-19 vaccinator status to all US dentists, dental students, and dental hygienists in 2021 (43). Similarly, the pandemic led to approval and expansion of telehealth services, including certain tele dentistry services.

Beyond vaccination, the broader concept of training pre- and/or postdoctoral students in additional skills for primary care has received national attention within the profession. The American Dental Education Association's (ADEA) 2021 Annual Session featured a Chair of the Board Symposium entitled *A Two-way Street: Primary Care and Oral Health Integration Training* with speakers from Harvard's Center for Integration of Primary Care and Oral Health. A key takeaway was that "the integration of oral health and primary care won't happen overnight, but it won't happen at all if we do nothing" (44). Previous ADEA panel sessions have examined curricular innovations to foster integrated mastery of biomedical concepts (45).

CODA determines the minimum competency standards that graduating dentists must meet but does not dictate how dental schools teach skills or measure competency (10). Thus, as long as it meets existing CODA Standards, an accredited predoctoral dental education program may require its graduates to demonstrate competency in standards that exceed this national benchmark–such as assuring competency in expanded roles in basic, primary healthcare. The intention of this project was to evaluate the feasibility of developing a new curriculum to provide such training in pre-doctoral dental programs, beginning at the level of expert opinion, the base of the evidence-based pyramid (46).

Purpose

The purpose of this study was to gain expert opinion about whether a pre-doctoral dental program could train its dental graduates as OP-PCP to competently provide primary healthcare in a specific set of proposed professional activities while the program remained in compliance with existing dental competency standards of the Commission on Dental Accreditation (CODA).

METHODS

Study Design

This expert opinion elicitation process (47) was a component of an Institutional Action Project for the Executive Leadership in Academic Medicine (ELAM) program at Drexel University by one author (SG). The study was deemed exempt from the institutional review board (IRB) human subject research review at UW.

Participants

The expert opinion elicitation took place between January and May 2018, engaging a convenience sample of educators in healthcare professions. The participant pool was structured to provide diversity by including different academic positions, areas of expertise, sex, and geographic location. Most participants were invited while attending the annual session of ADEA, where the chair-elect of the Section on Academic Affairs/Academic Deans (SG) was able to meet educational leaders face-to-face, explain the project, and request their participation. Some participants were added before and after the meeting to provide more range in expertise and teaching positions. Those who agreed to participate could respond in their preference of format: by email *via* questionnaire or discussion (SG), or through a verbal discussion (SG) by telephone or in-person.

Questionnaire Development

Sources representing expectations for dental and interprofessional competency were initially examined to create a list of professional skills an OP-PCP would need: *Standards of the Commission on Dental Accreditation* (10), *American Dental Education Association (ADEA) Competencies for the New General Dentist* (48), and *Interprofessional Education Collaborative (IPEC) Core Competencies for Interprofessional Collaborative Practice* (49). The competency statements in these three documents were grouped by content similarities. This revealed skills that an OP-PCP might need, which might not be covered or stressed in current dental education.

Each skill that a dental program could adopt to train OP-PCPs was restated in order to describe the level of competency proposed for new OP-PCP graduates. For some new skills, several alternative competency statements were proposed to determine how far the experts felt scope of practice should extend. All skills were examined to see whether they corresponded to any existing CODA standards. Then they were framed in a questionnaire, reviewed by study collaborators, and adjusted for content and clarity. In the final questionnaire, each respondent indicated whether they agreed with each proposed OP-PCP competency statement and optionally provided comments.

Data Analysis

As the intent was to collect qualitative data for a convenience sample of experts, the data were viewed at response distributions without statistical testing. These response distributions were categorized by two investigators as "agree/yes," "disagree/no," or "conditionally agree" (supported by comments). For questions requiring professional knowledge of clinical procedures (correlating with CODA Standard 24), only clinicians' responses were included. The investigators categorized comments into one of three groups: editorial directions for rewording or rewriting the proposal; affirmative statements, in which the respondent expressed enthusiasm; and conceptual/contextual observations or questions. The investigators (LM and SG) discussed any disparate categorizations to finalize this classification.

RESULTS

All proposed OP-PCP competency statements corresponded with existing CODA standards. These statements, grouped with their related CODA Standards, are presented in **Tables 1**, **2**, separating Standard 2-24 from the others. Respondents proposed three additional OP-PCP competency statements that also corresponded with existing CODA standards.

The convenience sample of experts captured distributions by sex, US location, professional field, academic role, and survey method (**Table 3**). No statistically significant differences were found among the characteristics when assessed by sex, professional field, or academic role (data not shown).

TABLE 1 | CODA Standards (CS) except CODA 2-24, and related Proposed Competency Statements (PCS) for Oral Physician - Oral Health Primary Care Provider (OP-PCP).

STD number	CODA Standard (CS) and Proposed Competency Statements (PCS)
CS 2-10	**Graduates must be competent in the use of critical thinking and problem-solving, including their use in the comprehensive care of patients, scientific inquiry and research methodology.**
PCS 2-10-1	OP-PCP graduates must be competent in performing clinical case reviews individually and in interprofessional healthcare teams.
CS 2-11	**Graduates must demonstrate the ability to self-assess, including the development of professional competencies and the demonstration of professional values and capacities associated with self-directed, lifelong learning.**
PCS 2-11-1	OP-PCP graduates must be competent in routinely self-assessing progress toward overall competency and individual competencies, considering needs for interprofessional as well as oral health knowledge.
PCS 2-11-2	OP-PCP graduates must be competent in educating others about health, including clinicians from other health professions, using critical thinking and feedback techniques.
CS 2-14	**In-depth information on abnormal biological conditions must be provided to support a high level of understanding of the etiology, epidemiology, differential diagnosis, pathogenesis, prevention, treatment and prognosis of oral and oral-related disorders.**
PCS 2-14	OP-PCP graduates must be competent to identify the etiology, epidemiology, differential diagnosis, pathogenesis, prevention, treatment and prognosis of oral, orofacial, and major systemic diseases that present in clinical care.
CS 2-15	**Graduates must be competent in the application of biomedical science knowledge in the delivery of patient care.**
PCS 2-15-1	OP-PCP graduates must be competent in describing a plan to regularly update their knowledge of advances and changes in modern biomedical sciences that apply to their clinical practice.
PCS 2-15-2	OP-PCP graduates must be competent in establishing a plan to regularly review "best practice" standards with their clinical team, including oral health standards with the general health team, and all relevant health standards with the oral health team.
CS 2-16	**Graduates must be competent in the application of the fundamental principles of behavioral sciences as they pertain to patient-centered approaches for promoting, improving and maintaining oral health.**
PCS 2-16-1	OP-PCP graduates must be competent in the use of effective techniques to discuss sensitive or embarrassing topics with patients, in delivering difficult news in a respectful manner, and in communicating with patients who are angry, fearful, sad, or otherwise highly emotional.
PCS 2-16-2	OP-PCP graduates must be competent in the use of nutritional counseling to promote, improve, and maintain oral and systemic health.
PCS 2-16-3	OP-PCP graduates must be competent in the use of evidence-based methods, including referral, to help patients rid themselves of unhealthy habits or disorders including those related to food intake, habits, substance abuse, and addictions.
CS 2-17	**Graduates must be competent in managing a diverse patient population and have the interpersonal and communications skills to function successfully in a multicultural work environment.**
PCS 2-17-1	OP-PCP graduates must be competent in communicating and collaborating with patients, families, interprofessional team members, and the public in a respectful and responsible manner to communicate health information and to make healthcare decisions.
PCS 2-17-2	OP-PCP graduates must be competent in working together with local communities, subpopulations, and other members of the interprofessional team to develop, deliver, and evaluate patient/ population-centered care and population health programs and policies that are safe, timely, efficient, effective, and equitable.
CS 2-18	**Graduates must be competent in applying legal and regulatory concepts related to the provision and/or support of oral healthcare services.**
PCS 2-18-1	OP-PCP graduates must be competent in describing the boundaries between dental and medical licensure.
PCS 2-18-2	OP-PCP graduates must be competent in delegating professional responsibilities according to each oral health team member's individual competencies and licensure.
PCS 2-18-3	OP-PCP graduates must be competent in identifying when a patient problem requires consultation with or referral to a member of a different health profession.
CS 2-19	**Graduates must be competent in applying the basic principles and philosophies of practice management, models of oral healthcare delivery, and how to function successfully as the leader of the oral healthcare team.**
PCS 2-19-1	OP-PCP graduates must be competent in accessing and documenting patient information in medical and dental records.
PCS 2-19-2	OP-PCP graduates must be competent in describing how to use medical and dental billing to receive compensation for patient care, as allowed by the laws of the state.
CS 2-20	**Graduates must be competent in communicating and collaborating with other members of the healthcare team to facilitate the provision of healthcare.**
PCS 2-20-1	OP-PCP graduates must be competent in comparing and contrasting the scope of licensure, roles, and responsibilities of the dentist working as a primary care provider with that of the medical doctor, the physician assistant, the nurse, the nurse practitioner, and the pharmacist.
PCS 2-20-2	OP-PCP graduates must be competent in participating in an interprofessional team approach that integrates oral health for the promotion and maintenance of overall health, and the prevention and treatment of disease.
PCS 2-20-3	OP-PCP graduates must be competent in accessing and documenting patient care and communications in medical or dental health records in an organized, accurate, and complete manner.
PCS 2-20-4	OP-PCP graduates must be competent in performing and documenting clear and concise referrals and consultations with other health professionals and follow up in a timely manner.
PCS 2-20-5	OP-PCP graduates must be competent in negotiating consensus on a shared plan of treatment with the other members of the interprofessional healthcare team.

(Continued)

TABLE 1 | Continued

STD number	CODA Standard (CS) and Proposed Competency Statements (PCS)
CS 2-21	**Graduates must be competent in the application of the principles of ethical decision making and professional responsibility.**
PCS 2-21-1	OP-PCP graduates must be competent in describing the ADA ethical principles and applying them to patient cases involving interprofessional healthcare.
CS 2-22	**Graduates must be competent to access, critically appraise, apply, and communicate scientific and lay literature as it relates to providing evidence-based patient care.**
PCS 2-22-1	OP-PCP graduates must be competent in deciding whether new evidence-based advances in biomedical science are pertinent to oral healthcare in their practice, and if they are, creating "best practice" standards which members of their interprofessional health team can use.
PCS 2-22-2	OP-PCP graduates must be competent in explaining evidence-based oral healthcare decisions and policies to their patients and interprofessional colleagues in terms they can understand.
CS 2-23	**Graduates must be competent in providing oral healthcare within the scope of general dentistry to patients in all stages of life.**
PCS 2-23-1	OP-PCP graduates must be competent in assessing the systemic and oral health of infant, child, adolescent, adult, pregnant, and geriatric patients.
PCS 2-23-2	OP-PCP graduates must be competent in provision of appropriate preventive counseling and referrals for the systemic health needs of infant, child, adolescent, adult, pregnant, and geriatric patients.
CS 2-25	**Graduates must be competent in assessing the treatment needs of patients with special needs.**
PCS 2-25	OP-PCP graduates must be competent in assessing the unique care, communication, psychosocial and diagnostic considerations, and treatment needs of patients of any ability, gender, sex, or age, within the scope of general dentistry.
PCS 2-25-1	OP-PCP graduates must be competent in explaining how patients' lives have been shaped by both biologic and psychosocial factors and identify aspects of the patient's abilities and needs that require special consideration by the oral and/or general health team.
PCS 2-25-2	OP-PCP graduates must be competent in identifying and following legal guidelines for reporting neglect and/or abuse of people with intellectual and/or developmental disabilities, special physical health needs, children, elders, and other vulnerable people.
PCS 2-25-3	OP-PCP graduates must be competent in providing a safe and comfortable clinical atmosphere for all patients.
PCS 2-25-4	OP-PCP graduates must be competent in serving patients with special health and/ or psychosocial needs and considerations as the oral health expert on the healthcare team.
CS 2-26	**Dental education programs must make available opportunities and encourage students to engage in service learning experiences and/or community-based learning experiences.**
PCS 2-26	OP-PCP graduates must be competent in serving on the healthcare team in a community-based setting as a primary care dentist or as a general dentist, in order to appropriately assess and address the healthcare needs of patients, and to promote and advance the health of populations.
PCS 2-26-1	OP-PCP graduates must be competent in functioning as a team member in a primary care setting, adapting to the role of dentist or primary care dentist as patient, community, and clinic needs dictate.

Distribution of support for the proposed OP-PCP competency statements showed general acceptance by the experts (**Figure 1**). Diversity of opinion occurred in some proposals associated with CODA Standard 2-24. The broadest range of opinion was seen with alternative competency statements proposed within Standard 2-24-A-1. Respondents considered how far they recommended OP-PCPs should develop skills in patient assessment, especially concerning use of an otoscope (2-24-A-1g) or stethoscope (2-24-A-1i, k, and n), assessing the abdomen (2_24-A-1n and o) or limbs (2-24-A-1n), or performing a peripheral neurologic examination (2-24-A-1q).

Respondents provided 261 comments. Fifty percent were editorial directions, including recommendations for wordsmithing or combining the proposal with another or grouping it with a different CODA standard. Twenty six percent were affirmative statements, agreeing with the proposal. Twenty four percent were conceptual/contextual observations or questions. This third group of comments revealed lack of uniformity in current dental education. Some commentators said certain suggested skills are already being taught and assessed at some dental schools, while others commented that those same skills are unrealistic to teach or impossible to assess. Respondents mentioned obstacles such as scope of practice, lack of time in the curriculum, and challenges in achieving appropriate levels of competency.

Illustrative and notable comment examples particularly occurred regarding 2.24. Proposal 2.24A.1 suggests various elements of an expanded physical examination. One expert commented on their agreement with the entire list, "This will be a big part of training." Another agreed that OP-PCPs should learn to examine the abdomen and commented: "Yes, any relation to having swallowed crown etc.,?" A third's comment on examining the limbs was: "Yes, visual, only if exposed," meaning that the OP-PCP should not, for example, pull up a patient's sleeves or pant legs to examine their patient's arms or legs for dermatologic features supporting a diagnosis of lichen planus or lupus erythematosus.

Proposal 2.24D.1 is that OP-PCP be competent to *provide health promotion and disease prevention plans, strategies, and interventions for oral diseases and for common major systemic diseases*. Comments included, "I am not sure about breadth here either," "I agree with all except interventions for major systemic diseases. This is where referral comes in," and "As written–implies responsibility to treat primarily major systemic

TABLE 2 | CODA Standard (CS) 2-24 only, and related Proposed Competency Statements (PCS) for Oral Physician – Oral Health Primary Care Provider (OP-PCP).

STD number	CODA Standard (CS) and Proposed Competency Statements (PCS)
CS 2-24	**At a minimum, graduates must be competent in providing oral healthcare within the scope of general dentistry, as defined by the school, including:**
CS 2-24 PART A	**… patient assessment, diagnosis, comprehensive treatment planning, prognosis, and informed consent**
PCS 2-24A-1	OP-PCP graduates must be competent in gathering information about the patient and their health including: a. Expanded patient interview b. Generally assess patient status c. Assess of mental status (orientation x 4) d. Assess weight + BMI e. Review medical + dental health records f. Examine skin of face + neck g. Examine head, neck, nose, eyes, ears, throat, + neck *with* the use of specialized equipment (i.e. otoscope) h. Examine head, neck, nose, eyes, ears, throat, + neck *without* the use of specialized equipment i. Assess respiration *with* stethoscope j. Assess respiration *without* stethoscope k. Assess heart *with* stethoscope l. Assess heart *without* stethoscope m. No assessment of abdomen n. Assess abdomen *with* palpation, *with* stethoscope o. Assess abdomen *with* palpation, *without* stethoscope p. Assess limbs q. Peripheral neurologic examination
PCS 2-24A-2	OP-PCP graduates must be competent in selecting, obtaining, and interpreting appropriate clinical tests, blood tests, and diagnostic imaging including salivary testing and assessment, glucose testing, A1C testing, and others as appropriate, including rapid testing for HIV with referral for confirmation and appropriate behavior counseling.
PCS 2-24A-3	OP-PCP graduates must be competent in screening and providing basic counseling and referral for diseases and conditions such as (but not necessarily limited to) these examples listed below: *Blood and Immune:* allergic diseases; anemias; benign and malignant vascular tumors; bleeding disorders; HIV and other immune deficiencies; Kaposi sarcoma; leukemia; lymphoma; neutropenia; polycythemia; others. *Cardiovascular:* angina; arrhythmia; carotid artery calcification; dyslipidemia; hypertension; MI; stroke; transient ischemic attack; others. *Endocrine:* adrenal disease; diabetes mellitus (Perform chairside glucose, a1c); multiple endocrine neoplasia; polycystic ovarian syndrome; obesity; parathyroid pathology; thyroid pathology; Turner syndrome; others. *Genetic and Developmental:* inherited diseases and syndromes, especially those with craniofacial manifestations. *Genitourinary/Breast:* benign prostatic hyperplasia; breast health; candidiasis; family planning; herpes; HPV infection; kidney failure; kidney disease; prenatal care; prostate cancer; renal osteodystrophy; sexually transmitted infections of the oral cavity; urinary frequency; urinary tract infection; others. *Gastrointestinal:* atrophic gastritis; Barrett's esophagus; celiac disease; dysphagia; Gardner syndrome; GERD; inflammatory bowel diseases; others. *Hepatobiliary:* gallstones; hepatitis; jaundice; liver failure; pancreatitis; others. *Musculoskeletal:* bone fractures; bone tumors; muscle tumors; muscular dystrophy; osteogenesis imperfecta; osteopetrosis; osteoporosis; Paget disease; syndromes; others. *Nervous system:* cranial nerve defects; dementia; multiple sclerosis; nerve sheath tumors; neurodegenerative diseases; sensory disorders; syndromes; others. *Psychiatric:* anxiety and depression; cognitive disorders; eating disorders; psychiatric disorders; substance use disorders; suicidal ideation; others. *Respiratory:* asthma; COPD; lung malignancy; oropharyngeal and pharyngeal malignancy; sinonasal polyps; sinusitis; sleep apnea; others. *Dermatologic:* acne; actinic damage; allergic conditions; esthetics; rosacea; skin cancers; syndromes; vesiculobullous diseases; others. *Social:* food insecurity; gender identity dysphoria; homelessness; sexual, physical, self, or emotional abuse; others.
CS 2-24 PART B	**… screening and risk assessment for head and neck cancer**
PCS 2-24B-1	OP-PCP graduates must be competent in selecting and applying diagnostic tests for oral conditions.
PCS 2-24B-2	OP-PCP graduates must be competent in selecting, performing, and submitting simple oral biopsies.
PCS 2-24B-3	OP-PCP graduates must be competent in working with the oncology team to prevent and manage the oral complications of cancer treatment, including chemotherapy, immunotherapy, and radiotherapy.

(Continued)

TABLE 2 | Continued

STD number	CODA Standard (CS) and Proposed Competency Statements (PCS)
CS 2-24 PART C	**... recognizing the complexity of patient treatment and identifying when referral is indicated**
PCS 2-24C-1	OP-PCP graduates must be competent in using a systematic approach to identify a potential systemic condition and identify when consultation or referral is appropriate.
CS 2-24 PART D	**... health promotion and disease prevention**
PCS 2-24D-1	OP-PCP graduates must be competent in providing health promotion and disease prevention plans, strategies, and interventions for oral diseases and for common major systemic diseases.
PCS 2-24D-2	OP-PCP graduates must be competent in providing basic nutritional, safety, and other lifestyle counseling, including administration of vaccinations where permitted by law.
PCS 2-24D-3	OP-PCP graduates must be competent in screening and providing interventions and prevention for patients with addictions and drug dependency, including alcohol, nicotine, and opioids. This includes recommendations regarding availability of opioid reversal agents.
PCS 2-24D-4	OP-PCP graduates must be competent in assessing the patient's medication profile to achieve medication optimization, including consultation with pharmacists, and refer for adjustment of medications not prescribed by dentists.
PCS 2-24D-5	OP-PCP graduates must be competent in detecting and managing patient abuse and neglect, and contributing to prevention efforts.
PCS 2-24D-6	OP-PCP graduates must be competent in functioning effectively as a medical team member in disaster relief efforts.
CS 2-24 PART E	**... local anesthesia, and pain and anxiety control, including consideration of the impact of prescribing practices and substance use disorder**
PCS 2-24E-1	OP-PCP graduates must be competent in diagnosis, prevention, and management of substance use disorder, including that which may arise in association with prescribing practices.

diseases–practicing medicine under current laws." Similarly, 2.24D.4 proposes that OP-PCP be competent to *assess the patient's medication profile to achieve medication optimization, including consultation with pharmacists, and refer for adjustment of medications not prescribed by dentists.* One expert's reaction was, "Too far outside scope." 2.24D.6 proposes that OP-PCP be competent to *function effectively as a medical team member in disaster relief efforts.* One expert commented, "Already should be doing this." Another commented "Must define the role. They cannot do emergency amputations, for example, ☺ [sic]. Need to define this carefully."

Proposal 2.24B.3 for OP-PCP competency is to *work with the oncology team to prevent and manage the oral complications of cancer treatment, including chemotherapy, immunotherapy, and radiotherapy.* One comment hinted at potential for antagonism between specialists and those choosing expanded scope of practice for OP-PCPs: "This is now overlapping with the specialty of Oral Medicine."

DISCUSSION

Expert opinion indicated proposed OP-PCP training is rooted in existing ADEA, CODA, and IPEC competencies, especially interprofessional practice. Experts supported teaching and assessing these skills within the existing framework of pre-doctoral dental education, and felt it was realistic to do so to the "competency" level. They agreed OP-PCPs would require extra education in critical thinking, patient assessment, diagnosis and treatment planning, prevention and health promotion, medical management of conditions already within the scope of dental care, and in certain primary care medical tasks. The respondent's comments, made in 2018, demonstrated a lack of agreement on some details related to scope of practice.

But factors beyond expert opinion are also influencing the practice of dentistry and the shape of dental education. Changes wrought by the pandemic and the evolving recognition of oral-systemic interactions (3, 50) support increased interest in expanding the role of dentists. A growing emphasis on IPE and integration of oral health into primary care is evident in curriculum development, specific funding programs, and other efforts (51–55). Ongoing changes in dentistry and dental education are in keeping with these OP-PCP competency statement proposals: 2.20.2, *participate in an interprofessional team approach that integrates oral health for the promotion and maintenance of overall health, and the prevention and treatment of disease*; 2.24D.2, *perform basic nutritional, safety, and other lifestyle counseling, including administration of vaccinations where permitted by law*; and 2.24D.6, *function effectively as medical team members in disaster relief efforts.*

Barriers to Change: Market Factors

Difficulty obtaining compensation for medical screening and counseling could potentially discourage dentists from primary care despite the obvious benefits to patient's health. Medical insurance coding is different from the claims coding used in dental insurance (56). The range of allowable diagnoses and procedures that can be billed to medical insurance is limited (57). Even if dentists could potentially bill medical insurance for some services, they and their staff are usually not trained to do so. Without compensation, dentists could not feasibly screen for hypertension, diabetes, obesity, missed vaccinations, and other timely primary care tasks. Therefore, Proposal 2-19-2 is that *OP-PCP graduates must be competent in describing how to use medical and dental billing to receive compensation for patient care, as allowed by the laws of the state.* Medical insurers would also need to be willing to compensate them for these additional services.

TABLE 3 | Characteristics of respondents.

Characteristics of respondents	*N*	Percentage
Total	**23**	**100%**
Sex		
Female	12	52.2%
Male	11	47.8%
Geographic location		
US East Coast	5	21.7%
Mid-US	9	39.1%
US West Coast	8	34.8%
Non-North American	1	4.3%
Professional Field		
Dentistry	18	78.2%
Anesthesiology	1	4.3%
Dental Hygiene	1	4.3%
Dental Public Health	2	8.7%
General Practice Dentist	4	17.4%
Oral Medicine w/wo Oral Radiology	4	17.4%
Oral Pathology w/wo Pediatric Dentistry	5	21.7%
Pediatric Dentistry	1	4.3%
Non-Dentistry	5	21.7%
Medicine (GI, Internal Med, Pediatrics, Psych)	4	17.4%
Educational Psychology	1	4.3%
Academic Role		
Administrator	14	60.9%
Faculty Member	9	39.1%
Survey Method		
Written Form	11	47.8%
Email Contact	7	30.4%
Verbal Interview	5	21.7%

Integrated dental and medical systems may provide the ideal setting for the OP-PCP (14, 54, 58–61). Large systems can institute value-based care models that incentivize desired changes; such models already occur in the dental marketplace. The rise of dental service organizations can also facilitate value-based changes, and their acquisition by larger health insurers. Larger health systems can feature interoperable electronic health records (E.H.R.) which improve collaboration and communication, reduce discrepancies and misunderstandings, and facilitate medical billing for dental care (62). Proposals 2-20-1, 2-20-2, 2-20-3, 2-20-4, and 2-20-5 describe competencies an OP-PCP must have to function successfully in such an integrated care setting.

Barriers to Change: Professional Identity

The self-identity of dentists is a barrier to change, whether by a new label or changing dentist's roles without re-branding them (63, 64). The increasing medical complexity of patients and broad calls for action to address systemic conditions such as hypertension (65) and diabetes (66) point to issues in which dentists could play a larger role. Nevertheless, dentistry retains a relative emphasis on technical skills (evident in the lengthy

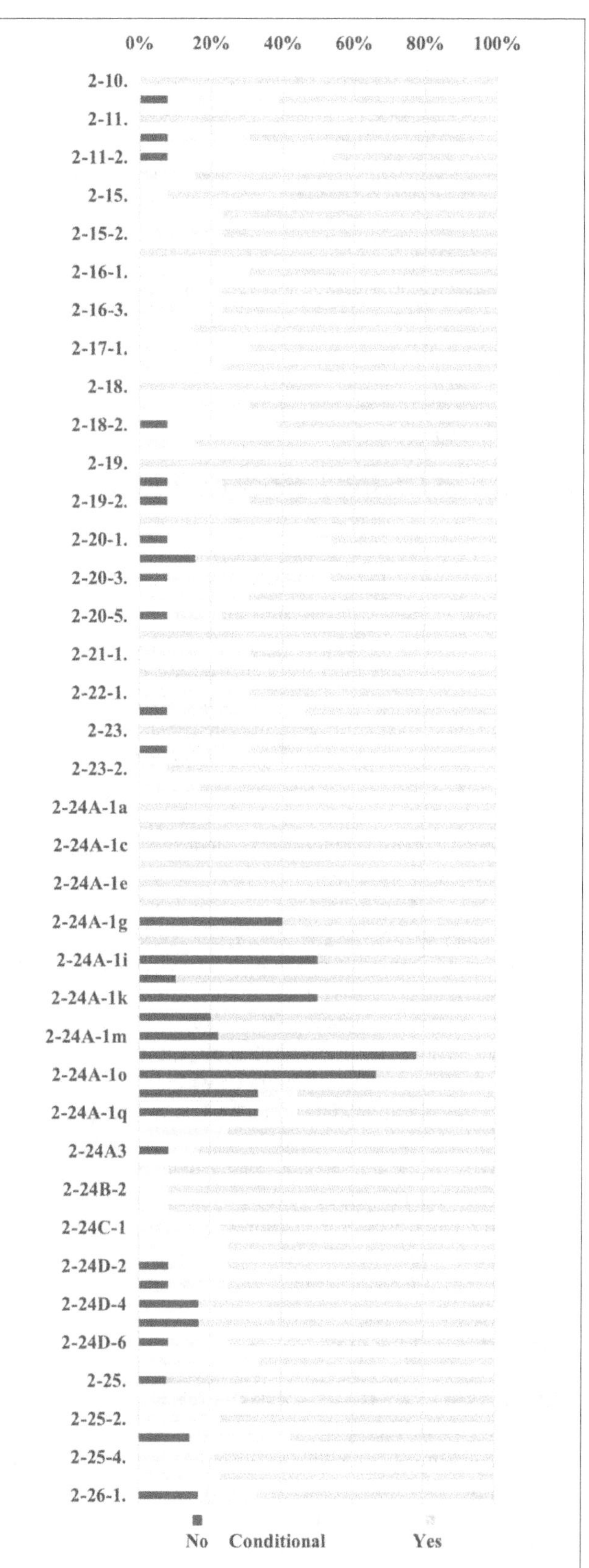

FIGURE 1 | Distribution of support for Proposed Competency Statements (PCS) for OP-PCP related to CODA Predoctoral Standards 2–10 to 2–26 [-separate file].

CODA Standard 2-24). Reluctance to cut any traditional skills to make way for new ones is likely.

It may be more difficult to convince dental students of the value of OP-PCPs than it would be to convince their patients (21, 36, 67, 68). Students enter school with expectations about being a dentist that don't include "primary care" tasks. They may say to themselves, "If I wanted to do that, I would have gone to medical school" (63, 64). Over the years, ADEA student surveys have shown that the top reasons students choose dentistry are personal dental experiences (54%), the influence of a family member or friend who is a dentist (38%) and the influence of their family dentist (33%) (69). Current models of dental practice, which have been slow to change, set expectations for students. However, recent events described already could influence a change in public and student expectations.

Barriers to Change: Cost of Dental Education

Given the high costs of dental education (reflected in tuition and high student debt), funding new programs will always be challenging. Dental school clinics operate primarily to train students and require a high faculty-to-student ratio. This model is less fiscally efficient than medical training that is embedded within hospitals and other clinical practice sites.

Dental schools are also typically safety net providers. While Medicaid covers pediatric dental care, adult dental benefits under Medicaid vary substantially between states, some states lacking them entirely. When money is tight, states often discontinue adult dental benefits. Traditional Medicare has no general dental benefit and Medicare Advantage Plans vary in coverage. Dental residencies with significant hospital-based training such as oral surgery or pediatric dentistry receive Graduate Medical Education (GME) funding but that money goes primarily to the hospitals, not the hospitals (70).

Students may be reluctant to participate in OP-PCP training if it would require additional time in dental school because 83% of dental students graduate with educational debt, averaging $304,824 in 2020 (71). Therefore, this proposal adapts predoctoral education within existing length of training. IPE could also advance this goal. If medical, dental, and nursing students all learned blood pressure measurement together, they would have greater confidence in each other's skills as future health professionals. Among others, Proposal 2-11-2, *educate others about health, including clinicians from other health professions, using critical thinking and feedback techniques* promotes this collaboration.

Barriers to Change: Scope of Practice

State laws govern the scope of practice of dentistry and other health professions. Changes in law allow healthcare practitioners, including faculty and students under their supervision, to perform tasks such as vaccinations and point of care diagnostic testing and counseling for systemic diseases (19).

For an expanded scope of dental practice to be successfully implemented, the profession would need to clearly define the desired scope of practice for the OP-PCP and achieve consensus on that definition. As Mathews [(72) Mathews 2010] mentions, this requires buy-in from all specialties. It would also be more likely to succeed if the change were supported by medical colleagues and those in other health professions. Such a conversation needs to begin somewhere, and the proposals presented to the experts in this project were aimed to begin such a discussion. Standard 2–24, the group of competency statements that lists specific clinical procedures, sparked the greatest diversity of opinion among the experts, as it was designed to do. Examples of comments provided by the experts, shared in the results, illustrate the need for further discussion and consensus on the scope of practice. Issues to be addressed include boundaries with dental specialties and other healthcare professions. Graduates would need to be cognizant of those limits, hence Proposal 2-18-1 is that *OP-PCP graduates must be competent in describing the boundaries between dental and medical licensure.*

Of relevance, historical changes that allowed advanced practice registered nurses (APRNs) and nurse practitioners (NP) in several states to be recognized as primary care providers are instructive. Such changes occurred in Massachusetts through legislation that recognized NPs as primary care providers (73). In Hawai'i, APRNs successfully introduced legislation to remove "barriers to full utilization of APRNs as primary healthcare providers with global signature authority and with prescriptive authority for controlled substances, medical equipment and therapeutic regimens in accordance with their scope of practice" (72). Key factors for a successful collaborative initiative were a comprehensive approach including all APRN specialties; key political champions who grasped the healthcare issues; the excellent reputation of APRNs; continuous communication and willingness to compromise on issues; and the support of nursing educators (72).

Limitations

This assessment is limited in its very nature, by design. Baseline expert opinion is challenging to acquire, especially using a grassroots, unfunded mechanism, yet it is valid to elicit opinions from a group of experts at the beginning of a bold new educational endeavor. The convenience sample is not generalizable to "population" but represents a valuable range of opinions. The expert opinion participant group had representation from females, males, deans, faculty members, and experts with geographic dispersion. The group included various ADA recognized dental specialty areas (74) whose definitions emphasize focus on patients or populations as opposed to procedures or specific anatomy.

Limitations of expert opinion are multifold. Foremost is the reliance on opinion versus synthesis of peer-reviewed scientific evidence. A high level of consensus was achieved in this one-round process, lending prima facie credibility to the findings. Nevertheless, this expert opinion assessment's function is simply to provide a starting point from which to define competencies for the OP-PCP, as demonstrated in similar processes in other professions (75). Further independent work based on this study is needed to progress toward finalizing OP-PCP educational competencies.

Next Steps

To become competent OP-PCPs, dental students would need authentic clinical experiences (76). Thus IPE must extend beyond didactic, simulation, and project-based learning, to include immersion in authentic collaborative clinical care settings where dentists function as OP-PCP (76–78).

Dental educators would need appropriate knowledge, skills, and attitudes to teach potential OP-PCPs. Many dental specialists in oral medicine, oral pathology, and oral surgery already have this expertise. Collaboration with other health professions education programs could help meet this need. Video teleconferencing could allow for more efficient faculty development across sites (76, 77).

Pilot projects could tackle key questions related to the modified curriculum's effectiveness and financial viability. Endpoints should include outcome measures that are student-centered (i.e., pass rates on national licensure examinations or alumni surveys), patient-centered (i.e., satisfaction of patients treated by these students), clinic-centered (i.e., satisfaction of health professionals who work with these students), finance-centered (i.e., differences in their clinical productivity as well as added training costs), and eventually community-centered (for example, improved healthcare outcomes in populations treated by these students and graduates).

CONCLUSIONS

No previous efforts have defined additional spheres of competency that should be required for dentists to function as OP-PCPs. These initial findings by 23 experts provide a platform for further discussion and action among dental and medical educators, policymakers, funders, health systems, patient groups and others. The healthcare system could gain high-quality capacity by using dentists as primary care providers within the scope of dental licensure to improve oral and overall health outcomes and achieve health equity.

AUTHOR CONTRIBUTIONS

SG conceived and designed the study and wrote the first draft of the competency statements and questionnaire. JB and WM reviewed the study design. LK, WM, PB, and CM-K reviewed the competency statements and questionnaire. SG recruited participants and collected comments. LK organized the database and analysis. SG and LK wrote the introduction, methods, results, and conclusions. SG, LK, and WM wrote the abstract. WM, PB, JB, and CM-K wrote sections of the discussion. LK, WM, and SG contributed to manuscript revision. All authors read and approved the submitted version.

REFERENCES

1. Myers-Wright N, Lamster IB. A new practice approach for oral health professionals. *J Evid Based Dent Pract.* (2016) (Suppl. 16):43–51. doi: 10.1016/j.jebdp.2016.01.027
2. Nasseh K, Vujicic M, Glick M. The relationship between periodontal interventions and healthcare costs and utilization. Evidence from an integrated dental, medical, and pharmacy commercial claims database. *Health Econ.* (2017) 26:519–27. doi: 10.1002/hec.3316
3. Borgnakke WS, Poudel P. Diabetes and oral health: summary of current scientific evidence for why transdisciplinary collaboration is needed. *Front Dent Med.* (2021) 2:709831. doi: 10.3389/fdmed.2021.709831
4. Kleinman DV, Horowitz AM, Atchison KA. A framework to foster oral health literacy and oral/general health integration. *Front Dent Med.* (2021) 2:723021. doi: 10.3389/fdmed.2021.723021
5. Nasseh K, Greenberg B, Vujicic M, Glick M. The effect of chairside chronic disease screenings by oral health professionals on healthcare costs. *Am J Public Health.* (2014) 104:744–50. doi: 10.2105/AJPH.2013.301644
6. National Prevention, Health Promotion and Public Health Council. *National Prevention Strategy.* Washington, DC: U.S. Department of Health and Human Services, Office of the Surgeon General (2011). Available online at: https://www.hhs.gov/sites/default/files/disease-prevention-wellness-report.pdf (accessed April 27, 2021).
7. Joskow CR. Integrating oral health and primary care: federal initiatives to drive systems change. *Dent Clin North Am.* (2016) 60:951–68. doi: 10.1016/j.cden.2016.05.010
8. American State and Territorial Dental Directors (ASTDD). *White Paper: Opportunities to Improving Oral Health and Chronic Disease Program Collaboration and Medical-Dental Integration.* (2018). Available online at: https://www.astdd.org/docs/opportunities-for-improving-oh-and-cd-integration-white-paper.pdf (accessed September 23, 2021).
9. Somerman M, Mouradian WE. Field grand challenge: integrating oral and systemic health: innovations in transdisciplinary science, healthcare and policy. *Front Dent Med.* (2020) 1:15. doi: 10.3389/fdmed.2020.599214
10. Commission on Dental Accreditation (CODA). *Accreditation standards for dental education programs.* Chicago: American Dental Association 2018. Available online at: https://www.ada.org/~/media/CODA/Files/predoc_standards.pdf?la=en
11. Glurich I, Berg R, Panny A, Shimpi N, Steinmetz A, Nycz G, et al. Longitudinal observation or outcomes and patient access to integrated care following point-of-care glycemic screening in community health center dental safety net clinics. *Front Oral Health.* (2021) 2:670355. doi: 10.3389/froh.2021.670355
12. MacNeil RL, Hilario H. Input from practice: reshaping dental education for integrated patient care. *Front Oral Health.* (2021) 2:659030. doi: 10.3389/froh.2021.659030
13. Mays KA. Designing oral health curriculum that facilitates greater integration of oral health into overall health. *Front Dent Med.* (2021) 2:680520. doi: 10.3389/fdmed.2021.680520
14. Mosen DM, Banegas MP, Dickerson JF, Fellows JL, Pihlstrom DJ, Kershah HM, et al. Evaluating the effectiveness of medical-dental integration to close preventive and disease management care gaps. *Front Dent Med.* (2021) 2:670012. doi: 10.3389/fdmed.2021.670012
15. Mouradian W, Lee J, Wilentz J, Somerman M A perspective: integrating dental and medical research improved overall health. *Front Dent Med.* (2021) 2:699575. doi: 10.3389/fdmed.2021.699575
16. Nash DA. The oral physician. creating a new oral health professional for a new century. *J Dent Educ.* (1995) 59:587–97. doi: 10.1002/j.0022-0337.1995.59.5.tb02949.x
17. Giddon DB, Swann B, Donoff RB, Hertzman-Miller R. Dentists as oral physicians: the overlooked primary healthcare resource. *J Prim Prev.* (2013) 34:279–91. doi: 10.1007/s10935-013-0310-7
18. Kaste LM, Wilder JR, Halpern LR. Emerging topics for dentists as primary care providers. *Dent Clin North Am.* (2013) 57:371–6. doi: 10.1016/j.cden.2013.02.002
19. American Dental Association. *Dentists: Doctors of Oral Health.* Available online at: https://www.ada.org/en/about-the-ada/dentists-doctors-of-oral-health (accessed April 27, 2021).
20. Gordon SC, Beemsterboer P, Berg J, Kaste LM, Murdoch-Kinch CA, Mouradian W. *The Other Doctors: Dentists in Primary Care.* Philadelphia, PA: Executive Leadership in Academic Medicine 2018 Leadership Forum (2018).
21. Barasch A, Safford MM, Qvist V, Palmore R, Gesko D, Gilbert GH. Random blood glucose testing in dental practice: a community-based feasibility study from the dental practice-based research network. *J Am Dent Assoc.* (2012) 143:262–9. doi: 10.14219/jada.archive.2012.0151

22. Herman WH, Taylor GW, Jacobson JJ, Burke R, Brown MB. Screening for prediabetes and type 2 diabetes in dental offices. *J Public Health Dent.* (2015) 75:175–82. doi: 10.1111/jphd.12082
23. Glurich I, Bartkowiak B, Berg RL, Acharya A. Screening for dysglycaemia in dental primary care practice settings: systematic review of the evidence. *Int Dent J.* (2018) 68:369–77. doi: 10.1111/idj.12405
24. Grigoriadis A, Räisänen IT, Pärnänen P, Tervahartiala T, Sorsa T, Sakellari D. Prediabetes/diabetes screening strategy at the periodontal clinic. *Clin Exp Dent Res.* (2021) 7:85–92. doi: 10.1002/cre2.338
25. Glick M, Greenberg BL. The potential role of dentists in identifying patients' risk of experiencing coronary heart disease events. *J Am Dent Assoc.* (2005) 136:1541–6. doi: 10.14219/jada.archive.2005.0084
26. Jontell M, Glick M. Oral healthcare professionals' identification of cardiovascular disease risk among patients in private practice in Sweden. *J Am Dent Assoc.* (2009) 140:385–91. doi: 10.14219/jada.archive.2009.0075
27. Singer RH, Feaster DJ, Stoutenberg M, Hlaing WM, Pereyra M, Abel S, et al. Dentist's willingness to screen for cardiovascular disease in the dental care setting: Findings from a nationally representative survey. *Community Dent Oral Epidemiol.* (2019) 47:299–308. doi: 10.1111/cdoe.12457
28. Parish CL, Pereyra MR, Pollack HA, Cardenas G, Castellon PC, Abel SN, et al. Screening for substance misuse in the dental care setting: findings from a nationally representative survey of dentists. *Addiction.* (2015) 110:1516–23. doi: 10.1111/add.13004
29. Davis JM, Arnett MR, Loewen J, Romito L, Gordon SC. Tobacco dependence education: A survey of US and Canadian dental schools. *J Am Dent Assoc.* (2016) 147:405–12. doi: 10.1016/j.adaj.2015.12.012
30. Faine MP. Recognition and management of eating disorders in the dental office. *Dent Clin North Am.* (2003) 47:395–410. doi: 10.1016/S0011-8532(02)00108-8
31. Debate RD, Tedesco LA. Increasing dentists' capacity for secondary prevention of eating disorders: identification of training, network, and professional contingencies. *J Dent Educ.* (2006) 70:1066–75. doi: 10.1002/j.0022-0337.2006.70.10.tb04179.x
32. Bhandari M, Dosanjh S, Tornetta P. 3rd, Matthews D. Violence Against Women Health Research Collaborative Musculoskeletal manifestations of physical abuse after intimate partner violence. *J Trauma.* (2006) 61:1473–9. doi: 10.1097/01.ta.0000196419.36019.5a
33. Tam S, Joyce D, Gerber MR, Tan A. Head and neck injuries in adult victims of intimate-partner violence. *J Otolaryngol Head Neck Surg.* (2010) 39:737–43.
34. Femi-Ajao O. Perception of women with lived experience of domestic violence and abuse on the involvement of the dental team in supporting adult patients with lived experience of domestic abuse in England: a pilot study. *Int J Environ Res Public Health.* (2021) 18:2024. doi: 10.3390/ijerph18042024
35. Greenberg BL, Glick M, Frantsve-Hawley J, Kantor ML. Dentist's attitudes toward chairside screening for medical conditions. *J Am Dent Assoc.* (2010) 141:52–62. doi: 10.14219/jada.archive.2010.0021
36. Andrews EA. The future of interprofessional education and practice for dentists and dental education. *J Dent Educ.* (2017) 81:eS186–92. doi: 10.21815/JDE.017.026
37. Bin Mubayrik A, Al Dosary S, Alshawaf R, Alduweesh R, Alfurayh S, Alojaymi T, et al. Public attitudes toward chairside screening for medical conditions in dental settings. *Patient Prefer Adherence.* (2021) 15:187–95. doi: 10.2147/PPA.S297882
38. Burger D. *Dentists Administering Vaccines Gaining Acceptance in States.* ADA News (2021). Available online at: https://www.ada.org/en/publications/ada-news/2021-archive/february/dentists-administering-vaccines-gaining-acceptance-in-states (accessed September 30, 2021).
39. Dental Quality Assurance Commission. *Coronavirus Screening in Dental Offices. State of Washington Department of Health.* (2020). Available online at: https://www.doh.wa.gov/Portals/1/Documents/2300/2020/COVID-DentalCommScreening.pdf (accessed April 23, 2021).
40. Dental Quality Assurance Commission. *Novel Coronavirus Disease 2019 (COVID-19) Vaccine Ordering and Administration.* (2021). Available online at: https://www.doh.wa.gov/Portals/1/Documents/2300/CovidVaccineIS.pdf (accessed April 23, 2021).
41. Colvard MD, Vesper BJ, Kaste LM, Hirst JL, Peters DE, James J, et al. 3rd. The evolving role of dental responders on interprofessional emergency response teams. *Dent Clin North Am.* (2016) 60:907–20. doi: 10.1016/j.cden.2016.05.008
42. Oregon Immunization Program. *Immunization Information for Dentists.* Available online at: https://www.oregon.gov/oha/PH/PREVENTIONWELLNESS/VACCINESIMMUNIZATION/IMMUNIZATIONPROVIDERRESOURCES/Pages/Dentists.aspx (accessed April 25, 2021).
43. White House. *Fact Sheet: President Biden Expands Efforts to Recruit More Vaccinators.* (2021). Available online at: https://www.whitehouse.gov/briefing-room/statements-releases/2021/03/12/fact-sheet-president-biden-expands-efforts-to-recruit-more-vaccinators (accessed April 23, 2021).
44. American Dental Education Association. *Key Takeaways from the 2021 Annual Session and Exhibit.* (2021). Available online at: https://www.adea.org/uploadedFiles/ADEA/Content_Conversion/2021Annual_Session/AS21_KeyTakeaways_FINAL.pdf (accessed April 21, 2021).
45. American Dental Education Association. *ADEA Chair of the Board of Directors Symposia.* (2017). Available online at: https://www.adea.org/2016/program/chair-symposia.aspx/ (accessed April 21, 2021).
46. Hujoel PH. Grading the evidence: The core of EBD. *J Evid Base Dent Pract.* (2009) 9:122–4. doi: 10.1016/j.jebdp.2009.06.007
47. Fink A, Kosecoff J, Chassin M, Brook RH. Consensus methods: characteristics and guidelines for use. *Am J Public Health.* (1984) 74:979–83. doi: 10.2105/AJPH.74.9.979
48. American Dental Education Association. Competencies for the new general dentist (as approved by the 2008 ADEA House of Delegates). *J Dent Educ.* (2008) 72: 823– 6. doi: 10.1002/j.0022-0337.2008.72.7.tb04552.x
49. Interprofessional Education Collaborative (IPEC). *Core competencies for interprofessional Collaborative practice: 2016 Update.* Washington, DC: Interprofessional Education Collaborative (2016). Available online at: https://ipec.memberclicks.net/assets/2016-Update.pdf (accessed September 30, 2021).
50. Kleinstein S, Nelson K, Freire M. Inflammatory networks linking oral microbiome with systemic health and disease. *J Dent Res.* (2020) 99:1131–9. doi: 10.1177/0022034520926126
51. Institute of Medicine (IOM). *Advancing Oral Health in America.* Washington, DC: The National Academies Press (2011). Available online at: https://www.hrsa.gov/sites/default/files/publichealth/clinical/oralhealth/advancingoralhealth.pdf (accessed April 27, 2021).
52. Clark M, Quinonez R, Bowser J, Silk H. Curriculum influence on interdisciplinary oral health education and practice. *J Public Health Dent.* (2017) 77:272–82. doi: 10.1111/jphd.12215
53. Park SE, Saldana F, Donoff RB, A. New integrated oral health and primary care education program in the dental student clinic. *J Mass Dent Soc.* (2016) 64:26–30.
54. Atchison KA, Rozier RG, Weintraub, JA. Integration of oral health and primary care: communication, coordination and referral. In: *NAM Perspectives.* Washington, DC: Discussion Paper, National Academy of Medicine (2018). doi: 10.31478/201810e
55. Health Resources and Services Administration (HRSA). *Primary Care Dental Faculty Development Program.* (2021). Available online at: https://www.hrsa.gov/grants/find-funding/hrsa-21-018
56. Napier RH, Bruelheide LS, Demann ET, Haug RH. Insurance billing and coding. *Dent Clin North Am.* (2008) 52:507–27. doi: 10.1016/j.cden.2008.02.008
57. California Dental Association. *Dental Benefit Plans News. Billing Medical Plans for Dental Treatment.* (2016). Available online at: https://www.cda.org/Home/News-and-Events/Newsroom/Article-Details/billing-medical-plans-for-dental-treatment-1 (accessed September 30, 2021).
58. Patel J, Mowery D, Krishnan A, Thyvalikakath T. Assessing information congruence of documented cardiovascular disease between electronic dental and medical records. *AMIA Ann Symp Proc.* (2018) 18:1442–50. Available online at: https://europepmc.org/article/med/30815189
59. MacNeil RL, Hilario H. The case for integrated oral and primary medical healthcare delivery: An introduction to an examination of three engaged healthcare entities. *J Dent Educ.* (2020) 84:917–9. doi: 10.1002/jdd.12286
60. Gesko DS, Worley D, Rindal BD. Creating systems aligned with the triple-aim and value-based care. *J Public Health Dent.* (2020) 80:S109–13. doi: 10.1111/jphd.12409

61. Santa Fe Group Webinar, Hinde W, Irving K, Baenen B; Murphy EA, Stenzel C. *Learning from the Convergence of Medical and Dental Insurance: Who's Driving the Change.* (2021). Available online at: https://santafegroup.org/webinars/learning-from-the-convergence-of-medical-and-dental-insurance-whos-driving-the-change/ (accessed June 30, 2024).
62. Feldman SS, Buchalter S, Hayes LW. Health information technology in healthcare quality and patient safety: literature review. *JMIR Med Inform.* (2018) 6:e10264. Erratum in: *JMIR Med Inform.* (2019) 7:e11320. doi: 10.2196/10264
63. Giddon DB. Should dentists become oral physicians? Yes, dentists should become oral physicians. *J Am Dent Assoc.* (2004) 135:438–49. doi: 10.14219/jada.archive.2004.0208
64. Giddon DB, Donoff RB, Edwards PC, Goldblatt LI. Should dental schools train dentists to routinely provide limited preventive primary medical care? two viewpoints viewpoint 1: dentists should be trained to routinely provide limited preventive primary care viewpoint 2: dentists should be trained in primary care medicine to enable comprehensive patient management within their scope of practice. *J Dent Educ.* (2017) 81:561–70. doi: 10.21815/JDE.016.023
65. Bakris G, Hill M, Mancia G, Steyn K, Black HR, Pickering T, et al. Achieving blood pressure goals globally: five core actions for health-care professionals. A worldwide call to action. *J Hum Hypertens.* (2008) 22:63–70. doi: 10.1038/sj.jhh.1002284
66. Reusch JEB. The Diabetes story: a call to action: 2018 presidential address. *Diabetes Care.* (2019) 42:713–7. doi: 10.2337/dci18-0050
67. Beazoglou TJ, Chen L, Lazar VF, Brown LJ, Ray SC, Heffley DR, et al. Expanded function allied dental personnel and dental practice productivity and efficiency. *J Dent Educ.* (2012) 76:1054–60. doi: 10.1002/j.0022-0337.2012.76.8.tb05358.x
68. Blue CM, Funkhouser DE, Riggs S, Rindal DB, Worley D, Pihlstrom DJ, et al. National Dental PBRN Collaborative Group. Utilization of non-dentist providers and attitudes toward new provider models: findings from the national dental practice-based research network. *J Public Health Dent.* (2013) 73:237–44. doi: 10.1111/jphd.12020
69. Istrate EC, Slapar FJ, Mallarapu M, Stewart DCL, West KP. Dentists of tomorrow 2020: an analysis of the results of the 2020 ADEA survey of U.S. dental school seniors. *J Dent Educ.* (2021) 85:427– 40. doi: 10.1002/jdd.12568
70. Committee on the Governance and Financing of Graduate Medical Education. Board on Healthcare Services. Institute of Medicine. In: Eden J, Berwick D, Wilensky G, editors. *Graduate Medical Education That Meets the Nation's Health Needs.* Washington, DC: National Academies Press (US) (2014). Available online at: https://www.ncbi.nlm.nih.gov/books/NBK248024/ (accessed September 30, 2021).
71. American Dental Education Association. *Trends in Dental Education 2020-21.* (2020). Available online at: https://www.adea.org/DentEdTrends (accessed April 24, 2021).
72. Mathews BP, Boland MG, Kim Stanton B. Removing barriers to APRN practice in the state of Hawai'i. *Policy Polit Nursing Pract.* (2010) 11:260–5. doi: 10.1177/1527154410383158
73. The Medical News. *New Legislation Addresses Massachusetts Primary Crisis.* (2008). Available online at: http://www.news-medical.net/news/2008/11/10/42685.aspx (accessed September 27, 2021).
74. American Dental Association. *Specialty Definitions: Approved and Adopted by the National Commission on Recognition of Dental Specialties and Certifying Boards.* Available online at: https://www.ada.org/en/ncrdscb/dental-specialties/specialty-definitions
75. Janke KK, Kelley KA, Sweet BV, Kuba SE. A modified Delphi process to define competencies for assessment leads supporting a doctor of pharmacy program. *Am J Pharm Educ.* (2016) 80:167. doi: 10.5688/ajpe8010167
76. Donoff RB, Daley GQ. Oral healthcare in the 21st century: It is time for the integration of dental and medical education. *J Dent Educ.* (2020) 84:999–1002. doi: 10.1002/jdd.12191
77. Giddon DB, Seymour BA, Swann B, Anderson NK, Jayaratne YS, Outlaw J, et al. Innovative primary care training: the Cambridge Health Alliance Oral Physician Program. *Am J Public Health.* (2012) 102:e48–9. doi: 10.2105/AJPH.2012.300954
78. MacNeil RL, Hilario H, Ryan MM, Glurich I, Nycz GR, Acharya A. The case for integrated oral and primary medical healthcare delivery: Marshfield Clinic Health System. *J Dent Educ.* (2020) 84:924–31. doi: 10.1002/jdd.12289

Permissions

All chapters in this book were first published by Frontiers; hereby published with permission under the Creative Commons Attribution License or equivalent. Every chapter published in this book has been scrutinized by our experts. Their significance has been extensively debated. The topics covered herein carry significant findings which will fuel the growth of the discipline. They may even be implemented as practical applications or may be referred to as a beginning point for another development.

The contributors of this book come from diverse backgrounds, making this book a truly international effort. This book will bring forth new frontiers with its revolutionizing research information and detailed analysis of the nascent developments around the world.

We would like to thank all the contributing authors for lending their expertise to make the book truly unique. They have played a crucial role in the development of this book. Without their invaluable contributions this book wouldn't have been possible. They have made vital efforts to compile up to date information on the varied aspects of this subject to make this book a valuable addition to the collection of many professionals and students.

This book was conceptualized with the vision of imparting up-to-date information and advanced data in this field. To ensure the same, a matchless editorial board was set up. Every individual on the board went through rigorous rounds of assessment to prove their worth. After which they invested a large part of their time researching and compiling the most relevant data for our readers.

The editorial board has been involved in producing this book since its inception. They have spent rigorous hours researching and exploring the diverse topics which have resulted in the successful publishing of this book. They have passed on their knowledge of decades through this book. To expedite this challenging task, the publisher supported the team at every step. A small team of assistant editors was also appointed to further simplify the editing procedure and attain best results for the readers.

Apart from the editorial board, the designing team has also invested a significant amount of their time in understanding the subject and creating the most relevant covers. They scrutinized every image to scout for the most suitable representation of the subject and create an appropriate cover for the book.

The publishing team has been an ardent support to the editorial, designing and production team. Their endless efforts to recruit the best for this project, has resulted in the accomplishment of this book. They are a veteran in the field of academics and their pool of knowledge is as vast as their experience in printing. Their expertise and guidance has proved useful at every step. Their uncompromising quality standards have made this book an exceptional effort. Their encouragement from time to time has been an inspiration for everyone.

The publisher and the editorial board hope that this book will prove to be a valuable piece of knowledge for researchers, students, practitioners and scholars across the globe.

List of Contributors

Wendy Mouradian
School of Dentistry, University of Washington, Seattle, WA, United States
The Santa Fe Group, New York, United States

Janice Lee
National Institute of Dental and Craniofacial Research, National Institutes of Health, Bethesda, MD, United States

Joan Wilentz
Independent Researcher, New York, United States

Martha Somerman
National Institute of Dental and Craniofacial Research, National Institutes of Health, Bethesda, MD, United States
National Institute of Arthritis and Musculoskeletal and Skin Diseases, National Institutes of Health, Bethesda, MD, United States

Moti Moskovitz, Sarit Faibis and Diana Ram
Department of Pediatric Dentistry, Faculty of Dental Medicine, Hadassah Medical Center, The Hebrew University of Jerusalem, Jerusalem, Israel

Doron Steinberg
Biofilm Research Laboratory, Faculty of Dental Medicine, Institute of Dental Sciences, The Hebrew University of Jerusalem, Jerusalem, Israel

Mira Nassar
Department of Pediatric Dentistry, Faculty of Dental Medicine, Hadassah Medical Center, The Hebrew University of Jerusalem, Jerusalem, Israel
Biofilm Research Laboratory, Faculty of Dental Medicine, Institute of Dental Sciences, The Hebrew University of Jerusalem, Jerusalem, Israel

Nadav Moriel, Avital Cher and Moran Yassour
Microbiology and Molecular Genetics Department, Faculty of Medicine, The Hebrew University of Jerusalem, Jerusalem, Israel

David Zangen
Division of Pediatric Endocrinology, Hadassah Medical Center, The Hebrew University of Jerusalem, Jerusalem, Israel

Ingrid Glurich, Aloksagar Panny, Neel Shimpi and Annie Steinmetz
Center for Oral and Systemic Health, Marshfield Clinic Research Institute, Marshfield, WI, United States

Richard Berg
Office of Research Computing and Analytics, Marshfield Clinic Research Institute, Marshfield, WI, United States

Greg Nycz
Family Health Center of Marshfield, Inc., Marshfield Clinic Health System, Marshfield, WI, United States

Amit Acharya
Center for Oral and Systemic Health, Marshfield Clinic Research Institute, Marshfield, WI, United States
Family Health Center of Marshfield, Inc., Marshfield Clinic Health System, Marshfield, WI, United States
Advocate Aurora Research Institute, LLC, Advocate Aurora Health, Inc., Downers Grove, IL, United States

Eija Könönen and Ulvi K. Gursoy
Institute of Dentistry, University of Turku, Turku, Finland

Noah Fine
Faculty of Dentistry, University of Toronto, Toronto, ON, Canada

Elaine O. C. Cardoso, Michael Goldberg and Howard C. Tenenbaum
Faculty of Dentistry, University of Toronto, Toronto, ON, Canada
Department of Dentistry, Centre for Advanced Dental Research and Care, Mount Sinai Hospital, University of Toronto, Toronto, ON, Canada

Michael Glogauer
Faculty of Dentistry, University of Toronto, Toronto, ON, Canada
Department of Dentistry, Centre for Advanced Dental Research and Care, Mount Sinai Hospital, University of Toronto, Toronto, ON, Canada
University Health Network (UHN), Toronto, ON, Canada

Francis Johnson
Department of Pharmacological Sciences, School of Medicine, Stony Brook University, Stony Brook, NY, United States

Lorne M. Golub
Department of Oral Biology and Pathology, School of Dental Medicine, Stony Brook University, Stony Brook, NY, United States

Vivianne Cruz de Jesus, Kangmin Duan and Prashen Chelikani
Manitoba Chemosensory Biology Research Group, Department of Oral Biology, University of Manitoba, Winnipeg, MB, Canada
Children's Hospital Research Institute of Manitoba (CHRIM), Winnipeg, MB, Canada

Mohd Wasif Khan
Children's Hospital Research Institute of Manitoba (CHRIM), Winnipeg, MB, Canada
Department of Biochemistry and Medical Genetics, University of Manitoba, Winnipeg, MB, Canada

Betty-Anne Mittermuller
Manitoba Chemosensory Biology Research Group, Department of Oral Biology, University of Manitoba, Winnipeg, MB, Canada
Children's Hospital Research Institute of Manitoba (CHRIM), Winnipeg, MB, Canada
Department of Preventive Dental Science, University of Manitoba, Winnipeg, MB, Canada

Pingzhao Hu
Children's Hospital Research Institute of Manitoba (CHRIM), Winnipeg, MB, Canada
Department of Biochemistry and Medical Genetics, University of Manitoba, Winnipeg, MB, Canada
Department of Computer Science, University of Manitoba, Winnipeg, MB, Canada

Robert J. Schroth
Manitoba Chemosensory Biology Research Group, Department of Oral Biology, University of Manitoba, Winnipeg, MB, Canada
Children's Hospital Research Institute of Manitoba (CHRIM), Winnipeg, MB, Canada
Department of Preventive Dental Science, University of Manitoba, Winnipeg, MB, Canada
Department of Pediatrics and Child Health, University of Manitoba, Winnipeg, MB, Canada

David M. Mosen, Matthew P. Banegas, John F. Dickerson, Jeffrey L. Fellows, Jason L. Scott and Erin M. Keast
Center for Health Research, Kaiser Permanente Northwest, Portland, OR, United States

Daniel J. Pihlstrom
Permanente Dental Associates, Portland, OR, United States

Hala M. Kershah
Dental Administration, Kaiser Permanente Northwest, Portland, OR, United States

Jean-Luc C. Mougeot, Micaela F. Beckman, Holden C. Langdon, Michael T. Brennan and Farah K. Bahrani Mougeot
Carolinas Medical Center—Atrium Health, Charlotte, NC, United States

Rajesh V. Lalla
Section of Oral Medicine-University of Connecticut Health, Farmington, CT, United States

Dushanka V. Kleinman
Department of Epidemiology and Biostatistics, School of Public Health, University of Maryland, College Park, MD, United States

Alice M. Horowitz
Department of Behavioral and Community Health, School of Public Health, University of Maryland, College Park, MD, United States

Kathryn A. Atchison
Division of Public Health & Community Dentistry, School of Dentistry, Fielding School of Public Health, University of California, Los Angeles, Los Angeles, CA, United States

Carolina F. F. A. Costa
Instituto de Ciências Biomédicas Abel Salazar, Universidade do Porto, Porto, Portugal
Nephrology & Infectious Diseases R&D Group, INEB - Instituto de Engenharia Biomédica, i3S - Instituto de Investigação e Inovação em Saúde, Universidade do Porto, Porto, Portugal

Andreia Garcia
Nephrology & Infectious Diseases R&D Group, INEB - Instituto de Engenharia Biomédica, i3S - Instituto de Investigação e Inovação em Saúde, Universidade do Porto, Porto, Portugal

Ana Merino-Ribas
Nephrology & Infectious Diseases R&D Group, INEB - Instituto de Engenharia Biomédica, i3S - Instituto de Investigação e Inovação em Saúde, Universidade do Porto, Porto, Portugal
Nephrology Department, Hospital Universitari Doctor Josep Trueta, Girona, Spain

Catarina Ferreira, Raquel B. R. Mesquita, António O. S. S. Rangel and Célia M. Manaia
Universidade Católica Portuguesa, CBQF - Centro de Biotecnologia e Química Fina - Laboratório Associado, Escola Superior de Biotecnologia, Porto, Portugal

Carla Campos
Instituto Português de Oncologia do Porto Francisco Gentil (IPO), Porto, Portugal

Luciano Pereira
Nephrology Department, Centro Hospitalar Universitário de São João, Porto, Portugal
Nephrology & Infectious Diseases R&D Group, INEB - Instituto de Engenharia Biomédica, i3S - Instituto de Investigação e Inovação em Saúde, Universidade do Porto, Porto, Portugal

Nádia Silva
Nephrology Department, Centro Hospitalar Universitário de São João, Porto, Portugal

Benedita Sampaio-Maia
Nephrology & Infectious Diseases R&D Group, INEB - Instituto de Engenharia Biomédica, i3S - Instituto de Investigação e Inovação em Saúde, Universidade do Porto, Porto, Portugal
Faculdade de Medicina Dentária, Universidade do Porto, Porto, Portugal

Álvaro Azevedo
Faculdade de Medicina Dentária, Universidade do Porto, Porto, Portugal
Laboratório para a Investigação Integrativa e Translacional em Saúde Populacional (ITR), Porto, Portugal

Raphael Osugue, Cassia F. Araujo and Mauro P. Santamaria
Division of Periodontics, Institute of Science and Technology, UNESP - São Paulo State University, São José dos Campos, Brazil

Flavio X. de Almeida and Magda Feres
Dental Research Division, Guarulhos University, Guarulhos, Brazil

Nidia C. Castro dos Santos
Division of Periodontics, Institute of Science and Technology, UNESP - São Paulo State University, São José dos Campos, Brazil
Dental Research Division, Guarulhos University, Guarulhos, Brazil

Irene Soffritti, Maria D'Accolti and Elisabetta Caselli
Section of Microbiology, CIAS Research Center and LTTA, Department of Chemical and Pharmaceutical Sciences, University of Ferrara, Ferrara, Italy

Chiara Fabbri and Maurizio Franchi
Section of Dentistry, Department of Biomedical and Specialty Surgical Sciences, University of Ferrara, Ferrara, Italy

Angela Passaro and Giovanni Zuliani
Unit of Internal Medicine, Department of Translational Medicine, University of Ferrara, Ferrara, Italy

Roberto Manfredini
Medical Clinic Unit, Department of Medical Sciences, University of Ferrara, Ferrara, Italy

Marco Libanore
Unit of Infectious Diseases, University Hospital of Ferrara, Ferrara, Italy

Carlo Contini
Section of Infectious Diseases and Dermatology, Department of Medical Sciences, University of Ferrara, Ferrara, Italy

Darya Dabiri, Donya Dabiri and Carol Wiese
Department of Dentistry, Division of Pediatric Dentistry, University of Toledo, Toledo, OH, United States

Samuel Richard Conti and Heather Raquel Conti
Department of Biological Sciences, University of Toledo, Toledo, OH, United States

Niloufar Sadoughi Pour, George Choueiri and Omid Amili
Department of Mechanical, Industrial and Manufacturing Engineering (MIME), University of Toledo, Toledo, OH, United States

Andrew Chong
Department of Cariology, Restorative Sciences & Endodontics, University of Michigan, Ann Arbor, MI, United States

Shaahin Dadjoo
Department of Orthodontics and Dentofacial Orthopedics, The Eastman Institute for Oral Health, University of Rochester, Rochester, NY, United States

Joyce Badal
Department of Medicine, University of Toledo, Toledo, OH, United States

Margaret Arleen Hoogland
Mulford Health Sciences Library, University of Toledo, Toledo, OH, United States

Travis Roger Taylor
Department of Medical Microbiology and Immunology, University of Toledo, Toledo, OH, United States

Lihua Peng, Bin Yan, Zhengpeng Li and Fei Pan
Department of Gastroenterology and Hepatology, The First Medical Center, Chinese PLA General Hospital, Beijing, China

Wanyue Dan
Department of Gastroenterology and Hepatology, The First Medical Center, Chinese PLA General Hospital, Beijing, China
Medical School of Nankai University, Tianjin, China

Anne O. Rice
Oral Systemic Seminars, Conroe, TX, United States

Selvasankar Murugesan, Dhinoth Kumar Bangarusamy, Annalisa Terranegra and Souhaila Al Khodor
Mother and Child Health Department, Sidra Medicine, Doha, Qatar

Mohammed Elanbari
Clinical Research Center Department, Sidra Medicine, Doha, Qatar

Xiang Qi and Bei Wu
Rory Meyers College of Nursing, New York University, New York, NY, United States

Xiaomin Qu
School of Social Development, East China University of Political Science and Law, Shanghai, China

Florence Carrouel, Claude Dussart and Denis Bourgeois
Health, Systemic, Process, UR4129 Research Unit, University Claude Bernard Lyon 1, University of Lyon, Lyon, France

Emilie Gadea
Equipe SNA-EPIS, EA4607, University Jean Monnet, Saint-Etienne, France
Clinical Research Unit, Emile Roux Hospital Center, Le Puy-en-Velay, France

Aurélie Esparcieux
Department of Internal Medicine and Infectious Diseases, Protestant Infirmary, Caluire-et-Cuire, France

Jérome Dimet
Clinical Research Center, Intercommunal Hospital Center of Mont de Marsan et du Pays des Sources, Mont de Marsan, France

Marie Elodie Langlois
Department of Internal Medicine and Infectious Diseases, Saint Joseph Saint Luc Hospital, Lyon, France

Hervé Perrier
Clinical Research Unit, Protestant Infirmary, Lyon, France

Alisa E. Lee, Iris R. Hartley, Kelly L. Roszko, Rachel I. Gafni and Michael T. Collins
National Institute of Dental and Craniofacial Research, National Institutes of Health, Bethesda, MD, United States

Chaim Vanek
Division of Endocrinology, Diabetes and Clinical Nutrition, Oregon Health and Science University, Portland, OR, United States

Yirui Xie, Caiqin Hu, Bing Ruan and Biao Zhu
State Key Laboratory for Diagnosis and Treatment of Infectious Diseases, Department of Infectious Diseases, National Clinical Research Center for Infectious Diseases, Collaborative Innovation Center for Diagnosis and Treatment of Infectious Diseases, School of Medicine, The First Affiliated Hospital, Zhejiang University, Hangzhou, China

Jia Sun
Ningbo Medical Center Lihuili Hospital, Ningbo, China

R. Lamont (Monty) MacNeil and Helena Hilario
University of Connecticut School of Dental Medicine, Farmington, CT, United States

Yuchen Zhang, Xiao Cao, Yu Jin and Qin Zhou
Key Laboratory of Shaanxi Province for Craniofacial Precision Medicine Research, College of Stomatology, Xi'an Jiaotong University, Xi'an, China
Department of Implant Dentistry, College of Stomatology, Xi'an Jiaotong University, Xi'an, China

Yinhu Li
Shenzhen-Hong Kong Institute of Brain Science-Shenzhen Fundamental Research Institutions, The Brain Cognition and Brain Disease Institute, Shenzhen Institutes of Advanced Technology, Chinese Academy of Sciences, Shenzhen, China

Yuguang Yang
Department of Advanced Manufacturing and Robotics, College of Engineering, Peking University, Beijing, China

Yiqing Wang
Department of Prosthodontics, School and Hospital of Stomatology, Peking University, Beijing, China

Yue Xu
Key Laboratory of Shaanxi Province for Craniofacial Precision Medicine Research, College of Stomatology, Xi'an Jiaotong University, Xi'an, China
Department of General Dentistry and Emergency Room, College of Stomatology, Xi'an Jiaotong University, Xi'an, China

Shuai Cheng Li
Department of Computer Science, City University of Hong Kong, Kowloon, Hong Kong SAR, China

Priyam Jani, Olivier Duverger and Janice S. Lee
Craniofacial Anomalies and Regeneration Section, National Institute of Craniofacial and Dental Research, National Institutes of Health, Bethesda, MD, United States

Rashmi Mishra
Craniofacial Anomalies and Regeneration Section, National Institute of Craniofacial and Dental Research, National Institutes of Health, Bethesda, MD, United States
Department of Oral Medicine, University of Washington School of Dentistry, Seattle, WA, United States

Pamela A. Frischmeyer- Guerrerio
Food Allergy Research Unit, National Institute of Allergy and Infectious Diseases, National Institutes of Health, Bethesda, MD, United States

Sara C. Gordon
Department of Oral Medicine, School of Dentistry, University of Washington, Seattle, WA, United States

Linda M. Kaste
Department of Oral Biology, College of Dentistry, University of Illinois Chicago, Chicago, IL, United States

Joel H. Berg
Department of Pediatric Dentistry, School of Dentistry, University of Washington, Seattle, WA, United States

Wendy E. Mouradian
Department of Pediatric Dentistry, School of Dentistry, University of Washington, Seattle, WA, United States
The Santa Fe Group, New York, NY, United States

Phyllis L. Beemsterboer
Center for Ethics in Healthcare, School of Dentistry, Oregon Health & Science University, Portland, OR, United States

Carol Anne Murdoch-Kinch
School of Dentistry, Indiana University, Indianapolis, IN, United States

Index

Printed in the USA
CPSIA information can be obtained
at www.ICGtesting.com
JSHW061300110324
58991JS00005B/77